Surgical Endocrinology

Surgical Endocrinology
Clinical Syndromes

Edited by

STANLEY R. FRIESEN, M.D., Ph.D. (Surg.)

Professor of Surgery, Department of Surgery, University of Kansas School of Medicine, University of Kansas College of Health Sciences and Hospital, Kansas City, Kansas

Editorial Consultant

ROBERT E. BOLINGER, M.D.

Professor of Medicine and Consultant in Endocrinology, Department of Medicine, University of Kansas School of Medicine, University of Kansas College of Health Sciences and Hospital, Kansas City, Kansas

With 28 Contributors

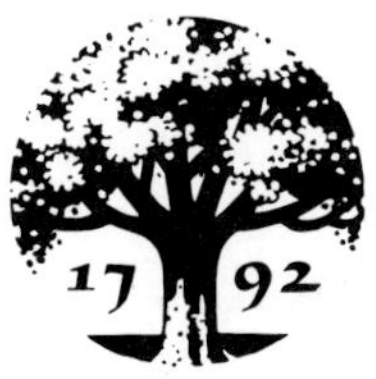

J. B. Lippincott Company

Philadelphia • Toronto

ISBN 0-397-50384-9

Library of Congress Catalog Card Number 78-68

Printed in the United States of America

1 3 5 4 2

Library of Congress Cataloging in Publication Data

Main entry under title:

Surgical endocrinology: clinical syndromes.

Bibliography: p.
Includes index.
1. Endocrine glands—Surgery. 2. Endocrine glands—Diseases. I. Friesen, Stanley Richard, [DNLM: 1. Endocrine glands—Surgery. 2. Nervous system diseases. WK100 S959]

RD599.S95 617′.44 78-68
ISBN 0-397-50384-9

To Students of All Ages
Who Ask
"Why?"

Contributors

Keith W. Ashcraft, M.D.
Pediatric Surgeon, Children's Mercy Hospital; Clinical Associate Professor, University of Missouri, Kansas City, School of Medicine, Kansas City, Missouri

Stephen R. Bloom, M.A., M.B., M.R.C.P.
Honorary Consultant and Senior Lecturer in Clinical Endocrinology, University of London, Royal Postgraduate Medical School, Hammersmith Hospital, London, England

Orlo H. Clark, M.D.
Assistant Professor of Surgery, University of California, San Francisco, School of Medicine; Staff Physician, Veterans Administration Hospital; Attending Surgeon, University of California Hospitals; Consultant Surgeon, Letterman Army Medical Center, San Francisco, California

Timothy S. Harrison, M.D.
Professor of Surgery and Physiology, The Pennsylvania State University College of Medicine, Hershey, Pennsylvania

Robert C. Hickey, M.D.
Professor of Surgery, and Executive Vice-President and Director, The University of Texas System Cancer Center; Staff Physician, M.D. Anderson Hospital and Tumor Institute, Houston, Texas

Thomas M. Holder, M.D.
Clinical Professor of Surgery, University of Missouri, Kansas City, School of Medicine, Kansas City, Missouri

Thomas K. Hunt, M.D.
Professor of Surgery and Ambulatory and Community Medicine, University of California, San Francisco, School of Medicine, San Francisco, California

Bernard M. Jaffe, M.D.
Professor of Surgery, Washington University School of Medicine, St. Louis, Missouri

Edwin L. Kaplan, M.D.
Professor of Surgery, University of Chicago, The Division of the Biological Sciences and the Pritzker School of Medicine, Chicago, Illinois

James E. McGuigan, M.D.
Professor and Chairman, Department of Medicine, University of Florida College of Medicine, Gainesville, Florida

Christopher Mallinson, B.A., M.B., F.R.C.P.
Consultant Physician, Lewisham Hospital; Lecturer in Medicine, Gastrolenterology Unit, Department of Medicine, Guy's Hospital Medical School, London, England

Walter H. Moran, Jr., M.D.
Professor of Surgery and of Physiology and Biophysics, West Virginia University School of Medicine, Morgantown, West Virginia

Jeffrey A. Norton, M.D.
Resident in Surgery, Duke University School of Medicine, Durham, North Carolina

Edward Passaro, Jr., M.D.
Professor of Surgery, University of California, Los Angeles, School of Medicine; Acting Chief, Surgical Service, Veterans Administration Wadsworth Hospital Center, Los Angeles, California

A. G. E. Pearse, M.A., M.D., F.R.C.P., F.R.C. Path.
Professor of Histochemistry and Consultant Pathologist, University of London, Royal Postgraduate Medical School, Hammersmith Hospital, London, England

William H. ReMine, M.D., M.S. (Surg.), D.Sc.
Professor of Surgery, Mayo Graduate School of Medicine; Consultant in Surgery, Mayo Clinic, Rochester, Minnesota

R. Neil Schimke, M.D.
Professor of Medicine and Pediatrics, and Chief, Division of Metabolism, Endocrinology and Genetics, University of Kansas School of Medicine, University of Kansas, College of Health Sciences and Hospital, Kansas City, Kansas

H. William Scott, Jr., M.D., D.Sc.
Professor and Chairman, Department of Surgery and Director of the Section of Surgical Sciences, Vanderbilt University School of Medicine; Surgeon-in-Chief, Vanderbilt University Hospital, Nashville, Tennessee

Laurence H. Smith, M.D.
Central Cardiology Medical Group, Inc., Santa Barbara, California

Selwyn Taylor, D.M., M.Ch., F.R.C.S.
Surgeon, University of London, Royal Postgraduate Medical School, Hammersmith Hospital; Vice President, Royal College of Surgeons, and Consultant to the Royal Navy, London, England

J. Blake Tyrrell, M.D.
Assistant Clinical Professor of Medicine, Metabolic Research Unit and Department of Medicine, University of California, San Francisco, School of Medicine, San Francisco, California

Jonathan A. van Heerden, M.B., Ch.B. (Cape Town), M.S., F.R.C.S.(C)
Assistant Professor of Surgery, Mayo Graduate School of Medicine, Rochester, Minnesota

Lawrence W. Way, M.D.
Professor of Surgery, University of California, San Francisco, School of Medicine; Chief, Surgical Service, Veterans Administration Hospital, San Francisco, California

Samuel A. Wells, Jr., M.D.
Professor of Surgery, Duke University School of Medicine, Durham, North Carolina

Charles B. Wilson, M.D.
Professor and Chairman, Department of Neurological Surgery, University of California, San Francisco, School of Medicine, San Francisco, California

Stuart D. Wilson, M.D.
Associate Professor of Surgery, The Medical College of Wisconsin, Milwaukee, Wisconsin

Bernard Zimmermann, M.D., Ph.D.
Professor of Surgery, West Virginia University School of Medicine, Morgantown, West Virginia

Robert M. Zollinger, M.D.
Emeritus Professor and Chairman, Department of Surgery, The Ohio State University College of Medicine, Columbus, Ohio

Foreword—a Look Back

This splendid and impressive monograph on the Neuroendocrine System by Stanley Friesen and his active coworkers and collaborators in the broadly erupting field of neuroendocrinology is indeed timely and will be welcomed by all segments of the profession. The endocrine system, with long if not deep historical roots in many medical disciplines, has been emerging for decades as a special field of study and investigation. Over the past two decades progress in the field has been phenomenal leading to histologic and chemical identification of responsible hormonal secreting cells, a truly remarkable achievement.

Dr. Friesen, distinguished surgeon of the alimentary tract, has schooled himself on the hormonal activities of cells in many organs and glands, and is well qualified to undertake the difficult task of integrating and correlating many recent new observations and discoveries for the clinician. His observation that complete gastrectomy in the patient with a malignant pancreatic gastrinoma will sometimes ablate metastases was a bold and enlightening innovation (*Surgery,* 62:609, 1967). Over long years, Friesen has followed the work of the London pathologist and histochemist, A.G.E. Pearse, with whom he collaborated on genetic aspects of the Zollinger-Ellison syndrome (*Ann. Surg.* 176:370, 1972).

It would take the experience of an accomplished molecular biologist to do justice to a worthy and critical appraisal of the many exciting and significant developments in the broad sweep of this rapidly expanding discipline, a competence to which this surgeon cannot lay the feeblest claim. Even so, Dr. Friesen very generously maintained that I could come up with something appropriate for the occasion.

In the third edition of his two-volume work on the Innere Sekretion (1916), Artur Biedl of Prague listed more than 350 pages of references, definitely suggesting that endocrinology has a long historical background.

Robert Graves, a brilliant Dublin physician, described the clinical syndrome of exophthalmic goiter that has come to be known as Graves' disease with such accuracy that the modern reader would recognize the entity readily from his account (*London Med. Surg. J.,* 7:516, 1835). Thomas Addison of Guy's Hospital, a colleague of Richard Bright, lived for his students; Addison described atrophy of the cortical portion of the adrenals, subsequently known as Addison's disease (*London Med. Gaz.,* 43:517, 1855). His demonstration that atrophy and disease of the capsular portion of the adrenals in patients resulted in anemia and death led Charles Brown-Séquard to excise both adrenals in dogs and other animals; the effect was uniformly lethal (*C.R. Acad. Sci.,* Paris, 43:422, 1856).

The London physiologists George Oliver and Edward Sharpey-Schäfer demonstrated the presence of a substance in the medulla of the adrenal that elevated blood pressure in dogs, which they called adrenalin (*J. Physiol.,* 18:230, 1895). This finding was reaffirmed by The Johns Hopkins pharmacologist John Abel, which agent he labeled epinephrine (*Johns Hopkins Hosp. Bull.,* 8:151, 1897). In a series of papers, the chemist Edward Kendall and colleagues at the Mayo Clinic (1934-49) isolated cortisone from the cortical portion of the adrenal, providing an effective therapeutic answer to the treatment of Addison's disease.

The skeleton of the Irish giant, Charles Byrne, one of the most exciting exhibits at London's Hunterian museum, has always captivated the interest of visitors. To lessen the risk of detection of the stealth of the body, John Hunter, unfortunately, found it necessary to destroy all the soft tissues, thus removing the many striking features of soft tissues of tongue, hands and feet of gigantism that Pierre Marie described so vividly under the title, Acromegaly (*Rev. Méd.,* 6:297, 1886), a condition not inherited, but owing to abnormal secretory influences occasioned by enlargement of the pituitary body. The otologist, Oskar Hirsch (1911), Harvey Cushing (1912) and the Vienna pathologist Jacob Erdheim (1916) added much to the understanding and management of some of the manifestations of acromegaly. For several decades up until quite recently it has often been said that the pituitary gland is the master gland in the hormonal symphony, a statement that recently has been seriously challenged by Roger Guillemin and other modern-day endocrinologists.

Claude Bernard (1849) noted in his doctoral thesis, that cane sugar ingested by rabbits and dogs did not appear in the urine; when injected intravenously, in similar amounts, however, sugar appeared regularly in the urine. This occurrence suggested to Bernard the glycogenic function of the liver constituting the first demonstration of the presence of an internal secretion, the name by which Bernard characterized the phenomenon.

Bayliss and Starling discovered the role of HCL in releasing from the upper jejunal mucosa a chemical reflex that stimulated the flow of pancreatic juice (*J. Physiol.,* 28:325, 1902). In an ingenious experiment, Starling destroyed the mesenteric nervous connections to an isolated upper jejunal loop, leaving the isolated segment suspended only by its blood vessels. On the spot, Starling correctly concluded that stimulation of pancreatic secretion from the denervated loop was a chemical reflex, an inference he was able to validate by rubbing sand and dilute HCL into the mucosa of another jejunal loop; upon filtering the solution and injection into a jugular vein, a strong pancreatic secretion was elicited. Bayliss and Starling subsequently labeled the chemical reflex a hormone.

In an obituary note on Ernest H. Starling, C. J. Martin of London related (*Br. Med. J.,* 1:900, 1927) that he was present in the laboratory when Starling performed the telling experiment just described. This observation lent a new concept to the regulation of the secretion of the digestive glands. Prior thereto, the prevailing opinion of workers in the field, including Pavlov and his coworker Popielski, and the Belgian physiologists, Wertheimer and LePage was a peripheral neural reflex. When Pavlov repeated and verified the Starling experiment, his interest in the physiology of the digestive tract waned; after some years he devoted the remainder of a long professional life to the study of conditioned reflexes.

Shortly after Bayliss and Starling's demonstration of a messenger in the mucosa of the upper jejunum which, on contact with HCL, released a hormone that stimulated secretion of pancreatic juice, Edkins demonstrated the presence of a hormone in the antral mucosa which he called gastrin (*J. Physiol.*, 34:133, 1906). Its presence was doubted by many physiologists for many years, until the London surgeon Heneage Ogilvie (1936-38) verified its existence by comparing the effects of antral excision and antral exclusion in gastric resection for duodenal ulcer (*Edinb. Med. J.*, 43:61, 1936; *Lancet*, 2:295, 1938). Leaving a segment of the antrum attached to the duodenum, Ogilvie observed, invited neostomal ulcer at the site of the gastrojejunal anastomosis, an occurrence that could have been foreseen in the heightened secretion of HCL in dogs fed meat after such an operation, a finding observed by Hans Smidt of Jena (*Arch. f. klin. chir.*, 130:307, 1924). Today the role of Edkins' gastrin in stimulating gastric secretion is a major concern of gastric physiologists and clinicians.

Ivar Sandström, a Swedish medical student, described the parathyroid glands. He sent his paper initially to Rudolph Virchow, who declined its publication in his Archiv, whereupon Sandström published it in a little known Swedish journal (*Upsala Läkaref Förhandl.*, 15:441, 1880). The function of the parathyroid glands remained a matter of considerable speculation until the Austrian surgeon Felix Mandl excised a small tumor of the left inferior parathyroid gland in a patient with fibrous cystic osteitis in 1925, followed by considerable relief to the patient and great improvement of the concomitant osteoporosis (*Wien. klin. Wschr.*, 38:1343, 1925). Mandl, a young surgeon in Professor Hochenegg's clinic at the University of Vienna's Allgemeines Krankenhaus, reported his interesting story at the December 4, 1925 meeting of the Vienna Congress of Physicians. Mandl had first implanted a parathyroid gland freshly obtained at necropsy from a patient who died in the emergency admittance ward, which procedure was without effect. Mandl noted that the patient's excreted urine was rich in calcium and white in color. No tumor was palpable in the neck but at operation a definite tumor of the left inferior parathyroid gland was found and excised. The patient's chronic bone pain relented immediately and his fractures healed. There was an observed 80 percent decrease in calcium excretion in the urine, attending the excision. Professor v. Eiselsberg, a keen student of ductless glands (*Wien. klin. Wschr.*, 5:81, 1892), was the presiding officer but strangely had nothing to say relative to this remarkable achievement; nor did the five well-known Vienna surgeons and physicians who discussed Mandl's presentation appreciate its significance. In defense of his thesis on conclusion of the discussion Mandl indicated that Siegfried Hoffheinz (*Virch. Arch.*, 256:705, 1925), an assistant to Professor Otto Lubarsch of the Pathologic Institute in Berlin, had observed hypertrophy of the parathyroid glands in more than 50 percent of patients with generalized osteitis fibrosa that had come to autopsy.

Adolph Hanson (*Milit. Surg.*, 52:280, 1923), a general surgeon of Faribault, Minnesota was the first to isolate an active parathyroid extract with helpful advice from Arthur Hirschfelder, professor of pharmacology at the University of Minnesota. Two years later, James Collip isolated parathormone (*J. Biol. Chem.*, 63:395, 1925), the active secretory principle of the ductless parathyroid gland.

The Canadian orthopaedic surgeon Frederick Banting of Toronto read Moses Barron's account (*Surg. Gyn. Obstet.*, 30:350, 1920) describing atrophy of the acinar cell portion of the pancreas attending obstruction of the duct of Wirsung by calculi. He then ligated the excretory ducts of the canine pancreas, producing atrophy of the trypsinogen-secreting area without injury to the cells of Langerhans located primarily in the tail of the pancreas (*J. Lab. Clin. Med.,* 7:251, 1921-22). These islets had been described in a Berlin Inaugural thesis by Paul Langerhans (1869) a medical student. By this means, Banting, with the assistance of Charles Best, also a medical student, isolated insulin, a useful agent in the control of diabetics and the only hope for juvenile diabetics.

In 1955 the University of Ohio surgeons Robert Zollinger and Edwin Ellison (*Ann. Surg.,* 142:709-29, 1955) described patients with gastric hypersecretion who proved to have pancreatic gastrinomas for whom total gastrectomy became the operation by choice. Their report has constituted the primary incentive and stimulus to the great forward thrust lent gastrin studies by Roderick Gregory and his associates in Liverpool (*J. Physiol.,* 169:18, 1963).

Since antiquity differences between male and female have been recognized as owing to dissimilarities in the sex glands. In his *Animal Oeconomy* (1786), John Hunter observed that in the male, the secondary sex organs, prostate, seminal vesicles and the penis depend upon the testes for maturation. Hunter used gross measurement and excision to establish the relationship. Microscopy was yet not in general use by biologists, and Hunter employed no magnification larger than a hand lens. In the "land-mouse" and the mole, the seminal vesicles are scarcely discernible in winter, said Hunter, but very large in summer, and the seminal vesicles vary in size according to the size of the testes. Hunter did not attempt castration of patients in the hope of diminishing urinary obstruction from prostatic hypertrophy.

A century after Hunter, Joseph Griffiths of Edinburgh (1890) reported that when a young bull was castrated, the prostate gland remained small. Griffiths extended Hunter's inquiry to the dog and cat, also studying the histologic changes attending castration. In a three-year-old dog, castrated a year earlier, Griffiths found the prostate small, firm, tough and fibrous, unlike the large soft gland of the normal male dog. A very similar situation attended castration of the male cat, especially when done at three weeks of age (*J. Anat. Physiol.,* 24:27, 1890).

Robert A. Moore reported the autopsy findings of a man 39 years of age who had undergone castration at 34 years in the hope of escaping the social stigma of being a homosexual. The prostate was considerably smaller than normal for his age, observed Moore, and the "seminal vesicles are exceedingly small" (*Am. J. Pathol.,* 12:620, 1936). There are few if any other published accounts of the condition of the prostate some years after castration in adult men.

Eunuchs, castrated as young boys before puberty, retain preadolescent soprano voices and have beardless faces. Eunuchs are free from enlargement of the prostate, common to aging men. Eunuchs were known in China 1100 years before Christ and were highly prized servants in households and government in the Orient and Eastern Mediterranean countries in antiquity. Oriental princes placed eunuchs in charge of the bedchamber and in the seraglios of their harems. Eunuchs are mentioned in both the Old and New Testaments.

Emasculation of young slave boys was common, for they commanded a considerably higher price than other boys in the slave market. They were sold as eunuchs for Moslem harems into the twentieth century. "A clean sweep" operation was usually done of scrotum, testes and penis.

In a succession of papers (1893-1904), J. William White of Philadelphia advocated excision of the testes as a solution for urinary retention occasioned by an enlarged prostate, a suggestion debated vigorously at the time. The mortality was surprisingly high, varying from 13 to 18 percent in the hands of its advocates, probably a reflection of application in terminal cases. Probably a third of White's patients upon whom orchiectomy was performed suffered from cancer of the prostate. Strangely enough, neither White nor any of his successors followed up with an account of the nature of the histology of prostatic tissue removed in patients undergoing orchiectomy for urinary retention (*Trans. Am. Surg. Assoc.*, 11:197, 209, 1893; *Ann. Surg.*, 40:788, 1904).

White's innovation preceded that of George T. Beatson (1896) of Glasgow, who performed excision of the ovaries in females for advanced cancer of the breast (*Lancet*, 2:104, 162, 1896), an operation that has been revived in recent decades and found often to be an effective palliative hormonal attack upon the problem of late breast cancer. Over the past three decades, orchiectomy has been endorsed by Charles Huggins (*Cancer Res.*, 1:293, 1941) as a therapeutic measure for cancer of the prostate. Whether castration will cause regression of benign prostatic hypertrophy in older men and animals is not definitely known. For cancer of the prostate current conventional professional advice is administration of agents to suppress plasma testosterone or orchiectomy. A few reserve all treatment until the appearance of metastases causing symptoms.

The interest and concern of physiologists, biochemists, and endocrinologists in more recent years in the function of ductless glands has added significantly to progress in this once very obscure field. The significant observations of the physicians Graves and Addison, and the surgeons Banting, Mandl, Hanson, Zollinger and Ellison have been illuminated by methodical studies in the hands of basic biological scientists and chemists.

The Galveston symposium of 1974 on gastrointestinal hormones (University of Texas Press, 1975) under the able supervision of the surgeon James C. Thompson served to point up the growing complexity of the problem of gastrointestinal hormones. The few hormones of that tract recognized 20 years ago have multiplied, indicating definitely that the field today is primarily one for the biochemist, chemist, endocrinologist, pharmacologist and physiologist.

The observant physician and surgeon of the Graves, Addison, Banting, Mandl and Hanson types will still continue to identify syndromes yet unrecognized, but their identification and clarification will need the attention of erudite representatives of the disciplines just enumerated. Definition of the nature of hormonal imbalances will serve to indicate the optimal mode of management.

The important contributions of three American scientists, Rosalyn Yalow, Roger Guillemin and Andrew Schally, working in diverse medical disciplines on broad aspects of endocrinology, fully justified their being named Nobel Laureates in October, 1977. Their significant work has opened new vistas for chemical identification of hormones, suggesting new methods for the control and management of neuroendocrine disorders. For decades, the hypophysis and the hypothalamus have been looked upon as the leaders of the hormonal symphony. Today, neuroendocrine secreting cells are known to be widely dispersed over the cerebral cortex and in the mucosa of the upper gastrointestinal canal. An abnormal secretion of somatostatin, secreted by both brain cells and mucosal cells of the upper gastrointestinal canal, may be a responsible inhibitory factor in many disorders, perhaps including peptic ulcer and mental disorders. Neuroendocrinology is offering renewed and promising challenges and a fertile field for investigators as well as clinicians, opening new vistas and lighting the way to important advances in practical medicine.

The recent startling progress in endocrinology suggests that it may not be out of place to ask whether the tools and contributions of endocrinologists may not come in time to supplant the surgeon's knife in dealing with some endocrine disorders.

OWEN H. WANGENSTEEN, M.D.
Regents' Professor Emeritus
University of Minnesota
Minneapolis, Minnesota

Preface

Within the last two decades there has been such a massive proliferation of basic and clinical information relating to the rapidly expanding dimensions of the neuroendocrine system that it seems necessary to examine the directions and the diversities of these discoveries in order to bring them into focus. There has been a virtual "explosion" of newfound endocrine cells, newly identified humoral products and newly described syndromes. The increasing variety of clinical presentations of these syndromes which result from hypersecretion of neuroendocrine tumors and hyperplasias demand early diagnostic recognition and require sophisticated surgical management. Some of the original observations concerning the systemic effects of hyperfunctioning tumors have been made by surgeons who are the appropriate ones to whom treatment is usually entrusted. Intelligent surgical treatment is based on accurate diagnosis and a conceptual understanding of the pathophysiology of such syndromes. Accordingly, this book is directed specifically to these three goals: The unification of basic and clinical concepts, the simplification of diagnostic criteria, and the presentation of therapeutic options in surgical management. To accomplish these aims the material is presented with a functional approach in which diagnostic and management flowcharts, as well as diagrams of the pathophysiology for each syndrome are employed; there is, in addition, editorial bridging of basic and clinical observations for increased understanding of the many syndromes that involve surgical management.

The neuroendocrine cells from which hypersecreting dysplasias arise and from which circulating hormones are elaborated have presumably always existed, having survived countless centuries of evolutionary influences, but the recent detection and identification of them has been an exciting scientific accomplishment, as judged by the profusion of published articles about them. The sheer numbers of these publications, however noteworthy, would suggest that some revelations would be remembered and others would go unnoticed or forgotten, just as the sparks of a volcanic eruption remain vivid in our memory while the ashes are lost to the winds. This book is a presentation of many of the illuminating "sparks" and some of the overlooked "debris" as a compilation of usable knowledge for general and specialty surgeons about this dynamic neuroendocrine system, in health and disease.

It has been my good fortune to observe at firsthand this rediscovery of the neuroendocrine system. My initial work with A. G. E. Pearse, during a sabbatical leave, concerned the role of the pyloric ganglion cells in the pathogenesis of congenital pyloric stenosis. At that time some of the histochemical characteristics of these myenteric cells were observed which would later become applicable to the developing APUD concept. Although other investigators considered these neural cells as the possible source of gastrin, it remained for James E. McGuigan to positively identify the gastrin cell to be within the mucosa. Shortly thereafter, I again had the opportunity to work with Pearse as the APUD concept was being formulated and was on the scene when a host of new endocrine cells in the gastrointestinal mucosa were found and described. The cytochemical similarities of these mucosal endocrine cells to the myenteric neural cells were confirmed and now, after more studies, the functional interrelationships of the autonomic nervous system and the diffuse endocrine system are firmly established, even to the extent that some of the same hormones have been found in both gastrointestinal and neural (brain) tissues. In the meantime, I had briefly observed Gregory and Tracy's monumental work on the isolation and identification of the gastrin polypeptides in hog antral mucosa and later, in human islet cell tumors. Many of the above milestone discoveries were prompted by the exciting clinical observations of Zollinger and Ellison that pancreatic islet cell tumors might be an unexpected source, other than the gastric antrum, of the ulcerogenic secretogogue, gastrin. At the present time it is the accumulation of *basic* scientific discoveries which is making the more recently described *clinical* syndromes understandable.

It is hoped that in this book the fusion of the discoveries in the basic sciences with the observations in the clinical sciences will clarify even the most complex endocrine syndromes. Only through a clear understanding of the basic concepts is it possible to sort out the extremely bizarre clinical presentations of some of the hyperfunctioning endocrine disorders. This is particularly relevant when we consider the wide spectrum of endocrinopathies, from the simple sporadic syndrome through a kaleidoscopic array of polyhormonal, pluriglandular, familial and "ectopic" phenomena.

I have observed that when physicians and surgeons have had occasion to talk and think about these so-called "rare endocrine syndromes" it frequently becomes apparent that the syndrome is not so rare after all. More often than not, such a possible "case" is suddenly recalled to memory, having been missed in diagnosis because of a lack of awareness of the syndrome or simply of lack of time to have read appropriate articles widely dispersed in many journals. More and more patients are now recognized as having endocrinopathies involving the gastrointestinal tract, and these are usually properly diagnosed and treated, but unexplainable clinical pictures are still occasionally observed, and these await future clarification. It is expected that this book, with its up-to-the-minute information, contributed by recognized authorities in their fields, will familiarize those physicians and surgeons who are already knowledgeable about most endocrinopathies with the most recent concepts of the pathophysiology, diagnosis and management of old and new syndromes. It should also provide a source of understanding for busy clinicians who care for patients of all ages who might have endocrine abnormalities.

There are a number of features which perhaps are unique to this book. In an attempt to unify conceptual and practical considerations, some of the basic information in the first part of the book is reintroduced in the clinical chapters, particularly in the editorial commentaries. Diagrams illustrating the pathophysiology of each syndrome, many of which are entitled mnemonically, further clarify the clinical presentations. There are, among the clinical chapters, practical applications of clinical concepts by means of management flowcharts which illustrate points of consideration and decision, from the presenting clinical situation to the final diagnosis of each syndrome. This book also departs from the traditional format of subjects by organ systems to a more functional grouping of syndromes based upon the type of hormone elaborated, such as those caused by secretion of the ubiquitous fast-acting *amines,* or of the newer but slower acting *polypeptides* and/or the familiar chronic-acting *steroids.* A composite table of useful information, matching syndromes with their humoral agents, biologic actions and diagnostic features is centrally placed in the book for ready reference to the key characteristics of each syndrome.

Certainly, as new information continues to develop, the present methods of diagnosis and treatment will necessarily be refined, but the fundamental concepts which are presented here are not likely to change. These modern-day concepts will continue to be applicable even to the newer approaches of target-cell modification and tumor therapy.

It is difficult to acknowledge fully the deep appreciation I have for the contributing authors, already exceedingly busy with ongoing work, who gave again of their time and expertise for this new book. I sincerely thank them and their associates and secretaries. The editors of J. B. Lippincott Publishing Company have been more than helpful and supportive. I am also grateful to Dr. Robert Bolinger, my long-time friend and editorial consultant on this book, for his abundant help and advice, and to my secretary, Mrs. Caroline Weaver, for her superb assistance from the inception of this book to its completion. The unselfish understanding of my wife, Beth, through many hours is more than I deserve and I thank her for that.

STANLEY R. FRIESEN, M.D.

Contents

PART 2: POLYPEPTIDES

PART 4: MISCELLANEOUS SYNDROMES

Surgical Endocrinology

SECTION ONE

BASIC CONCEPTS

1

Introductory Concepts of Clinical Endocrinology

Stanley R. Friesen, M.D., Ph.D.

In health, the functional integrity of the human organism seems to be maintained almost miraculously in a delicate balance, withstanding disruptive environmental forces by means of extremely efficient regulating mechanisms. This neurohumoral homeostasis is automatically achieved in response to controlling signals which, like thermostats, act as "biostats"; these sensitive mechanisms are seemingly inherent in the endocrine and autonomic nervous systems. All of the components of these systems are ultimately concerned with transferring "information" so as to regulate the internal environment of the body. Such internal communication involves intra- and intercellular messengers which bridge either short distances by means of local hormones and neurotransmitters, or greater distances through the humoral transmission of endocrine hormones or by neurochemical transmission along nerve fibers. It is becoming more and more evident that the autonomic nervous system and the endocrine system are so interdependent that their designation as a single system, the neuroendocrine system, might be more meaningful than as two separate systems. Even in disease, manifestations of abnormalities of both systems are frequently observed in the same clinical syndrome.

THE NEUROENDOCRINE SYSTEM

While Pavlov[16] was proposing that the regulation of various organs in the body was mediated by the nervous system, Bayliss and Starling[1] had developed evidence of a humoral regulatory mechanism such as the duodenal secretin influence on the exocrine pancreas. Each of these early investigators understood and acknowledged the presence of the so-called opposing mechanisms, but the closeness with which the neural and humoral regulatory mechanisms function has been fully appreciated only recently.

There are components within the overall nervous and endocrine systems which require definition and consideration of their interrelationships. The nervous system can be reasonably partitioned into three divisions: (1) *Somatic* (motor and sensory nerves), (2) *autonomic* (sympathetic and parasympathetic nerves), and (3) *neuroendocrine* (central and peripheral). Within the neuroendocrine division, the central hypothalamic-pituitary component is related to the peripheral component in a number of ways including: (a) Functionally by the trophic actions and feedback controls, (b) embryologically by the similar origins of many of the cells from the neuroectoderm (including the neural crest), (c) by the similar ancestral functions of amine storage and peptide synthesis, and (d) (based on recent findings) by the presence of the same humoral substances in both the hypothalamus and the gastrointestinal tract.[19] The peptides that are common to both sites are somatostatin, gastrin, vasoactive intestinal peptide and substance P (a neurotransmitter in Auerbach's and Meissner's ganglion cells). The neuroendocrine division is related to the autonomic division in many ways, including shared controls of vascular homeostasis by catecholamine release both as an endocrine hormone from the adrenal medulla and as a neurotransmitter from the sympathetic nerve endings—or in the shared regulation of acid secretion by vagal cholinergic cholinesterase and antral G cell gastrin on their own receptors on the parietal cell. Again both groups of cells have ancestral types which have in common the presence of cholinesterase and the storage of amines.

A large part of the endocrine system is in fact an effector arm of the nervous system, and changes in hormone secretion are one of the mechanisms by which the integrative function of the nervous system is effected. Furthermore, the development and function of the brain are affected by growth hormone, cortisol, thyroxine and insulin; conversely, the brain influences the entire endocrine system by means of the hypothalamus and the autonomic nervous system; even gonadal function and sexual behavior are reciprocal influences between the brain and the peripheral endocrine tissues.

Certainly the dimensions of the neuroendocrine system are expanding from what was once thought to consist almost entirely of the pituitary-thyroid-adrenal-gonadal axis to a larger scope of regulatory forces[18] (Fig. 1-1). Within that traditional axis of endocrine glands, which incidentally stem from different embryologic germ layers, the internal secretions are peptides and amines from the pituitary and thyroid glands and the very different chemical compounds, steroids, from the latter two organs. This axis is still classical of endocrine function in that the secreted hormones provoke biologic activity by their physiologic action on distant target cells and organs under feedback control.

Only recently has it been recognized that the endocrine cells of the gastrointestinal tract, including the pancreas, comprise an endocrine "organ" of such magnitude that in size and complexity it overshadows all the remaining endocrines put together.[17] The "clear cells" of the gastrointestinal tract were described first by Feyrter,[3] who considered them to be a "diffuse endokrine epitheliale organe" or a "peripheren endokrinen (parakrinen)" system as contrasted to the more central system centering around the pituitary gland. His use of the term paracrine has come to denote a diffuse system of cells that secrete hormones which have a local effect on neighboring cells. These so-called paracrine cells, situated as they are among and near potential target cells, constitute a large body of interacting and intercommunicating cells within another axis, the enteroinsular axis. For the most part, the stimulation and suppression of secretion and the response of target cells all occur in a localized region, but these paracrine cells seem also to have an endocrine (humoral) action, such as duodenal secretin action on the pancreas, and the effect of insulin and glucagon on the liver. In addition to the "paracrine" cells as those having a local effect and "endocrine" cells as those having an effect on distal target organs, one might further identify cells as "neurocrine" as exemplified by the portal stalk system of the hypothalamus and pituitary gland or those cells which release catecholamines and neurotransmitters, and possibly "ectocrine" cells of

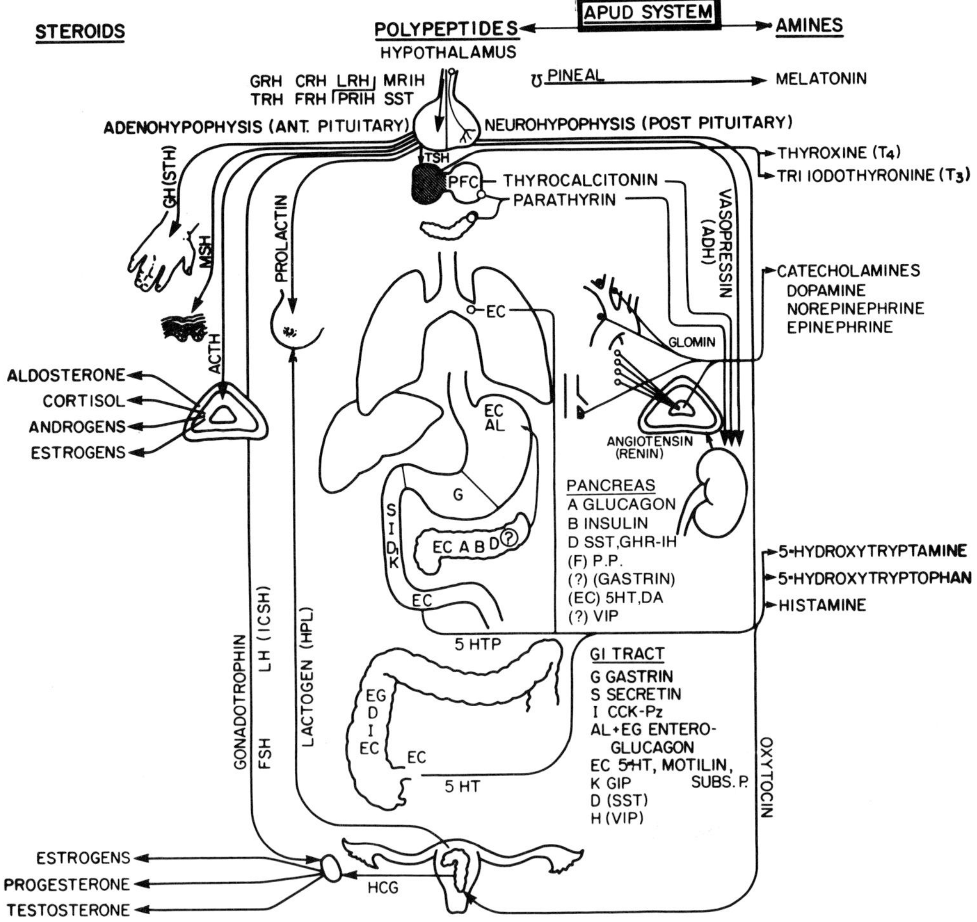

Fig. 1-1. This diagram illustrates dimensions of the neuroendocrine system. Note the cells and organs of origin, their humoral products and some of their target organs. The APUD system is composed of amine- and polypeptide-secreting cells and constitutes the larger part of the entire neuroendocrine system. Note also the fast-acting amines *(right)* and slow-acting steroid hormones *(left)*, with the interrelating central and peripheral polypeptide system between. Cell letters in parentheses indicate that cell and candidate hormones have not been definitely established as entopic. (Friesen, S. R.: Current dimensions of the endocrine system. *In* Longmire, W. P., Jr. [ed.]: Advances in Surgery. vol. 10. Chicago, Copyright © 1976 by Year Book Medical Publishers, Inc. Used by permission)

neural crest origin in the skin, such as melanocytes. Such explorations with semantic terminology can be expected when a vast new system of polypeptide and amine-secreting cells is uncovered and their prolific products are biochemically identified. The neuroendocrine system is thus composed of many components, in a central and peripheral pattern, which carry out a messenger function in several different ways.

THE ENDOCRINE CELLS

The APUD Concept

The embryologic derivation of many of the central and peripheral neuroendocrine cells to a large extent determines their humoral capacities. The peripheral steroid-secreting endocrine tissues of the adrenal cortex and the gonads differentiate from mesodermal origins, and their humoral products act generally on cytoplasmic (rather than membrane) receptors influencing the necessary biologic function of protein synthesis. Now they compose a smaller proportion of the neuroendocrine system than formerly, because of the inclusion of the gastrointestinal peptide and the amine-secreting cells. It was once thought that the origin of the latter group was entodermal, but it is now considered that most of the non-steroid-secreting cells, including those of the gastrointestinal tract and pancreas, are of neuroectodermal origin, including the neural crest. Furthermore, the important definition of cytochemical characteristics which are common to many of these cells has led to the APUD concept that has clarified many aspects of identification of neuroendocrine cells and their functional capabilities.[20] The acronym APUD refers only to a few of the many common characteristics of these cells; namely, **A**mine **P**recursor **U**ptake and **D**ecarboxylation leading to amine and polypeptide synthesis. The ability of these cells to take up precursor amines, to store amines, and to synthesize peptides is basic to their normal and abnormal potentialities and is probably attributable to their neural crest origin. The charter members of the APUD cell system, those having been shown first to be derived from the neural crest part of the neuroectoderm, are the C cells of the thyroid and the medullary cells (pheochromocytes) of the adrenal, and both in disease have been associated in a syndrome of multiple endocrinopathy, Type II; they secrete peptides and amines and are functionally involved in autonomic nerve activity. The parathyroid cells are presumed to be neuroectodermal in origin, though not from the neural crest, because comparative embryologic studies suggest their origin from neural placodes adjacent to pharyngeal pouches.[21] This origin, similar to that of the pituitary and hypothalamus, may account for the rather ubiquitous association of hyperparathyroidism with the two general types of multiple endocrinopathies. It can be observed in Figure 1-1 that the amine- and polypeptide-secreting cells (APUD cells) constitute a large proportion of the neuroendocrine system, except for the smaller steroid-secreting group; but it will also be noted that even the latter are intimately related and depend upon the presence of central trophic polypeptide products.

Regulation and Function

Just as most tissues of the body are regulated by neural and humoral influences, so the neuroendocrine cells themselves are controlled by at least four types of environmental influences.[7] (Fig. 1-2). The endocrine cell may be closed or "open" with microvilli with which to "sensor" the luminal environment. An example of the "open" cell is the gastrin (G) cell of the antral mucosa which is responsive to both chemical (pH) and physical (distention) influences. Other cells are presumed to be closed but are responsive, nevertheless, to chemical stimuli which diffuse into the cell and to tissue fluid osmolarity; an

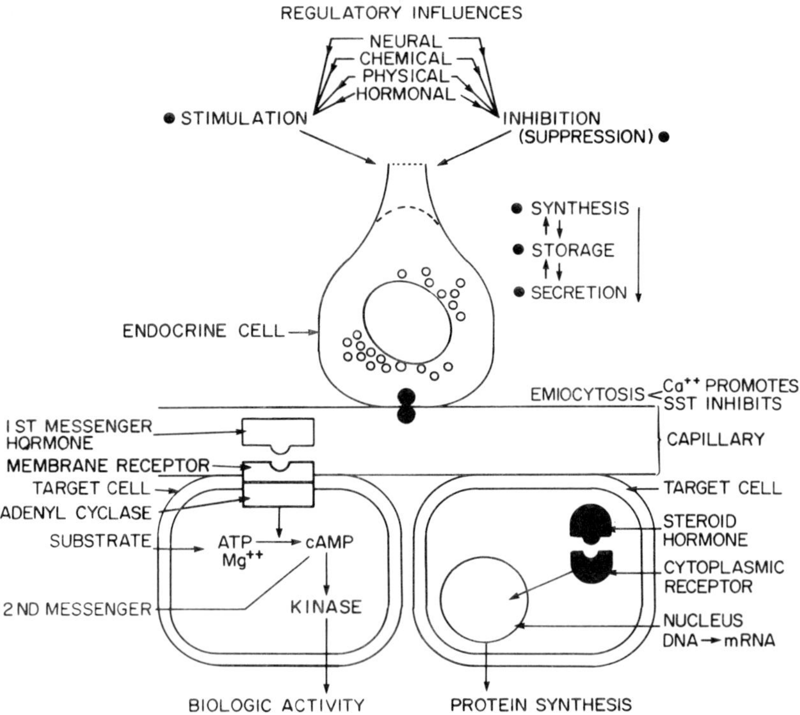

Fig. 1-2. This diagram illustrates humoral activity of endocrine cell and biologic activity of target cells at cellular and subcellular levels. The endocrine cell (with or without presumed microvilli) is responsive to four types of regulatory influences that stimulate or suppress its functions of synthesis, storage and secretion. The secretion of secretory granules into the bloodstream is by emiocytosis in which there is discharge of the humoral product across the cell-capillary interface. Amines and polypeptides activate their target cells by way of specific membrane receptors and the adenylcyclase enzyme system; the second messenger, cAMP, then promotes the biological activity of that target cell. The steroid hormone diffuses through the target cell membrane to activate its cytoplasmic receptor complex to initiate the specific biological function of protein synthesis. (Friesen, S. R.: Current dimensions of the endocrine system. *In* Longmire, W. P., Jr. [ed.]: Advances in Surgery. vol. 10. Chicago, Copyright © 1976 by Year Book Medical Publishers, Inc. Used by permission)

example of a closed cell is the beta islet cell in which the concentration of glucose influences the secretion or storage of insulin. Hormonal and chemical influences regulate the endocrine cell predominantly by means of feedback mechanisms within the neuroendocrine system. Neural and physical influences, on the other hand, may be instigated by systems other than the neuroendocrine system. Example of the latter might be the CNS stimulation by way of the autonomic vagus nerves that affect the G cells of the antrum at the sight of food; or the adrenal release of epinephrine triggered by the sight of danger; or the renal influence on circulating osmolarity of the blood, which in turn physically affects the posterior pituitary release of antidiuretic hormone.

The rate and direction of the endocrine cell functions of synthesis, storage and secretion (S-S-S) in either direction depend upon whether the cell's environment is stimulating or suppressing (-S-S) its action. Normal and hyperplastic endocrine cells are capable, generally, of responding to both stimulation and suppression, whereas autonomous tumor cells usually are not; these responses are useful as diagnostic tests. Unexplained exceptions include calcium or secretin stimulation of gastrinoma secretion and the calcium or pentagastrin stimulation of medullary carcinoma (thyroid C cells) release of thyrocalcitonin. It may be that these actions are mediated universally by the permissive effect of calcium ion on emiocytosis (the release of the secretory granules across the endocrine cell membrane into thc bloodstream).

The synthesis of the hormones in the endocrine cells is carried out by intracellular enzymes. The storage of the hormone within the secretory granules or the cytoplasm of the cells is variable. For instance, storage of parathyrin within parathyroid cells has not been observed (synthesis and secretion are apparently immediate or simultaneous); on the other hand, the thyroid gland stores large amounts of its amine hormone as thyroglobulin. Secretion or release of the humoral product from the endocrine cell appears to be influenced not only by its environment and calcium ion concentration at its membrane, but also can be inhibited specifically by a polypeptide, somatostatin;[22] this is true of the release of growth hormone (somatotrophin), gastrin, insulin, glucagon and perhaps other polypeptides, except thyrocalcitonin and parathyrin.

The Humoral Products

The first humoral substance to be recognized (1894) as having a messenger function was an amine, epinephrine; the first use of the word "hormone" (Greek hormaein, to excite or to arouse) was by Bayliss and Starling in 1902 to describe the action of secretin in an extract of duodenal mucosa on the exocrine pancreas. This hormone was later identified as a polypeptide. Thus the first two hormones, an amine and a polypeptide, are not only representative of APUD cell secretory products, but were identified originally by their function of provoking physiologic action, a biologic phenomenon. As a matter of fact, many additional humoral products have been identified by their function, physiologic or pharmacologic, before their molecular composition has been determined. The prototype of the third type of hormones, the steroids, was cortisol (hydrocortisone) which was isolated by Reichstein in 1937; its importance is suggested by the fact that it is the only steroid hormone that is essential to life.

Whereas most humoral substances have been identified with specific endocrine cells and specific physiologic actions on their target cells, some seem only to function as markers without a purpose; pancreatic polypeptide (PP) is such a circulating polypeptide.[23] Pancreatic polypeptide has been reported to be increased in association with endocrine neoplasms of the pancreas, such as insulinomas, gastrinomas, vipomas and glucagonomas. Furthermore, there are other humoral substances which sometimes circulate in association with known hormones which themselves have strong physiologic actions, such as the various prostaglandins and the kinins which are present in excess in patients with the carcinoid syndromes, pancreatic cholera and MCT syndromes.[12] The significance of these "extra"-humoral substances is still an enigma.

The humoral products, once secreted, circulate in physiologically minute amounts in different states: Thyroxine is bound to a carrier protein; epinephrine is in a free state; whereas cortisol circulates in both free and bound states. The fate of unused hormone is that of enzymatic degradation and excretion. When such control of its destruction is lost, this circumstance may in itself be a cause of secondary endocrine disease; for instance, renal failure may lead to secondary hyperparathyroidism and also to hypergastrinemia.

It is convenient to think of the circulating hormones, not only in terms of their chemical composition (amines, polypeptides and steroids) but also in terms of their functional interrelationships. Accordingly, insulin and glucagon have opposing actions and share their natural responsibility for carbohydrate metabolism with growth hormone, thyroxine, epinephrine and cortisol; parathyrin and thyrocalcitonin are antithetically involved in the divalent ion metabolism of calcium and phosphate and share one of their end-organs (the renal tubules) with another hormone (aldosterone) which is involved in the mineral metabolism of sodium and chloride; gastrin and the secretinlike hormones (GIP, CCK, VIP) have very dissimilar functions related to gastric acid and exocrine pancreatic secretion, but seem to compete for the same target cell receptors. However, another and more useful categorization is to consider the metabolic function in terms of being anabolic or catabolic. Those humoral agents with a general anabolic purpose are insulin, gastrin, growth hormone and the androgens; the remainder are generally catabolic, particularly glucagon, somatostatin, thyroxine and the secretinlike humoral agents.

The measurement of hormone content in blood, plasma or tissue has only recently become reasonably accurate quantitatively because of radioimmunochemical assay techniques, first accomplished for immunoreactive insulin by Yalow and Berson.[29] The biochemical definition of the molecular composition of the polypeptides and the synthesis of at least the active portions of them has led to the capability of producing antibodies for quantitative radioimmunochemical assays of many of the hormones. There is being developed a newer and possibly simpler technique for measurement of humoral substances by an enzyme-linked immunosorbent assay (ELISA) which employs enzymes rather than radioactive isotopes as markers of antibodies or antigens, the results of which can be read as a colorimetric change on a spectrophotometer. Whether this technique will be capable of the specificity which is required for the measurement of hormone molecules is unknown. The older bioassays for biologic activity of extracts of tissues containing humoral activity are still important for the qualitative and semiquantitative estimation of the functional capacity of a tumor or mucosa or blood concentrate. Although bioassays are often forgotten today and replaced by the radioimmune assay, it should be remembered that these different techniques may actually measure different portions of the hormone molecule—a biologically active principle and/or an immunoactive portion; such circumstances form the basis for occasional discrepancies in clinical data of patients.

The measurement of elevated levels of circulating hormones in the blood, by whatever method, must take into account the normal diurnal variations due to the inherent circadian rhythm, particularly of pituitary and adrenocortical elaboration, and also whether environmental factors (e.g., fasting, feeding, basal or active states) are influential at the time.

Although a hormone that is normally released from normal endocrine cells may be of the same molecular structure when elaborated from a hyperplastic or tumor cell, it is a general rule that when a malignancy of the endocrine cells elaborates that humoral product, the hormone is usually heterogeneous and of a larger molecular size, displaying altered biologic and immunologic capabilities. Some of these tumor products are the larger prohormones, such as proinsulin.

TARGET CELLS AND RECEPTOR MECHANISMS

The circulating hormones which are physiologically active in measurably miniscule amounts produce their effect by their action upon those specific and responsive target cells which in turn produce their biologic effect. The target cells may be specific glands, such as that part of the adrenal cortex which is responsive to the trophic polypeptide ACTH, or they may be diffusely scattered cells, as in response to growth hormone and thyroxine. Not infrequently several specific target areas may respond in a dose-related fashion to one polypeptide hormone, thus evoking more than one physiologic or pharmacologic response. Gastrin, for instance, physiologically stimulates parietal cell secretion of hydrogen ion (as gastric acid) and, by its trophic action, stimulates growth of the gastric parietal cells and Brunner's glands of the duodenal mucosa; pharmacologically it causes contraction of the distal esophageal sphincter. Other effects of gastrin, such as increased intestinal regurgitation and pyrosis, may be unmasked after total gastrectomy. Furthermore, a target cell may respond to more than one stimulus by virtue of the fact that it may possess more than one type of receptor; for instance there are three separate receptors on the gastric parietal cell: one for gastrin, one for acetylcholine and one for histamine.

Just as research has progressed to the molecular level of hormone identification and synthesis, so it has proceeded to the membrane and intracellular domain in search of receptor mechanisms. Investigators had noted that in many cases the effect of a given hormone appeared at some time after the stimulus was introduced and often at a time when the level of the hormone was minimal rather than maximal. These observations suggested that the hormone in some way evoked a second messenger which had its own time characteristics and that the hormone might be an *inducer* of enzymes, instead of a coenzyme. Receptors for at least 12 of the polypeptide hormones have now been identified and it appears that these receptors form an integral part of the target cell membrane (Fig. 1-2). When the hormone, the "first messenger," combines with its specific membrane receptor, the enzyme adenylcyclase is activated to catalyze the conversion of adenosine triphosphate (ATP) to cyclic adenosine monophosphate (cAMP), the "second messenger"; cAMP, together with its kinase, then calls forth the primary biologic function of that cell.[26] Such membrane receptors can be blocked pharmacologically (as with histamine-2 blockade of the gastrin receptor), or can be occupied by competing polypeptide hormones (as with CCK competitive attraction for the same receptor). The activity of the cAMP receptor mechanism can be measured; an important and unique biologic function of the polypeptide VIP is the stimulation of increased measurable cAMP receptor activity.[25]

The steroid hormone combines with its intracellular cytoplasmic receptor after diffusion through the target cell membrane. The hormone-receptor complex is then transferred into the target cell nucleus where gene transcription occurs and DNA is converted to messenger RNA, and specific proteins are synthesized.[15]

It can be considered that the membrane receptor with the adenylcyclase—cAMP complex constitutes a quantitative response to amine and peptide hormones, whereas the cytoplasmic receptor with its nuclear gene transcription for protein synthesis represents a qualitative response to steroids. The second messenger, cAMP, activated in common by many hormones which do not enter the cell, mediates a quantitative response, but the resulting biologic activity is still qualitatively specific for the first messenger; similarly, the steroid-activated gene transcription and messenger RNA qualitatively determine the specificity of the protein synthesis.

NEUROHUMORAL HOMEOSTASIS, NORMAL AND DECOMPENSATED

When all the mechanisms for the regulation of endocrine cell function and target cell response are in balance, a remarkable normal homeostasis is evident and purposeful not only for the efficient utilization and metabolism of energy, food, water and minerals, but also for the preservation of life by neurovascular responses and indeed, the preservation of the species by steroid hormone influences between the adrenals, the gonads, the placenta and the brain. The simple act of contemplating and consuming a meal initiates a domino effect of neurohumoral transmissions beginning with vagal stimulation of acid, through antral release of gastrin, duodenal secretin inhibition of gastric secretion and stimulation of pancreatic bicarbonate secretion, and including insulin and CCK-pancreozymin release after absorption of glucose, proteins and fats. The temporary fluctuations of the concentrations of polypeptides and exocrine products in the blood return almost immediately to stable basal levels. Even the rather strong challenge of 100 g. (100,000 mg.) of glucose during a glucose tolerance test in a normal individual is handled so that glucose and insulin homeostasis are attained within 2 hours. Also, when there is prolonged chronic stimulation, as in some abnormal disease states, compensatory regulation within normal bounds is the rule, at least for a time. But perhaps compensatory reactions to a chronic abnormal environment are possible only by the development of a reactive hyperplasia. It is not known what it is that disrupts the balance of homeostasis to the point of decompensation of neuroendocrine control, but the theoretical possibilities include the development of reactive hyperplasia in compensation for or response to a chronic abnormal environment, the development of hyperplasia or dysplasia upon genetic instigation, or by some unknown instigation toward neoplasia, de novo.

When the wide spectrum of clinical syndromes due to functional endocrinopathies are considered individually, some easily fall pathogenetically into a category of genetic instigation such as the familial multiple endocrine adenopathies; others, because of their sporadic incidence without preceding abnormalities or familial associations, seem to arise de novo, and still others may have no clinical explanation except to result, possibly, from abnormal environmental influences. Among the latter group are the increasing numbers of endocrinopathies which are based histologically on hyperplasia including:

1. The parathyroid hyperplasias (even tertiary hyperparathyroidism with tumor) which are associated with renal disease or with nonfamilial thyroid medullary carcinoma, or pancreatic apudomas, or those parathyroid hyperplasias and adenomas resulting from thiazide and glucocorticoid administration or irradiation[24]
2. The adrenocortical hyperplasias associated with abnormal cholesterol metabolism in the adrenogenital syndrome or resulting from chronic ACTH stimulation
3. The islet cell hyperplasias of nesidioblastosis (islet building) with hyperglucagonism which has been associated with "secondary" hyperinsulinism, hypergastrinism and even thyroid and parathyroid hyperplasias.[27]

It is easy to speculate that profound reactive changes can develop as a result of an abnormal environment lasting over a period of years. For instance, in patients with duodenal ulcer who have vagally induced acid hypersecretion of many months' duration, it might be expected that this continuous acid stimulation of the duodenal secretin mechanism could eventually provoke a breakdown in homeostasis. As a matter of fact, a long-standing history of duodenal ulcer disease seems to precede the development of the Zollinger-Ellison syndrome in many, but not all, patients; moreover, islet cell hyperplasia and antral G cell hyperplasia have been observed in duodenal ulcer patients. The intermediate type of hypergastrinism, due to antral gastrinosis in severe duodenal ulcer disease, may be an example of the result of an environment of chronic acid inhibition of antral release of gastrin with compensatory G cell hyperplasia.[10] It has also been hypothesized that chronic pyloric reflux of bile with its alkaline stimulation of the antral mucosa may lead to an abnormality of antral G cells and gastrin release.

Antral G cell hyperplasia has been hormonally induced experimentally in animals by the chronic administration of corticosteroids[14] (as has islet cell hyperplasia).[5] This is not surprising, since antral gastrinosis has been observed in patients in association with sporadic acromegaly, medullary thyroid carcinoma and hyperparathyroidism.[10] The G cells of the antral mucosa are the most accessible endocrine cells for study. When multiple endocrine organs are involved in a familial or genetic pattern, screening of relatives by endoscopic biopsy of antral mucosa has shown that G cell hyperplasia is of value in predicting the development of endocrinopathy in those patients.[11]

It is difficult, of course, to ascertain whether dysfunction precedes the development of hyperplasia. Certainly hyperplasia of any of the endocrine cells leads to endocrine dysfunction, and the development of autonomous neoplasia further disrupts homeostasis. But it is not known whether hyperplasia may proceed to dysplasia or neoplasia; in fact, whether hyperplasia, adenoma and carcinoma are histologically static or progressive in either direction is a controversial issue. The association of more than one type of these histologic patterns in the same gland, or in the same patient, for that matter, suggests a progression toward neoplasia. In patients who were at risk for hereditary medullary thyroid carcinoma and who had progressive increase of serum thyrocalcitonin levels in response to calcium infusion, C cell hyperplasia of the thyroid has been observed to precede the development of medullary carcinoma.[28] At the other end of the spectrum, remissions, exacerbations, and even spontaneous regression of endocrine tumors are sporadically reported, including melanoma of the skin (the melanocyte is an APUD "ectocrine" cell of neural crest origin). Occasional examples of objective regression of gastrin-secreting metastases to the liver and lungs after total gastrectomy have been observed;[6] these "embolic" metastases appear histologically to be composed of hyperplastic cells. It has been suggested that regression of such endocrine tumors can follow surgical correction of an abnormal feedback imbalance. Although no "gastrin factor" has been found in the stomach, there are investigations in progress in search of gastric or duodenal trophic influences on islet cells.[4]

CLINICAL SYNDROMES

One of the important diagnostic exercises with which the clinician must deal, even after the clinical syndrome and its humoral culprit are identified, is the determination of the histologic basis of the disease, therapeutic success depending to a large extent upon the pathologic changes which may be present. The clinician must consider numerous possibilities.

1. Is there hyperplasia with or without tumor?
2. Is the tumor single or multiple?
3. Is there microadenomatosis?
4. Is the tumor malignant, with or without functioning metastases?
5. Is the malignancy entopic or ectopic?
6. Finally, to make it even more difficult: Is there receptor failure or malfunction?

The judicious use of comparisons of inappropriate hormone levels with simultaneous exocrine determinations, and the appropriate evaluation of stimulation and suppression tests, will usually identify the pathologic basis of the hyperfunction and the receptor responsiveness. Angiography and selective venous sampling for hormonal assays are being employed increasingly for localization of the source(s) of humoral emanation, but radioactive scanning has not been helpful, with the possible exception of radioiodocholesterol scanning of the adrenal glands.

The finding of bilaterality and multiple foci of primary tumors, benign or malignant, and the detection of pluriglandular involvement should prompt endocrine screening of relatives in the family for a genetic connection. Multiple endocrine involvement in patients, and associated endocrinopathies in families, have occurred frequently and predictably enough to be grouped into several syndromes. The terminology of these arrangements is not settled, but there seems to be a preference for the term, "multiple endocrine neoplasia" (MEN) syndromes, in spite of the fact that hyperplasia is a more frequent histologic component of the syndrome than is either malignancy or adenomatous change; for this reason some prefer "multiple endocrinopathy" or "multiple endocrine adenopathy" (MEA), but not adenomatosis, as a more precise definition of the syndrome.

Some of the unique features of hyperfunctioning endocrine malignancies include a more fulminating clinical course, sometimes in crisis; disparately high or erratic plasma concentration values, suggesting heterogeneous hormones of large molecular size; nonsuppressibility, and the detection of polyhormonal manifestations.

The clinician must be continuously alert to the possibility that an apparently straightforward clinical endocrine syndrome, particularly if it has the above characteristics of a malignancy, might have an ectopic, rather than an entopic, source of hormone elaboration. Virtually all of these "ectopic" tumors are malignancies of either endocrine cells (organs) which elaborate an unexpected hormone, or of other organs which are not usually considered endocrine (paraendocrine syndromes—PES).[15] Various examples of ectopic syndromes are illustrated in Figure 1-3. In such instances the circulating hormone may have an action similar to a known hormone but may not be measurable by routine radioimmunoassay techniques; this is because the hormone molecule is usually larger than normal and is heterogeneous, requiring very special assay techniques. Furthermore, the entopic endocrine gland in a patient with ectopia is histologically normal, and its normal hormone is suppressible and at normal or undetectable levels. An example of such an instance is a patient with a severe

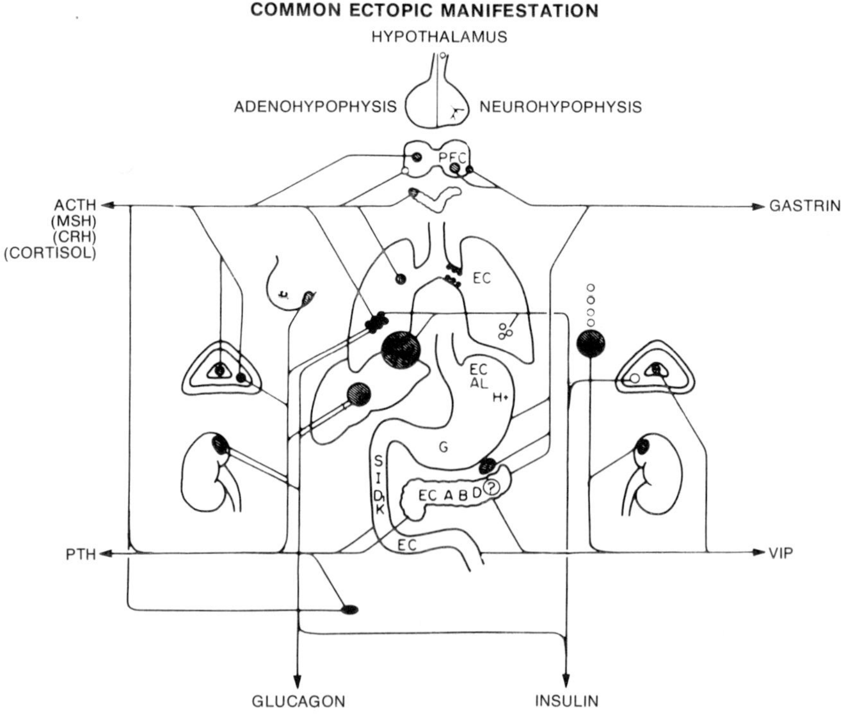

Fig. 1-3. This diagram illustrates the complex phenomena of "ectopia," in which increased elaboration of polypeptidelike activity from various sites has been reported. (Friesen, S. R.: Current dimensions of the endocrine system. *In* Longmire, W. P., Jr. [ed.]: Advances in Surgery. vol. 10. Chicago, Copyright © 1976 by Year Book Medical Publishers, Inc. Used by permission)

hypercalcemic syndrome due to ectopic elaboration of a heterogeneous hormone having parathyrinlike activity from an islet cell carcinoma;[9] the elevated blood calcium suppresses the PTH (which on the usual assays represents the hormone from the parathyroid gland) to undetectable levels which then rises to normal levels when the calcium ion level is brought down to normal by phosphate treatment. In another instance of ectopic hypercalcemia syndrome due to carcinoma of the breast or lung, for example, the absence of decalcifying bone metastases must be confirmed and excision of the so-called "ectopic" tumor should correct the hypercalcemia. The accepted differentiation between an ectopic endocrine tumor and an ectopic nonendocrine tumor rests only in the fact that the former contains secretory granules in the cytoplasm of the malignant cells on electron-microscopic study.

Realizing that most examples of "ectopia" involve the elaboration of polypeptides from APUD cells which have unique embryologic origins, common cytochemical functions and pluripotentiality, it is debatable whether there is, in fact, any example of true ectopia. It will be recalled that the APUD cells in their embryologic migration from the neural crest to the foregut take up habitat in any part of the entoderm, including the bronchi and lungs. These primitive cells, as they arrive at their new location, normally repress their multifunctional capacities and assume only their teleologic function for homeostasis in that location. With the development and onset of neoplastic change at a later time, there is a reactivation of the APUD cells' original capacities by a derepression of the primitive totipotentiality so that a malignant endocrine neoplasm, irrespective of its location, may elaborate a whole series of related humoral products that appear to be functionally and geographically "ectopic."[13] Furthermore, an ectopic location of a functioning tumor may be only a developmental anomaly, assuming that, in the course of migration, the APUD cells may have become "arrested" in mesenchymal tissues, or "deterred" in their course until neoplasia is somehow instigated.[10]

Thorough *clinical* evaluation of the patient's findings is still paramount in the diagnosis of any of the numerous endocrine syndromes; the laboratory confirmation usually allows the surgeon to proceed with surgical treatment in confidence with the aim of detection of the abnormality, possible excision of the source of hyperfunction, or elimination of the abnormal feedback mechanism. Some specific pharmacologic and chemotherapeutic agents, given systemically and selectively, are becoming available for alleviation of some of the syndromes. There are more options to come for the palliative treatment by receptor modification and for specific tumor therapy with and without surgical intervention.

There are neuroendocrine cells which become neoplastic to form rare tumors for which no function or hyperfunction has been identified or for which a function leading to a systemic effect is only speculative. Such clinical syndromes will be described after careful clinical observations are made and after appropriate candidate hormones, as yet unidentified, are defined and measured.

SUMMARY

Because an increasing majority of both entopic- and ectopic-functioning tumors arise from APUD cells, many of which have been shown to be derived from the neural crest of the neuroectoderm, this body of endocrine abnormalities has been grouped under the term neurocristopathies.[2,18] The APUD concept, conceived cytochemically, functionally and embryologically, is neither complete nor is it capable of being universally applied to the entire neuroendocrine system. However, there is a clearer understanding of many of the syndromes caused by these endocrinopathies because they have developed under the umbrella of the APUD concept.

Diagnostic capabilities center around the quantitative identification of the excessive circulating hormone(s), the resulting exocrine manifestations and the characteristic features of stimulation and suppression tests. As new information proliferates from the research laboratories and new syndromes are described, it is best to consider the endocrinopathies as disruptions of normal homeostasis by hyperfunctioning endocrine cells, hyperplastic or tumorous. In endocrine malignancy, the potential variety of humoral products is capable of producing a kaleidoscopic array of clinical endocrine syndromes.

REFERENCES

1. Bayliss, W. M., and Starling, E. H.: The mechanism of pancreatic secretion. J. Physiol., *28*:325, 1902.
2. Bolande, R. P.: The neurocristopathies, a unifying concept of disease arising in neural crest maldevelopment. Hum. Pathol., *5*:409, 1974.
3. Feyrter, F.: Über diffuse endokrine epitheliale Organe. Leipzig, Barth, 1938.
4. Fiddian-Green, R. G.: Is peptic ulceration a hormonal disease? Lancet, *1*:74, 1977.
5. Frenkel, J. K.: Pancreatic islet cell hyperplasia in hamsters treated with cortisone and chlorothiazide (Diuril). Fed. Proc., *19*:(1) 160, 1960.
6. Friesen, S. R.: The Zollinger-Ellison syndrome. *In* Ravitch, M. M. (ed.): Current Problems in Surgery, Chicago, Year Book Medical Publishers, 1976.
7. ——: APUD tumors of the gastrointestinal tract. *In* Hickey, R. C.: Current Problems in Cancer. vol. 1 [4], Chicago, Year Book Medical Publishers, 1976.
8. ——: Current dimensions of the endocrine system. *In* Longmire, W.: P., Jr.: Advances in Surgery. vol. 10, Chicago, Year Book Medical Publishers, 1976.
9. Friesen, S. R., and Allen, M. S.: Malignant hyperparathyroidism of pancreatic and parathyroid origins. Bull. Soc. Int. Chir., *34*:268, 1975.
10. Friesen, S. R., and McGuigan, J. E.: Ectopic apudocarcinomas and associated endocrine hyperplasias of the foregut. Ann. Surg., *182*:371, 1975.
11. Friesen, S. R., Schimke, R. N., and Pearse, A. G. E.: Genetic aspects of the Z-E syndrome: Prospective studies in two kindred; antral gastrin cell hyperplasia. Ann. Surg., *176*:370, 1972.
12. Jaffe, B. M., and Condon, S.: Prostaglandins E and F in endocrine diarrheagenic syndromes. Ann. Surg., *184*:516, 1976.
13. Levine, R. J., and Metz, S. A.: A classification of ectopic hormone producing tumors. Ann. N. Y. Acad. Sci., *230*:633, 1974.
14. Mejia-Michel, H., Bonsack, M. E., Eisenberg, M. M., and Delaney, J. P.: Gastrin cell hyperplasia induced by corticosteroids. Surg. Forum, *27*:421, 1976.
15. Montgomery, D. A. D., and Welbourn, R. B.: Medical and Surgical Endocrinology. Baltimore, Williams & Wilkins, 1975.
16. Pavlov, I. P.: The work of the Digestive Glands. Translated by W. H. Thompson. London, Charles Griffin & Company, 1910.
17. Pearse, A. G. E.: The endocrine cells of the G.I. tract: Origins, morphology

and functional relationships in health and disease. Clin. Gastroenterol., *3*:491, 1974.
18. ——: Neurocristopathy, neuroendocrine pathology and the APUD concept. Z. Krebsforsch. *84*:1, 1975.
19. ——: Brain polypeptides. Nature, *262*:92, 1976.
20. Pearse, A. G. E., and Polak, J. M.: Neural crest origin of the endocrine polypeptide (APUD) cells of the gastrointestinal tract and pancreas. Gut, *12*:783, 1971.
21. Pearse, A. G. E., and Takor, T. T.: Neuroendocrine embryology and the APUD concept. Proceedings of Endocrinology 1975. Clin. Endocrinol. [Suppl.]: 229, Feb., 1976.
22. Polak, J. M., Pearse, A. G. E., Grimelius, L., Bloom, S. R., and Arimura, A.: Growth-hormone release-inhibiting hormone in gastrointestinal and pancreatic D cells. Lancet, *1*:1220, 1975.
23. Polak, J. M., et al.: Pancreatic polypeptide in insulinomas, gastrinomas, vipomas, and glucagonomas. Lancet, *1*:328, 1976.
24. Prinz, R., et al.: Radiation associated parathyroid tumors: A new syndrome? Surgery, 1977 (In press).
25. Schwartz, C. J., et al.: Vasoactive intestinal peptide stimulation of adenylate cyclase and active electrolyte secretion in intestinal mucosa. J. Clin. Invest., *54*:536, 1974.
26. Steer, M. D.: Cyclic AMP. Ann. Surg., *184*:107, 1976.
27. Vance, J. E., et al.: Familial nesidioblastosis as the predominant manifestation of multiple endocrine adenomatosis. Am. J. Med., *52*:211, 1972.
28. Wolfe, H. J., et al.: C-cell hyperplasia preceding medullary thyroid carcinoma. N. Engl. J. Med., *289*:437, 1973.
29. Yalow, R. S., and Berson, S. A.: Assay of plasma insulin in human subjects by immunologic methods. Nature, *184*:1648, 1959.

Special Reading

Tischler, A. S., Dichter, N. A., Bialis, B., and Greene, L. A.: Neuroendocrine neoplasms and their cells of origin. N. Engl. J. Med., *296*:919, 1971.

2

The APUD Concept: Embryology, Cytochemistry and Ultrastructure of the Diffuse Neuroendocrine System

A. G. E. Pearse, M.D.

THE APUD CONCEPT

The term APUD is an acronym taken from the initial letters of the most constant cytochemical properties of a series of cells whose apparent common function is the synthesis and secretion of peptide or amine hormones. The letter *A* refers first to their (inconstant) content of endogenous amines and second, together with the letters *P* and *U*, to their potential for preferential uptake of the amino acid precursors of the two fluorogenic amines, dopamine and 5-hydroxytryptamine. The letter *D* refers to decarboxylation of the relevant precursors, 3,4-dihydroxyphenylalanine and 5-hydroxytryptophan. Ideally there should be an additional letter *S* at the end, to stand for storage, since once generated the amines are stored in or on membrane-bound "endocrine" granules. In addition to their lipoprotein membrane, and possibly matrix, these cells contain either endocrine peptides, or peptides having no apparent hormonal function. It is sometimes possible to demonstrate uptake and decarboxylation of amine precursors by cells having no granule content, but this is a transient phenomenon and demonstrable not only in endocrine cells but also in many other cells with high amino acid turnover. A certain amount of confusion, moreover, arises from the fact that a minority of the APUD cells can take up exogenously administered fluorogenic amines. By the same token, fluorogenic amines generated from exogenous precursors, by the action of extracellular amino acid decarboxylases, are also taken up.

Although the term APUD is derived from the amine-handling qualities of the cells which make up the series, it has always been understood to contain and express the remaining common cytochemical characteristics of the cells, together with their common ultrastructural features. In brief, these features are:

1. Exhibition of the property of masked metachromasia (and argyrophilia).
2. High content of nonspecific esterases or cholinesterases.
3. High levels of "mitochondrial" α-glycerophosphate dehydrogenase.
4. he presence of "specific" endocrine-type granules, usually round and 100 to 400 nm. in diameter, of various electron densities.

The Expansion of the APUD Concept

The idea which became the APUD concept[27,28] was formulated in 1966[25,26] when the observed common cytochemical and ultrastructural characteristics of a small group of endocrine cells, situated in different regions of the body, suggested that they shared a common origin from the neuroectoderm of the neural crest. Since that time elaborations of the concept have been made and the number of cells in the series has increased from the original six to approximately 40.

There are two principal reasons for this expansion. First, there has been an almost explosive increase in the number of endocrine cells identifiable in the gastroenteropancreatic (GEP) system. Second, despite earlier misgivings, it has become necessary to incorporate into the APUD series the endocrine cells of the hypothalamus and pineal gland. Together with the endocrine cells of the pituitary gland, these now constitute the central neuroendocrine division, leaving the remaining cells of the original series to represent the peripheral neuroendocrine division.[30] We can therefore present, in Tables 2-1 and 2-2, a full list of the members of the two division of the APUD series, together with their proven or presumptive products, both peptide and amine.

The Neuroectodermal Origin of the APUD Cells

The original formulation of the APUD concept stressed the position of the neural crest as the source of cells later transformed into the several varieties of the APUD cells. Subsequently, however, it became necessary to modify this narrow unitarian view, particularly when it was realized that the cells of the newly constituted central neuroendocrine division could not have such an origin.

The Central Division. Takor-Takor and Pearse[43] showed that Rathke's pouch, and at least a part of the floor of the diencephalon destined to become the hypothalamus, were derived not from the neural tube, neural crest or stomodeal ectoderm, but from specialized neuroectodermal thickenings, the neural ridges, situated in the midline and extending ventrally from the anterior neuropore. A number of embryologists view Rathke's pouch as a placode and, in the broadest sense, the brain itself, with its dorsal diencephalic pouch, the pineal gland, can properly be considered in the same category. Thus, the components of the central division of the APUD series, the hypothalamus, pineal and hypophysis, are all clearly established as neuroectodermal derivatives.

Table 2-1. The Central Neuroendocrine Division of the APUD Cell Series*

Pituitary	c	*ACTH*	(T)
	m	*MSH*	(T)
	s	*STH*	
	l	*PRL*	
Pineal	p	—	MT, 5-HT
Hypothalamus	Npv	Oxytocin	
	Nso	Vasopressin	
	Ndm	*TRF*	5-HT
	Nvm	*SRH*	DA
	Narc	*LHRF*	NA
	Nant	*MRF*	
	Nperiv	*SRIF*	

*See p. 20 for abbreviations used in this table.
Italics = Peptides and peptide hormones. Roman = Amine hormones. ( ) = Incompletely proven (peptides) or species variability (amines).

Table 2-2. The Peripheral Neuroendocrine Division of the APUD Cell Series

Pancreas	B	*Insulin*	
	A	*Glucagon*	(DA or 5-HT)
	D	*Somatostatin*	
	D_1	—	—
	F	*PP*	—
Stomach	G	*Gastrin*	—
	A(AL)	*Glucagon*	—
	ECL	—	(H)
	EC_1	*Subs.P.*	5-HT
Intestine	EC_2, EC_1	*Motilin, Subs.P.*	5-HT(MT)
	L	*Enteroglucagon*	
	S	*Secretin*	—
	D	*Somatostatin*	—
	D_1	—	—
	I	*CCK*	—
	K	*GIP*	—
	H	*VIP*	—
Thyroid	C	*Calcitonin*	(5-HT)
Parathyroid	Ch	*Parathyrin*	—
Carotid body	Type I	—	NA, DA
Skin	M'blast	—	Unidentified
Adrenal	A	—	A
	NA	—	NA
Lung	F	*(VLP)*	—
Urogenital	EC	—	5-HT
	U	—	—

Italics =Peptides and peptide hormones
Roman = Amine hormones

Abbreviations Used in Tables 2-1 and 2-2.

DA Dopamine
NA Noradrenalin
A Adrenalin
5-HT 5-Hydroxytryptamine
T Tryptamine
MT Melatonin
N Nucleus
pv Paraventricularis
so Supraopticus
dm Dorsomedialis
arc Arcuatus
H Histamine
GIP Gastric inhibitory peptide
VIP Vasoactive intestinal peptide
VLP Vasoactive lung peptide
STH Somatotropin
SRIF Somatotropin release inhibiting factor (Somatostatin)
CRF Corticotropin releasing factor
MRF Melanotropin releasing factor
PP Pancreatic polypeptide
Subs.P. Substance P
PRL Prolactin
SRH Somatotropin-releasing hormone
MSH Melanocyte-stimulating hormone
CCK Cholecystokinin
Ch Chief
M'blast Melanoblast
F Feyrter
ECL Enterochromaffinlike
EC Enterochromaffin
periv Periventricularis
U Urogenital

The Peripheral Division. It is a little more difficult to consider the evidence for and against a neural crest, neuroectodermal, or specialized ectodermal origin for the cells of the peripheral division of the APUD series. Studies using an allograft technique to produce quail-chick embryo chimeras, and a biologic marker system to identify the donor cells,[17] have completely validated the neural crest as the origin of the melanocytes, the two adrenomedullary cells, the Type I cell of the carotid body and the ultimobranchial C cell. Cytochemical marker experiments[30,33] have provided confirmation, and combined biological/ cytochemical marker experiments[38] have added additional support.

It is when we come to the GEP endocrine cells that the position becomes less clear. Cytochemical marker experiments, using both avian and rodent embryos, have provided circumstantial evidence in favor of their origin from neural crest, but there are a number of studies providing evidence for an endodermal (foregut) origin of all the endocrine cells of the gut and pancreas. These studies fall into four separate categories:

1. The finding of mixed endocrine-exocrine cells in the pancreas is held to confirm their common entodermal origin.[20,24,34]

2. Using the technique of chorioallantois-implanted grafts of rudimentary chick embryonic gut, Andrew[1] has found that enterochromaffin (EC) cells develop from foregut grafts taken before the presumptive arrival of the neural crest.

3. Pictet, Rall, Phelps and Rutter,[35] after presumptive removal with trypsin of all neuroectoderm and ectoderm from 3-somite rat embryos, have found on further culture that the developing pancreas contains both B cells and insulin.

4. On the basis of radioautographic studies indicating a similar turnover time (4 days) for "crypt-base" cells and endocrine cells alike, and on ultrastructural studies showing identical organelles (phagosomes) in both cell types, Cheng and Leblond[9,10] have proposed that the endodermal crypt-base cell is the progenitor of all cell types in gastrointestinal epithelium.

Observations made by conventional embryology show that in anuran, avian and mammalian (mouse, rat) embryos, the earliest dispersion of neurally programed ectodermal cells takes place before any form of operative interference could prevent their access to the developing gut. These studies do not prove that the GEP endocrine cells do indeed come from neuroectoderm, only that they could do so. Stronger, although still circumstantial, evidence is derived from studies that reveal the presence, in GEP endocrine cells, of neurotransmitter peptides or peptides closely related thereto. Similar evidence comes from the presence in epithelial tumors of indisputably neural origin of peptides cross-reacting with antisera to gut and pancreatic hormones. In the first of these categories is the revelation of somatostatin in the pancreatic D cell,[18] of the same hormone in the intestinal D cell,[36] and of a substance P in an intestinal endocrine cell subsequently identified as enterochromaffin.[31] In the second category are various reports of the presence of VIP in ganglioneuroblastomas, pheochromocytomas and other tumors.[14,32] Recently a gastrinlike peptide,[44] reacting with antigastrin sera, was identified in the cerebral cortex of a number of vertebrates. This finding provides further evidence of the essential similarity of peptide hormones and neurotransmitters and favors their common origin from neuroectoderm.

All these considerations accepted, the principal remaining example of a normal endocrine cell of presumptive endodermal origin producing a peptide hormone is the chief cell of the parathyroid gland. Its origin, in all vertebrate species, has been considered to be from the endoderm of the third and fourth visceral pouches. Comparative studies of parathyroid development in anurans, birds and mammals have shown that in the frog embryo the parathyroid gland arises from the ectoderm of the third and fourth visceral grooves and that it has no endodermal component. The situation in birds and mammals, in which at no stage is a proper gill chamber developed, are less easy to interpret. The gland, initially, contains both ectodermal and endodermal components but, presumably, the former predominate before the functional stage of hormone production begins. Thus the parathyroid is to be regarded as a placode, like the pituitary and, although its chief cells lack the amine-handling facility which is demonstrable in the majority of APUD cells, there is no longer any reason to exclude it from the series on this account.

IDENTIFICATION OF APUD CELLS

Cytochemical Identification

Of the three "histologic" methods for the demonstration of endocrine peptide cells (argyrophilia, lead hematoxylin, masked metachromasia), only the last can be described as cytochemical. The masked metachromasia reaction was first described by Manocchio,[19] and was originally thought to stain "practically all

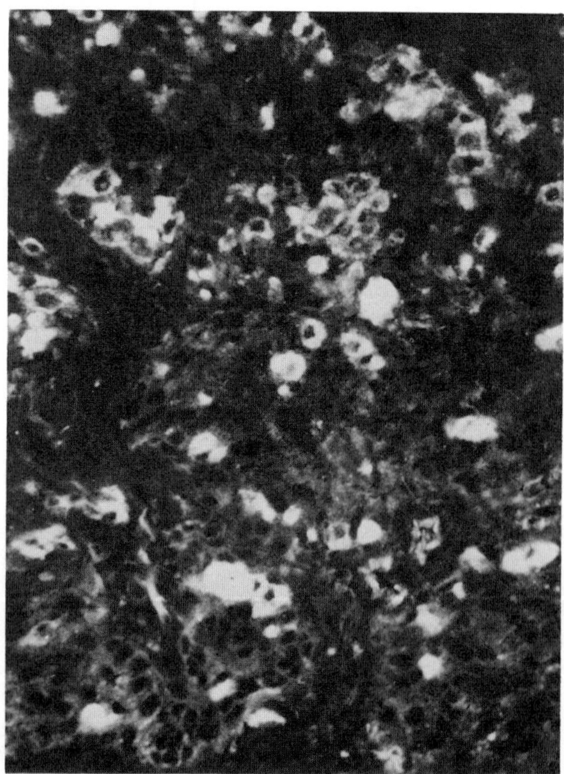

Fig. 2-1. Rat pituitary gland. Orange-red fluorescent cells demonstrated by the coriphosphine variant of the masked metachromasia technique are corticotropes. X 250

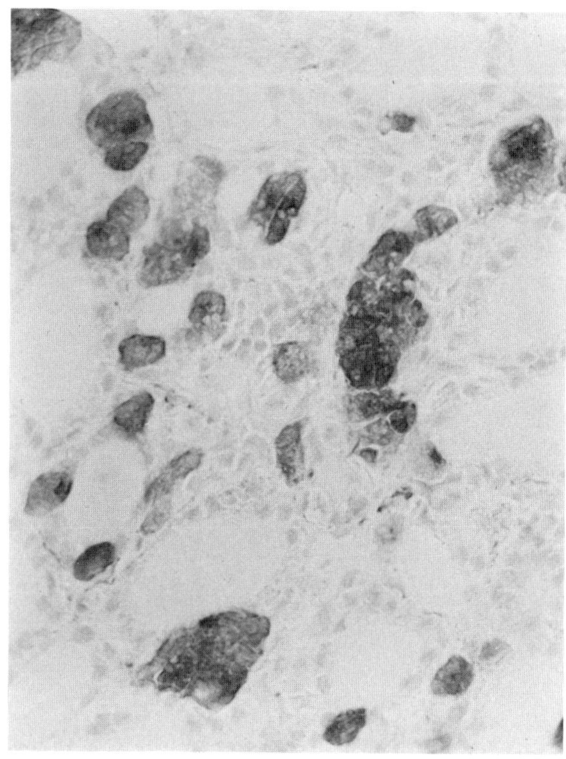

Fig. 2-2. Dog thyroid gland. The parafollicular C cells, source of calcitonin, possess a strong nonspecific cholinesterase. The enzyme is absent from the follicle cells. X 250

secretory granules of cells producing protein or peptide hormones."[42] Later it was considered to indicate first, the presence of a peptide containing a high proportion of side-chain acidic groups (aspartic and glutamic acids)[29] and, second, a predominantly random coil conformation. It has recently been shown[39] that removal of the lipoprotein membrane from the granules of thyroid C cells has no effect on the subsequent demonstration of masked metachromasia. Hence, their lipid component is unlikely to be making any significant contribution to staining.

An alternative, fluorescent, method for demonstrating masked metachromasia is shown in Figure 2-1.[8]

Three enzyme cytochemical techniques are used for indentification of APUD cells. These are for (1) the so-called mitochondrial *α-glycerophosphate dehydrogenase;* (2) the *nonspecific esterases* (usually by means of the azo dye and indoxyl methods), and (3) the *cholinesterases* (exceptionally the specific acetylcholinesterase). The significance of all three, in terms of hormone production, is unclear. The strong nonspecific cholinesterase of dog thyroid C cells is shown in Figure 2-2 and the very strong α-glycerophosphate dehydrogenase of the pancreatic B cells, of the same species, in Figure 2-3. A full list of the enzymic armament of the cells of the APUD series is not available. In the gastric fundus, for instance, Monga, Bonfanti and Bussolati[21] found cholinesterase in the histamine-containing ECL cells but not in the pancreatic glucagon-secreting A cells. Much more often present in neoplastic APUD cells, this cholinesterase is regarded by Drews[13] as a return to the embryonic form of the enzyme.

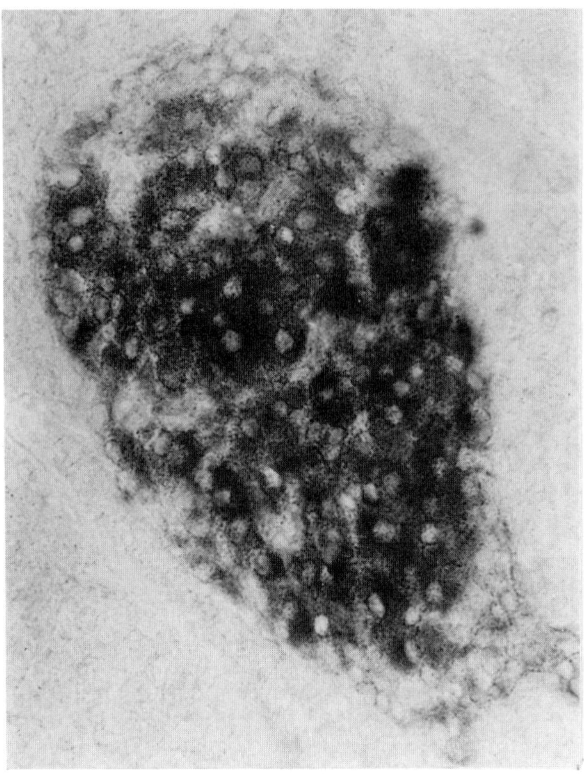

Fig. 2-3. Dog pancreatic islet. The menadione-linked (mitochondrial) α-glycerophosphate dehydrogenase activity of the B cells is extremely high; that of the surrounding A cells is much lower, and that of the peri-insular acinar cells lower still. X 300

The uptake and decarboxylation of the two amine precursors, 5-HTP and DOPA, and their subsequent demonstration by *formaldehyde-induced fluorescence* (APUD-FIF) is a satisfactory method for demonstrating the majority of cells in the APUD series. In contradistinction to the situation in tumors (apudomas), where the APUD-FIF method appears invariably to give a positive result, there may be difficulty in demonstrating the property in some normal cell types and in a few it is impossible. Fluorescence induced, after the exogenous application of L-dopa, in the mainly B cells of a dog pancreatic islet is shown in Figure 2-4.

The most satisfactory way of demonstrating a APUD cell is by immunocytochemistry, using an antiserum specific for the normal peptide product of the cell. Largely according to the preference of the operator, variations of an immunofluorescence procedure[11] or of the immunoperoxidase technique[23] are used. The type of result obtained is shown in Figures 2-5 and 2-6 for immunofluorescence and immunoperoxidase respectively.

Ultrastructural Identification

Provided that glutaraldehyde is used as the primary fixative, endocrine cell granules are uniformly well preserved for electron-microscopy. Lead citrate and uranyl acetate are normally used as counterstains. In organs in which there is apparently only a single endocrine peptide cell, such as the thyroid gland, its identification by electron-microscopy is deceptively easy. In organs such as the pituitary gland, gastrointestinal tract and pancreas, in which there are a number

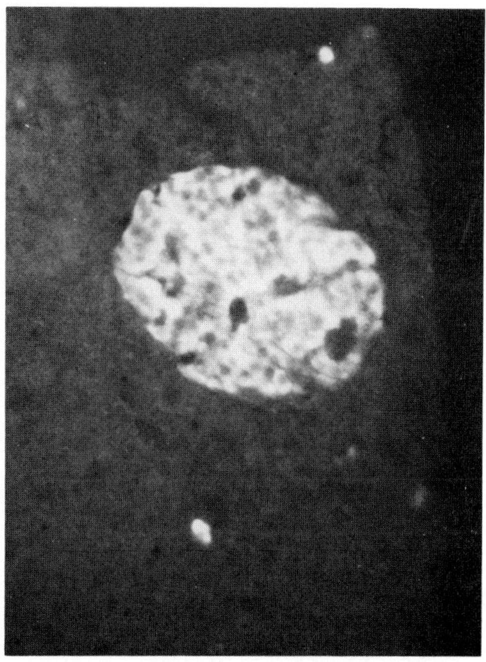

Fig. 2-4. Rat pancreatic islets. After intraperitoneal administration of L-dopa, the amino acid is taken up by both B and A cells, decarboxylated to dopamine, and stored in the endocrine granules. APUD-FIF technique. X 195

of endocrine cell types closely associated with each other, a stage is ultimately reached wherein it becomes necessary to make absolute correlation of cell type with peptide product (or amine).

In its simplest form this stage is exemplified by the identification as enterochromaffin cells of those having nonspherical, electron dense, granules (Fig. 2-7). As an ancillary technique, silver-staining methods are applied to ultrathin sections, as first shown by Häkanson, Owman, Sporrong and Sundler.[16]

The Masson-Fontana and similar reactions identify the nonspherical granules as argentaffin and hence as containing 5-hydroxytryptamine. Other silver reactions identify the nonspherical granules of these endocrine cells, and the spherical granules of the others, as argyrophil. The two techniques commonly used are those of Sevier and Munger,[41] and of Grimelius.[15] In Figures 2-8 and 2-9 the use of the former is illustrated, as a means of identifying the endocrine cell producing gastric inhibitory peptide (GIP). Figure 2-8 shows an immunofluorescent GIP cell (*A*, arrow) which exhibits argyrophilia (*B*, arrow), as do other EC cells in Figure 2-8*B*. At the ultrastructural level the two argyrophil cell types are revealed as K cells (Fig. 2-9, and upper inset) and enterochromaffin cells (Fig. 2-9, lower inset). Thus the K cells are to be regarded as the source of GIP.

Three other techniques which can be employed for the purpose of granule/hormone identification are each based on ultrastructural immunocytochemistry. The first uses a direct approach: the immune serum is applied to a fragment of tissue which is afterward fixed, processed and sectioned by standard procedures for electron-microscopy. In the second, antibody is again applied directly,[22] but this time to a thin section on the grid after a suitable degree of etching of the resin. As an alternative to these two the semithin-thin technique can be used.[7,32] Here a single 1 μm. section is cut, etched and processed for

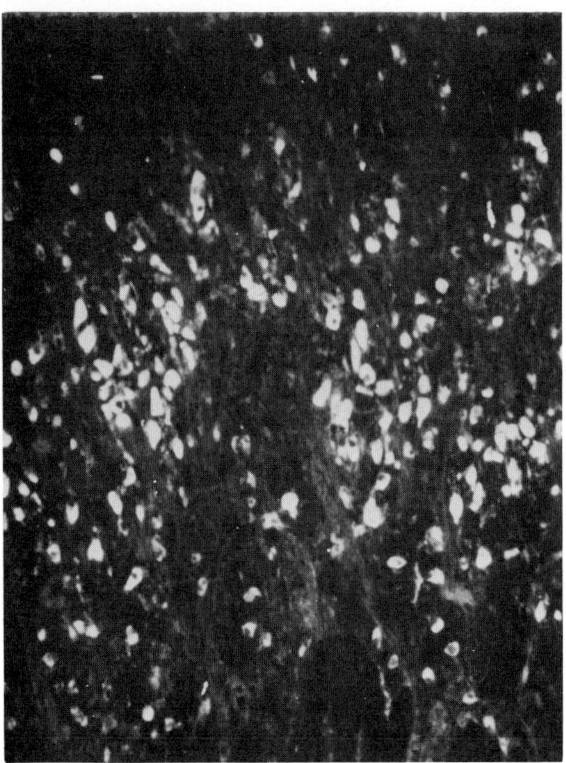

Fig. 2-5. Human gastric antrum. Immunofluorescence (indirect procedure) using antiserum to synthetic gastrin 2-17. The gastrin-containing G cells form a complete band across the midzone of the pyloric glands. X 100

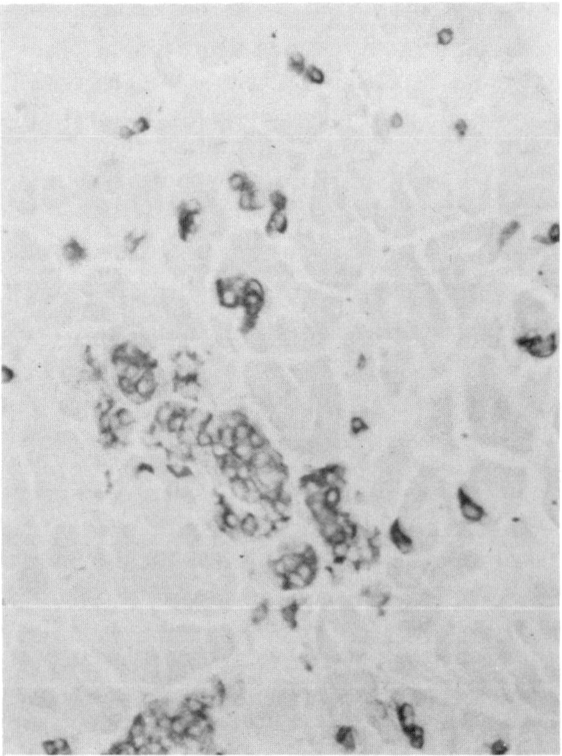

Fig. 2-6. Human pancreas. A child with nesidioblastosis was treated by subtotal pancreatectomy. The immunoperoxidase technique, using an antiserum to porcine insulin, reveals masses of insulin-containing B cells outside the islets and numerous scattered B cells in the acini also. X 120

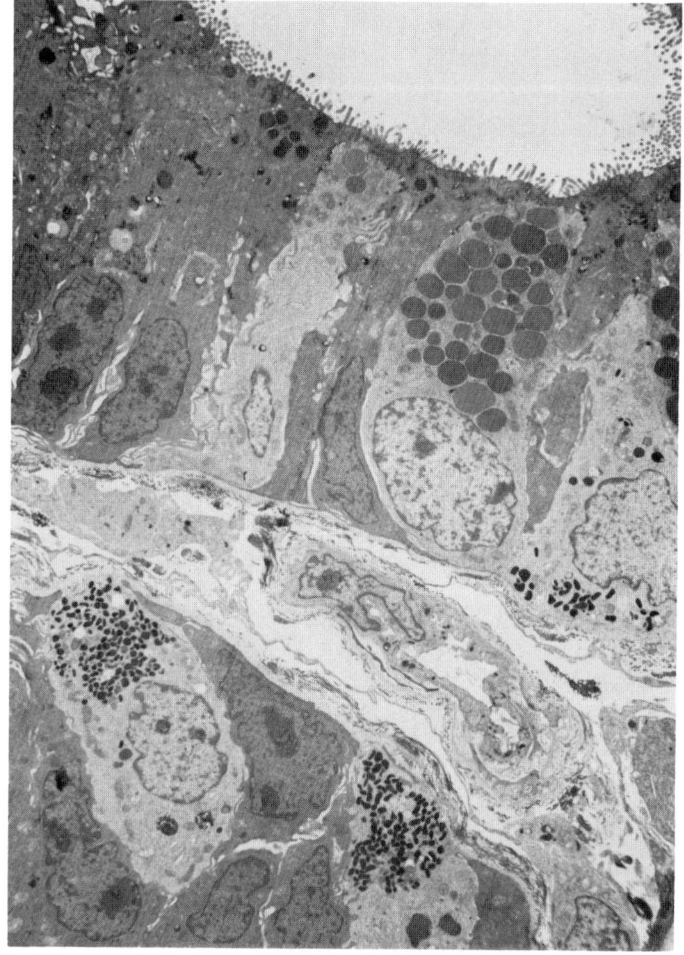

Fig. 2-7. Parts of two glands, human duodenal biopsy. Standard EM preparation, counterstained. Mucous-secreting goblet cells and three enterochromaffin (EC) cells are seen, the latter containing electron-dense nonspherical granules. The cell at lower left is an intermediate form. X 3′000

immunofluorescence (Fig. 2-10*A*). Succeeding (serial) thin sections are cut at 60 nm., and the first of these is used for conventional microscopy (Fig. 2-10*B* and *C*). These two procedures may be sufficient to permit absolute correlation to be made. Additional serial 60 nm. sections can be stained by appropriate silver methods to provide a further degree of identification (Fig. 2-10*D*). These illustrations show the localization of motilin to the EC cell of the small intestine by the semithin-thin technique but other gastrointestinal endocrine cells have been identified in the same way (e.g., cholecystokinin).[37]

CLINICAL IMPLICATIONS

Many endocrine syndromes and disorders can be reconciled with the APUD concept. Among them are the carcinoid, episodic hypoglycemia, Zollinger-Ellison, Cushing's and Verner-Morrison syndromes and, additionally, all varieties of the group of disorders classified as MEA (or MEN) and numbered, sequentially, I, II, IIb or III.

The cells, or rather their precursors, which are involved in these disorders

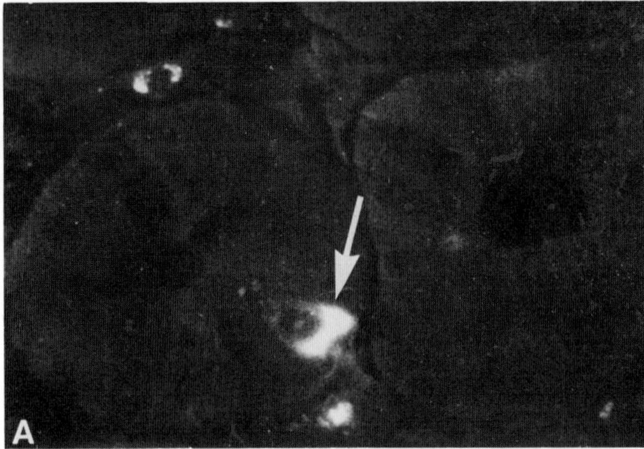

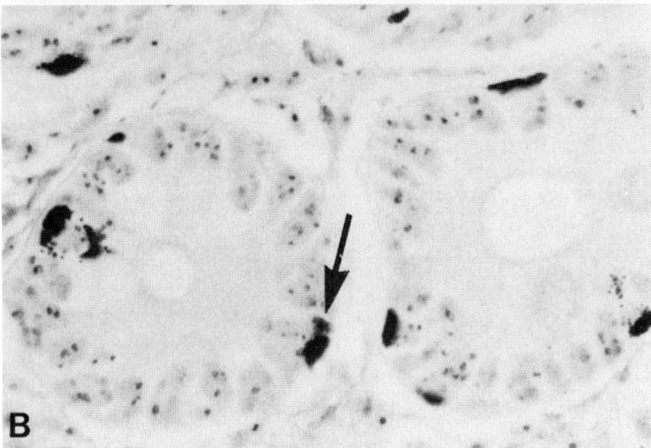

Fig. 2-8. Dog duodenum. *(A)* Immunofluorescence preparation shows a single GIP cell *(arrow)*. *(B)* The same cell *(arrow)* is argyrophil by the Sevier-Munger method. Several other cells (EC) are also argyrophil. X 600 (Buffa, R., et al.: Histochemistry, *43*:249, 1975)

must be considered to have at least a multipotential capacity for the production of hormonal peptides. This consideration, and the almost constant involvement of several different types of endocrine cells throughout the whole spectrum of disorders, is in general accord with the view that the cells have a common origin.

The term ectopic is used constantly to describe hormone production by abnormal or unusual sources and the syndromes caused thereby. If the site of production is removed only marginally from the normal one, this usage is topographically and morphologically correct. In terms of the APUD concept it is incorrect, or at least misleading, since none of the peptides produced by the cells of the APUD series is to be considered foreign to any of its members.

Pancreatic endocrine tumors are a case in point. Gastrin-secreting islet cell tumors, for example, are often described as ectopic, because the hormone is not normally found in adult pancreas. It is present in fetal pancreas, however, and one must presume that a precursor cell having the capacity for its production is present throughout life. A peptide reacting with antisera to VIP is likewise found, albeit infrequently, in endocrine cells in adult pancreas. In tumors of pancreatic origin, therefore, VIP is not ectopic and, because it is present in normal cells in autonomic ganglia and adrenal medulla, it is not to be regarded as ectopic in its alternative neoplastic site, the ganglioneuroblastoma.

Contrary to the usually accepted view, the source of carcinoid tumors is not the enterochromaffin cell but a multipotential precursor. These tumors may therefore produce and secrete any peptide or hormone normally produced by any one of the APUD cells of the gastroenteropancreatic system, without being deserving of the description "ectopic."

Little sense can be made of the rather constant participation of endocrine cells from different sources in relatively well-defined syndromes, with a single exception: Sipple's syndrome (MEA II). In this syndrome the thyroid C cell (medullary carcinoma), and the noradrenalin and adrenalin cells of the adrenal medulla (pheochromocytoma), sometimes accompanied by the Type I cell of the carotid body (chemodectoma), are regularly associated. All these cells are products of the rhombencephalic neural crest, arising in the embryo at much the same time from higher or lower segments of the column. For each the final program,

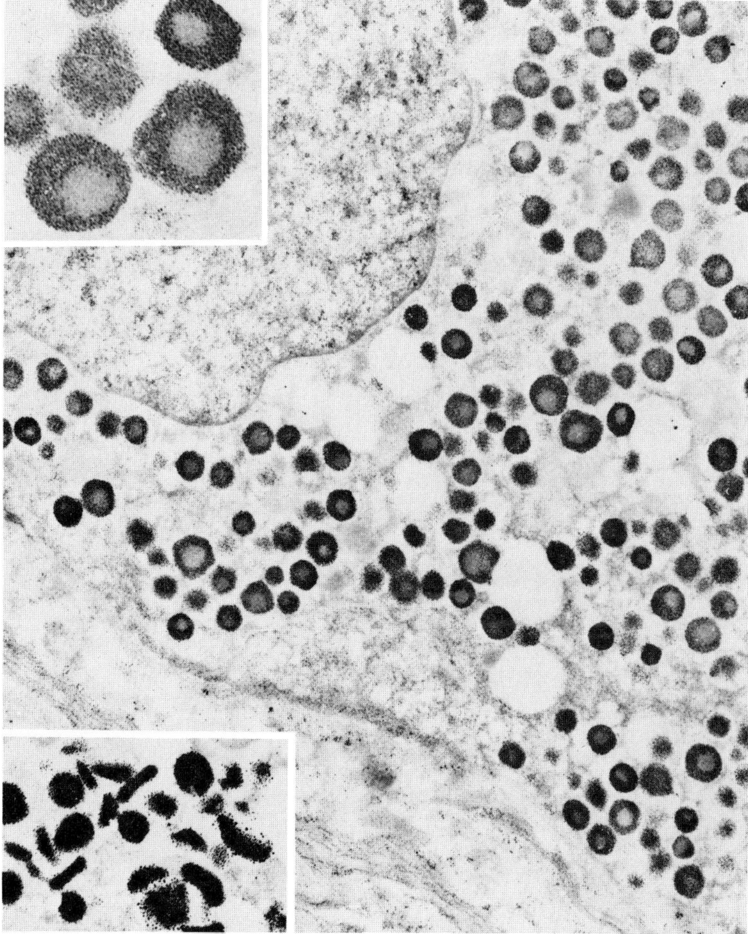

Fig. 2-9. Dog jejunum. Sevier-Munger silver impregnation shows the heavily stained granules of the K (GIP) cell (X 15'000). These are shown at higher magnification (*upper inset,* X 35'000) the polymorphic granules of an EC cell are shown (*lower inset,* X 15'500). (Buffa, R., et al.: Histochemistry, *43*:249, 1975)

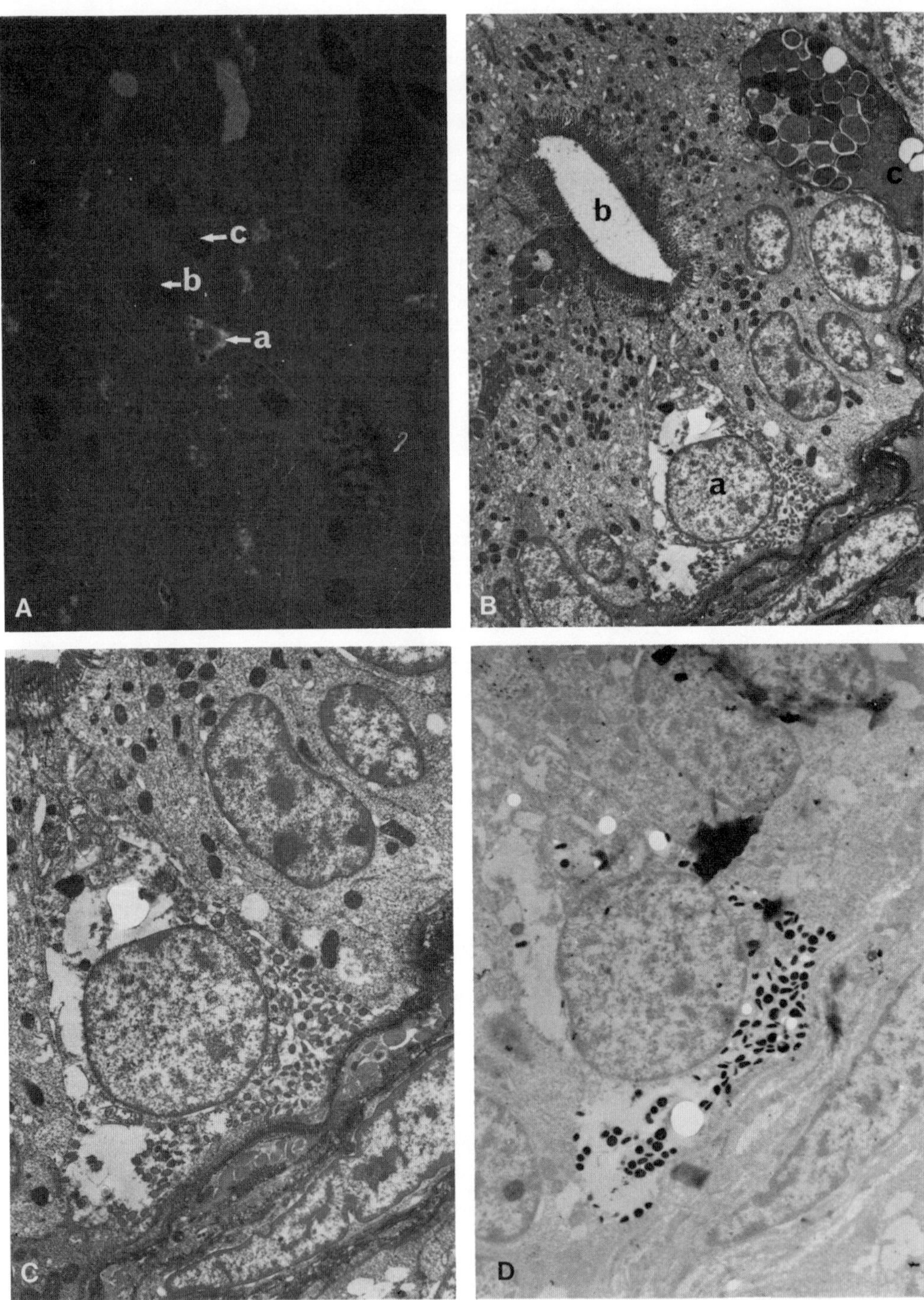

Fig. 2-10. (A) Dog, lower jejunum. Semithin (1μm.) section shows immunofluorescent motilin cell (a) with associated marker structures, gland lumen (b) and mucous cell (c). X 800 *(B)* Thin serial section of *A*. Shows motilin cell (a) containing nonspherical granules and the two markers (b and c). Counterstained E.M. preparation. X 3'250. *(C)* Higher magnification of *B* to show detail of the granules. X 5'750. *(D)* Thin section serial to *B* and *C*. Masson reaction shows that the granules are argentaffin. X 5'750.

producing the final hormonal product, is determined by the locus in which it finally resides. This has been shown, by the techniques of experimental embryology,[17] in which transposition of higher and lower portions of the neural crest is not accompanied by any change in the final function of the transposed cells. A recent observation by Baylin[5] and his associates is pertinent. These authors investigated a female patient with medullary thyroid carcinoma and associated pheochromocytoma who was a mosaic for the two forms of X-linked glucose-6-phosphate dehydrogenase. This fact allowed them to trace the clonal origin of the tumors. Their results suggest a single clone cell origin for both, a finding which fits very well the established embryology of the condition.

CONCLUSION

The identification of individual APUD cells of the peripheral division, outside the gastrointestinal tract and pancreas, is not a matter of great difficulty. Application of the method listed above, or usually of one or two only, will permit confident recognition.

In the central division the identification of individual hormone-producing cells of the pituitary gland has been made in a satisfactory manner largely by direct ultrastructural immunocytochemistry, often combined with light microscopic cytology.[3,12] In the hypothalamus, and perhaps in other regions of the brain, there are many difficulties to be overcome before complete identification of the cell types producing neuroendocrine, neurotransmitter and other peptides can be made with any degree of certainty. Because the "mountain" is there, if for no better reason, it will certainly be "moved," and there is no reason to doubt that success will be achieved. The level of technology is adequate, only the application is required.

REFERENCES

1. Andrew, A.: A study of the developmental relationship between enterochromaffin cells and the neural crest. J. Embryol. Exp. Morphol., *11*:307, 1963.
2. ———: Further evidence that enterochromaffin cells are not derived from the neural crest. J. Embryol. Exp. Morphol., *31*:589, 1974.,
3. Baker, B. L., and Jaffe, R. B.: The genesis of cell types in the adenohypophysis of the human fetus as observed with immunocytochemistry. Am. J. Anat., *143*:137, 1975.
4. Ballard, W. W.: Comparative Anatomy and Embryology. p. 158. New York, The Ronal Press, 1964.
5. Baylin, S. B., Gann, D. S., and Hsu, S. H.: Clonal origin of inherited medullary thyroid carcinoma and pheochromocytoma. Science, *193*:321, 1976.
6. Buffa, R., et al.: Identification of the intestinal cell storing gastric inhibitory peptide. Histochemistry, *43*:249, 1975.
7. Bussolati, G., and Canese, M. G.: Electron microscopical identification of the immunofluorescent gastrin cells in the cat pyloric mucosa. Histochemie, *29*:198, 1972.
8. Bussolati, G., Rost, F. W. D., and Pearse, A. G. E.: Fluorescence metachromasia in polypeptide hormone-producing cells of the APUD series and its significance in relation to the structure of the precursor protein. Histochem. J., *1*:517, 1969.
9. Cheng, H., and Leblond, C. P.: Origin, differentiation and renewal of four main epithelial cell types in the mouse small intestine. Am. J. Anat., *141*: 503, 1974.
10. ———: Origin, differentiation and re-

newal of four main epithelial cell types in the mouse small intestine. V. Unitarian theory of the origin of the four epithelial cell types. Am. J. Anat., *141*:537, 1974.

11. Coons, A. H., Leduc, E. H., and Connolly, J. H.: Studies on antibody production. I: Method for the histochemical demonstration of specific antibody and its application to a study of hyperimmune rabbit. J. Exp. Med., *102*:49, 1955.
12. Doerr-Schott, J.: Cyto-immunochemical study of the hypophysial cells of amphibians by light and electron microscopy. Fortschr. Zool., *22*:245, 1974.
13. Drews, U.: Cholinesterase in embryonic development. Prog. Histochem. Cytochem., *7* [No. 3]:1, 1975.
14. Fausa, O., Fretheim, B., Elgjo, K., Semb, L. S., and Gjone, E.: Intractable watery diarrhoea, hypokalaemia and achlorhydria associated with non-pancreatic retroperitoneal neurogenous tumour containing vasoactive intestinal peptide (VIP). Scan. J. Gastroenterol., *8*:713, 1973.
15. Grimelius, L.: A silver nitrate stain for α_2 cells in human pancreatic islets. Acta Soc. Med. Upsalien., *73*, 243, 1968.
16. Häkanson, R., Owman, C., Sporrong, B., and Sundler, F.: Electron microscopic classification of amine producing endocrine cells by selective staining of ultra-thin sections. Histochemie, *27*:226, 1971.
17. Le Douarin, N.: Particularités du noyau interphasique chez la Caille japonaise *(Coturnix coturnix japonica)*. Utilisation de ces particularités comme 'marque biologique' dans les recherches sur les interactions tissulaires et les migrations cellulaires au cours de l'ontogenèse. Bull. Biol. France et Belg., *103*:435, 1969.
18. Luft, R., Efendic, S., Hökfelt, T., Johansson, O., and Arimura, A.: Immunohistochemical evidence for localization of somatostatin-like immunoreactivity in a cell population of the pancreatic islets. Med. Biol., *52*:428, 1974.
19. Manocchio, I.: Metacromasia e basofilia delle cellule insulari alfa nel pancreas di mammiferi dopo metilazione e demetilazione. Arch. Vet. Ital., *15*:3, 1964.
20. Melmed, R. N., Benitez, C. J., and Holt, S. J.: Intermediate cells of the pancreas. I. Ultrastructural characterization. J. Cell Sci., *11*:449, 1972.
21. Monga, G., Bonfanti, S., and Bussolati, G.: Cholinesterase-rich cells in the rat fundic mucosa. A light and electron microscopical investigation. Histochem. J., *6*:559, 1975.
22. Nakane, P. K.: Application of peroxidase-labelled antibodies to the intracellular localization of hormones. Acta Endocrinol. (Kbh.) [Suppl.], *153*:190, 1971.
23. Nakane, P. K., and Pierce, G. B., Jr.: Enzyme-labelled antibodies for the light and electron macroscopic localization of tissue antigens. J. Cell Biol., *33*:307, 1967.
24. Orci, L., Ruffener, C., Pictet, R., Renold, A. E., and Rouiller, C.: Present state and evidence for mixed endocrine and exocrine pancreatic cells in spiny mice. *In* Falkmer, S., Hellman, B., and Täljdal, I. B. (eds.): The Structure and Metabolism of the Pancreatic Islets. pp. 37-52. Oxford, Pergamon Press, 1970.
25. Pearse, A. G. E.: 5-Hydroxytryptophan uptake by dog thyroid C cells and its possible significance in polypeptide hormone production. Nature, *211*: 598, 1966.
26. ———: Common cytochemical properties of cells producing polypeptide hormone with particular reference to calcitonin and the thyroid C cells. Vet. Rec., *79*:587, 1966.
27. ———: Common cytochemical and ultrastructural characteristics of cells producing polypeptide hormones (the APUD series) and their relevance to thyroid and ultimobranchial C cells and calcitonin. Proc. Roy. Soc. Bull., *170*:71, 1968.
28. ———: The cytochemical and ultrastructure of polypeptide-hormone producing cells of the APUD series,

and the embryologic, physiologic and pathologic implications of the concept. J. Histochem. Cytochem., *17*:303, 1969.

29. ———: Random coil conformation of polypeptide hormone precursor protein in endocrine cells. Nature, *221*:1310, 1969.
30. Pearse, A. G. E., and Polak, J. M.: Cytochemical evidence for the neural crest origin of mammalian ultimobranchial C cells. Histochemie, *27*:96, 1971.
31. ———: Immunocytochemical localization of substance P in mammalian intestine. Histochemistry, *41*:373, 1975.
32. Pearse, A. G. E., Polak, J. M., and Heath, C. M.: Polypeptide hormone production by "carcinoid" apudomas and their relevant cytochemistry. Virchows Arch. Abt. B. Cell Pathol., *16*:95, 1974.
33. Pearse, A. G. E., et al.: Demonstration of the neural crest origin of type I (APUD) cells in the avian carotid body using a cytochemical marker system. Histochemie, *34*:191, 1973.
34. Pictet, R. L., and Rutter, W. J.: Development of the embryonic endocrine pancreas. *In* Handbook of Physiology. vol. 1, pp. 25-66. Baltimore, Williams & Wilkins, 1972.
35. Pictet, R. L., Rall, L. B., Phelps, P., and Rutter, W. J.: The neural crest and the origin of the insulin-producing and other gastrointestinal hormone-producing cells. Science, *191*:191, 1976.
36. Polak, J. M., Pearse, A. G. E., Grimelius, L., Bloom, S. R., and Arimura, A.: Growth-hormone releasing inhibiting hormone (GH-RIH) in gastrointestinal and pancreatic D cells. Lancet, *1*:1220, 1975.
37. Polak, J. M., et al.: Identification of cholecystokinin-secreting cells. Lancet, *2*: 1016, 1975.
38. Polak, J. M., Pearse, A. G. E., Le Lièvre, C., Fontaine, J., and Le Douarin, N. M.: Immunocytochemical confirmation of the neural crest origin of avian calcitonin-producing cells. Histochemistry, *40*:209, 1974.
39. Rost, M. C. M., and Rost, F. W. D.: Storage granules of thyroid C cells in the dog: A cytochemical and ultrastructural study, in relation to the masked metachromasia reaction. Histochem. J., *7*:307, 1975.
40. Said, S.: Evidence for secretion of vasoactive intestinal peptide by tumours of pancreas, adrenal medulla, thyroid and lung: Support for the unifying APUD concept. Clin. Endocrinol., *5*:2015, 1976.
41. Sevier, A. C., and Munger, B. L.: A silver method for paraffin sections of neural tissue. J. Neuropathol. Exp. Neurol., *24*:130, 1965.
42. Solcia, E., Vassallo, G., and Capella, C.: Selective staining of endocrine cells by basic dyes after acid hydrolysis. Stain Technol., *43*:257, 1968.
43. Takor-Takor, T., and Pearse, A. G. E.: Neuroectodermal origin of avian hypothalamo-hypophyseal complex: The role of the ventral neural ridge. J. Embryol. Exp. Morphol., *34*:311, 1975.
44. Vanderhaejen, J. J., Signeau, J. C., and Gepts, W.: New peptide in the vertebrate CNS reacting with antigastrin antibodies. Science, *257*:604, 1975.

EDITORIAL COMMENTARY

No concept has influenced the understanding of modern-day endocrinology as much as has the APUD concept which developed out of the basic cytochemical investigations by Professor Pearse and his coinvestigators and which became immediately applicable to the clinical sciences. The incorporation of Feyrter's paracrine system into the overall neuroendocrine system by a broader acceptance of the APUD concept provided an enlightenment, not entirely without the heat of controversy, for both the basic and clinical sciences. As scientists of various persuasions examine cellular origins, cytochemically and embryologically, humoral biologic and immulogic capabilities and end-organ responses by virtually all scientific disciplines, the net result has been the addition, one by one, of new peptides to membership in the APUD fold, and finally, the identification of new clinical syndromes. The pathophysiologic characteristics of a cascade of new syndromes have been based on biochemical identification of new polypeptides and the synthesis of at least the active portion of them. There is a continuing unfolding of comparative embryologic findings concerning neural crest or neuroectodermal placodal origin of the APUD cells which have common cytochemical characteristics. The multipotentiality of these cells becomes evident as more and more clinically bizarre syndromes, including "ectopic" phenomena, are observed. Although the APUD system of cells constitutes an enlarging proportion of the neuroendocrine system, it is important to recognize that almost all endocrine tissue, except the steroid- and the thyroxine-secreting cells, stem from the same sources. Although the steroid-synthesizing endocrine cells, of a different embryologic derivation, have biologic functions which are absolutely essential for life, they ultimately depend on and are regulated by the trophic action of the polypeptides, the principal products of the APUD cell system. *S.R.F.*

3

Physiology of the Neuroendocrine System

Stephen R. Bloom, M.A., M.B., M.R.C.P.

COMPLEXITIES OF THE NEUROENDOCRINE SYSTEM

In the last century control of gastrointestinal function was considered to be mostly neural. Secretion of pancreatic juice, for example, was thought to be due to local nervous reflexes. With the discovery of secretin in 1902 by Bayliss and Starling the era of endocrinology began. Emphasis was given to the importance of hormones, released into the bloodstream and controlling distant organs. In the way of all scientific trends, these ideas became dominant and the earlier nervous reflex theories eclipsed. In spite of the early start of the gastrointestinal endocrine system with the discovery of secretin in 1902 and gastrin in 1904, the development of this branch of the endocrine system proceeded very slowly. The ease of investigation of endocrine glands, where all the hormone producing tissue is gathered together as a single mass, led to much earlier elucidation of their function. Thus knowledge of the physiology and pathology of the pituitary, thyroid, adrenals, pancreas and gonads has been long established. In contrast the understanding of the diffuse endocrine system has been far slower. This system is arranged to respond to a diffuse environmental stimulus. The gut provides a good example since here the usual stimulus, food, is non-homogeneous, and in order to get an integrated or average signal which truly reflects the total content of a particular nutriment, widespread analysis is required. Endocrine glands, on the other hand, sample only concentrations in the bloodstream and so can get all their information from a single blood vessel. As the diffuse endocrine system is spread throughout a considerable bulk of tissues, extraction of the active hormone is very difficult and extirpation of the endocrine cells impossible. Thus these two classical avenues to understanding the function of endocrine glands are not available. Another major difficulty is that since there are many different types of diffuse endocrine systems which all overlap, any crude extract of the relevant tissues will always contain an often considerable number of different hormonal principles. Therefore, progress on understanding the diffuse endocrine system had to wait the development of highly sensitive peptide purification techniques capable of pulling out tiny amounts of a single hormone. Such techniques (e.g., ion exchange, gel, affinity and hydrophobic chromatography, countercurrent distribution and isoelectric focusing, etc.) have been freely available only in the last decade. Thus we are at last beginning to appreciate the enormous complexity of an endocrine system that exists in every tissue.

So many new hormones have been found that the bewildered endocrinologist is now frequently heard to remark that the function of this or that new peptide is probably unimportant. The theory of evolution tells us, however, that any unimportant system is rapidly removed by the process of natural selection. It is reasonable to assume that almost all the components that are present across the mammalian species without significant change are essential for survival. Thus, the purification of hormonal peptides whose function is not yet understood is not a reflection on their lack of importance but rather on our own slowness to understand them.

NEWER CONCEPTS OF NEUROENDOCRINE PHYSIOLOGY

Particularly rapid advance has been made in the understanding of gut endocrinology, and this provides an excellent model in which to examine the newer concepts of neuroendocrine physiology. There are now seven well-characterized gut hormones which, it is widely agreed, act by way of the circulation.

Gut Hormones

The physiologic role of the following seven hormones is still subject to controversy:

Circulating Hormones

Gastrin	Motilin
Secretin	Gastric inhibitory peptide (GIP)
Pancreatic polypeptide (PP)	Enteroglucagon
Cholecystokinin (CCK)-pancreozymin	

Regarding the first hormone, the biologic significance of the multiple forms of *gastrin* released into the circulation is uncertain. So far the two major forms, G-34 and G-17, appear to have identical actions. The mechanisms of control for gastrin release, particularly the role of the vagus, are still under investigation. It has been shown that many early studies in animals are not applicable to man. A particularly important subject, the possible importance of gastrin excess in the etiology of duodenal ulcer, has been studied for nearly a decade without clear answer.

The major enigma of *secretin* is whether it plays any physiologic role at all. It has been shown pharmacologically to be a highly potent stimulus for pancreatic bicarbonate secretion. A good flow of alkaline pancreatic juice is seen after a meal. Unfortunately, no detectable rise of secretin occurs in the blood following a meal. Recent work, however, suggests that there may indeed be a rise but that it is extremely small and difficult to detect. If this is the case the next step is to prove that even a tiny rise might have biologic significance. Inital studies with secretin have been performed in the fasting state when secretin is, not surprisingly, rather inactive. Postprandially a number of other changes occur, for example elevation of plasma cholecystokinin (CCK). This latter hormone is known to potentiate the effects of secretin on the pancreas at least fourfold. This illustrates a general rule in physiology: that the actions of a hormone must be studied in its natural environment. Thus man's sensitivity to a small dose of secretin can only really be examined postprandially and this work has not yet been done.

Pancreatic polypeptide, one of the newest hormonal peptides to be isolated, is very easy to measure. This is partly because it circulates in high concentrations and partly because its discoverer, Dr. Chance of Eli Lilly, has made his highly sensitive and specific human pancreatic polypeptide antibodies freely available. Thus we know that there is a considerable release of PP (Pancreatic polypeptide) after a meal, and this is mediated by hormones released from the intestine and also by nervous reflexes mediated by the vagus. Direct intravenous infusion of nutriments has no effect on PP release. The release of PP from the pancreas, which is the only organ in which it is found in man, resembles that of insulin and the term entero-PP axis has been coined similar in concept to the enteroinsular axis. Pharmacologically, PP is most potent as an antagonist to cholecystokinin causing gall bladder relaxation, increasing choledochal tone and inhibition of pancreatic enzyme output. So far, however, physiologic quantities have not been shown to have any dramatic effects. Clearly PP must have some important role but it has so far eluded discovery.

The major problem with *cholecystokinin* is that it appears to circulate in even more forms than does gastrin. The several forms all have different biologic activity. Thus a radioimmunoassay which reliably reflects the biologic potency of circulating CCK is still not available. There have been several reports of successful estimations of plasma CCK-like immunoreactivity but not universal agreement on the results.

Motilin is another hormonal peptide which is still awaiting definition of its physiologic function. It is released from the jejunum and circulates in quite high concentration. Pharmacologically, it is extremely potent in influencing upper gastrointestinal motor activity. It appears particularly to enhance the tone of human antral and pyloric muscle and may therefore act to increase sphincter activity and thus delay gastric emptying. It has also been claimed, however, to increase myoelectric activity and thus enhance transit rates.

Gastric inhibitory peptide (GIP) was first isolated because of its action in preventing histamine-stimulated gastric acid. Subsequently it has been found to be more potent in its effects on the β cell as a potentiator of insulin release. Indeed the term Glucose-dependent Insulin-releasing Peptide has now been proposed as an alternative name. It seems that GIP is the main component of the enteroinsular axis, being released by glucose and fat and acting on the β cell to release insulin only when plasma glucose concentrations are elevated. Infusions of GIP in man which produce concentrations similar to those seen postprandially do indeed enhance insulin release very significantly. Thus the main research activity on GIP is concerning its pathology in man since it may have an important influence on carbohydrate metabolism.

Enteroglucagon which, unlike GIP and motilin is found low down in the small intestine and indeed in the colon as well, has still not been completely purified. There appear to be multiple forms both in tissue and in the circulation. Considerable argument exists as to whether enteroglucagon, or as it is also known glucagonlike immunoreactivity of intestinal origin, is one hormone or several and also concerning its exact relationship to pancreatic glucagon. Recent evidence suggests that it not only has similar immunoreactivity but also may contain the entire sequence of pancreatic glucagon within its structure. Evidence derived from a single tumor case which produced large amounts of enteroglucagon suggests that this substance may have a role in inhibiting intestinal transit and also a trophic action on the intestinal mucosa. There are many other circulating gut hormones which have been proposed. Only these seven are reasonably well established and even for them there is little agreement on their physiologic role. Although the gut is now well established as a major endocrine organ, research is still required to sort out its mode of action. Only then can its pathology be properly appreciated.

Pearse first proposed his APUD concept in 1966. This emphasized the similar characteristics of the endocrine cells and led to the precept that they might all be derived from a single embryologic source, the neuroectoderm and surrounding tissues. This in turn emphasized the similarities between the endocrine and the nervous systems which is stressed by the new term, the neuroendocrine system. Thus, similarities in the function of the two systems were to be expected. The discovery of many hormonal peptides in both brain and gut vindicated these theories which are listed below.

Brain Gut Peptides

Brain Gut Peptides

Substance P	Bombesin
Somatostatin	Neurotensin
Vasoactive intestinal peptide (VIP)	CCK-gastrin
Enkephalin	

In the brain these peptides have been localized to the synaptosome fraction and in the periphery have been found in fine nerve fibers. Therefore it seems likely that they act as peptidergic neurotransmitters. In addition in the gut they have also been localized to conventional endocrine cells. Thus they seem to act in a dual capacity. Indeed it has now become apparent that the control systems of the body may be divided roughly into three groups: (1) the nervous system, releasing neurotransmitters, (2) the paracrine system, releasing locally active substances affecting surrounding tissues only and (3) the classical endocrine system, with the active substance being released in the bloodstream to act at a distance. The second group, the locally acting hormones or paracrine system, has not been greatly emphasized. It is nonetheless important. A good illustration of this is the history of histamine in the control of gastric acid. It has long been known that histamine was the most potent stimulator of the parietal cell and that it was also found in high concentrations in the stomach. Its physiologic role, however, was very difficult to establish. The discovery of specific H_2 receptor blocking agents, however, has now demonstrated that histamine does indeed play an important role in the control of everyday gastric acid production. The paracrine system is by its very nature extremely difficult to investigate and only indirect phenomenon can be measured. Investigation of the effects of pharmacologic quantities of the local substance administered exogenously, the influence of specific blocking agents, the quantitation of tissue levels following dynamic stimuli, and the measurement of the active substance escaping into free tissue fluids and collected in lymph or luminal secretions provide some clue as to the normal physiologic functioning. A long list of paracrine substances can be drawn up but the importance of the individual components (e.g., nerve growth factor, epidermal growth factor, prostaglandins, serotonin, etc.) is difficult to estimate.

It is clear that a single active substance can play several different roles as is

Table 3-1. Some Actions of Brain Gut Peptides

Name	*Actions*
Somatostatin	Inhibits pituitary pancreatic and GI hormones Inhibits GI secretions
Enkephalin	Inhibits acid Constricts sphincter of Oddi Motor effects
Bombesin	Stimulates GI secretions
VIP	Inhibits acid Stimulates bicarbonate and intestinal juice Releases insulin and hepatic glucose
Neurotensin	Releases glucagon Inhibits acid

noted in Table 3-1. For example somatostatin may act as a peptidergic neurotransmitter in the brain but in the gut is most important in the paracrine system. Vasoactive intestinal peptide (VIP) is found in nerve fibers throughout the body and may be the main neurotransmitter of the system previously termed purinergic. However, high circulating concentrations of VIP sometimes occur and may be associated with endocrine pancreatic tumor (the Verner-Morrison syndrome). VIP is found in discrete endocrine cells in the mucosa of the gut where it appears to be acting as a local hormone. Neurotensin, which is present in high concentrations in the hypothalamus, is found in a specific large-granuled endocrine cell in the ileum. Its very precise localization suggests an equally precise physiologic function. It has been reported to be present in high concentrations in blood, and thus it may act as a peptidergic neurotransmitter and a circulating hormone. Similarly, the finding of CCK-gastrin immunoreactivity in the synoptosome fraction in the brain suggests that a member of this group may act as a neurotransmitter. One of the requirements for a neurotransmitter is rapid destruction, and it may well be that a small CCK octapeptidelike peptide, which is very much more quickly degraded in biologic fluids, is the main CNS form.

SUMMARY

It is now clear that hormones may be released by nerves, even into the bloodstream. Thus the original Pavlovian view of physiology is more correct than it recently seemed. The recent rapid increase in the understanding of the complexity, and yet unity, of the control system now offers an opportunity for the complete understanding of physiologic functions. It is clear that the old simple unitary ideas of control are wrong. Each bodily function is controlled by delicate balance of agonists and antagonists with the influence of numerous modifiers. The early discovery of insulin as a single powerful overriding hormone has provided a misleading model. It seems that for most systems there are several agonists, and the absence of any one can easily be compensated for. For example, although glucagon is believed to be an important influence on carbohydrate metabolism, patients without a pancreas, who thus have no circulating glucagon, still maintain a respectable hepatic output of glucose. An illustration of the complexity of the control of one function, the secretion of gastric acid, is given below. All 19 factors are important in the control of the acid content of the stomach. The naivete of the old view that the measurement of plasma gastrin would give true information on the potential output of acid can be clearly seen.

Factors Controlling Gastric Acid

Luminal	*Innervation*
1. Nutriments	11. Local
2. pH	12. Vagal
	13. Sympathetic
Paracrine	*Hormonal*
3. VIP	14. Gastrin
4. Enkephalin	15. CCK
5. Bombesin	16. GIP
6. Neurotensin	17. Secretin
7. Somatostatin	18. Bulbogastrone
8. Histamine	
9. 5 HT	19. Rate of gastric emptying and pyloric reflux
10. Prostaglandins	

When investigating the reasons for malfunction, it is necessary to look at all the factors involved. Though this may seem to be a hard task, we at last have an opportunity of properly understanding physiology and perhaps more important of finding out the cause of many diseases previously labeled "functional."

SPECIAL READING

Pearse, A. G. E., Polak, J., and Bloom, S. R.: The newer gut hormones. Gastroenterology, *72*:746, 1977.

Bloom, S. R.: Hormones of the gastrointestinal tract. *In* Baron, D. N., Compston, N., and Dawson, A. M., (eds.): Recent Advances in Medicine. ed. 17. London, Churchill-Livingstone, 1977.

——: Gastrointestinal hormones. *In* Crane, R. K. (ed.): Gastrointestinal Physiology. vol. 12, pp. 72-103. Baltimore, University Park Press, 1977.

EDITORIAL COMMENTARY

The evolution of the APUD concept from its cytochemical and acronymic inception developed hand in hand with embryologic revelations and with physiologic discoveries of the humoral potentialities of that expanding body of cells. These neuroendocrine-programed cells of the epiblast produce peptides which function as hormones or neurotransmitters. Although the biologic effects of extracts of gland and mucosa had been demonstrated by investigators such as Bayliss, Starling, Edkins, Heidenhain and Pavlov, there was a long lapse of time during which the mucosal cellular sources of the humoral products were not even seen, much less identified. All that was known of the physiology of the endocrine system was that the hormone was released from secretory granules of the endocrine cell into the bloodstream of the contiguous capillary to act as a messenger upon a target organ or cell. The synthesis, storage and secretion functions of the endocrine cell are influenced by neural, chemical, physical and hormonal factors which govern release of its hormone by stimulation or suppression. Moreover, the process of emiocytosis in which the secretory product is extruded from the cell into the bloodstream is also controlled by the presence of substances such as calcium ions as well as releasing and inhibiting hormones. Just as there are releasing and inhibiting factors in the hypothalamic-pituitary axis, it is now known that there are hormones such as somatostatin which inhibit the release of growth hormone, insulin, gastrin, glucagon, CCK, VIP and motilin, and there are also releasing hormones such as GIP which potentiates insulin release from the beta islet cell as a Glucose-dependent Insulin-releasing Peptide and bombesin which may be a more universal releasor of polypeptides in multiple endocrine adenopathy syndromes.

At the other end of the humoral circuit the target organ cell is known to be equipped with specific receptors which respond both physiologically and pharmacologically to neural and hormonal influences, that is, if these receptor sites are not already occupied or blocked. Specifically, these receptors are situated either on the membrane of the target cell (in response to polypeptides) or are intracellular (in response to steroid hormones). Several or many receptors may be located on one target cell to accomplish its biologic function; for example, the gastric parietal cell presumably has a receptor which responds to acetylcholine from the vagal nerve ending, one responding to the amine, histamine, and a third responsive to the polypeptide, gastrin. Modification of receptivity is pharmacologically practical; also physiologically, polypeptides having similar, but not identical, molecular structure, may occupy receptors, thus blocking the expected response of that receptor. The degree of response of some of the exocrine target cells can be measured by the determination of cyclic AMP activity after stimulation by some polypeptides (such as VIP) and other products (such as prostaglandins), and of course, the biologic effect is often measurable, for instance, as gastric acid (H+) output or serum calcium concentration, and so on.

The most remarkable developments, however, in the physiology of the neuroendocrine system have occurred in the elucidation of hormonal products related to that part of the system in the mucosa of the gastrointestinal tract originally described by Feyrter, in which the "messengers" appear to act more or less locally. The enteropancreatic paracrine cells interspersed with other paracrine cells, and among their exocrine cells, respond in dose-related fashion to their environment providing homeostasis between anabolism and catabolism by means of newly identified and confirmed amines and polypeptides. As a matter of fact, "new hormones" are being described almost daily. Some are even being identified without a clear idea of their physiologic action or purpose; for instance, pancreatic polypeptide (PP), originally found by Kimmel as "another peptide in the pancreas of the chicken," and now easily identified in humans because of the work of Chance, appears to be elevated in several types of apudomas and in the plasma of these patients. These observations raise the questions: Is PP solely a "marker" of pancreatic tumor activity or is it also functional as an antagonist of cholecystokinin? Some new hormone-candidates, as has been mentioned, appear to act only as mediators (releasors or inhibitors) of other established hormones. The fact that gut hormones have been found in the brain and nervous tissue and vice versa has linked the various functions of the entire neuroendocrine system and has expanded that system to immense proportions. Just as the autonomic system was labeled as having adrenergic and cholinergic functions, so the neurons are now described as being either secretory neurons or the more specialized synaptic neurons, having "peptidergic" or "purinergic" functions, respectively.

The functional potentiality of the neuroendocrine system involves yet other considerations. The molecular size of the humoral-candidate and the capacity for activity of its smaller molecular units depend upon its specific peptidase being present or absent or able to cleave the humoral molecule itself. In malignant tumors a peptidase for a large polypeptide or prohormone, for instance, may be missing or defective, resulting in elaboration of an abnormally large-sized molecule with bizarre activity. Furthermore, humoral products such as the enkephalins found in gastrin cells and as small molecular components of the larger endorphins found in the brain, have an opiate-like activity. Finally, abnormalities of elaboration of humoral products appear to be involved in abnormal mental states such as schizophrenia.

It is clear that the physiologic potentialities of the expanding neuroendocrine system are only beginning to surface in our understanding of our own physical and emotional homeostasis. *S.R.F.*

4

Immunochemistry of the Endocrine System

James E. McGuigan, M.D.

The present and continuing explosion of new information concerning the physiology and pathophysiologic significance of the gastrointestinal hormones was made possible by two investigational developments. The initial development was the purification and availability of pure gastrointestinal polypeptides. This enormously important contribution made possible the second development: The application of a wide variety of immunochemical techniques to important questions related to the hormones of the gastrointestinal tract including their organ, tissue and intracellular localization, their inhibition and stimulation of release and their degradation and inactivation. Immunochemical methods, utilizing antibodies to the gastrointestinal polypeptide hormones have proven powerful tools in the quest for answers to these questions and others. Immunochemical methods, because of their potential for specificity and sensitivity, provide unparalleled means for the detection, identification and measurement of the gastrointestinal peptide hormones.

Prior to the advent of radioimmunoassay measurements of the gastrointestinal peptides, all estimations of hormone levels depended upon bioassay techniques. For example, acid secretory responses of canine fundic pouches and rat stomachs were used to estimate serum gastrin levels, concentrations both in the clinical laboratory, in patients suspected of harboring the Zollinger-Ellison syndrome, and in investigative laboratories devoted to efforts to clarify the intricate interrelationships between gastrin and gastric acid secretion. Bioassay techniques have proven of limited value because of their lack of specificity of action and sensitivity, two prime assets of immunologic techniques.

RADIOIMMUNOASSAY

Radioimmunoassay measurements of many different types of molecules, including the gastrointestinal polypeptide hormones, were made possible by the pioneering investigations of Berson and Yalow.[3] These investigators were first to recognize and then to produce serum antibodies to insulin, and subsequently to use these antibodies in the construction of a radioimmunoassay method for measurement of insulin. From these landmark studies in which the technique of radioimmunoassay was developed and molded, radioimmunoassay has been applied widely to the measurement of substances too numerous to tabulate here.

In 1964, Gregory and Tracy[11,12] were successful in the purification and description of the primary structure of gastrin, isolated from the hog antral mucosa. This substance (gastrins) proved to be a pair of polypeptides, each containing 17 amino acid residues (heptadecapeptides), in one of which the tyrosyl residue was sulfated (gastrin II) and in the other it was nonsulfated (gastrin I). Repeated immunization of a variety of experimental animals with stringently purified porcine gastrin proved disappointingly unsuccesful, failing to produce antibodies to gastrin. It had been reasonable to proceed in immunization efforts with pure hormones, since there was prior evidence that some peptides, with as few as seven amino acid residues, could serve complete immunizing antigenic functions. As is known, however, the immunogenicity of different organic molecules including polypeptides may differ enormously; pure intact heptadecapeptide gastrins were insufficiently immunogenic in experimental animals to result in the desired antibody production. The carboxyl-terminal tetrapeptide amide of gastrin was shown by Gregory and Tracy to contain all of the biologic activities of the intact hormone; therefore, it seemed reasonable to assume that this peptide sequence possessed a high degree of functional and structural specificity. Antibodies were produced in rabbits and guinea pigs by immunization with the C-terminal tetrapeptide amide of gastrin covalently conjugated to bovine serum albumin. This technique is based on the well-established capacity for enhancement of the immunogenicity of small organic molecules, which are able to serve haptenic immunogenic functions when conjugated to large carrier macromolecules. Antibodies to the gastrin tetrapeptide amide exhibited equivalent immunologic reactivity with the tetrapeptide amide and with heptadecapeptide gastrin. The tetrapeptide amide sequence of gastrin proved not to be unique, inasmuch as the final five amino acid residues in cholecystokinin-pancreozymin were found to be identical with those of gastrin. Immunologic reactivity of antibodies to the tetrapeptide amide of gastrin was virtually equivalent for cholecystokinin-pancreozymin and gastrin. Therefore, because of the high degree of immunologic cross-reactivity with cholecystokinin-pancreozymin, antibodies to the gastrin tetrapeptide are of little value in the specific estimation of tissue or serum gastrin concentrations.

Subsequently, however, it has been possible to produce antibodies to gastrin with a high degree of specificity and negligible immunologic cross-reactivity with cholecystokinin-pancreozymin. This has been accomplished by the application of either of two techniques: (1) This has consisted of immunization of rabbits with human gastrin I (either residues 2 through 17, or less commonly, residues 1 through 17) covalently conjugated to bovine serum albumin. This method, which is used widely, results uniformly in the production of antibodies to gastrin, usually with high degrees of specificity and sensitivity. (2) This consists of immunization of guinea pigs with partially purified porcine gastrin. This technique, although less successful in producing antibodies in each injected animal, does, in those animals producing antibodies, produce antibodies of highly satisfactory specificity and sensitivity.

The major objectives in producing antibodies to gastrin were to utilize antibodies in the development of radioimmunoassay for measurement of the hormone and to use antibodies for cellular localization of the hormone; subsequently both objectives have been achieved.

THE SPECIFICITY AND SENSITIVITY OF ANTIBODIES

It is worth emphasizing some of the characteristics of antibodies which make them of unique value in the measurement and localization of gastrointestinal peptides. In response to immunization, whether it be with a small organic haptenic determinant, a polypeptide hormone, or a large protein molecule, antibodies are produced with specificity for limited and defined structural portions of immunizing molecules. These portions are designated as antigenic determinants. Most experimental data indicate that the antigenic determinant, therefore, the region of specificity for a single antibody molecule, does not exceed a structural region equivalent to six amino acid residues. Therefore, in response to immunization with a large protein antigen or polypeptide, antibody molecules are produced each with specificity for a limited region of the immunogen. With this concept in mind, it is possible to understand and predict that different antibodies produced in response to immunization with hormones such as gastrin, parathyroid hormone, insulin, cholecystokinin-pancreozymin, secretin, etc., would vary in respect to the specific region (carboxyl-terminal portion, mid-portion, or amino terminal portion of the parent molecule) at which they are directed and for which they are specific.

Differences among specificities of antibody molecules is often of great importance. Several examples may serve to emphasize the importance of these considerations. A variety of investigations have demonstrated the molecular heterogeneity of gastrin, both in the circulation and in tissues. Although the major form of gastrin in the antral mucosa and in Zollinger-Ellison tumors is heptadecapeptide gastrin (G-17), the predominant circulating species in normal man and in the Zollinger-Ellison syndrome is big gastrin, a polypeptide containing 34 amino acid residues (G-34) which also shares the original heptadecapeptide gastrin. Antibodies produced by immunization with heptadecapeptide gastrin which have principal specificity for the carboxy-terminal region of the molecule, and lack specificity for the amino-terminal region of the heptadecapeptide, usually exhibit similar immunologic reactivity (and, therefore, immunoassayability) for G-17 and G-34 gastrins. In contrast, antigastrin antibodies with specificity directed to the amino-terminal region of the gastrin heptadecapeptide usually demonstrate minimal immunologic reactivity with G-34 gastrin. The explanation for this difference is not known but may be due to steric hindrance; however, the impact of regional specificity on immunoreactivity is evident and extremely important in the consideration of the applicability of an antibody for radioimmunoassay for gastrin. A second example of the importance of specificity of antibodies can be understood on the basis of the necessity for correlation between biologic activity and immunologic reactivity by radioimmunoassay. It has been shown that removal of the carboxyl-terminal amide group from the gastrin heptadecapeptide group abolishes biologic activity. With antibodies to gastrin which have substantial specificity for the carboxyl-terminal region of the heptadecapeptide, this alteration in the gastrin molecule also results in almost complete loss of immunologic reactivity, resulting in the desirable failure to detect immunologically these structurally modified and biologically inactive molecules. Another example of the importance of specificity in the radioimmunoassay of gastrin is the production of antibodies with regional specificity for the polypeptide portion of gastrin (mid-portion) which contains the tyrosine residue. Antibodies to gastrin I with this type of specificity have been shown to recognize human gastrin I but to fail to recognize human gastrin II. Most antibodies to gastrin in wide use today do possess the capacity to detect and measure both gastrins I and II. The use of antibodies which recognize only gastrin I by radioimmunoassay result in low estimations of gastrin concentrations.

A second characteristic of antibody molecules, in addition to *specificity,* which makes them enormously important in measuring peptide hormone concentrations, is that of the enormous affinity which antibody molecules develop for their antigens. Affinity is a measurement of the strength of binding of an antibody molecule with its antigen. In general, the higher the affinity of antibodies, the greater the *sensitivity* achievable in the radioimmunoassay when these antibodies are used. Antibodies produced early after immunization are of lower affinity, and antibody affinity for the immunogen increases with time, thereby increasing potential radioimmunoassay sensitivity with antibodies produced after repeated immunization as opposed to one or two early immunizations. This characteristic of antibodies may be of great functional importance, especially when the sensitivity of the radioimmunoassay is crucial because of low circulating hormone concentrations.

PEPTIDE LOCALIZATION BY IMMUNOCHEMICAL METHODS

Immunochemical methods have proven of great value in the localization of gastrointestinal peptides. It has been possible to extract hormones from tissues, such as by the use of the rapid and effective method of boiling extraction of gastrin, and to measure immunoreactive peptide concentrations in the tissue extract by radioimmunoassay. In addition, it has been possible to utilize immunochemical techniques in the specific localization of intracellular hormones. In general, at the light microscopic level, this has been achieved by the use of fluorescein-labeled antibodies. The two principal techniques are those of direct and indirect immunofluorescence, with its several modifications. In direct immunofluorescence, appropriately prepared tissue sections are overlain with fluorescein-labeled antibodies to the hormone. In the indirect immunofluorescent method, the tissue is overlain with rabbit antibodies directed against the hormone and, after washing, fluorescein-labeled goat antibodies to rabbit gamma globulin are added as a second layer. With both techniques ultraviolet excitation makes it possible to identify the fluorescein label, and thereby to define the location of the polypeptide within tissues and individual cells. Using these techniques it has been possible to localize a variety of gastrointestinal hormones in their intracellular sites of residence. These have included gastrin, secretin, CCK, GIP, VIP and glucagon. In each instance these hormones have been found to be contained in cytoplasmic secretory granules in differentiated endocrine cells in the gastrointestinal mucosa. The distribution and density of these hormone-containing endocrine cells is variable. (There is also some evidence that VIP may be located within neural elements.) The precise localization of VIP remains to be resolved. It is also possible to localize gastrointestinal polypeptides at the ultrastructural level by use of antibodies labeled with horseradish peroxidase, with the identification of electron-dense particles overlying the hormone-containing granules. These immunologic techniques have proven enormously useful in defining the location, distribution, classification and intracellular granule pattern of the numerous gastrointestinal peptides.

THE TECHNIQUES OF RADIOIMMUNOASSAY

Radioimmunoassay techniques depend upon competitive binding of radiolabeled and non-radiolabeled peptide by antibody molecules. Unlabeled hormone competes with radiolabeled hormone for a finite number of receptor sites. The distribution of antibody-bound and antibody-free radioactivity provides the index of estimation of hormone concentration. Multiple techniques have been applied to the separation of antibody-bound and antibody-free radioactivity. The peptide hormones are radiolabeled with a gamma-emitting radioisotope, usually ^{125}I. The methods used for the identification of antibody-bound and antibody-free radioactivity involve the physical separation of these two portions of the radioimmunoassay incubation medium. Techniques have included the use of double-antibody methods, in which the original antibody to the gastrointestinal peptide is produced by immunization of an experimental animal such as a rabbit, and these rabbit antibodies can be subsequently precipitated by addition of excess goat anti-rabbit gamma globulin. Thus, after the addition of goat antibodies to rabbit gamma globulin radiolabeled hormone bound by rabbit antibody is separated from radiolabeled hormone free in solution. Another widely applied technique is that of charcoal absorption. Charcoal, when coated with protein, dextran or dextran and protein, possesses the capacity to bind small organic molecules and does not bind antibody-bound peptides. The ready precipitation of charcoal and the absorbed peptide, with the antibody-bound peptide in the supernatant solution, provides an effective mechanism for the separation of antibody-bound from antibody-free hormone. Other methods which have been applied include the exploitation of the net electrical charge characteristics of the gastrointestinal peptide hormones and the alteration in net charge when the peptide is bound by antibodies. An example is the use of anion-binding resins such as CG-4B which is able to bind avidly the negatively charged gastrin molecule, but exhibits negligible binding of gastrin when it is bound by gastrin antibodies.

There is wide application of radioimmunoassay measurement of many hormones, which include gastrin among the gastrointestinal hormones. The development of radioimmunoassays for secretin has proven more difficult than that for gastrin, reflecting both the fragility of the secretin molecule and the limited capacity to achieve satisfactory radioiodination of the secretin molecule. Great efforts have been expended in the attempts to produce a satisfactory radioimmunoassay for cholecystokinin-pancreozymin. There are substantial differences in the specificities and behavior of the limited number of radioimmunoassays which have thus far been described for cholecystokinin-pancreozymin. It is not possible to interpret the significance of these differences at the present time. More recently, radioimmunoassay methods have been developed for vasoactive intestinal peptide and for the gastric inhibitory peptide, as well as for motilin.

LIMITATIONS AND VALUE OF IMMUNOCHEMICAL METHODS

The use of immunochemical methods for the study of the gastrointestinal hormones requires understanding of the limits and requirements of interpretation of data, resulting from differences in specificity and sensitivity. It also requires the appreciation of the experimental difficulties that may lead to spurious interpretation of results, both because of unappreciated demands of specificity and nonspecific inhibition of binding which may be interpreted as immunologic reactivity. Extraction methods, separation methods, modes of calculation, estimation, selection of controls, incubation media and many other factors all present potential variables and pitfalls in the interpretation of results from immunochemical estimations of hormone concentrations. All of these factors must be assiduously examined in the acquisition of new data concerning the gastrointestinal hormones by application of immunochemical techniques.

The use of immunochemical methods has proven of great value in the diagnosis and clarification of certain endocrine disorders and it is certain that these uses will be more widely applied. A vivid current example is that of the Zollinger-Ellison syndrome in which radioimmunoassay techniques can be used to demonstrate the fasting hypergastrinemia which characterizes the syndrome as well as the responses to feeding, secretin and calcium which serve to distinguish patients with Zollinger-Ellison gastrinomas from other patients who may have clinically similar acid hypersecretory states. Immunochemical techniques involving antibodies to gastrin have also been of great value in the ongoing elucidation of the endocrinopathic state in patients with duodenal ulcer disease, a more subtle and complexly interrelated abnormality than that of the flagrant excess of circulating gastrin seen in gastrinoma patients. Identification of increased plasma levels of vasoactive intestinal peptide in most patients with the pancreatic cholera syndrome has also been of great value in recognizing these patients and distinguishing them from patients with nonendocrinopathic diarrheas. Immunochemical methods for estimation of gastrointestinal hormone concentrations are also of great value in the detection of latent hormonal disturbances in patients with multiple endocrine adenomatosis; for example, the latent gastrinoma in the patient with the MEA I syndrome. It is certain that these and other enormously powerful immunochemical methods will be brought to bear on the elucidation of the complex interactions between the many gastrointestinal hormones, their physiological roles and interrelationships, and their abnormalities both in primary endocrinologic disorders and secondary to nonendocrinologic diseases of the gastrointestinal tract. Immunochemical methods have indeed answered many questions concerning these subjects. However, as in many other areas of biologic investigation, they have also asked many questions. Their future application, I am sure, will not only answer many of these questions but also will ask many more.

REFERENCES

1. Basso, N., and Passaro, E. P., Jr.: Calcium stimulated gastric secretion in the Zollinger-Ellison syndrome. Arch. Surg., *101*:399, 1970.
2. Becker, H. D. , Reeder, D. D., and Thompson, J. C.: Extraction of cir-

culating endogenous gastrin by the small bowel. Gastroenterology, *65*:903, 1973.

3. Berson, S. A., and Yalow, R. S.: Radioimmunoassay in gastroenterology. Gastroenterology, *62*:1061, 1972.
4. Bloom, S. R., and Ogawa, O.: Radioimmunoassay of human peripheral plasma secretin. J. Endocrinol. *58*:24, 1973.
5. Boden, G., and Chey, W. Y.: Preparation and specificity of antiserum to synthetic secretin and its use in a radioimmunoassay (RIA). Endocrinology, *92*:1617, 1973.
6. Brown, J. C., and Dryburgh, J. R.: Current status of motilin. *In* Gastrointestinal Hormones. pp. 549-554. Thompson, J. C. (ed.): Austin, University of Texas Press, 1975.
7. Davidson, W. D., Springberg, P. D., and Falkinburg, N. R.: Renal extraction and excretion of endogenous gastrin in the dog. Gastroenterology, *64*:955, 1973.
8. Dockray, G. J., and Walsh, J. H.: Amino terminal gastrin fragment in serum of Zollinger-Ellison syndrome patients. Gastroenterology, *68*:222, 1975.
9. Friesen, S. R., Bolinger, R. E. Pearse, A. G. E., and McGuigan, J. E.: Serum gastrin levels in malignant Zollinger-Ellison syndrome after gastrectomy and hypophysectomy. Ann. Surg., *172*:504, 1970.
10. Ganguli, P. C., et al.: Antral-gastrin-cell hyperplasia in peptic ulcer disease. Lancet, *1*:583, 1974.
11. Gregory, R. A., and Tracy, H. J.: Isolation of two "big gastrins" from Zollinger-Ellison tumour tissue. Lancet, *2*:797-799, 1972.
12. Gregory, R. A., Tracy, H. J., and Agarwal, K. L.: Amino acid constitution of two gastrins isolated from Zollinger-Ellison tumor tissue. Gut, *10*:603, 1964.
13. Isenberg, J. I., et al.: Unusual effect of secretin on serum gastrin, serum calcium, and gastric acid secretion in a patient with suspected Zollinger-Ellison syndrome. Gastroenterology, *62*:626, 1972.
14. Kolts, B. E., and McGuigan, J. E.: Radioimmunoassay measurement of secretin half-life in man. Gastroenterology, *72*:55, 1977.
15. Kolts, B. E., Herbst, C. A., and McGuigan, J. E.: Calcium and secretin-stimulated gastrin release in the Zollinger-Ellison syndrome. Ann. Intern. Med., *81*:758, 1974.
16. Kuzio, M., Dryburgh, J., Malloy, K., and Brown, J. C.: Radioimmunoassay for gastric inhibitory polypeptide. Gastroenterology, *66*:357, 1974.
17. McGuigan, J. E., and Trudeau, W. L.: Immunochemical measurement of elevated levels of gastrin in the serum of patients with pancreatic tumors of the Zollinger-Ellison variety. New Engl. J. Med., *278*:1308, 1968.
18. Rehfeld, J. F., Stadil, F., and Vikelsoe, J.: Immunoreactive gastrin components in human serum. Gut, *15*:102, 1974.
19. Said, S. I., and Faloona, G. R.: Elevated plasma and tissue levels of vasoactive intestinal polypeptide in the watery-diarrhea syndrome due to pancreatic, brochogenic and other tumors. New Engl. J. Med., *293*:155, 1975.
20. Straus, E., and Yalow, R. S.: Differential diagnosis in hyperchlorhydric hyper-gastrinemia. Gastroenterology, *66*:867, 1974.
21. Trudeau, W. L., and McGuigan, J. E.: Effects of calcium on serum gastrin in the Zollinger-Ellison syndrome. New Engl. J. Med., *281*:862, 1969.
22. Yalow, R. S., and Berson, S. A.: Size and charge distinctions between endogenous human plasma gastrin in peripheral blood and heptadecapeptide gastrins. Gastroenterology, *58*:609, 1970.
23. ———: Radioimmunoassay of Gastrin. Gastroenterology, *58*:1, 1970.
24. Zollinger, R. M., and Ellison, E. H.: Primary peptic ulcerations of the jejunum associated with islet cell tumors of the pancreas. Ann. Surg., *142*:709, 1955.

EDITORIAL COMMENTARY

When it became possible to identify the molecular structure of polypeptide hormones, and then to purify and synthesize those peptides as antigens for the production of specific antibodies, a new dimension in endocrine research unfolded. Prior to the availability of these immunologic techniques, the study of endocrinopathies was approached by the observation of the exocrine end-organ effects of the candidate hormones and the qualitative estimations of their biologic action with bioassay preparations. Although bioassays were and still are important in the identification of the physiologic actions of hormones, the quantitative measurement by bioassay is imprecise and nonspecific. Furthermore, the biologic actions of secretin, gastrin and insulin, for instance, in extracts of the tissue in which they are native, have been known for several decades, yet until immunochemical techniques were developed it was impossible to accurately measure their concentration in blood or tissue, or to identify their normal cell of origin, much less their intracellular localization, or to differentiate the varieties of molecular structure of the hormones secreted from neoplastic endocrine cells. Radioimmunoassays and immunofluorescent techniques have made such basic investigations possible and have spawned remarkable advances in our understanding of the pathogenesis and the diagnosis of newly described and rediscovered endocrinopathies.

Recent milestones in polypeptide research surely include the development of radioimmunoassay of insulin by Berson and Yalow, the purification and the structural identification of gastrin by Gregory and Tracy, and the immunofluorescent localization of the gastrin (G) cell of the gastric antrum by McGuigan and his ingenious development of methods for the production of specific antibodies for gastrin and his refinements of immunochemical measurement of gastrin in the serum and tissues. The use of immunologic techniques has led to many additional discoveries of critical importance to modern understanding of endocrinopathies such as the separation of portions of molecules having different degrees of both functional capabilities and capacities for immunogenicity. The finding of "large" and "small" molecular forms of the hormones and portions of them demonstrating molecular heterogeneity has clarified some of the problems of disparate results and unexpected and capricious clinical pictures in patients. Moreover, refinements of radioimmunologic methods have lent clarity of understanding of the normal release of hormones under the influence of stimulation and inhibition, their output from hyperfunctioning hyperplasias and benign tumors, and finally, of the elaboration of more complex hormones having apparently similar functions but dissimilar immunogenic capabilities from neoplastic and ectopic tumors.

The development of unique methods of enhancement of weak immunogenicity of an organic molecule was an important improvement of the sensitivity of assays and the measurement of circulating peptides. Thus, more sensitive measurements have allowed greater precision of diagnosis of endocrinopathies, especially in the clinical development of stimulation and suppression tests and in the observations of the effects of surgical and medical treatment and of pharmacologic receptor-blocking.

There very likely will be further developments in assay techniques of the measurement of known as well as yet undefined hormones. It remains to be seen whether assays in which enzyme components are used instead of radioisotopes will meet the requirements for specificity and sensitivity. There are still some problems with variability of assay results and universal availability of these laboratory techniques to many clinicians. In the meantime it is more necessary than ever that there be clinical correlations of the measurements of the endocrine humoral concentrations and the exocrine end-organ effects with the pathologic and cytologic findings in patients who present well-defined clinical syndromes. *S.R.F.*

5

Genetics and the Endocrine System *

R. Neil Schimke, M.D.

Heritable factors play an exceedingly important role in the pathogenesis of disorders of the endocrine glands.[5] Virtually every endocrine disease has at least a partial etiologic genetic component; in some, abnormal gene function is of paramount importance. There are a number of different ways whereby genetic factors may influence hormone hypo- or hypersecretion, and some of these are listed in Table 5-1. It is important to recognize that the same phenotypic effect (i.e., clinical presentation) may result from a number of different genetic alterations. For example, proportionate dwarfism secondary to isolated growth hormone deficiency can occur as a consequence of a structural mutation in the gene coding for the growth hormone peptide, and the growth hormone molecule will be intrinsically defective. A mutation in a regulator gene can result in decreased levels of a normally structured growth hormone with the same phenotypic consequences. One mutation might be recessive, the other dominantly inherited. Moreover, a polygenic or a chromosomal disorder that might be associated with a developmental malformation can also feature growth hormone deficiency (i.e., midline closure defects of the first brachial arch may extend to the adenohypophysis with resultant deficiency of growth hormone). Although such has never been described, excessive secretion of growth hormone release-inhibiting hormone (somatostatin) can also produce short stature and the metabolic features of growth hormone deficiency. It is important not to "lump" these various conditions together under the rubric of "growth hormone deficiency," since the genetics, and hence the recurrence risks for the subsequent affected children in the family, may be different. Further, the therapy should be individually tailored to the etiology of the growth hormone deficiency state.

DEVELOPMENT OF THE ENDOCRINE SYSTEM

There is considerable evidence supporting the neural crest origin of those endocrine cells that secrete simple amines and peptides; this data is reviewed in Chapters 1 and 2. However, all endocrine tissue need not stem from the same embryologic source. The adrenal cortex and the gonads are derived from mesoderm and secrete steroids. Moreover, unlike a peptide hormone which likely is encoded by only a single structural gene, the synthesis of cortisol

* This work was supported in part by a John E. Fogarty Senior International Research Fellowship and was accomplished while the author was a Visiting Professor, University Department of Human Genetics in Edinburgh, Scotland.

Table 5-1. Possible Mechanisms of Gene Action in Endocrine Dysfunction

Type of Alteration	*Result*
Structural mutation	Altered peptide hormone structure ± immunologically detectable Hormone deficiency state
Regulatory mutation	Increase or decrease in synthesis of peptide hormone of normal structure Hormone hyper- or hyposecretion
Enzyme deficiency	Decreased hormone synthesis
Developmental malformation	Decreased hormone synthesis
Neurostimulatory defect	Decreased hormone synthesis
Defect in secretory mechanism	Decreased secretion of hormone secondary to abnormal sensor response or defective release mechanism
Peripheral unresponsiveness	Endocrine deficiency state with increased plasma hormone levels
Degenerative disorder	Decreased hormone levels secondary to autoimmune, toxic, vascular, etc. factors
Hormone antagonist	Endocrine deficiency state
Glandular hyperplasia	Variable May show hyper- or hyposecretion

requires a number of different enzymes, each of which is the product of one or more structural genes. The pituitary gland which contains cells derived from neural crest harbors still other cells, whose origin is unknown, that secrete glycoprotein hormones such as TSH, FSH and LH. These latter cells express a more complex biosynthetic capacity, since they too require not only at least two genes for the alpha- and beta-polypeptide subunits of these hormones but also an unknown number of other genes coding for enzymes necessary to add the appropriate carbohydrate residues to the nascent polypeptide chain. It is likely an oversimplification to assume that all endocrine tissue, whether it produces simple peptides or complex steroid molecules or glycoproteins, is derived from a single embryologic source. It remains conceivable, however, that the ultimate regulation of hormone secretion of all types resides within neural crest-derived cells, either indirectly or by some direct cell-cell interaction.[9]

CLINICAL EXPRESSION OF GENETIC MUTATIONS

Multiple genes are involved in the ontologic development of any tissue as complex as the endocrine system. For example, genes are necessary in the derivation of the neural crest; they influence the migration of those cells and obviously control their ultimate fate and phenotypic expression (i.e., whether they become odontoblasts, melanoblasts or endocrine cells).[7] These various genes often must act sequentially within a relatively short embryologic time frame. It is not surprising to note then that a number of mutations can result in the same phenotypic effect. This concept is easily understood insofar as it applies to congenital genetic disease. Less easy to comprehend are those genetic abnormalities that result in disease later in life such as Graves' disease or the multiple endocrine neoplasia (MEN) syndromes. In such cases, the genetic defect remains latent until additional factors, some of which may be environmental whereas others are likely genetic, produce a suitable milieu for the abnormal gene to produce its effect. Some patients harbor a gene mutation that may never become clinically evident, and the gene is said to show decreased or incomplete penetrance. Penetrance in this sense is an all or none phenomenon. If the gene is penetrant, it may be variably expressed. Expressivity in this context is akin to clinical grade of severity. As an example, one can cite a family in which MEN, Type I is segregating. This autosomal dominant condition features adenomas, adenocarcinomas or hyperplasia of the pituitary, parathyroid and pancreatic endocrine cells, with the resultant symptomatology dependent on appropriate hormone secretion. Not all affected members of the family have tumors of all these endocrine glands at any one time; in fact such an occurrence is exceedingly rare. Longitudinal follow-up frequently reveals additional glandular involvement in each individual with time; hence, the gene is variably expressed. Nonpenetrance can only be diagnosed if the pedigree analysis showed that a subject transmitted the gene but never developed any symptomatology throughout his lifetime. Again such a phenomenon in the MEN syndromes is rare, although with other genetic disorders such as diabetes mellitus it may be more common. For example, if an individual with a diabetic genotype maintained a stable ideal body weight, he might never develop clinical or chemical diabetes.

INHERITANCE PATTERNS

There are three basic ways in which heritable disorders can be transmitted in a family: Mendelian or single factor inheritance comprising autosomal and X-linked dominant and recessive patterns; polygenic inheritance, and chromosomal transmission. Each pedigree must be examined with care to determine which mode of inheritance is operational. Occasionally, suitable texts must be consulted if no clear pattern emerges.[4,5] Adequate genetic counseling and calculation of recurrence risks within a family thus has two prerequisites: an accurate diagnosis and knowledge of the way the disease in question is inherited.

Autosomal Inheritance

In autosomal inheritance, the abnormal gene is located on one of the autosomes (i.e., not on the X or Y chromosomes). Very few human genes have been localized to any specific chromosome, but such studies are currently underway. Pedigree analysis determines whether a condition is autosomal or X-linked or whether it is dominant or recessive. Dominant inheritance indicates that only one of the two homologous genes is abnormal, but the defect is severe enough to cause clinical disease in the affected individual who is heterozygous. Since the two homologous genes (alleles) segregate in meiosis, any offspring of any affected individual has a 50 percent chance of being likewise affected, and both male and female children are equally at risk. By contrast, an autosomal recessive genetic defect requires that both alleles be abnormal (i.e., the affected individual is homozygous). Each parent of such an individual is an obligate heterozygote, but since the condition is by definition recessive, a single dose of the deleterious gene causes no clinical abnormality. Rather than vertical transmission of the genetic defect as is seen with dominant inheritance, family studies reveal affected male and female sibs. If the condition is sufficiently rare, the heterozygous parents may be consanguineous.

Examples of autosomal dominant endocrine disorders include the MEN syndromes, one form of isolated growth hormone deficiency, and probably one type of neurohypophyseal diabetes insipidus, although the most common type is X-linked. Autosomal recessive disorders are exemplified by the various forms of congenital adrenal hyperplasia and the familial goiters due to the inborn errors of thyroxine biosynthesis.

X-Linked Inheritance

Within X-linked (or sex-linked) dominant inheritance, both males and females are affected, but affected males transmit the disorder to all their daughters (sons receive the Y chromosome), whereas affected females have a 50 percent chance of passing the condition on to either sons or daughters. This type of inheritance pattern may resemble autosomal dominance with the critical exception that with X-linkage, no male-to-male transmission occurs. Vitamin D-resistant rickets is a good example of X-linked dominant inheritance.

Females heterozygous for an X-linked recessive disorder are usually unaffected unless they have the Turner syndrome and only one X chromosome which contains the mutant gene, or unless they are homozygous, a situation found only rarely. Males with the mutation have no counterbalancing normal X chromosome and hence are termed hemizygous and are affected. Again, no male-to-male transmission occurs, and affected males are related to one another through the maternal side of the family. Carrier females transmit the disorder to 50 percent of their male offspring. The testicular feminization syndrome, XY pure gonadal dysgenesis and one form of familial panhypopituitarism are X-linked recessive disorders.

Polygenic Inheritance

There are some disorders in which no one single gene of major effect can be identified. Yet familial aggregation of such conditions is often striking, and since affected individuals are frequently widely separated by time and space, heritable factors must be of some importance. Such conditions are termed polygenic or multifactorial. In this class of disorders, an interaction between the environment and multiple genes of small effect is assumed in such a way that the recurrence risk, although finite, is usually small. The relatively common birth defects best fit this classification. For example, the random risk to the unaffected couple of having a child with congenital heart disease (CHD) is about 1 in 500. After the birth of an affected child the risk increases to approximately 1 in 50. After two affected children the recurrence risk for a third is about 1 in 17. In other words, unlike the situation with mendelian inheritance in which the recurrence risk remains the same no matter how many affected or unaffected are born, the risk for polygenic disorders increases with the birth of each affected individual. Moreover, the presence of an affected parent increases the risk to a similar degree (i.e., if a parent is affected, the risk to the first child is about 1 in 50 and so forth). It appears that the more individuals who are affected in the family, the greater the potential number of abnormal cardiovascular genes present and the more hostile the intrauterine environment. The latter may simply provide a threshold. For example, a certain drug may be a cardiovascular teratogen only if enough genetic mutations exist to provide an appropriate substrate.

Developmental abnormalities of the central nervous system (which may have associated endocrinopathy) are probably the best examples of this type of inheritance. Some forms of diabetes mellitus, especially the juvenile onset variety, may also be polygenic. For example, patients with juvenile diabetes often show evidence of autoimmune phenomena such as thyroid or parietal cell autoantibodies with or without associated clinical disease.[1] Juvenile diabetes also has been found to be associated with the HLA-8 haplotype.[2] In lower animals, and presumably in man, the histocompatibility antigen gene system is linked (i.e., physically associated on the same chromosome) with certain genes that control immunologic reactivity, the so-called immune response genes. One might postulate that the immune response genes usually linked to HLA-8 are abnormal to the extent that an individual with such a gene or genes may be more selectively susceptible to an external agent, perhaps a virus. The viral infection may then cause more than the usual cellular damage to such organs as the thyroid or stomach, causing inordinate cell lysis and release of "forbidden" contents. The remainder of the immune system, including other immune response genes, may then respond appropriately to these "foreign" proteins with the subsequent production of autoantibodies. The proposed virus may be predominantly pancreaticotropic and diabetes then dominates the clinical picture. In this setting the immune response genes may be multiple (i.e., polygenes) but will be associated with disease only when in contact with an unfavorable environment (i.e., the infecting virus). This interpretation is obviously speculative and only represents an attempt to rationalize the known familial aggregation of an endocrine disease of a given type with other heritable factors, which in the case of juvenile diabetes are apparently immunologic.

Chromosomal Disorders

Chromosome abnormalities are usually associated with malformations in multiple tissues, simply because many genes are nonspecifically lost or gained, depending on the type of meiotic error. The most common defects result from nondisjunction or asymmetric separation of the chromosomes during meiosis with the production of gametes containing more or less than the usual number of chromosomes. Fertilization then gives rise to chromosomally unbalanced zygotes such as the familiar trisomy 21 (Down's syndrome), XO gonadal dysgenesis (Turner syndrome) or the XXY Klinefelter syndrome. Deletions or loss of parts of chromosomes also can occur as can more complex rearrangements (i.e., translocations). For the most part, these disorders have a low risk of recurrence save for some of the translocation trisomies in which one parent is a balanced carrier of the rearrangement. In this case, the risk may be significant.

Most of these conditions have little relevance for the endocrinologist-surgeon, save perhaps for the sex chromosome anomalies. Patients with the Turner syndrome have an increased incidence of diabetes mellitus and thyroiditis, and there is some suggestion that they may be unduly susceptible to nonendocrine neural crest tumors.[10] The streak gonads are not premalignant unless the individual is mosaic (i.e., has an XY ovarian cell line as in XO/XY mosaicism).[8] Certainly if spontaneous virilization occurs in these patients, an ovarian tumor should be suspected until proven otherwise. Similarily, intersex states, occurring on a chromosomal basis, in which an intra-abdominal gonad may have an XY karyotype should be operated on for the dual purpose of delineating internal anatomy for potential reconstructive surgery and also for gonadectomy because of the malignant potential of these glands.

GENETICS AND SURGICAL ENDOCRINOLOGY

The vast majority of endocrine conditions with which the surgeon deals are likely sporadic and thus of no genetic moment. On the other hand, all too frequently little attention is paid to the family history by the surgeon or his staff, save for a brief notation that the family history was positive for "cancer" or "hormone problems." Potentially, any endocrine neoplasia may be heritable, and the surgeon with knowledge of the total implications of the Zollinger-Ellison syndrome should logically embark on a more detailed endocrine evaluation of an affected patient seeking other signs of MEN, Type I. Moreover, other first-degree relatives of such a patient at risk should be considered for the syndrome until proven otherwise. Because disorders such as the MEN syndrome are dominantly inherited and therefore variably expressed, longitudinal follow-up of the patient and his family should be instituted, since, as mentioned previously, other facets of the syndrome may appear at varying intervals later in life. The problem then becomes one of recognizing the heritable tumor syndrome in order to focus attention on the high-risk family.

Obviously when one encounters a patient with MEN, Type III or the mucosal neuroma syndrome, the external appearance itself is virtually diagnostic. Although the other MEN syndromes rarely show glandular hyperfunction before the second or third decade, patients with MEN, Type III have been found to have medullary thyroid tumor or at least C cell hyperplasia in early childhood.[6] The presence of the pathognomonic facies probably warrants early, prophylactic total thyroidectomy.

Similarly, the presence of cutaneous lipomas may be indicative of MEN, Type I in a patient with hyperparathyroidism. As a working generalization, heritable tumors, whether in the endocrine system or elsewhere, tend to be bilateral or multifocal. In the case of parathyroids, diffuse hyperplasia of all glands is more likely genetic than is a sporadic adenoma. The reason for the multifocal nature of inherited tumors is not clear. Knudson has suggested that the development of a tumor requires two mutational events.[3] In the case of sporadic tumors both events would, of necessity, be somatic. With heritable tumors, the first event would be meiotic and thus every susceptible cell would be vulnerable; hence, bilateral or multifocal lesions are the rule with familial tumors.

Another characteristic of familial tumor syndromes is that symptoms begin on the average at a younger age than in patients with sporadic lesions. Familial tumors may produce ectopic hormones such as ACTH, serotonin and prostaglandins by the medullary thyroid carcinoma in MEN, Type II or III, but they are probably no more likely to do so than are nonfamilial tumors. Ectopic hormone production probably represents a limited form of gene derepression (i.e., limited in the sense that tumors derived from neural crest have the potential to elaborate peptides and amines and not more complex molecules such as glycoproteins, which generally are secreted by cells not neural crest in origin).

The type of diagnostic studies one undertakes in an individual and his family depends upon the disease in question. For example, there is no need to perform chromosome analyses on family members at risk for well-recognized single gene disorders such as the MEN syndromes, since the genetic abnormality is submicroscopic. Chromosome studies are indicated in inappropriate masculinizing and feminizing states and in intersex conditions because of the relationship of the Y chromosome to neoplasia in an intra-abdominal gonad. By the same token, there is little merit in embarking upon extensive pituitary function studies when a firm diagnosis of MEN, Type II (pheochromocytoma, medullary thyroid tumor, parathyroid adenoma) has been made, since involvement of the adenohypophysis does not occur in this condition. In other words, if sufficient clinical information is available, including the family history, the number and type of expensive tests performed can be minimized. The increasing availability of radioimmunoassays, which require small volumes of blood or urine, may eventually allow for family screening on an outpatient basis and greatly expedite longitudinal follow-up of affected families.

CONCLUSIONS

There are obviously many ways in which genes can influence the endocrine system. It is hoped that the preceding paragraphs have provided a brief introduction, both to the rudiments of clinical genetics and to the myriad ways in which heritable factors can influence the endocrine system. The better understood the genetic mechanisms involved, the more rational the therapeutic approach.

REFERENCES

1. Appel, G. B., and Holub, D. X.: The syndrome of multiple endocrine gland insufficiency. Am. J. Med., *61*:129, 1976.
2. Cudworth, A. G., and Woodrow, J. C.: Evidence for HL-A-linked genes in "juvenile" diabetes mellitus. Br. Med. J., *3*:133, 1975.
3. Knudson, A. G., Jr., Strong, L. C., and Anderson, D. E.: Heredity and cancer in man. Prog. Med. Genet., *9*:113, 1975.
4. McKusick, V. A.: Mendelian Inheritance in Man. ed. 4. Baltimore, Johns Hopkins University Press, 1975.
5. Rimoin, D. L., and Schimke, R. N.: Genetic Disorders of the Endocrine Glands. St. Louis, C. V. Mosby, 1971.
6. Schimke, R. N.: Phenotype of malignancy: the mucosal neuroma syndrome. Pediatrics, *52*:283, 1973.
7. ——: Tumors of the neural crest system. *In* Genetics and Cancer. p. 179. New York, Raven Press, 1977.
8. Simpson, J. L., and Photopulos, G.:

The relationship of neoplasia to disorders of abnormal sexual differentiation. Birth Defects, *12*:15, 1976.
9. Warner, T. F.: Cell hybridization in the genesis of ectopic hormone-secreting tumors. Lancet, *1*:1259, 1974.
10. Wertelecki, W., Fraumeni, J. F., Jr., and Mulvihill, J. J.: Nongonadal neoplasia in Turner's syndrome. Cancer, *26*:435, 1970.

EDITORIAL COMMENTARY

Genetic phenomena are of particular relevance to endocrinopathies which occur in combinations such as the familial multiple endocrine adenopathies and those in which there are inappropriate masculinizing and feminizing states. Moreover, an understanding of the genetic potential for multiple or familial involvement even in the more common sporadic endocrinopathies is also important for the detection of other endocrine adenopathies in the affected patient and his/her first-degree relatives. Diagnostic screening of reasonable simplicity of a so-called "sporadic" patient and close relatives may reveal that the patient, particularly if he is a young adult, harbors latent endocrinopathies and is a progenitor, the first in the family to surface with a clinical abnormality.

There are many ways that abnormal genes influence the resulting endocrine abnormalities, affecting the structure, synthesis and secretion of the hormones and responsivity of the end-organ, to name but a few. The genetic defect may assert itself at birth or be latent, being influenced by environmental conditions later in life. Genetic abnormalities are more prevalent in endocrinopathies involving the APUD system of cells, being involved and necessary in the derivation, migration, fate and clinical (phenotypic) expression of neural cells of neuroectoderm and neural crest origin. The ultimate regulation of hormone secretion of all types may reside in neural-derived cells; thus, for instance, the polypeptide-secreting hypothalamic and pituitary APUD cells affect and regulate the steroid-secreting endocrine cells by their trophic and inhibitory actions.

It is important to note that the genetic-based endocrinopathies are frequently bilateral and multifocal and occur in younger patients than is the case in sporadic involvement. Multiple endocrinopathies involve a variation of histologic patterns ranging from hyperplasias to neoplasias; hence, there are semantic discrepancies in terms which are in fact synonymous: Multiple endocrine adenopathy (adenomatosis, MEA, and multiple endocrine neoplasia, MEN).

In this chapter the syndrome complex of medullary carcinoma of the thyroid, adrenal medullary pheochromocytoma, with mucosal neuromas, is referred to as MEN, Type III (the mucosal neuroma syndrome), whereas in other chapters this combination is termed MEN, Type IIb, by other authors. *S.R.F.*

6

Current Concepts of Diagnosis

Edward Passaro, Jr., M.D.

CLINICAL FEATURES

The visible and measurable manifestations of endocrine disease can be arbitrarily but conveniently grouped into those affecting mineral metabolism, energy, growth, and homeostasis (Table 6-1). Whereas each of the individual disorders is discussed in detail in subsequent chapters, this grouping despite its limitations will give an indication of their numbers and the type of diagnostic maneuvers necessary.

Table 6-1. Endocrine Disease Groups

Category	*Clinical Parameter*	*Endocrine Parameter*	*Disease*
Group 1			
Mineral imbalance	↑ Ca^{++}	↑ Parathormone	Hyperparathyroidism
	↓ Ca^{++}	↑ Calcitonin	Medullary carcinoma of the thyroid
	Hypertension, ↓ K^+	↑ Aldosterone	Aldosteronism
	↑↑ Ca^{++}	(unknown)	Lung tumors
Group 2			
Energy	↑ Catabolism	↑ Thyroxine	Hyperthyroidism
	Syncope, ↓ Glucose	↑ Insulin	Hyperinsulinism
	↑ Glucose	↑ Glucagon	Hyperglucagonism
	↓ Glucose	(unknown)	Retroperitoneal tumors
Group 3			
Growth	↑ Bone enlargement	↑ Growth hormone	Acromegaly
	↑ Male sexual characteristics	↑ Androgens	Masculinizing
	↑ Female sexual characteristics	↑ Estrogens	Feminizing
Group 4			
Homeostasis	Obesity, Muscle wasting, ↑ Urine 17-OH Corticosteroids	↑ Cortisol	Hypercorticolism
	↑ Gastric acid	↑ Gastrin	Gastrinoma
	Diarrhea, ↓ K^+	↑ Vasoactive Intestinal Polypeptide	Vipoma
	↑ Urine U.M.A.	↑ Catecholamine	Pheochromocytoma
	↑ Urine 5-H1AA, Histamine	↑ Serotonin, Histamine	Carcinoid

A careful clinical history may also contain features which suggest the following hormonal disorders:

Features of Endocrine Disease

Young middle age	Medically unresponsive
Apparent good health	Skin manifestations
Family history	

The patients are generally below 50 years of age and in otherwise apparent good health. Skin manifestations are evident in more than half of the endocrine disorders. A family history of endocrine problems is not uncommon, since some syndromes are attributable to genetic factors. Most endocrine diseases have an insidious onset and remain occult for long periods of time; others produce obvious dramatic changes. However long it may take, once manifested the clinical signs and symptoms of these disorders are usually severe and with few exceptions (such as hyperthyroidism) cannot be effectively treated medically. In fact, even when treated by surgical extirpation, endocrine disorders as a group show a propensity to recur. Thus, early accurate diagnosis and careful long-term evaluation by the appropriate diagnostic maneuvers are of exceptional importance in the treatment of endocrine disease.

DIAGNOSTIC TESTS

The recent rapid advances in technology and immunochemistry have made possible the direct measurement of hormones in blood in concentrations as low as 10^{-9}M. Such assays permit rapid and accurate assessment of endocrine disease and render obsolete the laborious chemical extractions of hormones from blood or urine. Where possible, serum or plasma assays should be used in evaluating endocrine disorders. It must be borne in mind that the measurement of a hormone in the blood is just that. It does not tell what the effect of that hormone level might be. For example, hypergastrinemia, by itself, does not mean that the patient is secreting acid! Pernicious anemia patients with comparable hypergastrinemia may be achlorhydric.

Ideally, a single determination of the amount of a particular hormone in the blood should suffice to diagnose an endocrinopathy. A markedly elevated serum gastrin concentration in an unoperated duodenal ulcer patient, for example, is diagnostic of a gastrinoma (Zollinger-Ellison syndrome). However, only rarely is a single determination of hormone levels diagnostic. More often, several blood determinations will be required, since hormone release may be cyclic, the amount of circulating hormone being influenced by the time of day, fasting state, physical activity and menstrual cycle to name but a few factors. Thus, in most cases, the time and the conditions under which the blood is obtained are very important. This is particularly true for hormones which exert primarily a homeostatic effect (Table 6-1, Group 4). In contrast, hormones affecting mineral metabolism (Table 6-1, Group 1) generally do not show such fluctuations, and one or two assay samples may suffice.

Unfortunately, even when the blood sample is obtained under optimal circumstances, useful information may not be provided by the assay. This paradox occurs because tumor activity may vary independently of known factors. The characteristic episodic release of norepinephrine by pheochromocytomas comes to mind. In these circumstances further steps must be taken to disclose the endocrine disorder.

A provocative test which causes the prolonged and heightened release of the hormone in question greatly facilitates the diagnosis. The agent used may either stimulate or suppress the release of hormones.

Stimulation tests ideally should be safe, rapid, easy to perform and have a sharp end-point. Such tests serve to uncover occult or forme fruste endocrine disease. Occult metastatic medullary thyroid carcinoma can be detected, for example, by means of a calcium infusion which stimulates the tumor to elaborate calcitonin. These tests also can serve to measure the tumor activity or mass (burden) and may be useful in evaluating the results of surgical or medical therapy.

Calcium and secretin infusions have been shown to be effective in causing the serum gastrin concentration to become markedly elevated in patients harboring a gastrinoma. They are particularly of value in patients suspected of having a gastrinoma, but whose basal serum gastrins are consistently in the normal range.[12] Just how these agents work is not known. The prompt marked increase of the hormone in the blood suggests that most provocative agents cause a release of stored intracellular hormone rather than acting through a chemical intermediary. Calcium, in particular, because of its importance in hormone secretion and in cell membrane permeability, has been useful as a provocative agent in a variety of endocrine disorders. Agents such as secretin may work because of altered cell membranes and hormone receptors present in tumor cells.[1]

Suppression tests on the other hand give some indication of autonomous function, a salient feature of tumors. By demonstrating that the release of the hormone is no longer suppressed by the appropriate agent (e.g., the inhibition of parathyrin release by hypercalcemia) the abnormal autonomous activity characteristic of tumors can be demonstrated. In general, suppression tests are useful where hormone release is continuous rather than cyclical in nature.

ROENTGENOGRAPHIC DIAGNOSTIC PROCEDURES

A variety of roentgenographic procedures employing selective catheterization of vessels have proven useful in evaluating endocrine disorders. Arteriographic studies are useful in demonstrating not only the presence of the lesion but also its blood supply. For adrenal tumors such as pheochromocytoma, in which excessive tumor manipulation is hazardous and the blood supply multiple and variable, this technique has been particularly helpful. Highly vascular tumors which are otherwise difficult to locate, such as insulinomas and parathyroid adenomas, can be visualized in selective arteriograms. Further, the presence of unsuspected metastases in the liver can be shown by hepatic arteriography.

Selective catheterization of the venous drainage from an organ can be used for retrograde dye studies to demonstrate the presence of a tumor. More often, however, selective venous catheterization is useful in obtaining blood samples for assay. For example, differences in hormone concentrations in the venous system draining the neck and mediastinum can localize parathyroid glands missed at previous operations.[3] This technique has proved invaluable in these instances.

Last, newer, noninvasive techniques are in the offing. They include sonography, scintillation computerized tomography and photoscanning following the injection of radio-labeled compounds selectively concentrated by an endocrine gland. These techniques and other new ones which apply to specific disorders will be discussed in the following chapters.

REFERENCES

1. Kolata, G. B.: Microvilli: A major difference between normal and cancer cells. Science, *188*:819, 1975.
2. Morrow, D. J., and Passaro, E., Jr.,: Calcium infustion test before and after total gastrectomy in the Zollinger-Ellison syndrome. Am. J. Surg., *129*:62, 1975.
3. Shimkin, P. M., Feldman, M. G., and Health, D. A.: Parathyroid dysfunction, parathyroid hormone assay and the surgeon. Am. J. Surg., *126*:534, 1973.

EDITORIAL COMMENTARY

There are general principles and precepts of diagnosis which pertain to all of the endocrine syndromes, though technical modifications or minor exceptions may be applicable to the diagnostic confirmation of specific endocrinopathies. It is important to emphasize that the specific radioimmunoassay of elevated levels of circulating hormone is diagnostic of a specific endocrine syndrome; yet the clinical presentation of that endocrinopathy also depends upon the receptivity of the specific target cell/organ. For these reasons it is necessary to study, also, the exocrine manifestations of the biologic action of the target cells which result from the effect of the increased hormone, often with simultaneous measurements of each. For instance, synchronous determinations of blood glucose and plasma insulin or of serum calcium, phosphorus and plasma parathyrin are much more meaningful and diagnostic than if measured at different times under other influences. There are refinements in measuring certain exocrine functions when attempting to determine the effect of certain hormones. For instance, the capability of measuring increased intestinal mucosal secretion as contrasted to decreased mucosal absorption has led to the elucidation of the former as a biologic effect of vasoactive intestinal peptide (VIP). The finding of increased activity of the adenylcyclase—cAMP receptor complex may also reflect increased concentrations of VIP and other polypeptides. It is logically important to match the level of circulating hormones to the expected biologic (exocrine) activity, not only in order to detect receptor capability but also to determine the site of abnormality. In the instances of the effect of trophic hormones on the elaboration of other hormones, simultaneous measurements of central and peripheral hormones can be diagnostic. As an example of the latter, elevated cortisol levels without elevations of ACTH point to a primary adrenocortical tumor without hypothalamic or pituitary instigation. Also, failure of receptor function of the target cell may cause or be associated with inappropriate excesses of the appropriate hormone; a disparity between a lack of biologic effect and an excess of the appropriate hormone points to a receptor incapability. A case in point concerns the presence of hypergastrinemia associated with the achlorhydria of pernicious anemia, a situation in which the circulating gastrin is elevated without the expected presence of gastric acid secretion. The gastrinemia is most likely due to the lack of acid inhibition of antral G cell release of gastrin, and the achlorhydria is due to a failure of parietal cell receptor response to the circulating gastrin. In this clinical situation a suppression test involving intragastric administration of 0.1 normal hydrochloric acid will effectively suppress antral gastrin release, causing a decrease in serum gastrin concentrations; thus an autonomous tumor source of hypergastrinemia is further ruled out diagnostically. Failure of suppression tests to elucidate suppression of release of circulating hormones is tantamount to tumor autonomy as contrasted to either normal homeostasis or to compensatory hyperplasia when present.

Another concept in the appropriate use of diagnostic tests in patients with hypersecretion of polypeptide hormones concerns the failure of further provocation by an exogenous humoral substance to affect or accentuate the biologic effect at a time when the endogenous hormone is already working maximally. An example of such tests is the failure of exogenous glucagon to further elevate the blood glucose or circulating insulin in patients with glucagonoma; another example is failure of histalog to further increase gastric secretion of acid significantly in patients with gastrinoma.

True stimulation tests are valuable for accurate diagnoses, particularly in the ulcerogenic syndrome. Secretin, administered exogenously, will paradoxically further elevate the hypergastrinemia due to a pancreatic gastrinoma, as contrasted to its pharmacologic action in normal patients, duodenal ulcer patients or those with antral gastrinosis. Similarly, calcium infusion test of either the short challenge type or the longer infusion variety is of importance because it will significantly elevate borderline or intermediate levels of serum gastrin in patients with ulcerogenic tumor, but will not usually increase the gastrinemia in which the source is antral G cell hyperplasia. In such situations, the possible presence of associated hyperparathyroidism must be taken into account when using the calcium stimulation tests. Exogenous calcium and pentagastrin stimulation of the release of thyrocalcitonin from occult medullary carcinoma of the thyroid gland are exceedingly useful diagnostic procedures. The mechanism of calcium stimulation of the release of gastrin and other polypeptides is not known; one theory is that the calcium ion is permissive of the emiocytosis of the secretory granules through the endocrine cell membrane, thus apparently accentuating the release of the hormone from endocrine tumor cells.

Whereas the measurement of excessive circulating hormone and the corresponding exocrine abnormalities that are consistent with the presenting clinical picture are diagnostic, the ultimate confirmation must include biopsy for histologic diagnosis and for radioimmune assessment of the humoral content of the tumor. Further documentation of the tumor's immunofluorescent specificity and the electron-microscopic definition of its secretory granules is sometimes necessary.

Selective sampling for arteriovenous differences in hormone concentrations in the blood on either side of the tumor is occasionally helpful in solving some unusual clinical problems. Finally, the comparison of preoperative and postoperative concentrations of circulating hormones (before and after tumor or end-organ excision) are of diagnostic and prognostic importance in determining whether excision has been complete or whether metastatic tumor is still present and functioning. In patients with ectopia of hormone or tumor, an attempt to confirm the heterogeneity of the humoral substance by special radioimmunoassays and bioassays is a present-day possibility for refined diagnoses within our current concepts of endocrinology. *S.R.F.*

7

Future Concepts of Management

Edward Passaro, Jr., M.D.

Projections into the future, at least by the wary, are not intended to be rash predictions. They are a method of providing perspective, a way of seeing where matters stand. Occasionally, they serve to gather up the unraveled ends, to weave the main threads into a cohesive whole and to bridge the gaps of ignorance.

Hormones, their cell receptors and the responsible tumors are the elements of all endocrine abnormalities. In the past the surgeon's interest has almost always been held uniquely by the tumor itself. But no longer. Now hormones and their receptors also attract attention, and the surgeon is unsure which component is at fault and where energies should be directed. This is understandable, since information about the hormone, its receptor and the vagaries of the tumor is either missing or is scanty for most endocrine problems.

The projections here will seem even less sure. They are admittedly tenuous; based on premises for the most part uncertain and carried to extremes in almost all ways untried. But no one need protest or apologize; the fallibility of the exercise is recognized. Indeed, it would be disappointing if these projections were not exceeded or superseded, but, if they make the present information more comprehensible, or if they excite wonder at what the future will bring, they will have served their purpose.

HORMONES

The surprising thing about endocrine disease is that it turns out to be more of the same; that is, excessive production of naturally occurring hormone(s). One would expect an occasional aberration—a quirk of a hormone that might be exceptionally potent or long-lived. But that seems not to occur. It is not the cell's product that is at fault but rather the cell's activity or its numbers. The gastrins and insulins of tumors are the same in their diversity and potency as those found in normal sources. It seems unlikely, therefore, that in the future a hormone monster might be confronted. It is apt to be just more of the same.

The difficulty is that "the same" is no longer quite so sure. In the past, investigators noticed an effect and hunted for the cause, proceeding back from a phenomenon mediated through the blood, to the extraction of a factor from some remote tissue which would produce the same phenomenon. The tissue extract was then purified and identified. It is different now. Chemists provide chemically identified and purified biologicals to be tried for hormone action. Each day the list of hormone contenders grows, particularly gastrointestinal hormones.[5] The panoply already includes hormones that stimulate other hormones and that inhibit or otherwise modify their action. The expectation is that a plethora of hormones or hormone-pretenders will be evident in the future. Further, they cannot hide anymore. Every new cell type seen under the microscope is suspect as the source of a new chemical messenger, and the techniques are at hand to track the hormone suspect to its lair.

To the surgeon, the hormone should be a marker—an index of what the tumor is doing. For medullary carcinoma of the thyroid the situation is clear, the presence of a tumor will result in abnormal quantities of thyrocalcitonin in the blood.[3] With gastrinomas, the situation is less clear. Provoking this tumor provides a better idea as to how it is behaving.[6] With tumors of the Verner-Morrison group, the current situation is even more unclear. Some contain high concentration of a plausible hormonal culprit along with elevated blood levels, and others do not.[7] Nevertheless, the trend remains. Tumors *do* have footprints. They have but to be found and recognized.

Hormones have not begun to be used for what they are worth. You have need on occasion to contract the gallbladder, to start and stop gastric emptying or to increase intestinal peristalsis. All of these actions are mediated by known hormones. So when was the last time *you* used a hormone? Perhaps you have not, but you will. Soon postoperative ileus will be a thing of the past and patients will defecate on command. Hormone derivatives or analogues, made in test tubes or altered in the body, will be utilized to do a specific job for the surgeon.

RECEPTORS

It is helpful to know where hormones go. The receptor, it appears, is as unique, sensitive and complex in its interactions as its complimentary hormone. Assays employing receptors (or artificial analogues) are inherently more specific and sensitive than their immunochemical counterparts. Further, the receptor is the first step in understanding how a hormone does what it does. The future for receptor understanding looks bright.

It is startling, all right! You swallow a pill and then you cannot make acid. You have blocked the receptors on your parietal cells and all additional incoming messages are turned away, unanswered. As a result of this development the gastroenterologists are beside themselves; they have a "magic bullet"! You can take it from there. A given receptor's receptivity might soon be able to be blocked or modulated with either a drug or a modified form of its hormone. Better yet, dormant receptors might be unleashed, causing them to multiply and congregate in the appropriate area.

You may wonder what the effects of tampering with receptors might be. It is a safe bet that Mother Nature has already supplied the answer. The identification of receptor diseases looms on the horizon:[1] Diseases caused by receptors that are destroyed, that are unresponsive, or that are just plain lazy! Imagine the following: A patient with a hypersecretory hypertrophic gastropathy. A piece of the fundic mucosa is taken and the receptors scrutinized. Ah-ha! The gastric inhibitory polypeptide receptor shows diminished affinity for the polypeptide. An analogue of gastric inhibitory polypeptide with heightened affinity for the receptor is given. Acid secretion decreases and the exuberant mucosal growth is at first checked and then reverts to normal.

Improbable? Maybe, even seemingly impossible; but perhaps plausible enough for the model to be reality some day.

TUMORS

Endocrine tumors with few exceptions are not malignant in themselves. It is what they do that is malignant. The excess hormone, not the tumor mass, causes the problem. Control of the excess hormone production rather than the tumor mass itself would perhaps suffice in most instances—and for a surgeon that is saying a lot.

The question is: What turns on and off the excess hormone production? What is desperately needed is a good notion of how to answer this question. Current thinking is that the cells of a polypeptide hormone-producing tumor are capable of producing a host of other polypeptides. What the cell does or does not do is a matter of derepression and repression of the information encoded in its nucleus. It is certain that the switching mechanism code will be understood and manipulated someday, but "someday" is too far away. It has probably already been done by chance. Is there a patient who once suffered from hyperinsulinism which stopped and who then developed intractable ulcer disease and hypergastrinemia? Why do vipomas get switched off so well by streptozotocin? In tissue culture, can gastrinoma cells be induced to begin producing cholecystokinin instead? So far, the answers to these questions are not in hand, but some one will soon provide them. The factors that control derepression and repression (and, in effect, tumor growth activity) are probably underfoot but no one has stumbled upon them. How else can the surgeon explain why gastrinomas have occasionally gone away once the stomach is removed?[4]

REFERENCES

1. Brown, M. S., and Goldstein, J. L.: Familial hypercholesterolemia: A genetic defect in the low-density lipoprotein receptor. N. Engl. J. Med., *294*:1386, 1976.
2. Cuatrecasas, P.: Membrane receptors. Ann. Rev. Biochem., *43*:169, 1974.
3. Deftos, L. J.: Immunoassay for human calcitonin. I. Method. Metabolism, *20*:1122, 1971.
4. Friesen, S. R.: A gastric factor in the pathogenesis of the Zollinger-Ellison syndrome. Ann. Surg., *168*:483, 1968.
5. Grossman, M. I., (ed.): Candidate hormones of the gut. Gastroenterology, *67*:730, 1974.
6. Morrow, D. J., and Passaro, E. P., Jr.: Calcium infusion test before and after total gastrectomy in the Zollinger-Ellison syndrome. Am. J. Surg., *129*:62, 1975.
7. Verner, J. V., and Morrison, A. B.: Non-β islet tumors and the syndrome of water diarrhea, hypokalemia and hypochlorhydria. Clinics Gastroenterol., *3*:595, 1974.

EDITORIAL COMMENTARY

In this chapter Dr. Passaro has unleashed his inquisitive mind, making cautious but imaginative projections into future possible methods of endocrine manipulation. He seems to have picked up "unraveled ends" of information in order to weave a tapestry that is as interesting to contemplate as to look at.

Accepting the fallibility inherent in such predictive exercises, he directs our attention to each of the elements of an endocrine system—the hormone, the receptor and the tumor.

One can easily take issue with his statements regarding the "sameness" of the hormones which are released from tumors or from their natural sources, and that in endocrine disease there is merely an excessive production of naturally occurring hormone(s). He states, "The gastrins and insulins of tumors are the same in their diversity and potency as those found in normal sources"; this may be true of their biologic capabilities, but it certainly can be added that consistent with molecular heterogeneity, the proportions of the various molecular forms of the hormones circulating from malignancies are different from those from normal sources. He does admit that "the same" is no longer quite so sure.

Modification of hormone function or structure is a modality of the future, as is the more current modification of receptor responsiveness. New techniques using enzyme-linked immunoassays instead of the radioisotope techniques may lead to more universal availability of the assay and perhaps to modification of hormone function; also investigations into receptor function by cytochemical assays may be helpful in defining hormone-receptor interrelationships. Assays of hormone and receptor activity need to be biospecific, rather than just immunospecific. Receptor blocking is already an established therapeutic modality which has revolutionized the care of patients who have endocrinopathies in which circulating amines are excessive; the same will certainly be true of receptors which receive polypeptides, as is now possible with the parietal cell receptor of gastrin.

Modification of the tumor, traditionally within the realm of surgical activity, is possible by specific chemotherapeutic agents such as streptozotocin. Just as experience with intravenous and intra-arterial administration of streptozotocin is accumulating, more specific compounds that affect the integrity of neoplastic endocrine cells will surely become available for superselective intra-arterial administration to the tumor itself. Yet the surgical excision of endocrine tumors, which is so successful for most of the benign adenomas of the sporadic variety, will remain a viable method of therapy. It remains to be seen whether surgical excision of hyperplastic endocrinopathies will continue to be of lasting benefit—or whether it will be possible to reverse the hyperplastic (or neoplastic) process by modification of the environment of those cells or by surgical interference of their abnormal feedback mechanisms.

Perhaps the prevention of genetic aspects of tumor instigation by means of manipulation of the information encoded in the nucleus of the endocrine cell will be possible. At another end of the spectrum, perhaps the specific destruction of all abnormally growing endocrine cells by cytotoxic agents can be balanced by transplantation of viable and normally functioning endocrine cells.

S.R.F.

8

Transposition and Transplantation of Endocrine Tissues

Robert C. Hickey, M.D.

HISTORY OF TRANSPLANTATION

Transplantation of human tissues has attracted man's attention from time immemorial. Indeed, the first reported homotransplant was from the Garden of Eden, on the occasion of a rib transfer. Major European museums display canvases depicting a transplantation scene.[11] In this scene, a patient who had devoted himself to the service of the Holy Martyrs of the Church of the Saints Cosmas and Damian in Rome is portrayed. The brother saints, Cosmas and Damian, who were probably twins, had practiced the healing arts in Asia Minor, and in the year A.D. 287 were beheaded because of their devotion to Christ. Centuries later, the saintly brothers, carrying various drugs and instruments, appeared in the dream of the sick man. One of the brothers, so the dream goes, went to the cemetery of St. Paul-in-Chains and removed a lower extremity from a recently buried Black Moor. The patient's diseased leg was amputated and replaced by the leg removed from the corpse. The amputated limb was placed in the tomb with the Ethiopian, and on the following day, the patient awakened to discover that he had a healthy extremity, without pain. Upon relating his story, the tomb was opened, and the diseased specimen found therein. Under the sponsorship of the Medici, the scene of the patient has been painted by Fra Angelico (the painting is now in the Museo de' San Marco, Florence); by an unidentified artist (Museum of the Alhambra, Granada) and by Fernando Rincon (Prado Museum, Madrid) and perhaps by others.

Antedating the science of endocrinology, rejuvenation by way of the use of sexual organs from animals was an ancient belief. Three thousand years ago, priests and elders of India and China consumed the sexual organs of animals to improve their vigor and intellect. In the eighteenth century John Hunter experimented with testicular transplants in the chicken, and the scientific study of rejuvenation started with the reports of physiologist Charles Edward Brown-Sequard. In 1889, at the age of 72, he injected himself with an extract of crushed testicles, semen, blood from the testicular vein and distilled water. This material, obtained from dogs and guinea pigs, brought about, he claimed, a renewed vigor and enjoyment of life. The French surgeon, Sergei Vornoff, combined both animal and human experimentation. He transplanted young human or primate testicular tissue into the scrotal sacs of elderly men, being careful to match blood types. This reportedly resulted in a euphoria in these men, an increased mental alertness, muscle tone, skin elasticity and sexual potency, but these observations have not withstood the critical test of time.[10]

The earliest records of transposition, autologous tissue transfers, in the human being were about 1,500 B.C. when skin flaps were used to rebuild severed noses. The earliest transplantation of one human organ to another human probably took place in the Methodist Episcopal Hospital in Philadelphia in 1912; here a homologous testicle was transplanted into the scrotum of a 19-year-old boy to replace a removed testicle; however, this transplant was unsuccessful.

An understanding of immunologic rejection is essential in the science of transplantation. Other factors that need to be considered are the state of the tissue being transplanted (fragments or whole organ), the age of the donor (fetal, neonatal, or adult), species, site of implant and in particular the similarity of genetic makeup.

Also, a knowledge of the various kinds of transplants is important. For example, an *autograft* is a transplant in which the host and the recipient are one and the same; an *isograft* is a transplant between closely related members of the same species, with the same genetic makeup (i.e., highly inbred animal strains or identical twins); an *allograft* is a graft between members of the same species who are not closely related; and a *xenograft* or *heterograft* is a transplantation from one species to another.

GONADAL TRANSPLANTATION AND TRANSPOSITION

Historically, the gonads have been thought to contain a rejuvenating power, but there are no firm data which can specifically relate body structure in aging (other than possibly osteoporosis) to gonadal secretions.

In gonadal surgical techniques, the application of transposition is more applicable than transplantation. The first record of an avulsion injury with loss of the left testicle was reported in 1855.[6] In current clinical urologic practice, the relatively rare avulsion "power take-off" injury is encountered. The injury is handled by split-skin grafting the penile shaft and, if possible, reconstructing the scrotum to contain the testes. When this is impossible, the exposed testes are placed in subcutaneous pockets in the thigh. Transposition of the denuded testes into superficial subcutaneous thigh pockets allows for sufficient mobility and a temperature suitable for spermatogenesis. Huffman, Culp, and Flocks[13] have reported one patient so treated whose wife has since delivered two infants. Intra-abdominal temperatures are sufficiently high to interfere with spermatogenesis. With high bilateral funiculo-orchiectomy, secondary to an avulsion injury, conceivably if the testicles are found, portions might well be cleansed, diced into 1-mm. cubes, and implanted at any site. This is assuming that no reconstruction is possible. The hormone-producing testicular Leydig cells have no functional temperature liability, and this unused, theoretical application might be examined.

In brief, clinical testicular transplantation has been directed toward maintaining the integrity of the function of the seminiferous tubules and not for the androgenic secretion of the interstitial cells.

Ovarian transplantation has fallen from clinical use. Robert Tuttle Morris (1857-1945), a New York surgeon, pioneered ovarian transplants.[26] In 1895 hormonal extracts were not available for therapy, and Morris emphasized his rationale for an overall conservative ovarian management. In one technique, he surgically preserved the ovary and transplanted it into the uterus or fallopian tube. Placing the graft, raw surface to raw surface, his most spectacular success was in implanting the tissue intra-abdominally into the peritoneum of the broad ligament. Of the six patients who received this autotransplant, three menstruated, and one conceived. He commented also upon cystic degeneration of a transplant from a cystic ovary, known to be a clinical phenomenon today. In the instance of one ovarian homotransplantation and subsequent conception, a doubt remained regarding total removal of the extirpated autogenous ovary. In Paris, in the 1930's, Professor Douay of the Hospital Brocha performed a heterologic autotransplant of ovaries into a "friendly" environment, beneath the labia majora, seemingly with success (i.e., the woman was able to continue her nocturnal profession), and she continued to menstruate.*

The technique of oophoropexy or lateral transposition of the ovaries in young females who are to receive pelvic radiation therapy is useful.[21] The ovaries are freed from the uterus by dividing the utero-ovarian ligament and the mesovarium. The major blood supply is maintained through the blood vessels in the infundibulopelvic ligament. Upon dividing the insertions beneath the fallopian tube, the ligament is lifted from the retroperitoneal bed, providing the ovary with a long vascular pedicle. This permits the ovary to be swung laterally and retained so by suturing it to the parietal peritoneum just below the iliac crest. In this position, the ovary is shielded from direct radiation. Of 20 patients reported by Lewis and his colleagues,[21] the hormonal function was preserved in most (i.e., menses continued in 17), but no data are available with respect to fertility.

In animal strains in which a genetic similarity exists, both testes and ovaries have been isografted, and the animal is capable of becoming impregnated[25] or of impregnating.[20] It is interesting to note that the rapid allograft rejection reaction between the Lewis and the Brown Norway strains of rats used by Lee,[20] confirms the ape-to-man testicular transplant rejection. Also, inbred orthotopic transplants (into the scrotal sac) maintained histologic viability, and the animal maintained successful impregnating capabilities, whereas the heterotopic testes transplants (abdominal) underwent atrophy and exhibited aspermia. The technique of Lee and his colleagues[20] included vas deferens and vascular anastomoses. In Chinese hamsters with orthotopically transplanted half-ovaries, the animals resumed estrus and were capable of being impregnated.[25]

THYROID-PARATHYROID TRANSPLANTATION

Early studies done on the thyroid gland, in terms of transplantation and autografts, has proven, histologically, to be successful. The ease of handling myxedema with exogenous thyroid materials mitigates against the use of autografts of the thyroid, therapeutically. There is a possible application in transplantation of the undescended lingual and subhyoid thyroid in the absence of a thyroid gland in the lower neck.[29] The lingual or sublingual ectopic tissue is quantitatively deficient and may be subjected to excessive thyroid-stimulating hormone (TSH), with resultant hyperplasia. Because of the compensatory enlargement, attention may be attracted to the ectopic gland. In the subhyoid

*Clark, R. L.: Personal communication, 1976.

thyroid, surgery is done most frequently to correct undesirable cosmetic appearance. Hyoid masses are usually asymptomatic and must be differentiated from the frequent anomalies, thyroglossal-duct cysts. Lingual thyroids must be distinguished from other cysts, fibroma, hypertrophy of the lingual tonsil, lymphangioma, sarcoma and other tumors, and may be symptomatic as a sequel to the hypertrophy and cause dysphagia, dysphonia, or dyspnea. The lesion may become painful and severe hemorrhage may develop, but in general, they are relatively asymptomatic. At The University of Texas System Cancer Center M. D. Anderson Hospital and Tumor Institute, relatively few lingual tonsils have been treated, and those usually conservatively, but most have been observed. The supposition that 5 percent become neoplastic is probably a biased assumption. A neoplastic growth attracts attention, and there are more lingual tonsils than are recognized. Seemingly, it is more important to be aware of the lingual tonsil and to treat the myxedema. Admittedly, thyroid tissue can be transplanted, but in the writer's experience, transplanted thyroid tissue functions poorly. While carrying out neck dissections and transplanting thyroid biopsies into the thigh muscles, there was no subsequent evidence of ^{131}I uptake in the transplant site, although the autologous transplant was proven to endure histologically.

In the clinical surgical milieu, iatrogenic hypoparathyroidism may result in extirpative manipulations in the thyrocervical region. The frequency of the complication has been variously cited but is probably more frequent than thought and can be a devastating condition. Halsted[9] investigated the course to be pursued when a parathyroid gland was accidently removed or deprived of blood supply. Lahey[18] and Cattell[4] advocated a "seek and implant" method for handling parathyroid glands during extirpative surgery, and this practice has become almost a surgical tradition. The data on the efficacy of transplantation has been presented by Hickey and Samaan,[12] and Wells,[28] et al., in independent studies by placing diced autografts in the forearm and then measuring parathyroid hormone (IPTH) in the venous effluent with autografts of both normal glands and a parathyroid adenoma.* There is a differential level of IPTH, higher in the venous drainage from the implanted arm. A homograft study by Groth, et al.,[8] was done on a patient who had undergone subtotal parathyroidectomy while receiving chronic renal dialysis. After a successful renal graft from a cadaver, the immunosuppressed patient became severely hypocalcemic and received an homologous hyperplastic parathyroid from a donor patient also on renal dialysis. This graft had proved histologic integrity by biopsy at 8 months and has sustained calcium homeostasis for an observed 20 months.

An alternate method to radical subtotal parathyroidectomy in selective patients with primary parathyroid hyperplasia or secondary hyperplasia is that of total parathyroidectomy and implantation of diced grafts into muscular sites. If hyperfunction occurs, portions of the grafted parathyroid tissue may be removed. Further, at the time of parathyroidectomy, permanent hypoparathyroidism may be safeguarded against by retaining and storing for use several small parathyroid pieces of tissue by freezing in liquid nitrogen. In the rat, parathyroid isografts will function normally after cryopreservation for 8 to 12

* The parathyroid adenoma tissue in the forearm is now known to function for at least 3 years.

months,* and in the human being these isografts have been known to remain viable for 6 weeks. Raaf, et al.[24] used a model of two inbred rat strains with genetic incompatibility and found that isogeneic parathyroid tissue could be placed in tissue culture, kept for 60 days, and then successfully transplanted; homografts or xenografts were uniformly rejected.

PANCREAS AND ISLET CELL TRANSPOSITION AND TRANSPLANTATION

Diabetes mellitus remains an unsolved problem. The untreated sufferer secretes copious quantities of urine, and from this comes its name, diabetes, from the Greek word "diabainein," meaning syphon or water pipe. In 1922, Banting and Best[3] reported on an extract from a previously duct-ligated pancreas. This extract was found to lower blood glucose level in pancreatectomized dogs. Also in that year, such an extract was successfully tried in the treatment of diabetes mellitus in man. There is no known cure for this serious chronic disease which ranks fifth as a cause of death within the nation, and is a major and significant contributor to occlusion of the coronary arteries, cerebrovascular accidents, renal failure, peripheral vascular diseases, gangrene and blindness. Indeed, it is estimated that about 4 and a half million Americans have diabetes. Insulin does prevent death from diabetic coma, controls the overt symptoms and does provide an increased life expectancy; however, the life expectancy for diabetic patients is approximately one-third less than the general population. The frequency of diabetes mellitus appears to be increasing, and it is estimated that the number of people with diabetes will double every 15 years.[5]

Organ Transplantation

The methods for controlling diabetes are through insulin administration and diet, and the scientific means of preventing its devastating complications and providing a cure is with endogenous insulin. In appropriate animal studies with either immunosuppression or genetic control, whole pancreatic transplantation is associated with production of circulating insulin and normal plasma glucose levels following transplantation to the drug-induced diabetic or pancreatectomized animals.[19] Alloxan-treated rat recipients of pancreatic-duodenal or duct-ligated pancreatic isografts showed a similar effect. Orloff[23] observed, in the latter, that the sequelae of diabetes mellitus (i.e., ocular, renal, or neural lesions) did not develop.

In the past decade, 49 whole pancreatic human transplants in 47 recipients were reported in the American College of Surgeons—National Institutes of Health Transplant Registry.[1] Only one of these recipients is alive with a functioning graft, which indicates the severity of the problems of transplantation. Gliedman[7] placed segmental pancreatic grafts of six patients with anastomosis of a main pancreatic duct to the ureter. The exocrine pancreatic drainage by way of the bladder seems well tolerated. These same authors advocated that renal transplants in patients with end-stage diabetic disease have staged renal and pancreatic transplantation because of surgical complications and that the pancreatic transplantation be carried out without the duodenum (i.e., duct drainage into the ureter). One patient, the sole survivor, in the study,

*Wells, S. A.: Personal communications, 1976.

is considered "long term" and has received a renal allograft 145 days after the pancreatic transplant.

Islet Cell Transplantation

One other option for the diabetic patient is that of a successful islet cell transplantation.[2,19] Kemp[17] collected pancreatic islets after collagenous digestion of the pancreas and injected the islets into the portal veins of inbred, streptozotocin-induced diabetic Lewis rats; injection by way of the portal venous system was thought to be the site of maximal effectiveness. Further exploration by Kemp on isogeneic transplanted islets placed in subcutaneous tissue, peritoneum and portal veins indicated that direct injection into the portal vein provided the most pleasing environment.[16] Cultured monkey pancreatic fragments have been used to ameliorate diabetes when transplanted by way of the portal vein in diabetic monkeys.[14]

The frustrating aspect of islet transplantation resides in the observation that whereas transplantation of isologous islet tissue is uniformly successful, there is an increased susceptibility of islets to allograft rejection as compared to other tissues (e.g., skin, kidney, and heart). The impetus toward islet transplantation to ward off secondary lesions, as in experimental diabetes, is very great; but successful islet transplantation in a human diabetic patient has not been reported. Najarian et al.,[22] have performed 10 islet transplants in seven immunosuppressed patients each of whom had previously received a renal allograft. The tissue was transplanted intramuscularly, intraperitoneally, or into the portal vein, without complications. None of the patients was cured of the diabetes, although one patient has had a sustained reduction in insulin requirements. The experiments suggested that a critical mass of islet tissue must be transplanted. Future trials should include larger quantities of islet tissue and well-matched, donor-recipient pairs.[27]

Optimistic misinterpretations of data must be avoided. A significant deficit for the majority of patients with severe diabetes may be the limited number of pancreatic donors and the likelihood of total inapplicability of xenograft techniques. Whether through genetic engineering there exists a possibility of insulin production by an altered bacterium or autogeneous tissue culture or by recombinant DNA techniques, is an approach unexplored. Moreover, the disease itself may be an immunologic phenomenon and thus explain the susceptibility of islet cells to strong immunologic rejection.

ADRENAL TRANSPLANTATION

The clinical applicability of adrenal tissues to transplantation is largely theoretical. A grave danger rests with ectopic adrenal tissue not being recognized at the time of adrenalectomy or of crushing the adrenal and leaving residual adrenal tissue behind. There is little question that an adrenal can be transplanted; when staged adrenalectomies were carried out for metastatic breast cancer, the author implanted adrenal tissue at the incision site planned for the second adrenalectomy and found, at a later time, histologically intact and viable cortical tissue. On the other hand, more recently, when removing a pheochromocytoma, adrenal tissue was planted in the abdominal musculature, and upon subsequent examination by ^{131} 1-19-iodocholesterol it was found that all biologic activity resided in the normal undisturbed adrenal. During the 1950's a procedure was tried to selectively implant adrenal tissue in the spleen at the time of a bilateral adrenalectomy for metastatic cancer. The rationale was to protect the patient against hypocortisonism; and, with drainage through the portal vein, the estrogenic hormonal substances would be metabolized by the liver. This technique has not been continued. Kaplan and Shires[15] have treated one patient, a 19-year-old male with Cushing's disease, by adrenalectomy and implantation of the adrenal tissue. There was apparent control of the disease and endocrine balance. In general, however, exogenous hormonal substitution is used for metabolic balance with adrenal insufficiency.

SUMMARY

In the surgical arena of endocrine transplantation, the greatest applicability is that of autologous parathyroid implantation. The area of greatest need is that of continuing investigation against the ravages of diabetes mellitus; the isolation and utilization of pancreatic islets appears to be the avenue of greatest promise. Transplantation of thyroid, adrenal and gonadal tissue seems to have little applicability because of the readily available satisfactory hormonal therapy. In special circumstances, the transposition of the gonads, as with avulsion injuries in the male or the need for irradiation protection in the female, does have a selected place in the surgical armamentarium.

REFERENCES

1. ACS/NIH organ transplantation registry: first scientific report. JAMA, *217*:1520, 1976.
2. Ballinger, W. F., and Lacy, P. E.: Transplantation of intact pancreatic islets in rats. Surgery, *72*:175, 1972.
3. Banting, F. G., and Best, C. H.: The internal secretion of the pancreas. J. Lab. Clin. Med., *7*:251, 1922.
4. Cattell, R. B.: Parathyroid transplantation. A report of parathyroid gland removal during thyroidectomy. Ann. J. Surg., *7*:4, 1929.
5. Crafford, O. B.: Report of the National Committee on Diabetes to the Congress of the U. S. Dept. HEW. Publication No. 67-108 (NIH), Washington, Government Printing Office, 1975.
6. Gibbs, R. W.: A case where the entire scrotum and perineum, together with one testicle and its cord attached, and nearly all the integument of the penis were torn off. Recovery with preservation of sexual powers. Charl. Med. J. Rev., *10*:154, 1855.
7. Gliedman, M. L., et al.: Pancreatic transplantation. Trans. Proc., *7*:93, 1975.
8. Groth, C. G., et al.: Survival of a homologous parathyroid implant in an immunosuppressed patient. Lancet, *1*:1082, 1973.
9. Halsted, W. S.: Auto-and-isotransplantation in dogs of the parathyroid glandules. J. Exp. Med., *11*:175, 1908.
10. Haviland, T. N., and Parish, L. C.: An early 20th century testicular transplant. Trans. Stud. Coll. Physicians Phila., *38*:231, 1971.
11. Hickey, R. C.: Current therapy—transplantation (modern day saints Cosmas and Damian). Wisc. Med. J., 521, 1967.
12. Hickey, R. C., and Samaan, N.: Human parathyroid autotransplantation. Arch. Surg., *110*:892, 1975.
13. Huffman, W. C., Culp, D. A., and Flocks, R. H.: Injuries of the external male genitalia. *In* Converse, J. R.: Reconstructive Plastic Surgery. Princi-

ples and Procedures in Correction, Reconstruction and Transplantation. pp. 2057-2064. Philadelphia, W. B. Saunders, 1964, 5.

14. Jonasson, O. *In* Matas, A. J., et al: Current status of islet and pancreatic transplantation. Diabetes, *25*:785, 1976.
15. Kaplan, N. M., and Shire, T.: Apparent cure of Cushing's disease by bilateral adrenalectomy and autotransplantation. Am. J. Med., *53*:377, 1972.
16. Kemp, C. B., et al.: Effect of transplantation site on the results of pancreatic islet isografts in diabetic rats. Diabetologia, *9*:486, 1973.
17. Kemp, C. B., et al.: Transplantation of isolated pancreatic islets into the portal vein of diabetic rats. Nature, *144*:447, 1973.
18. Lahey, F.: The transplantation of parathyroid in partial thyroid. Surg. Gynecol. Obstet., *42*:508, 1926.
19. Lazarow, A., et al.: The Banting memorial lecture: islet differentiation, organ culture and transplantation. Diabetes, *22*:877, 1973.
20. Lee, S., et al.: Testicular transplantation in the rat. Trans. Proc., *3*:586, 1971.
21. Nahas, W. A., et al.: Lateral ovarian transposition. Obstet. Gynecol., *38*:785, 1971.
22. Najarian, J. S., Sutherland, D. E. R., and Matas, J.: *In* Matas, A. J., et al.: Current status of islet and pancreatic transplantation. Diabetes, *25*:785, 1976.
23. Orloff, M. J., et al.: Long-term studies of pancreatic transplantation in experimental diabetes mellitus. Ann. Surg., *182*:198, 1975.
24. Raaf, J. H.: Transplantation of fresh and cultured parathyroid glands in the rat. Am. J. Surg., *128*:478, 1974.
25. Schmidt, F. L., et al.: A microsurgical technique for orthotopic ovarian transplantation in the Chinese hamster. Surgery, *80*:595, 1976.
26. Simmer, H. H.: Robert Tuttle Morris (1957-1945): A pioneer in ovarian transplants. Obstet. Gynecol., *35*:314, 1970.
27. Summerlin, W. T., Miller, G. T., and Good, R. A.: Successful tissue and organ allotransplantation without immunosuppression. J. Clin. Invest., *52*:83, 1973.
28. Wells, S. A., et al.: Transplantation of parathyroid glands in man. Clinical indications and results. Surgery, *78*:34, 1975.
29. Wertz, M.: Management of undescended lingual and subhyoid thyroid gland. Laryngoscope, *84*:507, 1974.

EDITORIAL COMMENTARY

A natural extension of the expanding frontiers already evident in endocrine cell identification, synthesis of humoral products, their measurement by quantitative immunoassay, and more recent manipulation of receptor capabilities is the therapeutic possibility of endocrine transposition and transplantation. This chapter places these possibilities in appropriate historic perspective and suggests areas where the need for such advances is evident (i.e., particularly where substitution by administration of hormonal products is impractical, inconvenient, or impossible). These needs are in the fields of permanent hypoparathyroidism or in those clinical situations in which total excisions of the humoral source are necessary, such as for hyperplasias or some endocrine malignancies, or perhaps in patients with diabetes mellitus. Part of the problem with the latter condition is that the etiology of diabetes mellitus is not clearly identified, and the diabetes mellitus of adult onset is a different metabolic entity from the juvenile type. There may be a greater applicability and rationale for consideration of islet cell transplantation in patients with juvenile diabetes in which there appears to be an abnormality of the beta cells of the pancreatic islets, which is not the case in the adult-onset variety. It appears that the diabetes mellitus of adult onset may be due to an altered immunologic phenomenon, which might render further immunologic modification more difficult or even impossible. Certainly current investigative and clinical experiences suggest that there are more problems with *organ* transplantation of insulin- (and glucagon-) secreting tissues than there are with islet *cell* transfers. Organs for transplantation, being composed of multiple types of tissues, probably provoke greater problems of immunologic suppression than do relatively pure endocrine cells. Although xenograft techniques may be inapplicable, the author of this chapter offers three possible investigative approaches for the future. In the meantime it seems reasonable, at least in patients with juvenile diabetes mellitus, that the pursuit of investigations toward islet cell transfers is appropriate. There are at least three areas into which islet cells can be transposed: the liver, the spleen, or the muscles of the forearm. Experimental transposition of islet cells to the former sites has been reported and clinical transplantation to the latter site of fresh and frozen parathyroid tissue has already been successfully accomplished in terms of measurable function and support.

Another practical problem of immense proportions concerns the limited number of pancreatic donors. To achieve the needed critical mass of islet tissue in the face of an apparent paucity of donors and the additional problems of harvesting sufficient numbers of functioning islet cells, it may be appropriate to consider the pharmacologic production of islet hyperplasia by a process of nesidioblastosis (islet building) in either the donor pancreas or in the transplanted islet cells of the recipient. Such hyperplasia has been produced in hamsters by the administration of cortisone and hydrochlorothiazide. Chronic administration of the latter has been reported to be associated with but not necessarily the cause of recurrent parathyroid adenomas.

It is interesting to speculate on the possible future clinical application of the recent modification of DNA in bacteria for the purpose of their synthesis of protein, specifically the bacterial production of insulin. Will such a source of insulin, or other humoral peptides, make endocrine cell transplantation obsolete even before its universal application? The final chapter in this field, of course, has not been written.

S.R.F.

SECTION TWO

CLINICAL SYNDROMES

Humoral and Biologic Actions in Clinical Syndromes

Syndrome	*Usual Pathology*	*Hormone Abnormality*	*Normal Cell of Origin*	*Stimulated by**	*Suppressed by**	*Target*	*Biologic Activity*	*Clinical Picture*	*Ectopic Site*
					AMINES				
Hypermetabolic	Thyroid Hyperplasia Adenoma	↑ T_4 ↑ T_3 (↑ LATS)		TSH TRH	Iodine (Beta blocker) (Antithyroid drugs)	All tissues	↑ Catabolism ↑ 0_2 consumption ↑ CHO ↑ Glycogenolysis ↑ Ca^{++} loss ↑ Protein consumption	Hypermetabolic Weight loss Myopathy	Hypothalamus (TRH) Placenta Lung (TSH) Pituitary (TSH)
							Enhances catecholamines ↑ Inotropic ↑ Chronotropic ↑ Neuromuscular ↑ Thermogenic effect	Cardiac Tachycardia Tremor, "Stare" Heat intolerance	
Panic	Pheochromocytoma Ganglioneuroma Chemodectoma Glomus jugulare Zuckerkandl	↑ Epinephrine ↑ Norepinephrine	A NA	T_4 T_3 ↓ Glucose (ACTH) (Glucagon) (Histamine)	(Adrenergic blockers)	Alpha receptors	Vasoconstriction ↑ Pilomotor Pupillary dilation	Hypertension Headache Panic Anxiety	"Extra adrenal" (Dopamine)
						receptors	Beta Vasodilatation (heart/brain) ↑ Chronotropic ↑ Inotropic ↓ Bronchial and uterine sm. m.	 Tachycardia Palpitation	
						Metabolic tissues	↑ Glycogenolysis ↑ Lipolysis	↑ Glucose	
		(↑ Acetylcholine)				Sweat glands	↑ Cholinesterase	Sweating	

Humoral and Biologic Actions in Clinical Syndromes *(Continued)* [82]

Syndrome	*Usual Pathology*	*Hormone Abnormality*	*Normal Cell of Origin*	*Stimulated by**	*Suppressed by**	*Target*	*Biologic Activity*	*Clinical Picture*	*Ectopic Site*
Carcinoid	*Foregut* Carcinoid and APUDomas	↑ 5-HTP ↑ Histamine (+Polypeptides)	EC		(Glucocorticoids)	Skin	Vasodilatation	Flushing Hypotension Tachycardia Lacrimation	"Foregut" Lung Pancreas Duodenum
	Midgut Carcinoid	↑ 5HT ↑ Motilin ↑ Subst. P. (+Bradykinin)	EC	(Ca^{++})		Intestine	Hyperperistalsis	Diarrhea	
						Bronchi	Bronchospasm	"Asthma"	
						Right endocardium	↑ Fibrosis	Right valvular obstruction	
					POLYPEPTIDES				
Hypoglycemic	Pancreatic Adenoma Hyperplasia Carcinoma	↑ Insulin ↑ Proinsulin	B	↑ Glucose (Glucagon)	↓ Glucose (? Diazoxide) (Somatostatin)	Liver	Anabolic ↑ Glycogenesis ↓ Gluconeogenesis ↓ Lipolysis ↓ Ketogenesis	Cerebral Glucopenia Incoherence Headache Syncope	Pleural Mesothelioma (Somatomedin) Lung carcinoma
		↑ 2° Catecholamines				B receptors	Chronotropic (Compensatory ↑ glycogenolysis)	Tachycardia Trembling	
Hyperglycemic	Pancreatic Carcinoma Hyperplasia	↑ Pancreatic Glucagon ↑ Enteroglucagon	A AL-EG	↓ Glucose	↑ Glucose	Liver	Catabolic ↑ Glycogenolysis ↑ Gluconeogenesis ↑ Lipolysis ↑ Insulin ↑ Ketogenesis	"Diabeteslike" Dermatitis	Lung Liver Kidney
		↓ 2° Catecholamines				GI tract	↓ Secretion ↓ Motility ↑ Inotropic ↑ Chronotropic	Ileus Constipation Tachycardia	

Ulcerogenic (Z-E)	Pancreatic Carcinoma Hyperplasia Adenoma Duodenal Adenoma	↑ Gastrin	Antral G cell Fetal Islet Cell	↑ pH Distention (Ca^{++}) (Secretin) (Glucagon)	↓ pH (SST)	Stomach	↑ H^+ secretion ↑ EG tone (Pharm.)	Intractable ulcer Diarrhea	Thyroid Parathyroid Parapancreas Duodenum
Diarrheogenic (WDHA, Verner-Morrison, pancreatic cholera)	Pancreatic Carcinoma	↑ VIP	H			Intestine	⇅ Motility ↑ Secretions ↑ cAMP	Diarrhea ↓ K^+	Lung Adrenal medulla Kidney
						Stomach	↓ H^+ ↓↓ H^+	Hypochlorhydria Achlorhydria	
	Hyperplasia Ganglio-neuroma	↑ GIP ↑ Secretin-like	K S						
	APUDomas Islet hyperplasia	↑ PP ↑ CCK-P_2	F I	Food	Atropine Secretin	G-I tract Stomach Pancreas Intestine Stomach	↓ Motility ↑ H^+ ↑ H_2CO_3 ↓ Secretions ↓ H^+	Diarrhea with gastric hyper-secretion	
		↑ (Prostaglan-dins)							Thyroid (MCT) Islets
Hypercalcemic	Parathyroid Adenoma Hyperplasia Carcinoma	↑ PTH	Ch	↓ Ca^{++}	↑ Ca^{++}	Kidney	↑ Ca^{++} ↓ Tubular reabsorption of phosphate	"Stones"	Pancreas Lung Breast Kidney Liver
						Bone	↑ Resorption Ca^{++}	Bone cyst pain	
						Intestine	↑ Absorption Ca^{++}		
						(Antrum)	(↑ Gastrin?)	"Ulcer"	
						(Neural)	↓ Neuromus-cular	Weakness Stupor	
MEA-I	Pancreatic Hyperplasia Carcinoma Adenoma	↑ Gastrin	?	↑ pH (Ca^{++}) (Secretin) (Glucagon)	↓ pH	Stomach	↑ H^+	Familial Intractable ulcer	

Humoral and Biologic Actions in Clinical Syndromes *(Continued)*

Syndrome	*Usual Pathology*	*Hormone Abnormality*	*Normal Cell of Origin*	*Stimulated by**	*Suppressed by**	*Target*	*Biologic Activity*	*Clinical Picture*	*Ectopic Site*
		↑ Insulin	B	↑ Glucose	↓ Glucose	Liver	↑ Glycogenesis	Hypoglycemia	
		↑ Glucagon	A	↓ Glucose	↑ Glucose	Liver	↑ Glycogenolysis	Hyperglycemia	
	Parathyroid Hyperplasia	↑ PTH	Ch	↓ Ca^{++}	↑ Ca^{++}	Kidney Bone Intestine	↑ Serum Ca^{++}	Hyperparathyroidism	
	Pituitary tumor	↑ ACTH-MSH	c	↓ Cortisol	↑ Cortisol	Adrenal cortex	↑ Cortisol	Headache Cushing's disease	
		↑ GH	s	↓ Glucose	↑ Glucose	Ectoderm		Acromegaly	
		↑ PRL	L			Breast		Galactorrhea	
	Adrenocortical tumor or hyperplasia	↑ Cortisol				All tissues	↑ Cortisol	Cushing's syndrome	
Medullary carcinoma, thyroid (+MEN-II; Sipple's)	Thyroid Carcinoma Medullary	↑ TC	C	(↑ Ca^{++}) (↑ Pentagastrin)	↓ Ca^{++}	Kidney Bone	(↓ S. Ca^{++}) (↑ PTH, ↑ S. Ca^{++})	Mass in neck (Hyperparathyroidism)	
		↑ (Prostaglandins)				Intestine	↑ Secretions	Diarrhea	
		↑ (5 HT)	EC			Intestine Skin	↑ Motility ↑ Vasodilatation	Skin flushing	
		↑ (ACTH)				Adrenal cortex	↑ Cortisol	Cushing's syndrome	
	Pheochromocytoma	↑ Catecholamines				Adrenal receptors	Vasoconstriction	Hypertension (Panic)	
	Parathyroid hyperplasia	↑ PTH	Ch	↓ Ca^{++}	↑ Ca^{++}	Kidney Bone Intestine	↑ Serum Ca^{++}	Hyperparathyroidism	
Acromegaly or gigantism	Ant. pituitary Adenoma Hyperplasia	↑ HG (STH)	s	↓ Glucose Arginine	↑ Glucose	Ectoderm	↑ Growth ↑ Protein synthesis ↑ CHO metabolism	*Prepuberty* Gigantism *Postpuberty* Headache ↓ Visual fields Large extremities Thick skin Diabetes Visceromegaly	

Forbes-Albright	Pituitary Adenoma	↑ PRL ↓ PRIH	L	TRH	PRIH	Breast	Lactation	Galactorrhea (Nonpuerperal)	Placenta Lung Kidney
		↓ FSH				Ovary	↓ Menses	Amenorrhea	
Pituitary hyperthyroidism	Pituitary tumor	↑ TSH		↑ TRH	T_4	Thyroid	↑ T_4	Hyperthyroidism	
Sheehan's syndrome	Pituitary necrosis (postpartum)	↓ PRL				Breast	Hypopituitarism	Failure of lactation	
Cushing's disease	Pituitary tumor Basophilic Hyperplasia	↑ ACTH	c	↓ Cortisol	↑ Cortisol (Partial by dexamethasone 8 mg.)	Adrenal cortex	↑ Cortisol ↑ Androgens ↑ Aldosterone ↑ Prolactin ↑ Catabolism ↓ HPG	Truncal obesity Acne, hirsutism Hypertension Galactorrhea Muscle wasting Weakness Amenorrhea	
Nelson's syndrome	Pituitary tumor	↑ (ACTH)MSH	m			Skin	↑ Pigments	Hyperpigmentation after adrenalectomy Enlarged sella turcica	
					STEROIDS				
Cushing's syndrome	Adrenocortical tumor	↑ Cortisol ↓ ACTH				All tissues	↑ Steroids	Hypertension Truncal obesity	(Hypothalamus) (CRH) (Islets) (CRH + ACTH) (Lung) (ACTH)
Conn's syndrome	Adrenocortical adenoma (Hyperplasia)	↑ Aldosterone (↓ Renin) ↓ Angiotensin		↓ BP ↓ Blood volume ↓ Na^+ ↑ K^+ ↑ ACTH Angiotensin II (Na^+ loading)	↑ Na^+ ↓ K^+ (Upright position) (Spironolactone)	Kidney Intestine Sweat glands	↑ Na^+ retention ↑ Plasma volume ↓ Renin ↓ K^+ ↓ H^+	Hypertension Headache Polyuria Muscle weakness Alkalosis (Hypocalcemic tetany)	

Humoral and Biologic Actions in Clinical Syndromes *(Continued)* [86]

Syndrome	*Usual Pathology*	*Hormone Abnormality*	*Normal Cell of Origin*	*Stimulated by**	*Suppressed by**	*Target*	*Biologic Activity*	*Clinical Picture*	*Ectopic Site*
Virilizing	Pinealoma	?Melatonin	p			Pituitary	↑ ACTH		
	Pituitary Hyperplasia	↑ ACTH	c			Adrenal cortex	↑ Adrenal testosterone		
	Adrenal adenoma	↑ Adrenal testosterone				Genitals		Virilizing	
	Pituitary tumor	↑ ICSH				Testes	↑ Testosterone	Virilizing	
	Testicular (Leydig)	↑ Testicular testosterone				Genitals		Virilizing	
	Testicular choriocarcinoma	↑ ICSH				Opp. Testicle	↑ Testosterone	Virilizing	
	Adrenal tumor or hyperplasia (in female)	↑ Adrenal androgens			(Dexamethasone)	Genitals		Masculinizing	
	Arrhenoblastoma of ovary	↑ Ovarian androgens				Genitals		Masculinizing	
Feminizing	Pituitary tumor	↑ LH				Ovary	↑ Ovarian estrogens	Feminizing	
	Placental choriocarcinoma	↑ HCG				Ovary	↑ Ovarian estrogens	Feminizing	
	Ovarian granulosa cell tumor	↑ Estrogens				Genitals		Feminizing	
	Ovarian choriocarcinoma	↑ HCG				Opp. ovary	↑ Ovarian estrogens	Feminizing	
	Adrenal tumor (in male)	↑ Adrenal estrogens				Genitals		Feminizing	

*Without parentheses = Stimulation and suppression in *normal* state.
With parentheses = Stimulation and suppression in *abnormal* state.

PART 1
Amines

9

The Hypermetabolic Syndrome: Hyperthyroidism, Thyrotoxicosis, Graves' Disease

Selwyn Taylor, D.M., M.Ch., F.R.C.S.

The term thyrotoxicosis, although it is in general usage, is probably a misnomer, since in this condition the circulating thyroid hormones are of normal composition although present in excess; the hypothesis that the gland is producing a toxic secretion in this syndrome was long ago abandoned. The hypermetabolic state of hyperthyroidism can present in a variety of ways, the most common being best described as Graves' disease. Robert Graves of Dublin described three patients with this syndrome in 1835, and since we do not know the cause of the disease it is quite useful to use his name eponymously. He was, however, preceded by Caleb Parry of Bath England by some 10 years in giving an account of the condition published posthumously in 1825, but Graves' name is now in common usage both in the United Kingdom and in the United States. It is interesting to note that in most countries of Europe the name of Basedow is applied; Basedow was a German physician who did not write about hyperthyroidism and exophthalmos until 1840.

CLINICAL SYNDROMES OF HYPERTHYROIDISM

Hyperthyroidism associated with increased levels of circulating thyroid hormones may manifest itself by the following various clinical pictures.

Clinical Syndromes of Hyperthyroidism

1. Hypermetabolic syndrome
   - T_4 excess
   - T_3 excess
   - Graves' disease (Diffuse "toxic" goiter)
2. Thyrocardiac syndrome
   - Plummer's disease (Nodular "toxic" goiter)
3. Wasting syndrome (Proximal myopathy)
4. Tumor hyperthyroidism
   - Entopic
     - Thyroid carcinoma - T_4 excess
   - Ectopic
     - Anterior pituitary tumor - TSH excess
     - Gonadal tumors - TSH-like excess
5. Thyrotoxicosis factitia
6. Jod-Basedow's disease

The classic example of the hypermetabolic state, Graves' disease, usually the most florid of the clinical syndromes, presents typically in the young female patient with a diffusely enlarged goiter. A thyrocardiac syndrome, sometimes called Plummer's disease presents a clinical picture of cardiac failure with mild hyperthyroidism superimposed on nodular "toxic" goiter in older patients. The wasting syndrome is characterized by weakness and muscle atrophy (proximal myopathy) in mildly hyperthyroid patients. Rarely, hyperthyroidism results from excessive hormone production by tumors, both entopically and ectopically. Finally, the ingestion of large amounts of thyroid medication (thyrotoxicosis factitia) or of iodide by certain patients in goiter regions (Jod-Basedow's disease) produces symptoms and signs of hyperthyroidism.

GRAVES' DISEASE

Etiologic Considerations of Graves' Disease

Although the cause of Graves' disease is not known, it is useful to review its characteristics and also the accompanying changes in bodily systems, since they throw much light on the mechanism of hyperthyroidism. In Graves' disease there is hyperplasia of the thyroid gland, in many patients a distinctive protrusion of the eyeballs or exophthalmos, and in a minority of patients, an unusual localized thickening of the skin, especially over the lower leg, called pretibial myxedema. The disease is also characterized by a tendency to spontaneous remission which is true of many of the syndromes produced by endocrine gland hyperfunction. There is a strong hereditary tendency, and it is unusual to encounter a patient with Graves' disease who does not have some relative also affected. The disease is much more common in women than in men in a ratio of about 6:1. Hashimoto's thyroiditis, which is also genetically determined, is seen more commonly in association with Graves' disease than in the ordinary population. Thyroid autoantibodies were first demonstrated in Hashimoto's thyroiditis, and they are also present in many patients with Graves' disease although in much smaller amounts. Approximately 85 percent of patients with Graves' disease show antibodies to thyroid microsomal antigen; 65 percent have positive complement fixation; 46 percent have positive tanned red cell agglutination, using red cells coated with thyroglobulin.

The presence of autoantibodies in the serum of patients with Graves' disease shows that we are dealing here with some abnormality of the immune system, and a study of the various immunoglobulins found in this disease has provoked an enormous amount of research in recent years. One particular immunoglobulin of the IgG class is produced by lymphocytes in patients with hyperthyroidism and is generally referred to as LATS. These initials stand for long-acting thyroid stimulator to distinguish it from the more rapidly acting thyroid stimulator, TSH or thyrotropin, when using the mouse for its bioassay. McKenzie has perfected an assay using the mouse thyroid to measure LATS and has shown that approximately 50 percent of patients with Graves' disease have this abnormal immunoglobulin in their serum. In addition a further number of patients can have this immunoglobulin demonstrated in their serum by concentration techniques. It may be found in high concentration when severe exophthalmos and pretibial myxedema occur. The most striking evidence that LATS could be a causal factor in Graves' disease is the demonstration that mothers who have this circulating immunoglobulin occasionally give birth to a baby with neonatal hyperthyroidism, which gradually disappears over the subsequent weeks as the LATS is metabolized. Neonatal hyperthyroidism is as common in male babies as female. The fact that a large proportion of patients with Graves' disease do not have detectable levels of LATS in their serum makes it appear unlikely that it can be the cause of Graves' disease. Other abnormal circulating immunoglobulins are still being discovered and in particular, the human thyroid-stimulating globulins, often referred to as HTS, may well play an important role in the etiology of the disease.

Since in Graves' disease it is usual to see an enlarged thymus gland, lymph node hyperplasia in the neck and occasionally peripheral lymphocytosis, it is natural that an immune disorder of cellular type should have been implicated, and Volpe has proposed that it is a disorder of delayed hypersensitivity due to thymic lymphocytes stimulating the thyroid cells. I would postulate an abnormality produced by one of Macfarlane Burnett's forbidden clones of cells, which is inherited and which is augmented by the other autoimmune processes of the body. It is almost as if the thymus itself is at the root of this strange disease.

The association of hyperthyroidism with great mental stress or strain has been described for many years. How this can come about is hard to see, but undoubtedly it does occur. It may be that a vicious circle is started by way of the release of adrenal hormones or as a result of the central nervous system acting through the hypothalamus and causing an increase in thyrotropin-releasing hormone (TRH) with the resultant rise in TSH and a start in increased activity in the thyroid gland. Another apparent etiologic factor in hyperthyroidism is weight loss. There are many cases on record where a woman has gone on a strict diet and lost weight and then eventually is found to be hyperthyroid. Again, the mechanism is obscure.

The very delicate regulation of the thyroid gland by the amount of iodine in the diet may well bear some relationship to hyperthyroidism, and Ingbar has proposed that in this condition the gland loses its ability to sense its own iodine content. We know that the thyroid gland in a normal adult needs between 100 and 200 μg. of iodine daily to produce the hormones necessary for health. When the iodine falls below this level there is stimulation of the gland by TSH, hyperplasia, and eventually a "nontoxic" goiter is produced, well seen in areas of endemic goiter. In an opposite fashion, high concentrations of iodine in the diet lead to inhibition of thyroid stimulation and mechanisms are present to protect the thyroid gland in these circumstances. The effect of a high intake of iodide in inhibiting thyroid hormone production, which is usually called the Wolff-Chaikoff effect, is used in the preparation of patients for surgery. It is possible, as Ingbar suggests, that should the thyroid lose its ability to sense its own iodine content, and therefore to regulate the mechanisms which come into force in high and low iodine intake, the gland might well become overactive and produce what is called Graves' disease. Such a theory is in part supported by some recent observations in the field. In Tasmania where there is a generalized iodine deficiency, it was recently decided to introduce iodide into the diet by incorporating iodate in the flour used in bread manufacture. The introduction of the iodate coincided with an apparent epidemic of hyperthyroidism which slowly settled over the following years, and this has been interpreted as showing that there were a number of patients in the population who were potentially sufferers from Graves' disease but who did not demonstrate the symptoms of the disease because they were iodine deficient. Increasing the amount of iodine in the diet released the capacity to manufacture excess hormone. This phenomenon of hyperthyroidism occurring in individuals who have been starved of iodine, after they are given an excess of the element, has been long known in endemic areas and was given the name of Jod-Basedow by German authors.

No discussion of etiology of Graves' disease would be complete without mentioning the ophthalmopathy which accompanies it in many patients. There is pushing forward of the eye from the orbit which is accompanied by an infiltration of the ocular muscles and orbital fat with lymphocytes and fibroblasts. In addition there is a myopathy which results in poor coordination of the eye muscles and such phenomena as lid-lag. Unfortunately the eye changes of Graves' disease may precede, accompany or succeed the changes in the thyroid gland, thus making interpretation very difficult. Brown Dobyns has shown that an exophthalmos-producing substance, EPS, can be extracted from the serum of the patients with severe eye disease and when injected into fish, can be assayed. A substance resembling EPS has been extracted from the anterior pituitary. Final identification of EPS has yet to be clarified, but it appears to be distinct from LATS.

Diagnosis

In trying to arrive at a diagnosis, the first and most important task is to obtain a thorough and accurate case history from the patient. The discussion on etiology above reveals that certain specialized questions must be included. The patient must be asked place of birth and upbringing, since hyperthyroidism is common in some areas of the world and rare in others. In the endemic areas of the world thyroid enlargement may be almost universal. Next, a good family history should be obtained, since Graves' disease often affects various members of the family, the hereditary factor being probably a tendency to autoimmunity. Dietary habits should be enquired into, since a distaste for seafood and fish may result in low iodine intake.

Clinical Picture

It is convenient to consider the clinical picture of hyperthyroidism as the end product of accelerated metabolism by most of the body's tissues due to the excess production of thyroid hormones. In a typical case of Graves' disease as it occurs in a young woman, the diagnosis is rarely in doubt. The thyroid gland is typically two to three times its normal size and very soft with a bruit to be heard over it due to the increased blood flow. The pulse rate is increased and the pulse pressure very prominent due to the lowering of the diastolic pressure. The skin is moist, especially the palms of the hands, and the patient tends to throw away clothes from the shoulders and neck because everything feels so hot. The tendon reflexes are brisk and in addition, the patient is generally nervous and apprehensive and often short-tempered. Many of these features are due to overactivity of the sympathetic nervous system, and this accounts for the fact that they can be largely controlled by sympathetic blocking agents such as propranolol (Inderal). The staring of the eyes and protrusion of the eyeballs adds a most characteristic look to patients with this condition and rarely there is also thickening of the skin over the lower third of the front of the leg, pretibial myxedema, and there may be changes in the nails and even in the skin of the fingers. In addition there is almost invariably muscle weakness and the patient may have great difficulty in mounting the stairs. The toxic effect on the renal tubules is shown by increased thirst, polydipsia and frequent passage of urine, polyuria. In like manner the alimentary tract is overactive and patients show great hunger and frequently looseness of the bowels, which on occasion may be so severe as to be misdiagnosed as colitis.

Although a typical example of Graves' disease is readily recognized, on the other hand a patient with nodular toxic goiter may show few of these signs and complain of even less symptoms. In such patients there may have been thyroid enlargement present for many years, and the onset of hyperthyroidism is insidious. The first presentation to the doctor may be for the patient to have atrial fibrillation and congestive heart failure. Indeed the brunt of this disease falls on the myocardium, and the whole condition is referred to by some as thyrocardiac disease.

To generalize, the older the patient the less obvious the diagnosis, and this is not surprising because the tissues become less able to respond to the stimulus of increased thyroid hormones. Contrariwise, in childhood the disease is usually severe and obvious.

In addition to Graves' disease which is typically seen in young adults and toxic nodular goiter which is seen in an older population, there are a number of other pathologic states which are responsible for an increased level of peripheral circulating thyroid hormones. Some patients may take large doses of thyroid hormone by mouth, often denying this, and the resultant thyrotoxicosis factitia may be difficult to diagnose. Occasionally a patient is seen with a solitary nodule which becomes hyperactive, the whole of the disease being produced by the excessive hormone production of this one "hot" area in the gland. This syndrome is usually called after Plummer. An extremely rare cause of hyperthyroidism is hydatidiform mole and choriocarcinoma, but probably the rarest cause is a tumor of the anterior pituitary secreting increased levels of TSH.

Eye Signs

The classification of the eye changes of Graves' disease is a matter of some difficulty, and we are grateful to Werner for his simple approach to this problem. Below are shown the various degrees, from 0 to 6, which may be encountered, and there is a convenient mnemonic in the initial letters of each category adding up to the word "nospecs."

Degrees of Exophthalmos

"NOSPECS"
0 *N*o signs or symptoms
1 *O*nly signs, no symptoms
2 *S*oft-tissue involvement
3 *P*roptosis
4 *E*xtra-ocular muscle involvement
5 *C*orneal involvement
6 *S*ight loss

Many other metabolic upsets occur in the body in severe hyperthyroidism.

Liver function is impaired and in the male this may be so severe as to lead to increased steroid levels and gynecomastia. There may be a considerable loss of calcification in the skeleton, with pain in the back. The hair may become brittle and lackluster, quite unlike the change seen in myxedema. Frontal headache is common. Finally, both myasthenia gravis and migraine are more common in those with hyperthyroidism than in the rest of the population.

Tests of Function

There are today so many tests of thyroid function that it becomes a little bewildering, especially since many of them are sponsored by so much advertisement that the unfortunate physician is inundated with literature and finds it difficult to choose the most suitable for his work. Outlined here are the various kinds of tests of function which the laboratory can now determine and with a preference indicated for those we have found most useful for diagnostic purposes and a strategy for using them.

T_4 and T_3. Circulating thyroid hormones are bound to protein; a specific globulin, the thyroid-binding globulin (TBG), is by far the most important site, although a little is bound to prealbumin. The TBG is raised in such conditions as pregnancy, during the administration of the contraceptive pill and steroids, and this similarly raises the level of PBI. Protein-bound iodine was formerly the usual way of measuring circulating thyroid hormone, and the value of the test was not only limited by those factors mentioned above but was also elevated after administration of organic iodides as occurs in myelography and cholecystography. On the whole, it was a very useful test with a normal range between 4 and 8 μg./100 ml. of serum, but it has now been largely superseded by direct measurements of the thyroid hormones. Thyroxine or T_4 can be measured by competitive protein binding or by radioimmunoassay and the level, although it varies a little from laboratory to laboratory, has a normal range in our hospital of 70 to 150 nmol./1. It is also possible by radioimmunoassay to measure the level of triiodothyronine or T_3, and this reflects fairly well the level of thyroid hormone in the blood; the normal level in our laboratory is 1 to 2.5 ng./ml.

Resin uptake test of free binding capacity (FBC) of the serum is a very useful measure of the level of thyroid hormone in the patient and depends on the fact that if radioactive labeled T_3 or T_4 is added to some of the patient's serum, the fraction which is bound is inversely proportional to the concentration of thyroid hormone present, since it occupies the binding sites that have been left free. In other words, the sites which are not occupied by the patient's own circulating thyroid hormones are occupied by the added radioactive T_3, and thus a high uptake test means a low level of circulating thyroid hormone and vice versa.

FTI. The above test has led to a measure called the free thyroxine index (FTI) which is an index obtained from measurement of T_4 and FBC, and in our laboratory falls normally within the range of 45 to 160. It is useful because it is unaffected by the amount of change in the binding sites, such as occurs in pregnancy and taking the contraceptive pill, and is a very effective test of the amount of thyroid hormone available in the plasma. It is not a measure of the absolute amount of free thyroxine in the serum, but correlates well with it.

TSH. The measurement of TSH is also available now by radioimmunoassay and is of value in patients suspected of hypothyroidism.

TRH. The only value of testing the patient with thyrotropin-releasing hormone is to measure the responsiveness of the pituitary: 400 μg./square meter is administered intravenously and samples of serum taken to observe the peak level of TSH which normally reaches 4.5 to 20 mU/l. between 20 and 30 minutes. It is thus a sensitive test for hyperthyroidism in which there is no response.

Radioactive Iodine. The uptake of isotope by the thyroid gland was formerly the most common method of investigating its function. A small dose of ^{131}I (5-50 μCi) is given by mouth and the uptake in the thyroid measured directly at 24 and 48 hours; a blood sample taken at 48 hours is used to measure the level of protein-bound radioactive iodine. This test is very much at the mercy of the patient's diet, since an increase of iodine in the diet can give low levels, whereas patients from areas of endemic goiter show correspondingly high levels. The test is not now in common usage but the isotope ^{123}I, which gives a much smaller dose of radiation is becoming available. The isotope ^{130}I, with its much shorter half-life can be used intravenously followed by a 20-minute uptake. This has now been replaced by the use of radioactive technetium, in the form of pertechnetate 99, which is injected intravenously, and the gland can be scanned at 20 minutes and the overall uptake measured at the same time. The advantages of the ^{99}Tc are the very small dose of radiation involved, due to its short half-life and the quality of the scans obtained.

The Basal Metabolic Rate. Forty years ago this was the only direct measure of thyroid hormone activity in the body, and it is now more of historic value than any other. It consists of having the patient under basal conditions of fasting in a quiet room and then measuring the consumption of oxygen by a rebreathing technique. In expert hands it is extremely accurate, but finds no place in modern clinical diagnosis.

Scanning of the thyroid gland is extremely useful if nodules are present and it is necessary to know if they are functioning more actively or less actively than the rest of the gland. Either ^{131}I or ^{99}Tc is used for this purpose, and the scan is recorded graphically on a piece of paper and the data colored to show the intensity of activity in the various areas.

Strategy. With all the above tests it is necessary to have a plan for the investigation of any patient suspected of thyrotoxicosis. The most useful single test to ask for is the serum thyroxine measured by competitive binding and at the same time the resin uptake or so-called FBC. From these two measurements an FTC can be obtained, and it is a very good measure of thyroid function. A further refinement is the radioimmunoassay of serum thyroxine and also of serum triiodothyronine, the latter being relatively elevated in severe hyperthyroidism and in some examples of hot nodule. In addition, if the gland is nodular, scanning may be performed, otherwise the above laboratory tests will provide all the information reasonably necessary.

Other Tests. Echography or the use of ultrasonics to map out swellings in the thyroid gland is becoming more frequently used now that scanners are being developed capable of good definition. Cysts can be identified without difficulty and some solid tumors are well visualized.

Management

There are three distinct modes of treatment available; drugs which influence thyroid function or the symptoms it produces, surgery for the removal of overactive thyroid tissue and radioactive isotopes with which to destroy thyroid tissue by radiation.

Drug Therapy. This therapy started with the introduction by Astwood in 1943 of thiouracil which prevents the synthesis of thyroid hormones by the gland. Methylthiouracil is still sometimes prescribed in doses of 200 mg. at 8-hour intervals, and apart from toxic side reactions which include skin rashes, lowering of the white cell count, especially granulocytes, and occasionally depression of the bone marrow, excellent control of the overactive thyroid gland is obtained. Propylthiouracil and later the imidazoles, especially carbimazole, have been introduced because of their apparent lower toxicity in doses adequate to suppress thyroid function. In our clinic the usual treatment plan is to prescribe 10 to 20 mg. of carbimazole every 8 hours. Once the disease has come under control, in some 3 to 6 weeks, the dose is reduced and can then be maintained for up to 2 years to see if a remission of the symptoms can thus be induced. It is essential that the tablets be taken at 8-hour intervals, because of the excretion by the kidneys and conjugation in the liver which so rapidly destroy its effectiveness. Ideally this form of therapy is used for young patients with mild symptoms who appear likely to go into remission. A 2-year course is then administered, but not more than 50 percent of patients can be expected to have a long-term remission.

Surgery. Subtotal thyroidectomy in the control of hyperthyroidism was introduced in the beginning of this century by such pioneers as Dunhill in Australia and Crile in the United States. The operation had a considerable mortality and morbidity rate until the introduction by Plummer of the Mayo Clinic in the 1920s of Lugol's solution or a saturated solution of potassium iodide as a preoperative measure. Subsequently the introduction of the antithyroid drugs and more recently of the beta blockers such as propranolol (Inderal) has made preparation of the patient for operation even safer.

In general the patient is first of all rendered euthyroid either by giving an antithyroid drug such as carbimazole for 3 to 6 weeks and then brought into hospital for operation, or, especially in those patients who have vascular glands, by giving Lugol's iodine solution, 5 drops every 8 hours, for 2 weeks before surgery and this, by exerting the Wolff-Chaikoff effect, makes the gland both less productive of thyroid hormones and less vascular and therefore much more amenable to the surgeon's knife. More recently the use of beta blockers has been found to achieve many of the same results in far less time. Propranolol 40 mg. administered every 8 hours effectively controls all the sympathetic nerve symptoms including the tachycardia, nervousness, insomnia and tremor, while not affecting the thyroid gland directly in any way. It is thus possible to operate upon the patient safely, without any risk of postoperative thyroid crisis, after only a few days' preparation. Preferably the propranolol should be given for not less than 4 or 5 days, but the drug must be continued for at least a week postoperatively, until the excess thyroid hormone circulating has been metabolized.

The disadvantages of surgical treatment are that the patient must be admitted to hospital and have a general anesthetic, and there is a risk of damage to the recurrent laryngeal nerves which will cause hoarseness, or of the inadvertent removal of parathyroid glands which may then result in hypocalcemia.

The indications for thyroid surgery vary from country to country and in the

United Kingdom where there are many experienced thyroid surgeons and excellent training programs for residents, surgery is often the preferred method of treatment for toxic goiter. Unquestionably the number of complications after thyroid surgery is greater in the hands of less experienced thyroid surgeons. The mortality rate should be not more than 1/1000, permanent damage to a recurrent laryngeal nerve 1 percent and tetany 0.5 percent. Complications increase substantially when second or third operations are called for.

The incidence of hypothyroidism after thyroidectomy should be between 5 percent and 10 percent in the first year. Thereafter in our follow-up studies and in those of Brown Dobyns in Cleveland, the additional fall-off has been minimal. It in no way approximates that following radioiodine therapy. Hyperthyroidism persisting after operation usually indicates a technical fault but recurrence occurs in some 5 percent. I aim to leave a total of 8 g. of tissue, more if there is evidence of lymphocytic infiltration and prominent lymph nodes, less if the gland is dark and meaty or if the patient is a child. The great value of subtotal thyroidectomy is that it brings the thyrotoxicosis under control immediately, far quicker than by any other kind of therapy. For wage earners this can be important. It is desirable for all patients with large nodular toxic goiters; for children whom we believe are rarely well controlled by drugs and in whom radioactive iodine is dangerous, and also for pregnant mothers, especially those who wish to breast feed their babies.

The preparation of the patient should render him euthyroid by any of the methods described above. The level of calcium should be determined and repeated postoperatively. Radiographs of chest and neck are obtained and indirect laryngoscopy performed to note movement of the vocal cords. We do not routinely scan toxic goiters unless nodules are present, nor determine the level of thyroid autoantibodies.

Radioactive isotopes in the form of ^{131}I has been used for treating hyperthyroidism for 35 years. It is given orally and the amount is determined by the size of the gland and the severity of the disease. The average dose in a young adult is approximately 4 mCi, but it may vary from as little as three to very much larger doses in older patients with large multinodular toxic glands. The symptoms are not fully controlled for some weeks, and the full benefit of the isotope is not realized for 3 months, since the destruction of the gland is progressive. Unfortunately, the damage to the gland does not always end in 3 months, and there is a gradual fall off in the gland's function leading eventually to hypothyroidism in most patients. This is progressive year by year so that if the patients live long enough, they are quite likely to develop this complication. For this reason the dose of the isotope has been greatly reduced in recent years and the symptoms of hyperthyroidism controlled by propranolol or carbimazole for up to a year. The drug dosage is then tapered off and hopefully the patient remains euthyroid. The only other risk is the possibility of irradiating a fetus or a child with its attendant hazard of inducing a thyroid carcinoma. The isotope therefore must not be given to a pregnant woman or to patients under 20 years of age. In the United Kingdom in most clinics it is not usual to give the isotope to patients under the age of 40 years because of these fears. There seems very little, if any, risk however, of initiating carcinoma in the gland in adults, although there is a very real one in infancy and childhood.

Strategy for Treatment

With the facts outlined above a strategy has been evolved for treating patients with hyperthyroidism. Most patients when first seen are given a course of antithyroid drugs until the disease is controlled. In the case of young adults, more especially those with mild disease, this therapy is continued for 2 years in the hope that a long-term remission will be induced. Patients who are more toxic and especially those who are actively engaged and anxious to return to their work as soon as possible are treated either with radioactive iodine or by surgery. Radioactive iodine is never used in pregnant women or in those in the child-bearing period, nor is it ever used for children. It finds its greatest value in the older patient and also in those who have recurrent hyperthyroidism after other modes of therapy. It is not used in older patients where the gland is very bulky because very large doses are necessary and the results are not so predictable. Subtotal thyroidectomy is used for many more patients in the United Kingdom than in the United States and the advantage is considered to be the fact that patients are returned rapidly to full work with very little risk of hypothyroidism as a long-term complication. It is also particularly useful in pregnancy where the mother is anxious to breast feed her baby. If performed in the second trimester, the risk of inducing abortion is negligible.

Endocrine exophthalmos remains an enigma, although it has been in evidence for about 3,000 years, having been recorded by the Egyptians in their graphic stone carvings. The treatment of any disease when the cause is unknown must of necessity be empirical, and we are still far from understanding the mechanisms behind exophthalmos. The simple mnemonic of Werner, "nospecs," is useful in recording the severity, and although the condition is much more common in females than in males, one should beware of the man over 40 years of age who develops increasing exophthalmos, because the course of the disease in the male may be extremely rapid and severe. Upper lid retraction is the common accompaniment of Graves' disease, especially in the young patient, and appears to be due to sympathetic nerve activity, since it is largely controlled by giving guanethidine locally as eyedrops, or systemically by giving propranolol. Why the exophthalmos should so commonly start in only one eye is not known, but it usually progresses to involve both, although frequently not with the same severity. The major eye change is the increase in the volume of the orbital contents, and when this is very severe it is often referred to as malignant exophthalmos. In its final stages the extraocular muscles are paralyzed and eventually neuritis of the optic nerve can cause blindness. Before this occurs there may be damage to the cornea and infection may likewise destroy the patient's sight. The great excess of lymphocytes and fibroblasts which invade the eye muscles and orbital fat makes it seem likely that some upset of the normal immunologic processes is at the root of this condition, but such surmise does little to help us in management. In my clinic it is the rule to treat the hyperthyroidism first and then to keep the patient euthyroid or even mildly hyperthyroid by giving thyroxine so that the anterior pituitary secretion of TSH is suppressed. Patients, if at all obese, are encouraged to lose weight. They wear spectacles with broad side-pieces to protect the exposed cornea. Tarsorrhaphy is used to protect the cornea, and if the condition progresses further the patient is given large doses of prednisone, up to 60 or even 80 mg. per day. If it seems unlikely that the disease can be reasonably controlled in this way, and if the eyesight is threatened, orbital decompression is the final treatment preferably done by way of the maxillary antral approach.

Another form of therapy for exophthalmos was introduced in 1963 by Catz and Perzik. They used total thyroidectomy either by surgery, or surgery and radioiodine ablation, and claimed improvement in most patients. Other workers have not been so successful, but total thyroidectomy is not easily accomplished. The method is still on trial and this judgment also applies to the use of hypophysectomy for exophthalmos by surgical ablation, external irradiation or implantation by yttrium rods.

Long-Term Management

All patients who have been treated for hyperthyroidism need to be carefully followed for the rest of their lives and many methods have evolved in recent years using computers and postal services to arrange for the annual review of such patients. They are all at risk to develop hypothyroidism, much more than the remainder of the population. There is also the risk, though to a much lesser extent, of a recrudescence of the disease.

SELECTED READING

Beaugie, J. M.: Principles of Thyroid Surgery. London, Pitman Medical, 1975.

Burrow, G. N. (ed.): Current concepts of thyroid disease. Med. Clin. North Am., *59*: [No. 5], 1975.

Evered, D. C.: Diseases of the Thyroid. London, Pitman Medical, 1976.

deGroot, L. J., and Standbury, J. B.: The Thyroid and Its Diseases. ed. 4. New York, John Wiley & Sons, 1975.

Hamburger, J. I.: Diagnosis and Management of Common Thyroid Problems. Springfield, (Ill.), Charles C Thomas, 1969.

Irvine, W. J. (ed.): Thyrotoxicosis. Proceedings of the Edinburgh Symposium. Edinburgh, Livingstone, 1967.

Symposium on Graves' disease. Mayo Clin. Proc., *47*:801, 911, 1972.

EDITORIAL COMMENTARY

Because of its embryologic development, the thyroid gland, similar to the adrenal gland, plays at least a dual role in its influence on metabolic processes of the body. The dominant "thyroid hormones" emanate from that part of the thyroid gland which is formed and descended from the primitive pharynx in the region of the first and second branchial arches; on the other hand, thyrocalcitonin is secreted by the C cells of the thyroid gland (the ultimobranchial body, phylogenetically) which were the first cells to have been shown to be derived from the neural crest as charter members of the APUD system. The former hormones, thyroxine (T_4) and triiodothyronine (T_3) regulate metabolic processes in tissues related to energy, growth, actions of the cardiovascular system, the somatic nervous system, and particularly the sympathetic nervous system. An excess of these circulating thyroid hormones in hyperthyroidism produces several clinical pictures, the most dramatic of which is seen in Graves' disease, a typical example of the hypermetabolic syndrome. Other clinical pictures of hyperthyroidism include the thyrocardiac syndrome (Plummer's disease) and the wasting syndrome of proximal myopathy.

The thyroid hormones, T_4 and T_3, are synthesized from tyrosine in the gland and from circulating iodides, are stored, bound to thyroglobulin in the colloid of the gland, and through proteolytic hydrolysis are secreted into the bloodstream. The direction of action between synthesis and secretion and vice versa depends upon (1) an adequate supply of circulating iodides and glandular iodine, (2) the presence of glandular tyrosine and appropriate enzymes, (3) the trophic action of the anterior pituitary thyrotropin, TSH, and hypothalamic thyrotropin-releasing hormone, TRH (both polypeptides), and (4) the level of the thyroid hormones themselves. By feedback mechanisms an increase in the circulating thyroid hormones inhibits pituitary release of TSH, and a decrease in their levels stimulates hypothalamic release of TRH; environmental temperature also affects hypothalamic release of TRH.

The thyroid hormones act on target cells in a number of ways. They stimulate cyclic AMP (cAMP) activity (as do polypeptide hormones), and they also increase the transcription of messenger RNA and increase the synthesis of protein in mitochondria (similar to the action of steroid hormones). Specifically, the thyroid hormones activate energy-producing respiratory processes in cells as measured by increased oxygen consumption, a hypermetabolic effect. There are effects of increased glycogenolysis resulting in hyperglycemia, a mineral effect resulting in increased urinary calcium loss, a catabolic effect of muscle wasting with weakness; but the predominant effects are on the cardiovascular and nervous systems. These effects are demonstrable by an increase in the pulse rate, cardiac output and blood flow and, somatically, as nervousness, irritability and muscular tremors, and most interestingly on the autonomic system where there is vasomotor instability, sweating, gastrointestinal hypermotility and occasionally, hypertension. The hypermetabolic syndrome appears to be accountable to the fact that thyroxine enhances the metabolic, circulatory and neuromuscular actions of epinephrine and norepinephrine; thus many of the clinical features of "thyrotoxicosis" are explicable in terms of the actions of catecholamines. It is interesting to note that tyrosine is necessary in the synthesis of both thyroxine in the thyroid and norepinephrine at the sympathetic postganglionic nerve terminals. These associations thus are the basis of the therapeutic use of propranolol, a beta-adrenergic blocking agent, in the hypermetabolic syndrome; this therapy may effect a significant improvement in the peripheral symptoms and signs of "thyrotoxicosis" such as a reduction of pulse rate and blood pressure, an amelioration of lid retraction and digital tremor. This adrenoreceptor blocking agent has no effect on the thyroid gland itself, therefore this inhibition of the action of catecholamines is usually used as an adjunct to treatment which is otherwise directed to the underlying thyroid disease.

Historically, the relationship between sympathetic activity and hyperthyroidism has been recognized for more than a century; indeed, Poncet in 1897 recommended resection of the cervical sympathetic chain in preference to thyroidectomy in elderly patients with hyperthyroidism. More recently and over the course of time the need for surgical thyroidectomy has decreased because of prevalent iodine supplementation in foods and the development of effective nonoperative treatments of Graves' disease. However, surgical treatment with appropriate preoperative preparation is still advocated by some for Graves' disease which appears in children, in women who are of child-bearing age, or in patients such as wage earners requiring prompt resolution of their hypermetabolic state.

The problem of the etiology and treatment of the associated exophthalmos in Graves' disease appears unresolved. The "stare" or lid retraction of noninfiltrative exophthalmos is due to the effect of thyroxine stimulation of the sympathetic nervous activity of the levator palpebrae; the infiltrative type of exophthalmos is accountable to mucopolysaccharide infiltration of orbital tissues, apparently due to an elaboration of abnormal thyroid-stimulating substances of the gamma-globulin class (LATS, LATS protector). *S.R.F.*

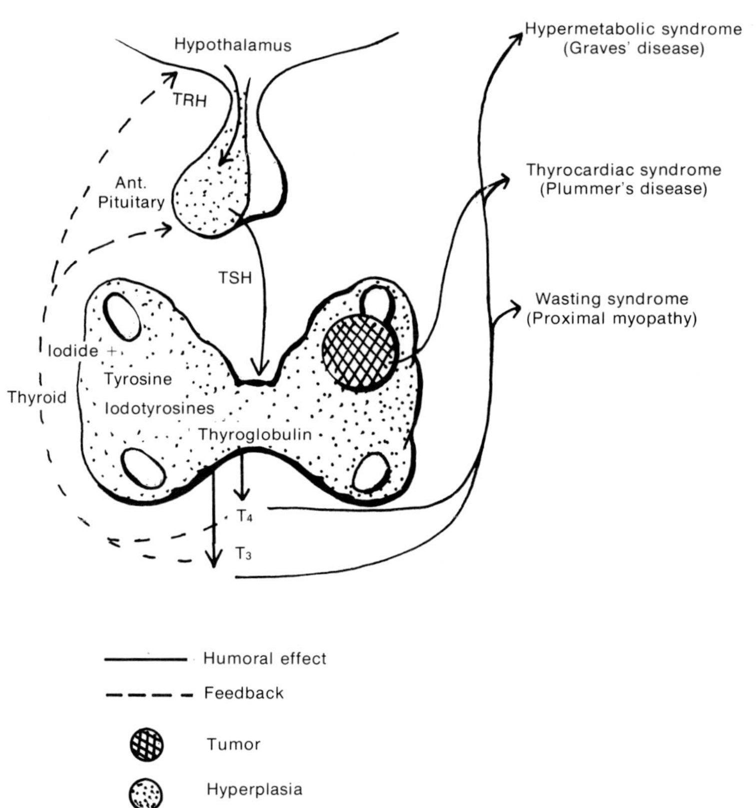

Fig. 9-1. Pathophysiology of the hypermetabolic syndrome.

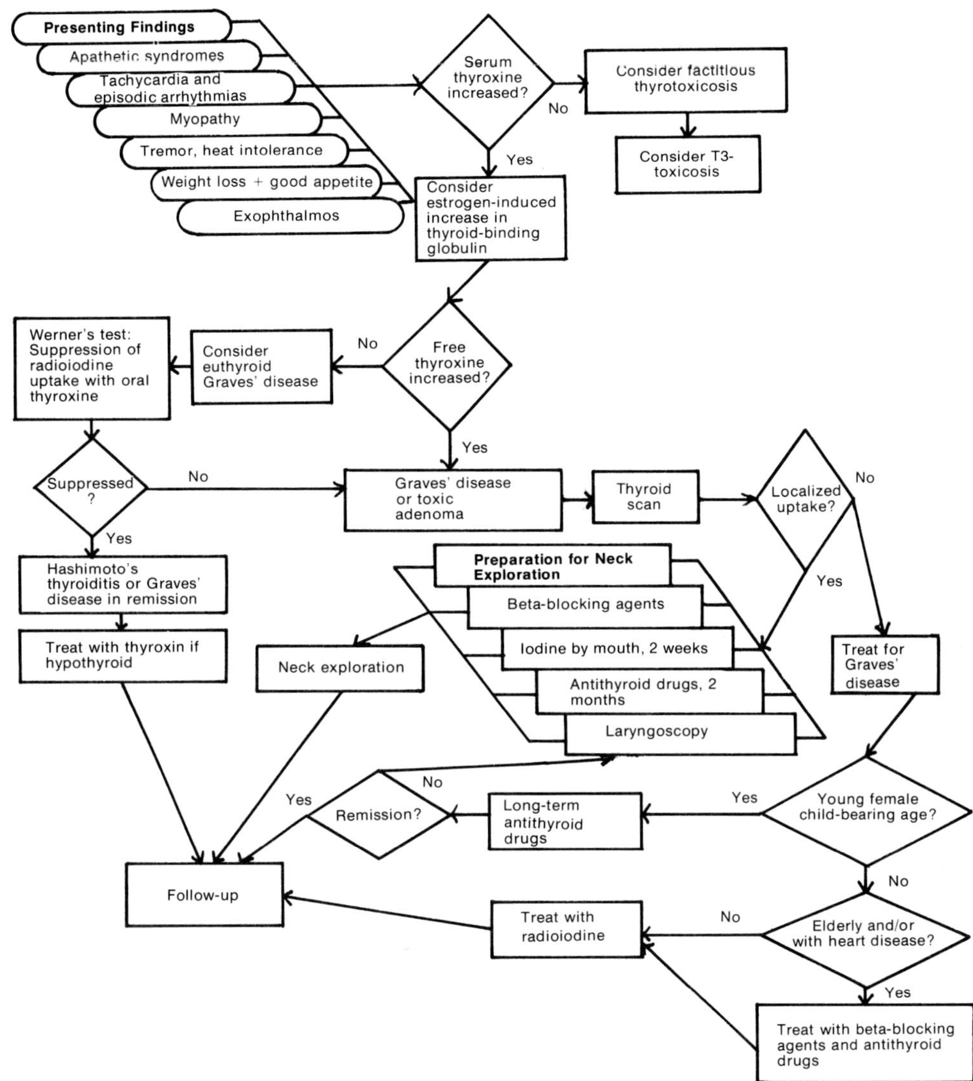

Fig. 9-2. Management flowchart of the hypermetabolic syndrome.

10

The Panic Syndrome: Pheochromocytoma

H. William Scott, Jr., M.D., D.Sc.

The late Walter B. Cannon,[4] one of Harvard's great physiologists, did much of the fundamental research which delineated the role of the sympatho-adrenal medullary system in the alarm reaction which releases catecholamines and, teleologically, prepares lower animals and man for "fight or flight." This physiologic response occurs pathologically with pheochromocytoma. The term "panic syndrome" is appropriately applied to the clinical manifestations of uncontrolled release of catecholamines from this potentially lethal tumor.

The tumor originates in a majority of cases in the adrenal medulla and less frequently in the cells of the extra-adrenal paraganglion system which are disseminated along the paravertebral axis from the pelvis to the base of the skull. The cell of origin is regarded by Pearse[16] as part of the neuroendocrine group of cells which he calls the APUD system. These cells are able to secrete polypeptide hormones and are, whether by origin or by functional similarity, very much alike. Multiple endocrine neoplasia, Type II, is a genetic disorder involving multifocal tumor formation in this system of polypeptide-secreting cells. Its expressions include pheochromocytoma, medullary carcinoma of thyroid, parathyroid tumors and multiple mucosal neuromas which may occur in combination or singly in several members of a kindred. Familial pheochromocytoma also occurs in association with neuroectodermal dysplasias which include von Recklinghausen's disease, tuberous sclerosis, Sturge-Weber's syndrome and Lindau-von Hippel disease. In these various familial syndromes, bilateral adrenal pheochromocytomas are prone to occur. However, in its most frequent form the tumor occurs as a single lesion of adrenal medullary origin without familial associations.

CLINICAL FEATURES

The incidence of pheochromocytoma has been variously estimated as 0.4 to 2 percent of all hypertensive patients. The majority of these tumors occur in adults, but about one-fifth of reported cases have been in children. The reported incidence is from 5 months to 82 years. Chong, ReMine, et al.[5] recently reported 138 patients with pheochromocytoma who were operated on at Mayo Clinic between 1926 and 1970. There were 63 males and 75 females. The tumor was extra-adrenal in 10 percent, bilateral in 4.4 percent, multiple in 7 percent and malignant (proven by metastases) in 18 patients (13.4 percent).

The symptoms and signs of pheochromocytoma are those resulting from the release of excessive amounts of catecholamines (epinephrine or norepinephrine). Epinephrine and norepinephrine are similar in metabolic action, but epinephrine is 30 to 100 times more potent than norepinephrine. Table 10-1 shows the most common symptoms and signs.

Table 10-1. Symptoms and Signs of Pheochromocytoma

	Approximate (%)	
Symptoms	*Adult*	*Child*
Persistent hypertension	65	92
Paroxysmal hypertension	30	8
Headache	80	81
Sweating	70	68
Palpitation, nervousness	60	34
Facial pallor	40	27
Tremor	40	0
Nausea	30	56
Weakness, fatigue	25	27
Weight loss	15	44
Signs		
BMR over +20%	50	83
Fasting blood sugar over 120 mg./100 ml.	40	40
Glycosuria	10	3
Eye ground changes	30	70

(Hume, D. M.: Pheochromocytoma. In Astwood, E. B., and Cassidy, C. E. (eds.): Clinical Endocrinology. vol. II, p. 519. New York, Grune & Stratton, 1968)

As indicated in Table 10-1, hypertension is the most common manifestation of pheochromocytoma. Three clinical patterns occur: (1) There is the classic pattern of paroxysmal hypertension with normal blood pressure between paroxysms. This was once thought to be the only manifestation of the tumor. (2) Blood pressure may be elevated in a sustained fashion without paroxysms and resembles essential hypertension. (3) Extreme fluctuation may be superimposed on constant elevation of blood pressure.[23]

Paroxysms of hypertension occur in 30 to 50 percent of patients with pheochromocytoma. These apparently represent episodes of massive release of hormone, either epinephrine, norepinephrine or both. Paroxysms are characterized by extreme levels of hypertension, severe headache, sweating, tachycardia, palpitation, pallor and anxiety. Occasionally, syncope, nausea, vomiting, angina and visual difficulties may occur. In children convulsions may occur during such attacks. Paroxysmal episodes may persist from a few minutes to several hours and may occur several times a day or much less frequently. Paroxysms may be spontaneous or may be precipitated by a variety of stimuli (see p. 104). Anesthesia and any form of operative procedure can readily precipitate a severe paroxysmal attack. The paroxysmal episodes often terminate in sweating and extreme weakness and are usually accompanied by hyperglycemia and elevation of the catecholamines in blood and urine.

In the absence of severe paroxysms, sustained hypertension may be accompanied by a variety of complaints including headache, nervousness, palpitation, nausea, weakness, pallor, anorexia, constipation, weight loss, dizziness and shortness of breath. Many of these symptoms probably reflect intermittent release of small amounts of catecholamines from the tumor.

Stimuli That May Precipitate Paroxysmal Attacks

Change of posture (bending, stooping, lateral flexion)	Carotid sinus pressure
Exertion	Change of temperature
Trauma to side or abdomen (including massage)	Sleep
Local heat	Laughing
Perirenal air insufflation	Sexual intercourse
General anesthesia	Shaving
Parturition	Gargling
Meals	Straining at stool
Alcohol	Sneezing
Histamine (as in gastric analysis)	Having blood pressure taken
Amobarbital sodium sedation	Urination (pheochromocytoma of the bladder)
Tetraethylammonium	Propylthiouracil
Pain	Corticotropin
Hyperventilation	Smoking
Emotional stress	Glucagon

(Moorhead, E. L. II, Caldwell, J. R., Kelly, A. R., and Monales, A. R.: The diagnosis of pheochromocytoma. JAMA, *196:* 1107, 1966 © American Medical Association, 1966)

Physical examination is often normal but may show findings related to the tumor. Most patients are thin; tremulousness and evidence of excessive sweating may be observed. Tachypnea and tachycardia may be present. The skin may exhibit neurofibromatosis, port wine stains, café au lait spots, and there may be conjunctival telangiectasis. Retinal manifestations of hypertension may be present. A large abdominal tumor may occasionally be palpable. The rare cervical tumors are said to be usually palpable. Coexisting thyroid tumors (medullary carcinoma) may be present in familial pheochromocytoma.

Abdominal palpation, especially if vigorous in the vicinity of a pheochromocytoma, may precipitate a paroxysmal hypertensive attack. At one time rough massage over the area of suspected tumor was advocated as a clinical diagnostic maneuver, but the hazard is obvious and should be avoided.

During paroxysmal episodes patients may present convulsive seizures, cardiac arrhythmias and systolic blood pressures in excess of 300 mmHg. and may sustain paralytic strokes. Blanching of face and extremities, Raynaud's phenomenon and profuse sweating may be observed during these attacks.

No single symptom and no set of symptoms is specific for pheochromocytoma, and the presence or absence of any symptom or group of symptoms neither makes nor excludes the diagnosis. In the following list of 11 distinct clinical pictures with which pheochromocytoma can present, the first five include the most frequent symptoms and signs which have been already outlined, the last six deserve special mention.[23]

There is a tendency for patients with pheochromocytoma to have elevation of blood glucose because of beta-adrenergic stimulation. This can be accompanied by glycosuria, and the picture thus can mimic diabetes mellitus. The glucose tolerance test is characteristically abnormal in pheochromocytoma, and the differential diagnosis must be made by careful observation of blood pressure and by measurement of catecholamines in blood and urine.

Patients with thyrotoxicosis are frequently thin, tremulous, nervous, diaphoretic and may have mild hypertension. All of these symptoms can be produced by pheochromocytoma, and the tumor can cause an elevated basal metabolic rate as well. Measurement of thyroid hormone which is not elevated in patients with pheochromocytoma and measurement of catecholamines in plasma and urine will differentiate the two diseases.

Patients with pheochromocytoma often have multiple vague complaints, appear nervous and anxious and sometimes have tachypnea. They may be diagnosed as having anxiety, hyperventilation syndrome, hypochondriasis or other forms of psychosomatic disease. According to Melmon,[13] actual psychotic reactions may occur.

Presenting Symptom Complexes in Patients With Pheochromocytoma

1. No symptoms; pheochromocytoma found incidentally or accidentally
2. Sudden death after minor trauma
3. Arrhythmias, tachycardia, unexplained hypotension or cardiac arrest following induction of anesthesia
4. Paroxysmal attacks: the "classic" presentation
5. Sustained hypertension, simulating benign essential hypertension
6. Polydipsia, polyuria, elevated fasting blood glucose and abnormal glucose tolerance test simulating diabetes mellitus
7. Weight loss, tremulousness, tachypnea and increased basal metabolic rate simulating thyrotoxicosis
8. Tachypnea, tremulousness and nervousness simulating an acute anxiety reaction
9. Nervousness, personality changes and psychotic reaction simulating psychosis
10. Fever, leukocytosis and sustained hypotension simulating gram-negative sepsis
11. Chronic congestive heart failure: catecholamine myocarditis

Hamrin,[7] and Fred, et al.[6] have published reports of patients with fever, leukocytosis and sustained hypotension who were initially diagnosed as having gram-negative sepsis and who were finally found to have pheochromocytoma.

A more catastrophic shock-state may suddenly occur with hemorrhagic necrosis of a pheochromocytoma as recently described by Van Way, et al.[22] This syndrome is typified by necrosis and hemorrhage within the tumor, rupture of the tumor's capsule and retroperitoneal hemorrhage. If unrecognized and untreated by emergent operation, the syndrome is usually fatal.

Other uniquely hazardous relationships of pheochromocytoma are the tumor's occurrence in childhood, in pregnancy and in the wall of the urinary bladder.

Pheochromocytoma is particularly dangerous in children because of its mimicry of other clinical conditions more commonly treated by pediatricians. Stackpole, et al.[21] have pointed out that the severe hypertension that usually develops is frequently followed by congestive heart failure, encephalopathy and death. This sequence of events can be prevented by early diagnosis and removal of the tumor. In both Hume's[10] review of pheochromocytoma in children (see Table 10-1) and that of Stackpole, et al.[21] (Table 10-2), hypertension was almost always sustained rather than paroxysmal. Whereas headache is common in both adults and children with pheochromocytoma, the children frequently have associated nausea and vomiting and visual complaints. In half of the children, tumors were bilateral, multiple or extra-adrenal. The incidence of malignancy in Hume's[10] series was 2.4 percent.

Table 10-2. Signs and Symptoms in 95 Children With Pheochromocytomas

	Number	Percentage
Hypertension	95	100
Sustained 84 (88%)		
Intermittent 11 (12%)		
Headache	71	75
Sweating	64	67
Nausea and vomiting	46	48
Weight loss	36	38
Visual disturbances	35	37
Abdominal pain	30	32
Polydipsia and polyuria	29	31
Convulsions	21	22
Acrocyanosis	21	22

*In five patients the clinical history was not given in sufficient detail for signs and symptoms. (Stackpole, R. H., et al.: J. Pediatr., *63*:315, 1963[21])

Stackpole and his associates have emphasized that the most important single cause of death in a child with pheochromocytoma during operation and the early postoperative period is the presence of an undiscovered tumor. The operative mortality rate in Stackpole's collected series was 22 percent.[21]

Pheochromocytoma in pregnancy produces, in addition to the usual clinical and metabolic manifestations of the tumor, an increased risk of spontaneous abortion, sudden shock and perinatal death. The lives of both mother and child are at risk. In the early months of pregnancy, the tumor must be differentiated from toxemia and later on from preeclampsia. According to Page and Copeland,[15] approximately half of the reported deaths have occurred in postpartum period rather than during the stress of parturition. The only accurate method of making the diagnosis of the tumor is to measure catecholamines and metabolites in all pregnant women who are hypertensive.

Pheochromocytoma occasionally occurs in the wall of the bladder, presumably arising from paraganglionic cells. It presents the striking symptom complex of headache, sweating and hypertension on micturition. However, the patient may have paroxysmal attacks which are precipitated by other causes; therefore, only a very careful history will confirm the fact that many of the paroxysms are initiated by voiding. The presence or absence of hematuria appears to determine how early the disease is identified. The earlier the hematuria, the earlier the diagnosis. The tumor may occur anywhere in the bladder from dome to trigone and can usually be diagnosed by cystoscopy. Although two out of 28 tumors in Sarman's[19] collected series were considered malignant, most vesical pheochromocytomas are small lesions (less than 3 cm. in diameter) and usually can be treated by partial cystectomy with good results.

PREOPERATIVE MANAGEMENT

Confirmation of the diagnosis of clinically suspected pheochromocytoma requires measurement of catecholamines and their metabolites in the patient's blood and urine. To understand the clinical symptoms produced and the laboratory tests used to establish diagnosis, it is helpful to consider three aspects of catecholamine biochemistry and physiology: (1) Their biosynthesis,

(2) metabolic breakdown and (3) physiologic and pathologic effects and pharmacologic antagonism by adrenergic blocking agents.

Catecholamine biosynthesis is outlined in Figure 10-1. In the normal adrenal medullary cell, the first three steps are carried out in the cytoplasm. Dopamine is then incorporated into granules within the cell. Dopamine is converted to norepinephrine by dopamine beta-hydroxylase found only in the granules, and the norepinephrine is then linked to binding protein. This protein-bound norepinephrine is the major storage pool within the cell. However, some of the norepinephrine in the granules is free and is in equilibrium with free norepinephrine in the cytoplasm. Cytoplasmic norepinephrine is converted by phenylethanolamine n-methyltransferase to epinephrine, which is then taken up and stored in separate granules. On stimulation of the medullary cell, the contents of the granules are released into the extracellular space by epicytosis.[3]

In the sympathetic nerve ending, norepinephrine is produced and released in a similar manner. However, the sympathetic nerve endings do not contain n-methyltransferase and do not make epinephrine. In adults, epinephrine is found only in the adrenal medulla where it is the predominant catecholamine and has a concentration four to six times that of norepinephrine. In infants and young children, epinephrine has been extracted from the organs of Zuckerkandl. This has very direct clinical applicability: an epinephrine-producing pheochromocytoma is nearly always an adrenal tumor or is located in the organs of Zuckerkandl.

The metabolic pathways for the catecholamines, as they pass from synthesis to degradation, are outlined in Figure 10-2. Primary interest in pheochromocytoma revolves around the metabolites of norepinephrine and epinephrine, specifically normetanephrine, metanephrine and vanillylmandelic

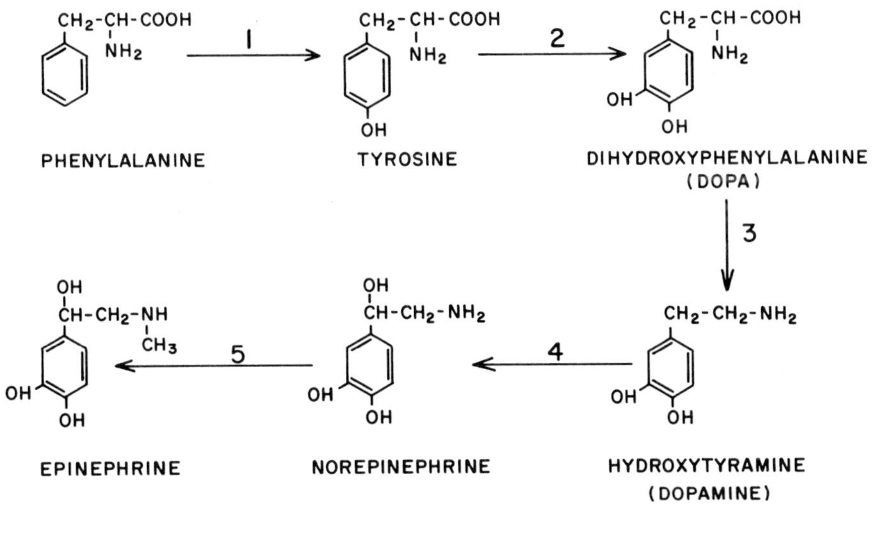

Fig. 10-1. Biosynthesis of norepinephrine and epinephrine.

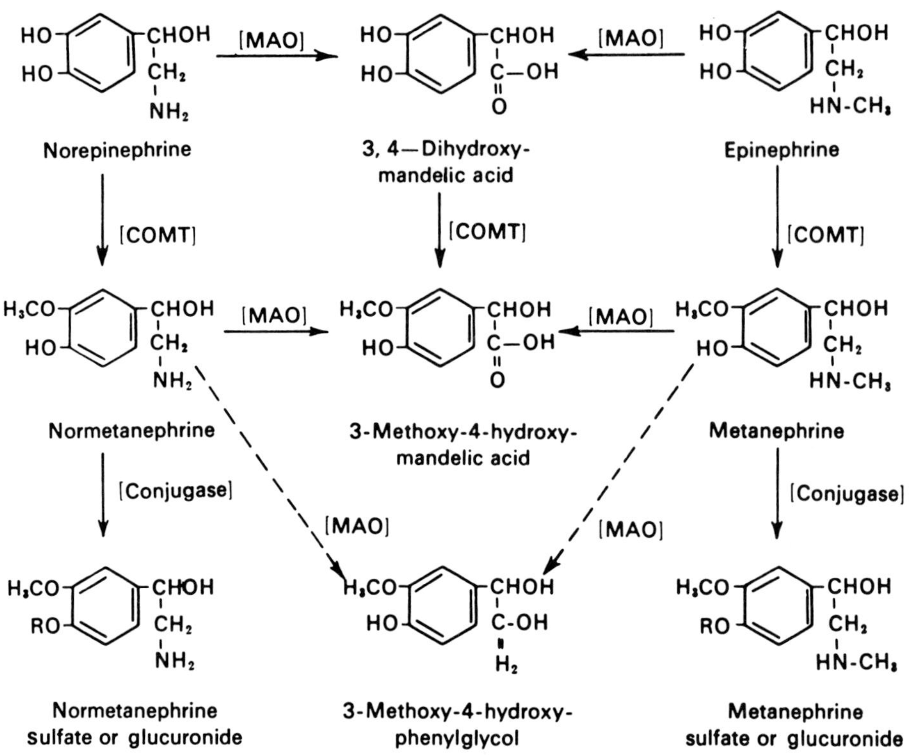

HO, HO, CHOH, CH_2, NH_2 — Norepinephrine → [MAO] → HO, HO, CHOH, C—OH, O — 3, 4—Dihydroxy-mandelic acid ← [MAO] ← HO, HO, CHOH, CH_2, HN-CH_3 — Epinephrine

[COMT] [COMT] [COMT]

H_3CO, HO, CHOH, CH_2, NH_2 — Normetanephrine → [MAO] → H_3CO, HO, CHOH, C—OH, O — 3-Methoxy-4-hydroxy-mandelic acid ← [MAO] ← H_3CO, HO, CHOH, CH_2, HN-CH_3 — Metanephrine

[Conjugase] [MAO] [MAO] [Conjugase]

H_3CO, RO, CHOH, CH_2, NH_2 — Normetanephrine sulfate or glucuronide

H_3CO, HO, CHOH, C-OH, H_2 — 3-Methoxy-4-hydroxy-phenylglycol

H_3CO, RO, CHOH, CH_2, HN-CH_3 — Metanephrine sulfate or glucuronide

Fig. 10-2. Steps in metabolic degradation of epinephrine and norepinephrine MAO-monamine oxidase. COMT = catechol-O-methyltransferase. (O'Neal, L. W.: Surgery of the Adrenal Glands. St. Louis, C. V. Mosby, 1968)

acid (VMA). The two enzymes involved are monamine oxidase, a mitochondrial enzyme, and catechol O-methyltransferase, a cytoplasmic enzyme. Monamine oxidase is found specifically in the sympathetic nerve endings and the adrenal medullary cell. However, circulating catecholamines are broken down by both enzymes.[14] LaBrosse, et al.[11] using tritium-labeled epinephrine, found that 40 percent was excreted as VMA and 40 percent as metanephrine, indicating activity of both pathways in the metabolism of circulating catecholamines. As indicated in the figure, all metanephrines are formed by the action of catechol O-methyltransferase on circulating catecholamines. Metabolism within a tumor is more likely to begin with monamine oxidase as a first step and proceed to VMA. Assays for metanephrine and VMA complement one another in diagnosis of pheochromocytoma. Normal values for excretion of urinary catecholamines and metabolites are shown in Table 10-3.

Ahlquist's[1] division of adrenergic responses into those of alpha and beta receptors has clarified the understanding of the action of epinephrine and norepinephrine. His work was verified by the discovery that adrenergic blocking agents are specific for either alpha or beta receptors. Alpha receptors are generally excitatory and beta receptors inhibitory in the periphery. Pure alpha stimulation causes peripheral arteriolar constriction with attendant rise in blood pressure. Cardiac effects of alpha stimulation are produced by reflex changes, most notably a vagal-mediated bradycardia. Beta stimulation causes

Table 10-3. Normal Values for Excretion of Catecholamines and Metabolites

	Normal Excretion Rate
Catecholamines	10—100 μg. per 24 hours
Norepinephrine	10— 70 μg. per 24 hours
Epinephrine	0— 20 μg. per 24 hours
Vanillylmandelic acid (VMA)	1.8— 7.0 mg. per 24 hours
Normetanephrine and metanephrine	<1.3 mg. per 24 hours

peripheral vasodilation with lowering of diastolic pressure. Cardiac receptors are purely of the beta variety and produce tachycardia and inotropism.

Norepinephrine is a relatively pure alpha stimulator, although it has some cardiac beta-stimulatory properties that are usually seen only after alpha blockade. Epinephrine has a mixed effect. It is a more potent alpha stimulator than norepinephrine, but it also has a strong beta-stimulant effect. Dopamine has an anomalous effect: cardiac beta stimulation with a specific renal vasodilation that is neither alpha nor beta.

The catecholamines produce a general hypermetabolic effect which seems to account for the feeling of "nervousness" common in patients with pheochromocytoma. The two more specific effects are glycogenolysis, primarily in the liver, and elevation of serum-free fatty acids from increased activity of a triglyceride lipase enzyme found in adipose tissue. Both of these effects have been shown by Robison and coworkers[18] to be mediated by stimulation of adenylcyclase, causing an increase in cyclic 3′,5′ adenosine monophosphate (cAMP) which acts as a secondary messenger to stimulate activity of the target enzyme.

Laboratory confirmation of the diagnosis of pheochromocytoma can usually be made quite easily by measurement of free catecholamines, VMA and metanephrines in 24-hour collections of the patient's urine (Table 10-3). Urinary free catecholamines were elevated above 100 μg. per 24 hours in 27 patients in the clinical series of 34 patients with pheochromocytoma studied at Vanderbilt University.[20] In all but two of these, the elevations were repeatedly in excess of 200 μg. per 24 hours, most commonly in the range of 300 to over 1,000 μg. per 24 hours. Urinary VMA was elevated above 12 g. per 24 hours in 15 patients and was below 10 mg. per 24 hours in three others in the series. Urinary metanephrines, elevated above 1.3 mg. per 24 hours, are considered to be the most accurate indicator of pheochromocytoma at Mayo Clinic,[5] whereas the endocrine laboratory at Vanderbilt[23] favors free catecholamines. Harrison[9] has emphasized the reliability and accuracy of measurement of urinary free catecholamines and metanephrine in the differential diagnosis of pheochromocytoma and the inaccuracy and unreliability of the commonly used colorimetric reaction for VMA which he considers to be a poor analytical test. Dopamine and its principal metabolite, homovanillic acid, are not generally elevated in patients with pheochromocytoma.

Vena caval catheterization with assay of plasma catecholamines at various levels was advocated in localization of pheochromocytoma as early as 1955 by von Euler and Strom.[24] The details of the technique have been recently described by Harrison and his associates.[9] It is their feeling that localization of pheochromocytoma by caval catheterization is particularly helpful in small ectopically located lesions which are not identified by other methods.

Roentgenographic studies which have been helpful in localizing the site of pheochromocytoma before operation include nephrotomography, intravenous urography, retroperitoneal pneumography, adrenal venography, flush aortography and selective arteriography of renal arteries and other aortic branches.[23] Each of these methods has limitations and none is totally reliable. Presacral gas insufflation can bring the contour of the adrenal glands into sharp relief and resolution can be improved further by laminagraphy. The use of gases soluble in blood, such as carbon dioxide or nitrous oxide, enhances the safety of the technique; however, it has not been used frequently in the United States in recent years. Retrograde adrenal venography was introduced in the United States by Reuter, Bookstein and their associates[17] who learned the technique from its originators in Sweden and England. It has been found widely useful by many radiologists in demonstrating a variety of adrenal lesions including pheochromocytoma. Concern about the hazard of extravasation of contrast media has limited its use in some clinics including our own. However, Harrison[9] points out that extravasation is rarely now seen as technical sophistication has developed, and it is uncommon to have a severe hypertensive reaction result from the study. During the past decade at Vanderbilt,[20,23] we have come to rely preferentially on contrast arteriography in most patients with suspected pheochromocytoma. Whereas rapid injection of hypertonic iodinated contrast medium is a powerful pharmacologic stimulus for catecholamine release from the pheochromocytoma, if the procedure is carried out with appropriate precautions, including monitoring of vital signs and electrocardiogram with full preparation for carrying out whatever resuscitation may be required, excellent results can be safely obtained.

An effective radioscanning technique for pheochromocytoma would be a great diagnostic asset. Beierwaltes and his associates[2] have worked on the problem for many years. Recently they demonstrated that ^{14}C-tagged dopamine given intravenously is concentrated in pheochromocytoma and a scanning method with a gamma-ray emitting isotope for the tumor may soon be available. They have adapted the ^{131}Iodocholesterol adrenal cortical scanning procedure[12] to demonstrate adrenal pheochromocytoma by a definite negative impression of the lesion. The technique is not applicable to extra-adrenal tumors.

Localization of pheochromocytoma before operation can be accomplished by one or more of these diagnostic procedures in a majority of patients. However, it must be emphasized that careful surgical exploration remains the most dependable localizing method of all.

Preoperative preparation of patients with pheochromocytoma during the last decade has usually included the use of adrenergic blocking agents. Of the various drugs which produce alpha-adrenergic blockade, the most widely used are phenoxybenzamine (Dibenzyline) and phentolamine. Beta-adrenergic blockade is produced by only a few drugs, all derivatives of the beta stimulator, isoproterenol; Propranolol is in general use for this purpose.[23]

Phenoxybenzamine produces alpha-adrenergic blockade with relatively minor side effects. Its action is slow. It appears to inactivate the alpha-adrenergic receptor by forming a stable bond with it. Peak effect occurs 1 to 2 hours after oral administration. The drug is generally given orally in daily doses of 20 to 200 mg. The effects of daily administration are cumulative for 5 to 7 days. Phentolamine is a 2-substituted imidazoline which causes rapid and transient alpha-adrenergic blockade. Onset of action after intravenous administration is within 30 seconds, peak effect is within 5 minutes and duration of action is 30 to 60 minutes. Absorption after oral administration is erratic. Accordingly, it is usually given by intravenous infusion. The initial dose is 1 to 5 mg., but the rate of administration may vary from 2 to 50 mg. per hour and must be titrated against blood pressure. Phentolamine is useful in the acute control of hypertension in pheochromocytoma but is inferior to phenoxybenzamine for long-term use.[23]

Propranolol induces a competitive beta-adrenergic blockade with a half-life of several hours. It is usually given orally in doses of 10 to 40 mg. every 6 to 8 hours. The intravenous preparation is used primarily for intraoperative administration; the dose is 1 to 3 mg. over several minutes with electrocardiographic monitoring.[23]

The clinical indications for use of alpha- and beta-adrenergic effector blockade outlined by Harrison, et al.[8] in 1968 have been summarized below, modified by the addition of increased hematocrit (low plasma volume) as another indication for alpha blockade.

Indications for Alpha-Adrenergic Blockade (Phentolamine, Phenoxybenzamine)

Blood pressure > 200/130	Use of beta-adrenergic blockade
Frequent, severe, uncontrolled hypertensive attacks	Hematocrit > 50%

(Harrison, T. S., et al.: Ann. Surg., *168*:701, 1968[8])

Indications for Beta-Adrenergic Blockade (Propranolol)

Pulse rate > 140 a minute	Persistent ventricular extrasystoles
Any history of arrhythmia	Pure epinephrine-secreting tumors

(Harrison, T. S., et al.: Ann. Surg., *168*:701, 1968[8])

These are useful clinical guides which are consistent with current clinical practice. Achievement of effective alpha blockade with phenoxybenzamine usually takes from 4 days to 2 weeks. The end-point of treatment is elimination of hypertension, sweating and weakness, and cessation of paroxysmal attacks. Control of hypertension for 1 to 3 weeks prior to operation is probably beneficial. Spontaneous restoration of normal plasma volume during this period should reduce operative risk. The extent to which operative intervention should be delayed to permit optimal alpha blockade remains a subject of controversy. Indications for beta-adrenergic blockade are even more controversial. The most common specific situation in which beta blockade is indicated is in a patient in whom tachycardia develops on alpha blockade. A second indication is severe tachycardia or atrial tachyarrhythmia as a presenting manifestation. Propranolol must be given only after alpha blockade has been established.

INTRAOPERATIVE MANAGEMENT

Anesthetic management in most clinics in recent years has begun with adrenergic blockade. It should be emphasized that complete blockade is not obtainable, and the patient must still be protected from excessive catecholamine release at operation. Thiopental and nitrous oxide are generally used for induction with deep halothane anesthesia for maintenance in most patients. A lidocaine drip is used to control arrhythmias with phentolamine supplementation if needed. Aggressive blood and fluid replacement are used during operation in anticipation of hypotension after removal of the tumor. Usually 50 to 75 g. of albumin and 2 to 3 liters of Ringer's lactate are given during operation. At Vanderbilt an effort is made to avoid the use of norepinephrine infusions during or after operation.[20,23]

Operative procedure has been based on the need for wide exposure and nonmanipulative dissection in removal of pheochromocytomas. An anterior transperitoneal approach which permits examination of both adrenal glands and a search of the paraspinal axis are desirable. With large (>6 cm. diameter) tumors, extension of the incision across the costal margin into the eighth or ninth intercostal space greatly improves exposure. At Vanderbilt we have used either a midline or transverse thoracoabdominal incision in the majority of patients with adrenal pheochromocytomas. There have been no deaths during operation. We believe the safety and excellence of the exposure justify the slight increase in morbidity.

At operation, even though the site of the tumor has been well-localized preoperatively, careful examination of the contralateral adrenal and the renal fossa, the paraspinal axis and the pelvis in search of additional tumors should be made. A left adrenal tumor may be approached by reflecting the mobilized spleen and the pancreatic tail medially and the splenic flexure inferiorly, or by dividing the gastrocolic omentum and retracting the tail of the pancreas, spleen and stomach upward. The right adrenal is approached by mobilizing the hepatic flexure of the colon, displacing it inferiorly and dividing the lateral peritoneal attachments of the duodenum to permit the latter and inferior vena cava to be retracted medially. Careful, gentle dissection with early control of the tumor's blood supply is highly desirable. A technique which "dissects the patient away from the tumor" and minimizes manipulation of the lesion will reduce the release of catecholamines and the risk of operation. When a large adrenal tumor (>6 cm. in diameter) presents, the possibility of carcinoma must be considered and wide exposure using a thoracoabdominal incision is mandatory to permit radical en bloc, nonmanipulative resection of the tumor with the ipsilateral kidney and, if necessary, in the case of left adrenal tumors the tail of the pancreas and spleen. An upper abdominal incision is first made, the abdomen and contralateral adrenal explored and the incision then carried across the costal margin into the eighth or ninth intercostal space with division of the diaphragm on the side of the tumor. This permits truly excellent exposure of a large pheochromocytoma (Fig. 10-3).

Postoperative complications are rather frequent. In general the hazards of operation combine those peculiar to pheochromocytoma with those of any large upper abdominal or thoracoabdominal procedure.

RESULTS AND PROGNOSIS

In the 138 patients with pheochromocytoma treated surgically at Mayo Clinic from 1926 through 1970, the mortality rate of the primary operation was 2.9 percent.[3] Two of the deaths were due to massive uncontrollable bleeding

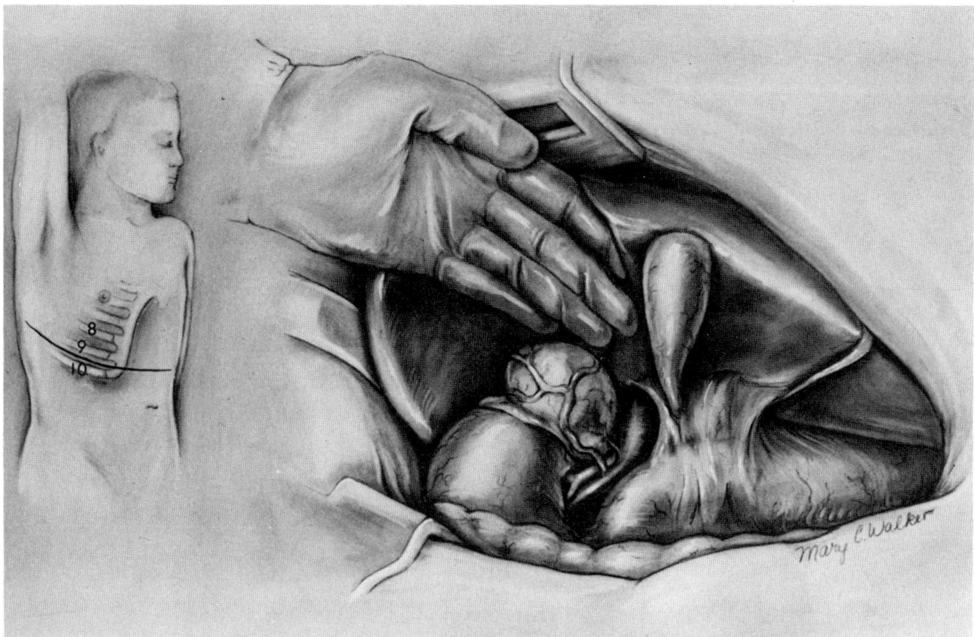

Fig. 10-3. Exposure of adrenal pheochromocytoma by thoracoabdominal incision *(right)*. (Scott, H. W., Jr., et al.: Ann. Surg., *183*:587, 1976[20])

from inferior vena cava or common iliac veins. In the other two deaths, cardiac arrest occurred during operation. These four deaths occurred prior to 1965. This enviable record illustrates the excellence of the screening program used by one group of clinicians and the fine cooperative efforts of physicians, anesthesiologists and surgeons in carrying these difficult patients safely through anesthesia and operative removal of the tumors.

In a 26-year period (1950-1976) at Vanderbilt University Affiliated Hospitals, 45 patients with pheochromocytoma were observed ranging in age from 9 to 78 years. There were 30 females and 15 males. Familial occurrence of tumors presented as multiple endocrine neoplasia Type II in two patients and two others had the associated findings of von Recklinghausen's cutaneous neurofibromatosis and Lindau-von Hippel disease respectively. The remainder had no familial or neuroectodermal dysplasic associations. In 11 patients seen in the earlier years of this period of study, clinical diagnosis of pheochromocytoma was not made and the tumor was discovered at autopsy by the pathologist. In four patients the pheochromocytoma was an incidental autopsy finding but in the other seven the tumor contributed to the death of the patient. Among the 34 patients in whom the clinical diagnosis was made, 32 had removal of primary pheochromocytomas with a single postoperative fatality (Table 10-4). In two patients with metastatic malignant tumors, only biopsy of metastases was done to establish pathologic diagnosis prior to chemotherapy.[20]

Pathologic classification of pheochromocytomas as benign or malignant is based on the presence or absence of proven metastases. This practice is followed because histologic pattern does not accurately predict biologic behavior.

Table 10-4. Pheochromocytoma: Early Survival (Vanderbilt University Affiliated Hospitals, 1950-1976)

	Patients	*Deaths*
Clinical diagnosis made (Surgical removal)	34*	1†
Clinical diagnosis not made (Autopsy)	11	11
Total	45	12

*Two patients had only biopsy of metastic tumor.
†Renal failure after removal of tumor and left kidney.

The results for patients who survived operative removal of pheochromocytoma have varied with age, familial relationships and the benign or malignant characteristics of the tumor. Patients with familial pheochromocytoma and those in the childhood age group have an increased tendency to have bilateral tumors as well as synchronous and metachronous multiple extra-adrenal tumors.

Follow-up has been completed to late 1976 in all but two patients of the Vanderbilt series (Fig. 10-4). In these exceptions, a single benign adrenal pheochromocytoma was removed in 1957 and 1963 and each patient remained normotensive and asymptomatic for a period of 11 years and 18 months respectively before they were lost to follow-up. Each of the four patients with malignant pheochromocytoma who were clinically managed received x-ray therapy and various chemotherapeutic agents and died with disseminated metastases 9 months, 2, 3, and 11 years after the diagnosis was made. In two

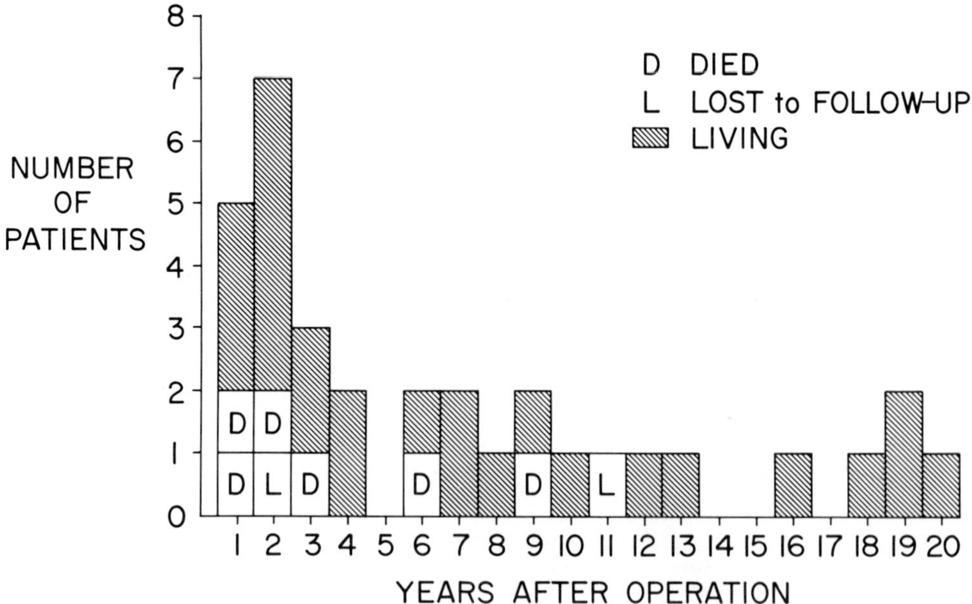

Fig. 10-4. Pheochromocytoma: late survival (1950-1975). Follow-up data in 34 patients with pheochromocytoma in whom clinical diagnosis was made and treatment instituted. (Scott, H. W., Jr., et al.: Ann. Surg., *183*:587, 1976[20])

of these patients an histologic benign pheochromocytoma had initially been removed 11 and almost 6 years, respectively, prior to death from metastatic disease. In the 26 remaining patients with benign pheochromocytoma, up-to-date follow-up extends from 1 to 20 years. In this group are two adults with MEN-II, and the only child in the series, a 9-year-old boy with no identifiable familial associations. Each had bilateral adrenal pheochromocytomas removed with satisfactory courses on maintenance steroids in the last 1 to 4 years. One of the two patients with MEN-II is known to have widely distributed metastases of medullary thyroid carcinoma. Each of these three patients is normotensive.

Among the 23 other patients who had a single benign pheochromocytoma removed, 14 who have been followed from 12 months to 20 years have remained normotensive and asymptomatic with no evidence of recurrence of pheochromocytoma. However, in the 9 other patients, hypertension has persisted or developed in the period of follow-up after excision of the tumor. One of these patients had malignant hypertension with diffusely severe renal arteriolosclerosis and nitrogen retention at the time her small para-aortic pheochromocytoma was excised. She sustained no improvement from removal of the tumor and died in uremia 3 months later. Catecholamines were normal after operation in this patient and have been in the normal range in each of the other eight patients who have developed hypertension during the follow-up period. In each instance hypertension has been controlled satisfactorily with antihypertensive drugs. Three of these patients are on digitalis preparations and one also has an enlarged heart which has been attributed to catecholamine myocardiopathy. Diabetic glucose tolerance tests which existed before operation in nine patients have reverted to normal in seven after removal of the pheochromocytoma.[20]

Pheochromocytoma can simulate any hypertensive syndrome. Although it is an uncommon cause of high blood pressure, all hypertensives should be screened for the tumor. Follow-up for life is mandatory in all patients with surgically treated pheochromocytoma.

REFERENCES

1. Ahlquist, R. P.: A study of adrenotropic receptors. Am. J. Physiol., *153*:586, 1948.
2. Anderson, B. G., Beierwaltes, W. H., Harrison, T. S., Ansari, A. N., and Buswick, A. A.: Labeled dopamine concentration in pheochromocytoma. J. Nucl. Med., *14*:781, 1973.
3. Axelrod, J., and Weinshilbaum, R.: Catecholamines. N. Engl. J. Med., *287:*237, 1972.
4. Cannon, W. B.: The Wisdom of the Body. New York, Norton, 1939.
5. Chong, G. C., ReMine, W. H., Van Heerden, J. A., Sheps, S. G., and Harrison, E.: Current management of pheochromocytoma. Ann. Surg., *179*:740, 1974.
6. Fred, H. L., Allrod, D. P., Garber, H. E., Retiene, K., and Lipscomb, H.: Pheochromocytoma masquerading as overwhelming infection. Am. Heart J., *73*:149, 1967.
7. Hamrin, B.: Sustained hypotension and shock due to an adrenalin secreting pheochromocytoma. Lancet, *2*:123, 1962.
8. Harrison, T. S., Bartlett, J. D., Jr., and Seaton, J. F.: Current evaluation and management of pheochromocytoma. Ann. Surg., *168*:701, 1968.
9. Harrison, T. S., Gann, D. S., Edis, A. J.,

and Egdahl, R. H.: Surgical disorders of the adrenal gland: physiologic background and treatment. New York, Grune & Stratton, 1975.
10. Hume, D. M.: Pheochromocytoma in the adult and the child. Am. J. Surg., *99*:458, 1960.
11. LaBrosse, E. H., Axelrod, J., Kopin, I. J., and Kety, S. S.: Metabolism of 7 H^3-epinephrine-d-bitartrate in normal young men. J. Clin. Invest., *40*:253, 1961.
12. Lieberman, L. M., et al.: Diagnosis of adrenal diseases by visualization of human adrenal glands with ^{131}I-19-iodocholesterol. N. Engl. J. Med., *285*:1387, 1971.
13. Melmon, K. L.: The Adrenals: Part II: Catecholamines and the adrenal medulla. *In* Williams, R. H. (ed.): Textbook of Endocrinology. p. 379. ed. 4. Philadelphia, W. B. Saunders, 1968.
14. O'Neal, L. W.: Surgery of the Adrenal Glands. St. Louis, C. V. Mosby, 1968.
15. Page, L. B., and Copeland, R. B.: Pheochromocytoma. Disease-a-Month, Jan. 1968.
16. Pearse, A. G. E.: The cytochemistry and ultrastructure of polypeptide hormone producing cells of the APUD series and their embryologic, physiologic and pathologic implications of the concept. J. Histochem. Cytochem., *17*:303, 1969.
17. Reuter, S. R., Blair, A. J., Schteingart, D. E., and Bookstein, J. J.: Adrenal venography. Radiology, *89*:805, 1967.
18. Robison, G. A., Butcher, R. W., and Sutherland, E. W.: Cyclic AMP. New York and London, Academic Press, 1971.
19. Sarman, K. P.: Tumors of the Urinary Bladder. New York, Appleton-Century-Crofts, 1969.
20. Scott, H. W., Jr., et al.: Pheochromocytoma: present diagnosis and management. Ann. Surg., *183*:587, 1976.
21. Stackpole, R. H., Melicow, M. M., and Uson, A. C.: Pheochromocytoma in childhood. J. Ped., *63*:315, 1963.
22. Van Way, C. W. III, Feraci, R. P., Cleveland, H. C., Foster, J. H., and Scott, H. W., Jr.: Hemorrhagic necrosis of pheochromocytoma associated with phentolamine administration. Ann. Surg., *184*:26, 1976.
23. Van Way, C. W. III, Scott, H. W., Jr., Page, D. L., and Rhamy, R. K.: Pheochromocytoma. Current Problems in Surgery. June, 1974, Chicago, Year Book Medical Publishers, 1974.
24. von Euler, U. S., Gemzell, C. A., Strom, G., and Westman, A.: Report of a case of pheochromocytoma with special regard to preoperative diagnostic problems. Acta Med. Scand., *153*:127, 1955.

EDITORIAL COMMENTARY

The clinical picture that is characteristically seen in patients with pheochromocytoma is related to the physiologic actions of excessive concentrations of local and circulating catecholamines upon specific adrenoreceptors. The panic syndrome is mnemonically descriptive of many such patients and can be further qualified as, the hypertensive syndrome with panic. In that case the syndrome would have to be differentiated from others in which endocrine-based hypertension is a frequent component, such as hypertension with hypokalemia in Conn's syndrome (hyperaldosteronism), hypertension with truncal obesity (Cushing's syndrome), hypertension with hypermetabolic syndrome (hyperthyroidism) and renal ischemic hypertension with excessive angiotensin. Furthermore, the syndrome associated with pheochromocytoma has also been called the great mimic, so that variations of the typical clinical picture include hypertension with hyperglycemia simulating diabetes mellitus and with symptomatology simulating thyrotoxicosis, myocarditis, acute anxiety reaction, psychosis and even hypotension simulating septic shock. The classic picture, however, is one of paroxysmal hypertension, but sustained hypertension is equally as common; either situation is hazardous and to overlook a diagnosis of pheochromocytoma is a potentially lethal circumstance for the patient.

Pheochromocytoma, meaning a tumor with "tawny-colored cells," occurs in the adrenal gland or in paraganglionic tissues as a neoplasm of cells which are classic members of the APUD series of the neuroendocrine system. Extra-adrenal sites of chromaffin tissue are normally in greatest number at birth and involute until puberty, which may explain why multiple tumors of the adrenal or extra-adrenal sites are more common in children; but three sites persist beyond childhood: the carotid body, the glomus jugulare and possibly, the aortic body. When there is a familial genetic component, the tumor may be bilateral, multiple, and even may be associated with thyroid medullary carcinoma of C cells (the prototype polypeptide-secreting APUD cell) and hyperplastic hyperparathyroidism, and is called Sipple's syndrome or multiple endocrine adenopathy (MEA, Type II), which is discussed in Chapter 18. Pheochromocytoma was first described in a patient in 1922 and the first successful removal was by C. H. Mayo in 1927; the isolation of the pressor substance was first reported by Beer, King and Prinzmetal in 1939. Long before that time, however, epinephrine was the first hormone to be recognized as such in 1894 by Oliver and Schafer, and isolated by Abel in 1898. In spite of this, the word, "hormone," was first applied by Bayliss and Starling in 1902 to the polypeptide, secretin. The adrenal medulla functions as a giant presynaptic sympathetic nerve ending which has the ability to synthesize not only norepinephrine but also epinephrine.

The secretory products involved in the panic syndrome, therefore, are epinephrine and norepinephrine; the former derives primarily from tumors of the adrenal medulla and circulates freely, whereas the latter is synthesized from tyramine in the medullary ganglia and also at the terminal synapses of the sympathetic ganglia and paraganglionic sites, and acts primarily as a local neurotransmitter. The actions of these amines are immediate, within seconds, much faster than the polypeptide actions, and the rapidity of action is best illustrated by the homeostatic preparation of the body for "fright, fight and flight"; such an example is the immediate palpitation and pilomotor reaction at the moment of crisis such as a near-accident. The nature of the actions of these catecholamines became clear after Ahlquist's elucidation[1] of the two types of adrenoreceptors. The alpha-adrenoreceptors are responsive to both epinephrine and norepinephrine and mediate vasoconstriction (hypertension), and stimulate the pilomotor apparatus and cause pupillary dilatation and eyelid retraction (appearance of panic). The beta-adrenoreceptors of the heart are responsive to epinephrine, mediating an increase in cardiac rate and output and by vasodilation of the vessels of the heart (a redistribution of blood thus occurring from skin and intestinal vessels to the myocardium, brain and skeletal muscles). Beta-adrenoreceptors also relax bronchial and uterine smooth muscles (epinephrine effect) and increase metabolism by stimulation of cAMP to affect glycogenolysis (hyperglycemia) and lipolysis. Epinephrine thus affects primarily the heart rate and metabolism by systemic effects on distal target organs, whereas norepinephrine acts to provide blood pressure homeostasis by local neurotransmitter effects on the heart and blood vessels.

It is evident then from these adrenoreceptor actions that the pharmacologic treatment by adrenoreceptor blocking agents is extremely important; in pheochromocytoma the alpha-receptor blockers are thus the primary agents to ameliorate hypertension and panic, together with the secondary use of beta receptor blockers for the unmasked tachycardia and arrhythmia. A generalization can be made that in pheochromocytoma the use of alpha blockers is of primary importance, whereas in hyperthyroidism the use of beta blockers is primary. The phenomenon of sweating and salivation which is sometimes seen in patients who have pheochromocytoma is not mediated by norepinephrine, but rather by acetylcholine in the cholinergic fibers of the sympathetic nervous system.

Related tumors of the sympathetic nervous system which may be functional also include the malignant neuroblastoma of infants from the primitive neural crest cell and the benign ganglioneuroma from the differentiated ganglion cell. Dopamine, a precursor and the neurotransmitter of the hypothalamus, may also be elaborated by the above tumors, as well as by the malignant pheochromocytoma. It is interesting to note that these neural tumors have also been reported to elaborate the polypeptide, vasoactive intestinal polypeptide (VIP), to produce the diarrheogenic syndrome (see Chap. 15). *S.R.F.*

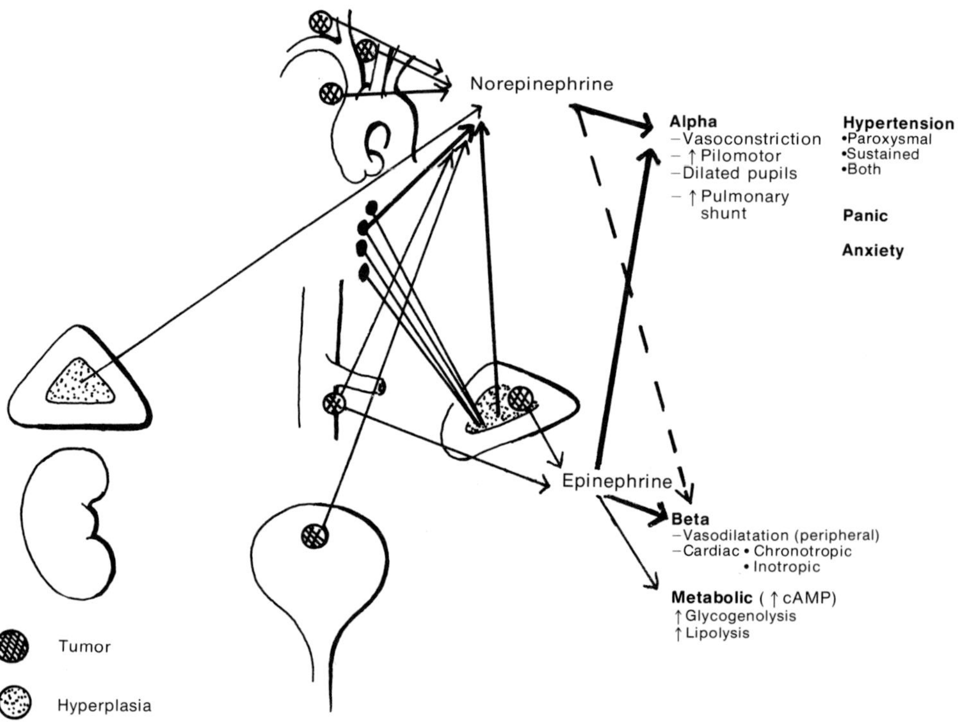

Fig. 10-5. Pathophysiology of the "panic" syndrome (pheochromocytoma and ganglioneuroma).

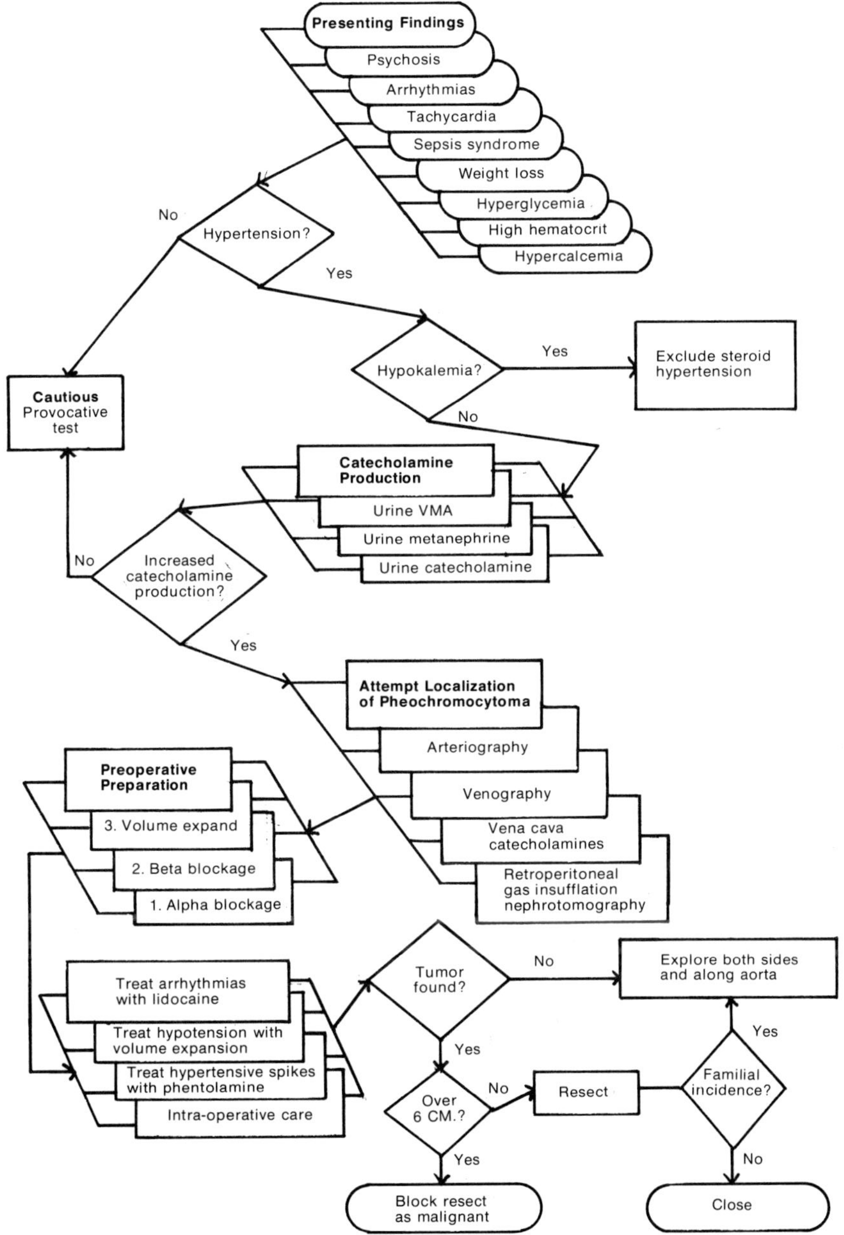

Fig. 10-6. Management flowchart of the "panic" syndrome.

11

The Carcinoid Syndromes

Edwin L. Kaplan, M.D.

Carcinoid tumors are interesting and unique both because of their variable malignant potential and the fact that they are part of the "apudomas," a group of endocrinologically active tumors which secrete amines and polypeptide hormones. It was first recognized in the early 1950's that when ileal carcinoids metastasize massively to the liver, they often produce a constellation of symptoms and signs called the carcinoid syndrome. At first serotonin excess was thought to be the cause of these symptoms; later kinins were implicated. It is now clear that a whole spectrum of syndromes and many variants of the classical carcinoid syndrome may occur. Especially foregut carcinoids may secrete multiple combinations of amine and polypeptide hormones, and the patient may present with symptoms related to one or more of these humoral products.

This review will focus on the preoperative diagnosis of these tumors and the syndromes which they cause, their intraoperative management and finally the long-term surgical, pharmacologic and chemotherapeutic treatment of patients with the various carcinoid syndromes. First, a brief discussion of carcinoid tumors is appropriate.

CARCINOID TUMORS

Historical Aspects

Although several descriptions of probable carcinoid tumors were published earlier, it is generally Lubarsch[31] who is credited with the first report of a patient with multiple ileal carcinoid tumors, in 1888. He called these, "little carcinomata." Oberndorfer,[40] in 1909, coined the name carcinoid (karzinoide) for these tumors (meaning, resembling carcinoma), for, although they appeared to be carcinomas, he pointed out that they often had a benign course.

Kulchitzky,[27] in 1897, recognized that some cells of the crypts of Lieberkühn of the intestines contained granules. Ciaccio, 9 years later, called these *enterochromaffin cells* since they stained with chromium or chrome salts. In 1910, Hübschmann[21] first proposed that carcinoid tumors arise from these Kulchitzky cells. Four years later Gossett and Masson[17] demonstrated that the granules of carcinoid tumors had an affinity for silver. Hence, the name, *argentaffinoma*, has been used interchangeably with carcinoid tumors at times.

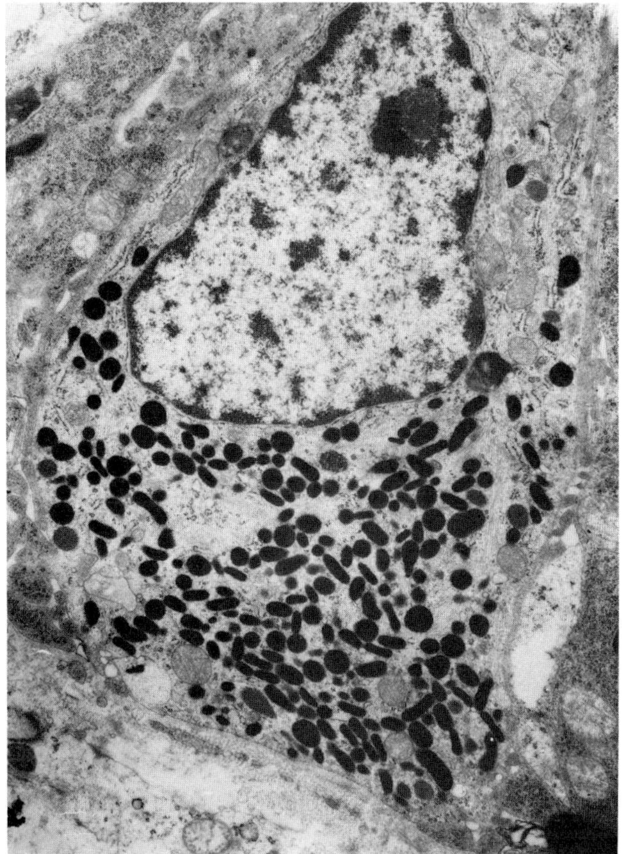

Fig. 11-1. A typical enterochromaffin (EC) cell from the ascending colon, with subnuclear granules which are uniformly electron dense. The granules are round and cigar shaped. Uranyl acetate and lead citrate. X 14,000. (Courtesy Michael C. Rosner, and Robert H. Riddell, M.D.)

Embryology and Derivation

It is now accepted that carcinoids are tumors of enterochromaffin cell (EC) origin (Fig. 11-1). These cells are rather ubiquitous and are found in most tissues derived from endoderm—gastrointestinal tract, pancreas, gallbladder, bronchial epithelium and urogenital tract. Until recently it was assumed that the EC cells also are derived from endoderm. However, now it is generally accepted that they are a part of the APUD system of cells described by Pearse.[44] As such, they are derived from neuroectoderm. They share common cytochemical and ultrastructural characteristics with other APUD cells, all of which secrete amines and polypeptide hormones.[43]

Pathology

Carcinoid tumors occur throughout the gastrointestinal tract from the esophagogastric junction to the anus (Table 11-1). They also arise frequently from the bronchus[14] or from an ovarian teratoma[50] and, in rare instances, from the testis,[63] urethra,[57] larynx,[15] thymus[22] and sacrococcygeal teratomas. About three-quarters of all abdominal carcinoid tumors are of midgut origin. Forty-five percent arise from the appendix and 28 percent from the small intestine, usually the ileum (Fig. 11-2). Carcinoids are, in fact, the most common tumor of the small intestine. The rectum is the third most common site for these tumors. Bronchial carcinoids comprise 10 percent of all carcinoids in some series[14] (Fig. 11-3).

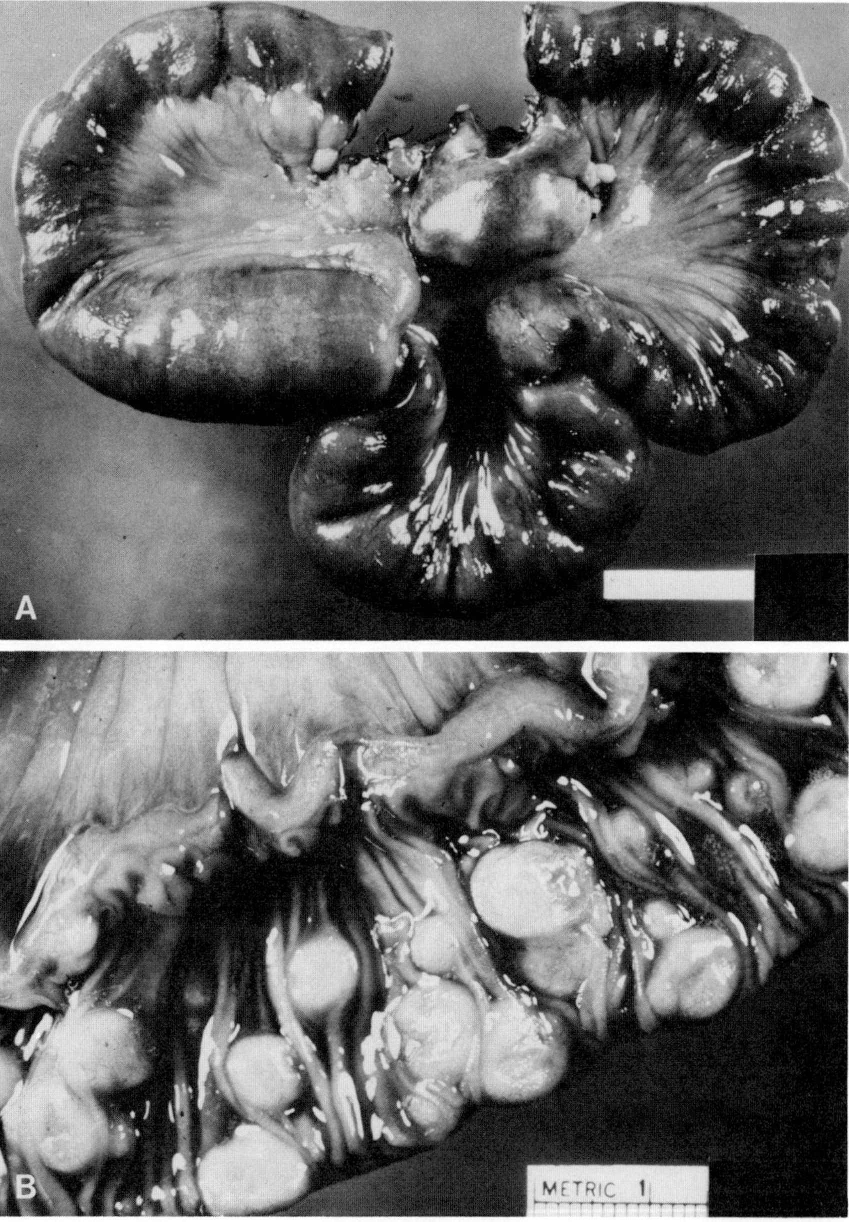

Fig. 11-2. Ileal carcinoid tumor with metastases. *(A)* The resected small bowel specimen demonstrates partial intestinal obstruction and massive nodal metastases. *(B)* The mucosal surface is studded with multiple submucosal carcinoid tumors. (Courtesy Francis H. Straus II, M.D.)

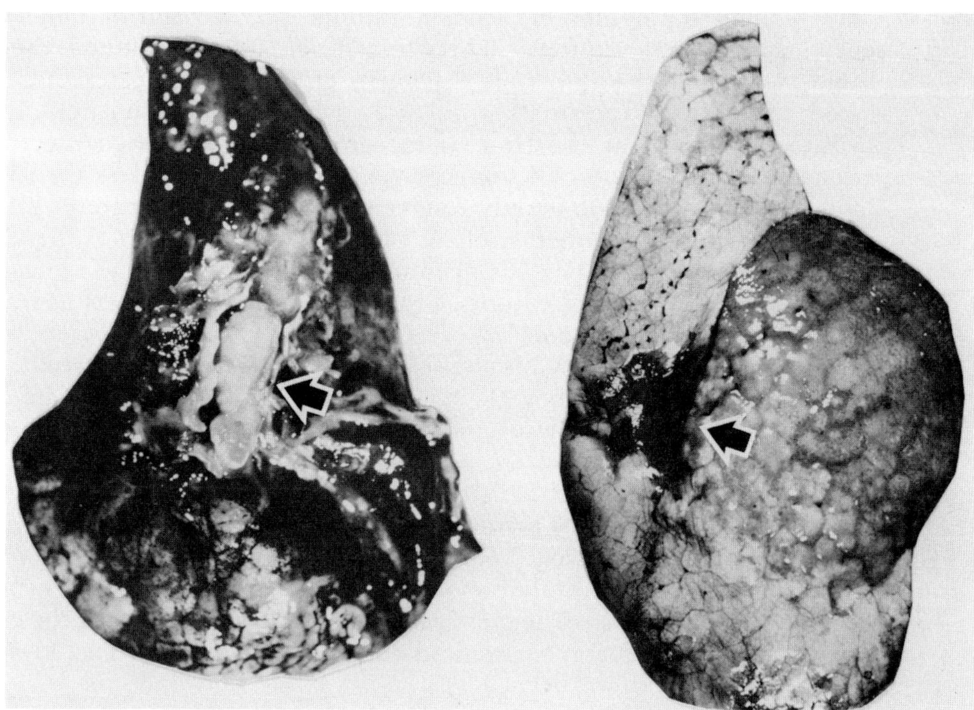

Fig. 11-3. (Left) An opened bronchus demonstrates a large bronchial carcinoid tumor *(arrow). (Right)* This lesion plugged the bronchus and resulted in an area of atalectasis *(arrow).* (Courtesy Francis H. Straus II, M.D.)

Two important characteristics of carcinoid tumors which have important clinical implications are their tendency for multicentricity and their frequent association with other concurrent malignancies. Twenty-nine percent of ileal carcinoids are multiple.[37] Separate malignancies were noted in 13 percent of appendiceal, 7 percent of rectal and 29 percent of small intestinal carcinoids in the Mayo Clinic series.[36,37] Many of these associated lesions are endocrine-secreting tumors; however, others are routine adenocarcinomas of the bowel and elsewhere.[53]

Table 11-1. Collected Series of 3,718 Abdominal Carcinoid Tumors

Primary Site	*Site of Tumor Percent of All Cases*	*Average Percent Metastasis*	*Carcinoid Syndrome, Percent of All Cases*
Esophagus	0.03	—	0
Stomach	2	23	6
Duodenum	5	20	3
Jejuno-ileum	28	34	67
Meckel's diverticulum	1	19	2
Appendix	45	2	4
Colon	2	60	4
Rectum	16	18	1
Ovary	1	6	12
Biliary tract	0.3	30	0
Pancreas	0.05	—	1

(Adapted from Wilson, H., et al. Curr. Probl. Surg., 7:1, 1970[62])

The malignant potential of carcinoid tumors and their ability to metastasize depend upon several factors. The *site of origin* of the tumor is important (Table 11-1). For example, only 2 percent of appendiceal carcinoids, but 34 percent of lesions of the small bowel and 60 percent of colon carcinoids demonstrate metastases at the time of recognition. The *size* of the tumor is perhaps most important. Of small bowel carcinoids, those less than 1 cm. in diameter were metastatic in only 2 percent of cases. Those tumors 2.0 cm. or greater were found to be metastatic in 100 percent of instances.[37] In 307 cases of rectal carcinoids, 1.7 percent of tumors less than 1 cm. had metastasized, compared to 10 percent of tumors 1 to 2 cm., and 82 percent of tumors with diameters greater than 2 cm.[2]

Carcinoid tumors of the GI tract present grossly as slightly elevated, smooth, yellow or tan nodules. They are submucosal lesions and usually are covered with an intact mucosa. Microscopically midgut tumors often appear as sheets of monotonous polygonal cells, whereas foregut carcinoids typically have a more trabecular pattern. (Fig. 11-4). The cytoplasm of midgut tumors contains granules which stain black with ammoniacal silver nitrate. This is called a positive *argentaffin* reaction. Foregut and rectal carcinoids are *argyrophil* in nature. They will accumulate cytoplasmic silver deposits only in the presence of reducing agents. The electron microscopic appearance of the cells of a typical midgut and foregut carcinoid tumor differs greatly (Fig. 11-5). The

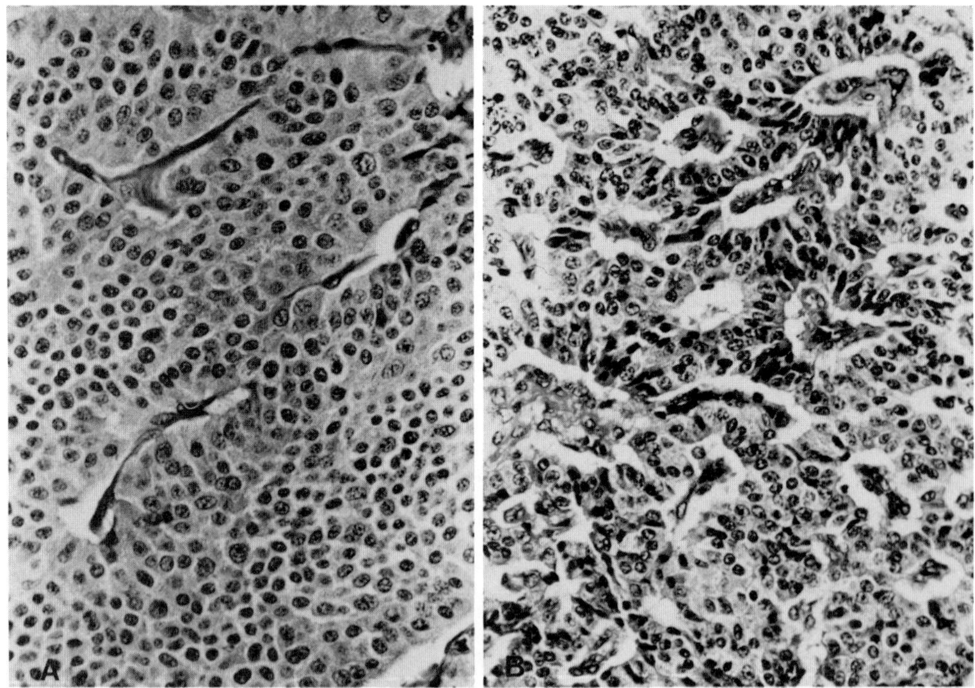

Fig. 11-4. The light microscopic appearance of a typical midgut and foregut carcinoid tumor. *(A)* Ileal carcinoid; solid nests of relatively small, uniform cells. H. & E., X 300. *(B)* Bronchial carcinoid; a trabecular pattern of anastomosing ribbons of tumor cells. H. & E., X 300. (Courtesy Wilbur A. Franklin, M.D.)

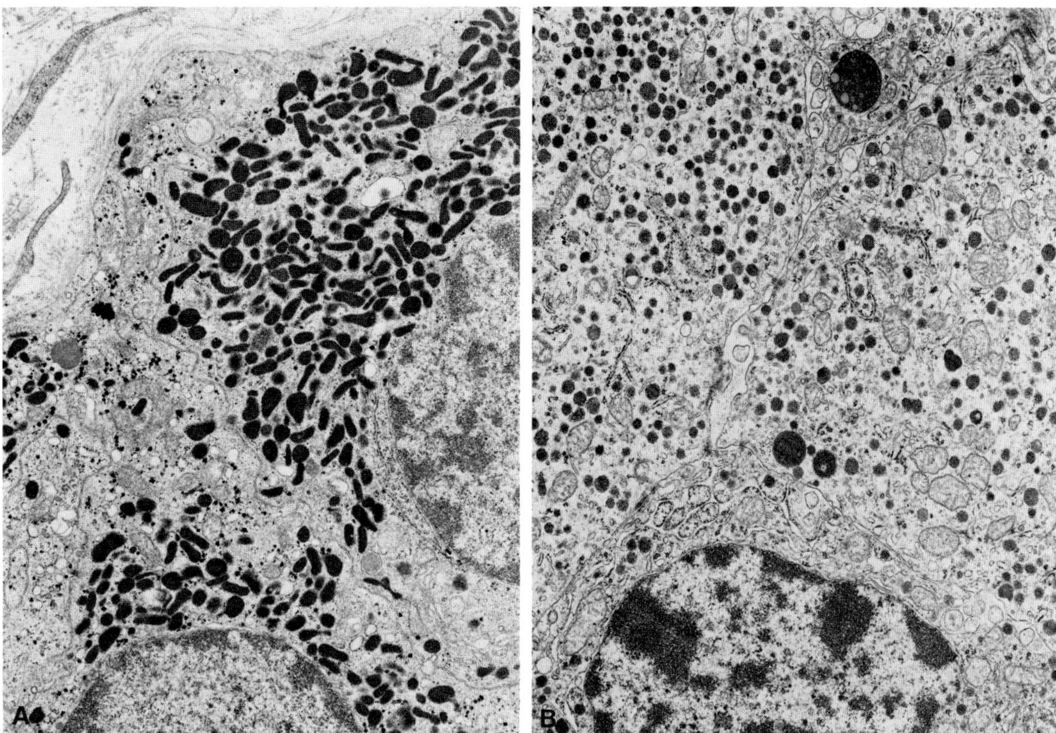

Fig. 11-5. (A) Electron micrograph of an ileal carcinoid tumor. Several cells are seen that contain cytoplasmic secretory granules which are round, oval or dumbbell shaped and measure up to 3,500 Å in greatest dimension. Note the similarity of these tumor cells to the normal midgut enterochromaffin (EC) cell. Uranyl acetate and lead citrate. X 18,000. *(B)* Electron micrograph of several cells of a bronchial carcinoid tumor. The cytoplasmic granules are round and measure up to approximately 1,800 Å. Uranyl acetate and lead citrate. X 18,000. (Courtesy Andrew M. Churg, M.D.)

cells of rectal carcinoids, although generally thought of as being hormonally inactive, may contain granules which are similar in appearance to those of medullary carcinomas of the thyroid.[16]

For many years carcinoid tumors were divided into benign and malignant categories. Now most pathologists agree that all carcinoids, or certainly all extra-appendiceal carcinoids, should be considered to be potentially malignant lesions. The usual criteria of cell anaplasia and mitoses are not applicable to carcinoids, and definite evidence of malignancy must be determined by the demonstration of gross or microscopic invasiveness.

Carcinoid tumors invade the bowel locally involving first the muscularis and then the serosa (Fig. 11-6). Regional lymph node metastases almost never occur in the absence of local invasion. Massive metastases to lymph nodes are common, the liver being the most common site of distant metastases. The presence of lung metastases indicates far-advanced disease. Other metastases are unusual but include bone (osteoblastic and osteolytic), skin, brain, ovary, breast, pancreas, etc.

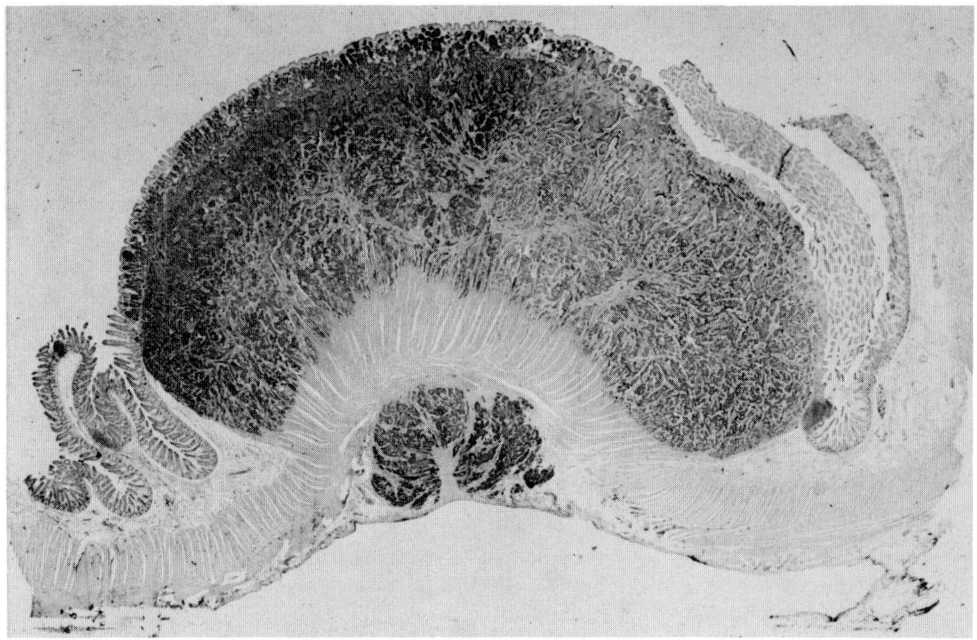

Fig. 11-6. The light microscopic appearance of an ileal carcinoid tumor from a patient with massive liver metastases and a carcinoid syndrome. The primary tumor has invaded the muscularis propria and a serosal implant is clearly seen.

THE CLASSIC CARCINOID SYNDROME

It was long known that human serum but not plasma contained a vasoconstricting substance. In 1948, Rapport and coworkers[49] isolated this and called it *serotonin*. By 1952 it was determined that the origin of this aminc was the Kulchitsky cells.[11] In the next 2 years serotonin was isolated from a carcinoid tumor,[28] elevated levels of this amine were found in the blood and urine of two patients with carcinoid tumors,[46] and the malignant carcinoid syndrome was clearly delineated by groups in the United States, Switzerland and Sweden.[23,54,58]

Serotonin

Since serotonin plays a role in the pathogenesis of the carcinoid syndrome, it is appropriate to briefly examine its properties and metabolism. Serotonin is an indolealkylamine which has potent pharmacologic effects. In man, its biosynthesis is accomplished almost exclusively by the enterochromaffin cells, by some other APUD cells and by some elements of the central nervous system. It is synthesized from the amino acid tryptophan (Fig. 11-7). Normally only about 2 percent (10 mg.) of the daily ingested tryptophan is converted to serotonin. In patients with carcinoid tumors, however, much larger quantities of this amino acid (up to 60 percent) are converted to serotonin at the expense of protein and niacin production.

Most serotonin in the body is found in the cells which produce it. In the bloodstream, platelets actively concentrate serotonin, so that virtually all of the normal blood level of 0.1 to 0.3 μg./ml. is found in these cells.

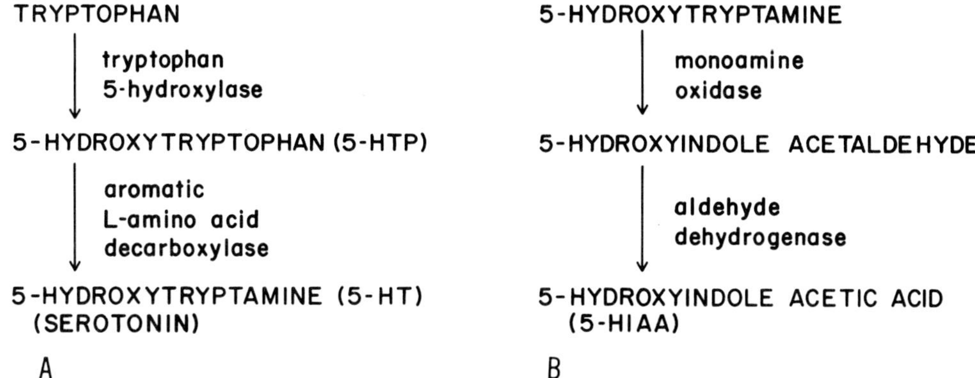

Fig. 11-7. The major metabolic pathway for *(A)* synthesis and *(B)* degradation of serotonin (5-hydroxytryptamine).

The major organs which metabolize serotonin are the liver and the lung. This is due to their high levels of monamine oxidase. Up to 80 percent of this amine in portal blood is degraded by the liver, whereas up to 98 percent of serotonin which gains access to the systemic circulation is removed during one passage through the lungs.[60] The major pathway of metabolism for serotonin is illustrated in Figure 11-7.

Clinical Presentation and Pathogenesis

The classic carcinoid syndrome is caused by the humoral secretions of carcinoid tumors which originate in the midgut—the jejunum, ileum, Meckel's diverticulum and the appendix. In its complete form it involves several different organ systems—vasomotor, cardiopulmonary and gastrointestinal (Table 11-2).

Table 11-2. Symptoms and Signs of the Classical Carcinoid Syndrome

Major Manifestations	*Mean Incidence (%)*
Hepatomegaly	70
Cutaneous flushing	75
Vasomotor changes	
Hypotension	
Diarrhea	70
Endocardial lesions	50
Bronchoconstriction	20
Venous telangiectasis	50
Edema	52
Minor Manifestations	
Pellagra	5
Peptic ulcers	5
Arthralgias	6
Fibrosis	
Retroperitoneal	
Peyronie's disease	
Myopathy	

(Adapted from Thörsson,[58] Rosenberg[55] and Levine[29])

Hepatomegaly. Most carcinoids are of gastrointestinal origin and are consequently drained by the portal venous system to the liver. Since the liver metabolizes most of the serotonin to which it is exposed, the carcinoid syndrome does not occur from a GI primary tumor until massive liver replacement by tumor has occurred. At that time serotonin or other active hormones can reach the systemic circulation and symptoms occur. Thus, hepatomegaly is common in these instances. On the other hand, bronchial carcinoids, ovarian teratomas and other rare carcinoids which drain directly into the systemic circulation may result in a carcinoid syndrome before any metastases are present. Two-thirds of all carcinoid syndromes are caused by tumors of small bowel origin (see Table 11-1).

Cutaneous Flushing. Flushing of the skin occurs early in most patients with a carcinoid syndrome (Fig. 11-8). The flush may be deep red or even simulate cyanosis, but more commonly, patients present with flushing that looks like the blush of nervousness or of alcohol excess. The face and neck is involved first. Later the upper trunk and extremities may be affected as well. Flushes tend to be precipitated by ingestion of certain foods such as cheese or alcohol or by exertion, pain, straining at stool or emotional stress in some individuals. In most patients the flushes only last for several minutes; however in some patients, particularly those with bronchial or other foregut variant syndromes, it may last for several days and be accompanied by facial edema.[18]

Although serotonin was the original humoral agent found in carcinoid tumors, it soon became apparent that hypersecretion of this one agent cannot explain all of the manifestation of the carcinoid syndrome. In most patients whose flush was induced by epinephrine, hepatic vein serotonin was found to be unaltered.[52] Furthermore, intravenous infusion of serotonin produces hypermotility of the gut and hypotension but not a typical flush.[30] It is now felt that bradykinin, a nine-amino acid polypeptide may play the major role in these flushes.[33] Some carcinoid tumors have been demonstrated to contain

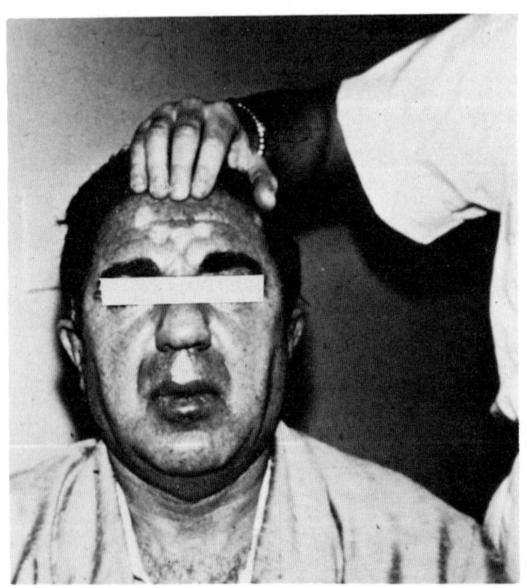

Fig. 11-8. A patient with a bronchial carcinoid tumor shows a severe vivid cutaneous flush characteristic of a foregut carcinoid tumor. Just prior to taking this picture, the physician at his side pressed the patient's forehead with his hand. Note the pale imprint of his fingers, further demonstrating the magnitude of the flushing. (Courtesy Richard R. P. Warner, M.D. The Gastrointestinal Division of the Department of Medicine, The Mount Sinai School of Medicine of the City University of New York, and the Carcinoid Tumor and Serotonin Research Foundation, Inc.)

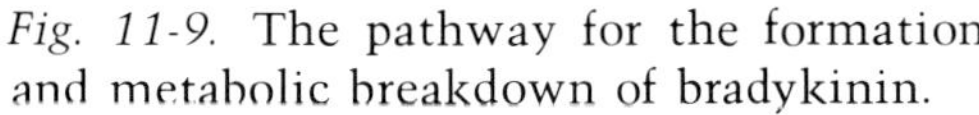

Fig. 11-9. The pathway for the formation and metabolic breakdown of bradykinin.

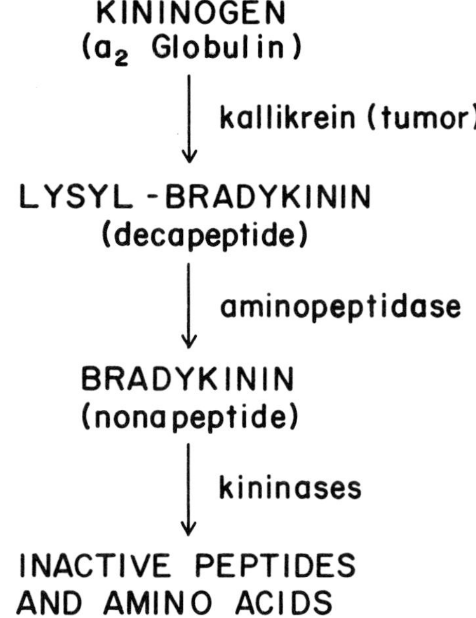

kallikrein, an enzyme which catalyzes the formation of bradykinin from a serum $\alpha_2$globulin (Fig. 11-9). Serum bradykinin has been found to be elevated in some patients with carcinoid tumors.[39] This peptide is one of the most potent vasodilators known. It also produces increased intestinal motility and bronchoconstriction. When administered to normals or to patients with carcinoid tumors it produces a flush which is sometimes indistinguishable from spontaneous flushes. Endogenous epinephrine release and alcohol ingestion have been demonstrated to release kinins.

Prostaglandin E has also been found to be elevated in the serum of most patients with carcinoid tumors and in others with medullary carcinoma of the thyroid who may flush as well.[24] Infusion of these fatty acids into man also results in flushing and hypermotility of the GI tract.

Finally, serotonin or one of its metabolites has not been entirely ruled out as a cause for some flushing. It has been demonstrated in several patients with carcinoid syndrome that flushing and hypotension followed calcium infusion. At the time of symptoms serotonin was markedly elevated.[25] Thus, each of these agents or a combination of them may play a role in the pathogenesis of the classical carcinoid flush.

Venous Telangiectasia. This pattern develops in about half of the patients during the course of their disease. Telangiectasia is most prominent over the nose, upper lip and cheeks and a "butterfly" pattern may occur. It is very similar in appearance to the acne rosacea of alcoholics.[29] The pathogenesis of this lesion is unknown.

Vasomotor Changes. Hypotension (not hypertension) frequently accompanies the attacks of flushing. The kinins, serotonin, prostaglandins and histamine may each produce this effect.[29]

Diarrhea. Severe borborygmus or diarrhea occurs in a large majority of patients with the carcinoid syndrome and is often the most disabling part of the disease. Urgency, with frequent passage of watery diarrhea or flatus is common. Increased bowel motility (i.e., shortened transit time) is usually stated as the cause. However, recent studies of patients with carcinoid tumors and with medullary carcinoma of the thyroid, who have a carcinoid syndrome, have demonstrated that abnormal fluid and electrolyte fluxes of the small intestine are commonly present and may be the cause for the watery diarrhea.[3] Occasionally patients may develop a malabsorption syndrome, as well.

Bradykinin and prostaglandin E may each cause hypermotility. Calcitonin, elevated in many cases of carcinoid tumors, has also been demonstrated to result in the secretion of fluid and electrolytes into the small intestine of the experimental animal.[19] Motilin, a newly described peptide, may also play a role. However, diarrhea correlates best to hyperserotoninemia. In addition, this symptom is frequently well controlled by anti-serotonin drugs.[29]

Endocardial Lesions. About 50 percent of patients with the classic carcinoid syndrome develop characteristic endocardial lesions during the course of their disease. Fibrous tissue, similar to collagen, is deposited on the endocardium and valve cusps. These lesions are most prominent on the right side of the heart except when a right-to-left shunt or a bronchial carcinoid is present. Then, similar lesions may occur in the chambers of the left heart. The most common valvular lesions are tricuspid insufficiency and pulmonary stenosis. Clinically these patients may present with right-sided congestive heart failure. A high incidence of supraventricular extrasystoles and tachyarrhythmias may occur. High cardiac output may be present in patients who flush.

The pathogenesis of the fibrosis is unknown. Serotonin, and for that matter methysergide, a serotonin antagonist, each has resulted in retroperitoneal fibrosis. However, strong evidence against the role of this amine has also been compiled.[51] Some investigators feel that bradykinin effects may be causative, due to increased capillary permeability.

Bronchial Constriction. Asthma occurs in only 10 to 20 percent of patients with the classic carcinoid syndrome. Serotonin, prostaglandins, bradykinin and histamine are each known to be potent bronchoconstrictors.

Edema. Half of the patients with the carcinoid syndrome develop edema.[18] This may be due to right-sided heart failure; however, hypoproteinemia, found in most of these patients, generally plays a role.

Pellagralike Skin Lesions. Since tryptophan is diverted by the tumor from the biosynthesis of niacin, 5 percent of patients develop classic pellagra (i.e., pigmented skin lesions in areas of exposure to sunlight), diarrhea and organic brain syndrome.[29]

Fibrosis. Retroperitoneal fibrosis accompanies some carcinoid tumors and may cause intestinal obstruction in some patients by kinking the bowel; ureteral obstruction has also occurred. Several instances of Peyronie's disease, dense fibrosis of the dorsal shaft of the penis, have also been reported in patients with the carcinoid syndrome.[5] This may represent a further manifestation of the fibrosis.

Arthropathy. Stiffness of the hand joints, pain on movement of the joints and pain on releasing an object that was tightly gripped, have been reported.[48] Loss of bone density, multiple cystic areas of the phalanges and erosions of the interphalangeal joint surfaces occur in these patients. Chronic serotonin excess has been proposed as a possible cause.

Myopathy. Several cases of carcinoid syndrome with proximal myopathy and another with ocular myopathy have been reported.[4] This lesion may be reproduced in rats by injection of serotonin. The incidence of myopathy may be much higher than currently described since weakness is generally attributed to overall debilitation.

Peptic Ulcers. It is unclear whether or not a true increase in peptic ulceration occurs in patients with the classical carcinoid syndrome.

VARIANT CARCINOID SYNDROMES

Carcinoid tumors, especially of the foregut, have the potential for secreting numerous amine and polypeptide hormones and producing syndromes which deviate from the classic carcinoid syndrome. Two patterns are seen with sufficient frequency to be called variant syndromes. These are associated with bronchial[34] and gastric[38] carcinoids. Whereas many individuals with these two lesions manifest parts of the classic syndrome, others present with these specific variant syndromes.

Bronchial Carcinoid Syndrome

Rather than having frequent transient flushes, individuals with these tumors may have prolonged and severe flushing attacks often lasting up to 3 or 4 days.[18,34]. The flushes are accompanied by periorbital and facial edema, marked lacrimation, salivation, sweating and an increased temperature and pulse rate. Marked diarrhea, hypotension, nausea, vomiting and asthma frequently accompany the flush. Anxiety and disorientation may precede the attack. Patients with bronchial carcinoids often have left-sided endocardial lesions. Mitral and aortic valvular disease may result in left heart failure with pulmonary edema.

The cause of this distinct syndrome is unknown. However, it is thought by some to represent the effects of kinin release.[29] Patients with this syndrome frequently respond to treatment with glucocorticoids, which are of no benefit in the classical syndrome. Prednisone treatment results in a marked decrease in flushing and other signs and symptoms in many of these patients. Corticosteroids have been demonstrated to prevent kallikrein release in in-vitro systems; the same may hold true for bronchial carcinoids.

Bronchial carcinoids tend to be more aggressive than their midgut counterparts. They metastasize to bone (osteolytic and osteoblastic), skin, brain, heart, lungs, thyroid, kidneys and lymph nodes. Finally, they are more frequently associated with multiple endocrine adenomatoses, acromegaly and Cushing's disease than are other carcinoid tumors.

Gastric Carcinoid Syndrome

Patients with these tumors frequently have a distinctive flush which starts as vivid red patches with sharply defined, serpentine borders and often occurs after meals.[38] As time passes, these patches become confluent. Diarrhea may not be prominent. There is an increased incidence of peptic ulcer associated with gastric carcinoids. The atypical flush and peptic ulcerations may be caused by the secretion of histamine from some of these tumors. In addition, most gastric carcinoids, as well as some other foregut carcinoids and a rare midgut carcinoid, lack the enzyme decarboxylase and thus, they secrete 5-hydroxytryptophan.[29] These patients excrete increased amounts of serotonin, 5-hydroxytryptophan and 5-hydroxyindoleacetic acid (5-HIAA) in their urine. Methyldopa (Aldomet) administration frequently benefits those patients whose tumors lack decarboxylase, whereas it is of little or no value in the classic syndrome.

CARCINOID SYNDROME FROM NONCARCINOID TUMORS

Lesions other than carcinoid tumors may at times secrete serotonin or 5-hydroxytryptophan and present with symptoms of the carcinoid syndrome. These include medullary carcinomas of the thyroid (which also secrete kallikrein and prostaglandins), oat cell carcinomas of the lung, pancreatic islet cell cancers, neuroblastomas and other chromaffin tumors. Very rarely, squamous cell cancers of the lung, hepatoma and biliary duct tumors may be associated with increased 5-HIAA as well.[29]

CARCINOIDS AND OTHER ASSOCIATED ENDOCRINOPATHIES

Carcinoid tumors are associated with other tumors, both hormonally active and inactive, in as many as 25 to 50 percent of cases. Often these tumors are derived from other APUD cells. Carcinoids may be associated with both types of multiple endocrine neoplasia syndromes, MEN-I and MEN-II. Among all carcinoids, those of foregut origin are most likely to secrete endocrinologically active peptide substances and to be associated with pluriglandular syndromes, (especially bronchial carcinoids). When several carcinoid tumors are present one may secrete one substance whereas another secretes a different peptide or amine.

The biologically active substances which are known to be secreted from or associated with carcinoid tumors are listed below.

Biologically Active Substances Produced by or Associated With Carcinoids and Carcinoid-Islet Cell Tumors

Frequently	*Less Frequently*	
Serotonin	ACTH	Gastrin
Kallikrein	MSH?	Calcitonin
Histamine	Growth hormone (GH) or GH-releasing factors	Parathyroid hormone
Prostaglandins		Catecholamines?
	Insulin	ADH?
	Glucagon	Substance P

Acromegaly may accompany bronchial and other carcinoids. When a pituitary adenoma is present, this combination is thought to represent a genetic disorder of neuroectodermal origin. However, several recent studies suggest that growth hormone or a growth hormone-releasing factor may be secreted from the carcinoid tumor, itself.[7] Feldman and associates[12] found that 45 percent of patients with active carcinoid syndromes had elevated basal growth hormone levels. Hyperserotoninemia may possibly be the cause of the increased secretion of growth hormone as well.

Cushing's Syndrome. Carcinoid tumors, most commonly of bronchial origin, have been demonstrated to secrete ectopic ACTH and to produce Cushing's syndrome with adrenocortical hyperplasia.[41] Extrapulmonary sites which have been implicated include carcinoids of the appendix, stomach, pancreas, thymus and ovary. Hyperpigmentation has been considered by some to be due to secretion of melanocyte-stimulating hormone (MSH).

Peptic Ulcers. Pancreatic carcinoids and carcinoid-islet cell tumors of the duodenum frequently secrete gastrin.[13,61] Patients often present with the Zollinger-Ellison (Z-E) syndrome with or without a concurrent carcinoid syndrome.

Hyperglycemia. Hyperglucagonemia resulting in mild diabetes mellitus has been reported in combination with hyperserotoninemia in several tumors.[13]

Hypoglycemia. Hyperinsulinism and hyperserotoninemia may occur together in the same patient resulting in simultaneous hypoglycemia and a carcinoid syndrome.[13]

Hyperparathyroidism. Parathyroid hyperplasia has been reported to be present in association with bronchial and thymic carcinoids as part of the MEN-I syndrome. Hyperparathyroidism has been proved in several cases of ileal carcinoids[56] as well. Increased serum parathyroid hormone (PTH) without hypercalcemia has been detected in patients with an ovarian, rectal and ileal carcinoid.[26] Ectopic secretion of PTH by a gastric carcinoid has been reported.[9]

Hypercalcitoninemia. Increased serum calcitonin has been reported in patients with carcinoid tumors of foregut, midgut and hindgut origin in the absence of medullary carcinomas of the thyroid.[9,26]

It thus appears that many carcinoid tumors secrete one or more peptide or amine substances with the resultant development of many combinations of clinical syndromes. To illustrate this point, Pearse and associates[45] recently demonstrated by immunohistochemistry that of 46 tumors with the morphologic appearance of carcinoid or carcinoid-islet cell tumors, only 16 contained no evidence of peptide production. The remainder included 10 gastrinomas, 6 insulinomas, 5 calcitoninomas, 4 corticotrophinomas (ACTH-producing), 1 vipoma (VIP-producing) and 4 tumors which produced more than one peptide.

PREOPERATIVE DIAGNOSIS OF CARCINOID SYNDROMES

Carcinoid tumors which are totally asymptomatic may be found on physical examination as an abdominal, testicular or ovarian mass. A submucosal mass is often felt on rectal examination. A routine chest roentgenogram may show a superior mediastinal mass or a lung nodule. Other carcinoid tumors may produce symptoms related to their tumor mass. Patients with these tumors present with atelectasis, pneumonia or hemoptysis in cases of bronchial carcinoids, or intestinal obstruction, intussusception or biliary obstruction in gastrointestinal carcinoid tumors. Pain in the abdomen may be due to peptic ulceration, necrosis of hepatic metastases, or rarely to infarction of the intestines. Many appendiceal carcinoids are found incidently, however, and acute appendicitis from blockage of the lumen by tumor may occur.

Techniques for preoperative localization of tumor are well known and include barium studies, scintigraphy with isotopes, angiography, ultrasound and

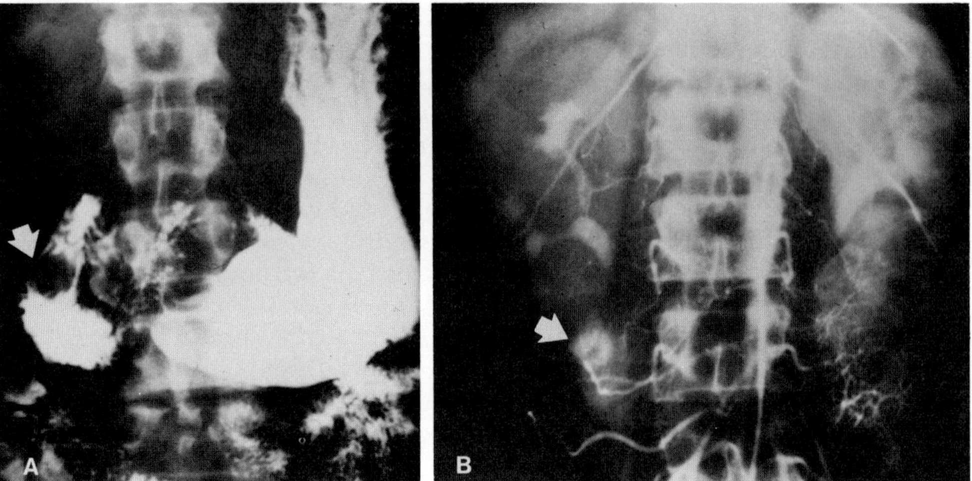

Fig. 11-10. Successful localization of a carcinoid, islet-cell tumor of the duodenum. *(A)* A barium meal study demonstrates a filling defect in the second part of the duodenum *(arrow)*. *(B)* Angiographic visualization. The characteristic tumor blush is present in the same location *(arrow)*.

endoscopy with biopsy (Fig. 11-10). Sound judgment in the use of each procedure is essential since, for example, massive bleeding may occur if a bronchial carcinoid is biopsied through the bronchoscope.

Other patients may be diagnosed first because of the effects of hormones secreted from the tumor or the recognition that a polyglandular syndrome is present. It is important that physicians be aware of the manifestations of the classic and variant carcinoid syndromes and of the effects of ectopic peptide secretions. These symptoms are often subtle and insidious in onset and development. Patients with early carcinoid syndrome may be thought to have a more common problem. Flushing and diarrhea occurring with drinking, for example, might be considered to be the effect of the alcohol itself; facial telangiectasia and even hepatomegaly could be considered further evidence of chronic alcoholism.

Chemical Tests

Urinary 5-Hydroxyindoleacetic Acid (5-HIAA). The single most useful chemical test for diagnosing a carcinoid is the proper measurement of urinary 5-HIAA. Most patients with carcinoid syndrome excrete increased amounts of 5-HIAA in the urine; however, rarely this measurement is normal although a carcinoid syndrome is present. This is especially true if diarrhea is not a prominent symptom.

The normal value of 5-HIAA in most laboratories is 2 to 9 mg. in 24 hours. Levels above 15 mg. in patients without malabsorption and above 30 mg. in patients with malabsorption provide strong evidence for the diagnosis of a carcinoid or some other serotonin-producing tumor. Proper collection of the specimen is important.[29] If the jar contains acid (as is used for catecholamines) the result of 5-HIAA will be falsely low. During collection of the urinary specimen, no fruits, fruit juices or nuts should be eaten since it is known that bananas, tomatoes, avocados, red plums, walnuts and eggplants contain serotonin and may falsely elevate the 5-HIAA values. The following drugs also interfere with the assay and cause elevated values: glyceryl guaiacolate, phenacetin and mephenesin. Falsely low values of 5-HIAA may be caused by phenothiazines and methenamine mandelate. Methyldopa, ethanol and MAO inhibitors also give low values. Thus, for correct results, a proper diet and the avoidance of these drugs are essential.

Other 5-Hydroxyindoles. Urinary serotonin and 5-hydroxytryptophan may be measured by paper chromatography. These assays are particularly helpful in identifying patients whose tumors lack decarboxylase.[29] Such patients excrete increased urinary serotonin and 5-hydroxytryptophan as well as elevated urinary 5-HIAA. Most midgut carcinoids contain decarboxylase and excrete only 5-HIAA, whereas foregut tumors sometimes lack this enzyme and excrete this different pattern. Thus, the urinary metabolites may aid both in the diagnosis of a carcinoid tumor and in its anatomic localization.

Other Screening Tests

Blood serotonin, measured in a basal state or following provocative tests may aid in the diagnosis of carcinoid tumors. Normal values for this amine are 0.1 to 0.3 μg./ml. in most laboratories. The presence of polyglandular disease or ectopic hormone production may be detected by the following screening tests: blood glucose, serum calcium, electrolytes and cortisol; urinary 17-hydroxycorticosteroids, gastric acidity and an x-ray of the skull. When appropriate, serum gastrin, glucagon, insulin, ACTH, growth hormone, parathyroid hormone and calcitonin may be determined by radioimmunoassay techniques. Histamine, prostaglandin and bradykinin measurements are available in some research laboratories.

Provocative Tests

When a carcinoid syndrome is suspected, either alcohol ingestion or several specific tests may be used to aid in the diagnosis.

Epinephrine Test. Agents with beta-adrenergic receptor-stimulating activity, such as epinephrine, have been found to induce flushes in most but not all patients who flush spontaneously from the carcinoid syndrome.[59] This is thought to be mediated by release of active kallikrein from the tumor. The patient, under strict control, is given 1 μg. of epinephrine. Subsequent doses of 2, 5 and 10 μg. are given at intervals of 10 minutes or until a flush occurs. A positive result is the appearance of a flush 45 to 90 seconds after administration of the epinephrine. Hypotension and tachycardia frequently accompany this response. A negative result is facial blanching or transient hypertension.

Calcium Provocative Test. Calcium infusion has been reported by Kaplan and associates[25] to result in a severe, typical carcinoid attack in several patients with a carcinoid syndrome. Flushing, weakness, hypotension, nausea and the passage of stool or flatus occurred. Kinin levels were not determined in these patients; however, blood serotonin increased markedly and correlated with symptomatology in these patients (Fig. 11-11).

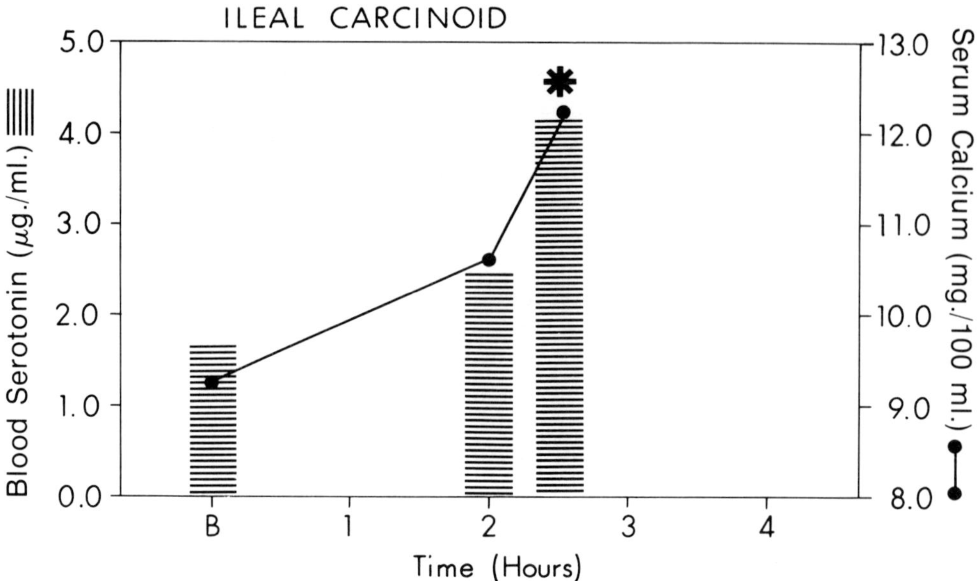

Fig. 11-11. Calcium infusion into a patient with a classic carcinoid syndrome resulted in severe flushing and other symptoms at 2½ hours after its onset (*). Blood serotonin concentrations, elevated in the basal state, increased markedly at the time of the carcinoid attack. (Kaplan, E. L., et al.: Am. J. Surg., *123*:173, 1972)

Localization of a Carcinoid Tumor

Once it is established that a patient has a carcinoid syndrome, the localization of the tumor may be of utmost importance. It is well known that most carcinoid tumors occur in the GI tract and that the presence of the carcinoid syndrome usually signifies massive liver involvement with tumor. However, special attention should be directed to rule out the presence of a medullary carcinoma of the thyroid, and carcinoids of the testes, ovary, bronchus, larynx and mediastinum which are potentially completely curable.

TREATMENT OF CARCINOID TUMORS WITHOUT CARCINOID SYNDROME

Although an average of 15 percent of all gastrointestinal carcinoids will metastasize, only 6 percent of those tumors with metastases will ever result in a carcinoid syndrome.[62] Hence, treatment of the tumor, per se, is of considerable importance.

Surgical Considerations

In this group, anesthesia presents no difficulties since no humoral factors are involved. At operation, a careful exploration is imperative because of the known high incidence of associated APUD tumors or other carcinomas. The operative approach differs from site to site but always depends upon an assessment of the size of the tumor, the degree of local invasion and the presence or absence of regional or distant spread. In most areas, lesions greater than 1 cm. in diameter should be treated as frank carcinomas, and the principles of a curative cancer resection should apply if no distant metastases are identified. In lesions less than 1 cm. in diameter, complete local resection may be adequate if no invasion of the muscularis propria or lymph node spread is demonstrated.

Tumors of the jejunum or ileum should be removed by segmental resection even if they are small. If they are larger than 1 cm., are multiple, or show local invasion or lymph node spread without distant metastases, a wide resection should be performed excising all areas of lymph node drainage. In lesions of the terminal ileum a right hemicolectomy should be performed as well in order to encompass the lymph node-bearing area. *Appendiceal* carcinoids are a special case since they are generally small and rarely have true metastatic disease.[36] Appendectomy with removal of the mesoappendix should suffice for most small incidental lesions. If lymph node involvement is recognized, if the lesion is larger than 1 cm., or if local spread is apparent, a right hemicolectomy and node resection should be performed.

Rectal carcinoids are frequently small and generally asymptomatic. They present a special problem because of their anatomic position, since an abdominal perineal resection is necessary, in many instances, if an aggressive tumor is demonstrated. Most authors[42,47] agree that if a rectal carcinoid is less than 2 cm., it should be completely excised transanally and examined for local invasion of the muscularis. If none is present, frequent proctoscopic examinations should be performed. If the lesion is 2 cm. or greater in diameter or if it shows evidence of invasion, it should be treated as a frank carcinoma. An appropriate cancer operation should be performed in these patients since lymph node metastases will be present in most.[2] Other *colon* carcinoids should be treated aggressively because of their high malignancy potential.

Gastric carcinoid tumors generally require gastrectomy with node dissection. The duodenal or gastric ulcers which accompany them should be treated by a standard ulcer operation if hypergastrinemia is not present. *Duodenal* carcinoids or *carcinoid islet-cell* tumors may be treated by local excision if they are very small. However, a radical pancreatoduodenectomy (Whipple operation) should be performed if the tumors are demonstrated to invade the muscularis or if local node involvement without hepatic metastases is present.

Ovarian carcinoids should be resected and a careful examination of the bowel should be performed. Whereas most of these tumors are primary teratomas of the ovary, others represent metastases from bowel lesions.[50] *Bronchial* carcinoids should be treated by lobectomy or pneumonectomy depending upon the location and size of the lesion. Finally, rare lesions of the mediastinum, testes or urogenital tract should be treated by wide excision and appropriate node dissections. Palliative resection or bypass operations of abdominal carcinoids are sometimes necessary in patients with widespread metastases because of bowel obstruction or bleeding.

TREATMENT OF CARCINOID TUMORS

Anesthetic Considerations

The availability of a skilled anesthesiologist who is familiar with the pharmacology of the carcinoid syndrome is imperative. The anesthesiologist must be prepared to deal with a number of emergencies related to the release of serotonin, bradykinin or other substances during induction and operation.

The most important consideration of anesthetic management is the parodoxic response of these patients to endogenously or exogenously administered beta-adrenergic receptor agonists. These agents cause what has been called "bradykinin shock" (i.e., flushing and hypotension). Thus, all drugs and anesthetic agents which stimulate endogenous release of catechols should be avoided. An endotracheal tube is imperative since bronchospasm may occur. Curare should be avoided since this may result in bronchoconstriction of its own. If hypotension occurs, colloids and crystalloids should be administered to fill the intravascular space, since the fall in blood pressure may be due to vasodilation. If a vasoconstrictor agent is required, an alpha-receptor agonist such as phenylephrine (Neosynephrine) or methoxamine (Vasoxyl) should be used since they will not cause flushing. Finally, these patients may be slow in awakening because of the central nervous system effects of serotonin.

Surgical Considerations

All patients with the carcinoid syndrome should be studied and probably explored so that potentially curable lesions outside of the GI tract can be resected. Hepatomegaly, per se, is not a contraindication to exploration since this may be due to congestive heart failure. In abdominal carcinoids, although a curative resection is most unlikely, the following operative principles should apply: (1) As much tumor mass as possible should be safely removed. Carcinoids are often slow-growing tumors and for long periods of time, patients may be more troubled by systemic humoral symptoms than by tumor growth itself. Removal of significant tumor bulk may greatly ameliorate these symptoms. (2) The primary tumor should be excised, whenever possible, to prevent intestinal obstruction, intussusception or bleeding. If this cannot be done an intestinal bypass procedure may be considered.

Local enucleation of multiple tumor metastases from the liver has been tried with some benefit. Formal hepatic lobectomy should be reserved for those unusual instances in which all or most metastatic tumor is localized to one lobe of the liver. One must be certain that sufficient normal functioning hepatic parenchyma is present in the other lobe before embarking upon this procedure.

Hepatic artery ligation has been tried as a treatment for liver metastases with limited success. Hepatic dearterialization (i.e., ligation of the hepatic artery and all of its collateral circulation and division of the gastrohepatic omentum) has resulted in tumor necrosis and a beneficial initial relief of symptoms in several patients who were recently reported.[1,32] This mode of therapy should be used only in patients with good hepatic reserve.

Some patients with carcinoid heart disease may benefit from valvular reconstruction or replacement if they are in heart failure. A patient with severe tricuspid valve disease was operated upon 14 years after the onset of the carcinoid syndrome. Replacement of her tricuspid valve resulted in the resolution of ascites and edema which had been previously refractive to chemotherapeutic therapy.[20]

Nutritional Therapy

Patients with carcinoid syndrome are generally nutritionally depleted due to diversion of tryptophan from its role in protein and niacin synthesis.[29] Niacin, 50 mg. or more must be added to the diet of each person with a carcinoid syndrome. A therapeutic multivitamin pill daily will suffice. Removal from the diet of all food which incites a flush is imperative. Intravenous albumin therapy may be necessary to treat the edema which is due to hypoproteinemia, in severe cases of nutritional debility. The control of diarrhea and malabsorption will usually benefit the general nutritional status of the patient.

Pharmacologic Therapy

Diarrhea. Diarrhea will often respond to sufficient doses of various narcotic preparations: paregoric, codeine, tincture of opium or Lomotil. However, certain specific agents may be especially beneficial and include the following:

1. Methysergide (Sansert). This serotonin antagonist is begun with a dose of one 2-mg. tablet twice a day with meals. The maximal dose is generally 16 mg. daily. Fibrosis of the retroperitoneum, lungs and heart valves has occurred. These complications are minimized by suspending treatment for 3 to 4 weeks after every 6-month course of therapy.
2. Cyproheptadine (Periactin). An antiserotonin and antihistaminic drug. The average effective dose is 1 or 2, 4-mg. tablets, 4 times daily.
3. Parachlorophenylalanine (PCPA), an inhibitor of tryptophan hydroxylase, is available only on an experimental basis. It is effective in doses of 2 to 4 g. per 24 hours.[10] Harmful side effects have occurred, however, which include an eosinophilic syndrome, behavior disorders and hypothermia.
4. 5-Fluorotryptophan. An experimental drug which is an analog of 5-hydroxytryptophan has been reported to be safe when given in a dose of 200 mg., 3 times daily, for a year. Diarrhea abated and 5-HIAA levels dcreased in these patients, although tumor growth was unchanged.[6]

Flushing. This symptom is usually not benefited by the antiserotonin drugs that control diarrhea. The following drugs may be beneficial:

1. Phenoxybenzamine (Dibenzyline). Drugs that block adrenergic alpha-receptors may be effective in controlling flushes. Dibenzyline 10 to 20 mg. per day is the average effective dose, but some patients may require as much as 60 mg. daily.
2. Glucocorticoids. Prednisone in low and moderate doses is often highly effective in reducing the frequency and severity of flushing associated with bronchial carcinoid syndrome. These drugs are not generally efficacious in other carcinoid syndromes.
3. Methyldopa (Aldomet). A known decarboxylase inhibitor, it may produce substantial symptomatic relief in patients with carcinoids that secrete 5-hydroxytryptophan.
4. Phenothiazines (i.e., Thorazine) may benefit the flushing of patients with foregut carcinoids but also may be helpful in some midgut carcinoids.

Bronchoconstriction. The administration of epinephrine and isoproterenol (Isuprel) parenterally to these patients commonly leads to adverse and dangerous effects (e.g., flushing and hypotension). Cautious use of these agents by inhalation may be tried and may be beneficial without producing harmful effects.

Chemotherapy of Carcinoid Tumors

Several single or multiple drug regimens have been recently reported and appear to be effective and include the following:

Cyclophosphamide, Methotrexate or Both. Mengel and Shaffer[35] found that 31 percent of 41 patients exhibited a 50 percent shrinkage of liver size while on this regimen. Eleven additional patients (26%) demonstrated a 20 to 50 percent shrinkage of liver size.

5-Fluorouracil, Streptozotocin or Both. The Mayo Clinic group[8] demonstrated a 43 percent response rate to 5-fluorouracil, a 50 percent response to streptozotocin and a 66 percent response rate to combinations of these two agents.

Both groups emphasize that an exacerbation of symptoms of the carcinoid syndrome frequently occurs during and after treatment with chemotherapeutic agents. It is the policy at the Mayo Clinic to defer systemic chemotherapy until the patient is experiencing significant symptoms that can not be relieved by simpler and safer means.

Because of the favorable responses in these studies, the Eastern Cooperative Oncology Group is currently undertaking a prospective study of streptozotocin combined with either 5-FU or cyclophosphamide in the treatment of metastatic carcinoid tumors.

TREATMENT OF ASSOCIATED ENDOCRINOPATHIES

Cushing's Syndrome

Glucocorticoid excess has been completely reversed, in some instances, by removal of the primary carcinoid if metastatic disease was not present. Resection of the bulk of tumor may ameliorate symptoms. Bilateral adrenalectomy may be necessary if resection, tumor chemotherapy or drug therapy directed to the adrenal cortex is ineffective.[41]

Acromegaly

Surgical resection of the pituitary or irradiation to this organ is usually necessary. However in two recently reported cases, amelioration of symptoms of acromegaly followed the removal of the primary bronchial carcinoid.[7]

Zollinger-Ellison Syndrome

Two-thirds of the tumors which secrete gastrin are known to be malignant. Others may be multiple or may be associated with islet cell hyperplasia. For these reasons, total gastrectomy should be the overall aim of operative therapy whenever hypergastrinemia results in a severe ulcer diathesis. Whenever possible, however, all of the tumor or the bulk of it should be removed as well. Small carcinoid-islet cell tumors of the duodenum should be searched for when a patient with Z-E tumor is explored; they should be excised when they are found.

Hyperparathyroidism

In carcinoid syndromes, as in the MEA syndromes, multiglandular disease of the parathyroids is the rule. When hyperparathyroidism is present, both sides of the neck should be explored. In cases of hyperplasia a subtotal parathyroidectomy should be performed, removing all parathyroid tissue except 40 to 60 mg. of the most normal-looking parathyroid gland. One must be certain that this remaining gland has a normal blood supply and is viable before removing the remaining parathyroids. Parathyroid transplantation of this remnant to the arm muscles has not been utilized by the author at the initial neck exploration.

PROGNOSIS

The survival of patients with carcinoid tumors clearly depends upon the site of origin, the stage of disease at which it is treated and finally upon the completeness of surgical excision. The 5-year relative survival rates of 2,837 cases of carcinoid tumors are listed in Table 11-3. With tumors manifesting only local invasiveness, the overall 5-year-survival was 94 percent and ranged from 75 percent in the small bowel to 99 percent in the appendix. Regional node involvement decreased the survival of each lesion except that of appendiceal carcinoids; the mean 5-year-survival for all carcinoids of this stage was 64 percent. When distant spread was present, however, as is the case in most patients with carcinoid syndrome, the overall 5-year-survival was only 18 percent.

It has been further pointed out that when the carcinoid syndrome is present, patients are generally more debilitated than others with the same degree of tumor spread.[8] The prognosis of patients with the carcinoid syndrome has been shown to correlate with the urinary 5-HIAA output. In a recent Mayo Clinic study,[8] patients with urinary elimination of 5-HIAA between 10 and 49 mg. per 24 hours survived for an average period of 29 months; between 50 and 149 mg., for 21 months; and 150 mg. and over, for only 13 months. Thus, although some patients survive for long periods of time with metastatic tumor, it is well to note that in others, the disease is quite aggressive.

Table 11-3. Five-Year *Relative* Survival Rates (%) by Site and Stage

	Stage			
Site	*Local*	*Regional*	*Distant*	*All Stages*
Stomach	93	23	0	52
Small intestine and ileocecum	75	59	19	54
Appendix	99	100	27	99
Colon except appendix	77	65	17	52
Rectum and rectosigmoid	92	44	7	83
Lung and bronchi	96	71	11	87
All sites	94	64	18	82

(Godwin, J. D. II: Cancer, *36:*560, 1975[14])

REFERENCES

1. Aune, S., and Schistad, G.: Carcinoid liver metastases treated with hepatic dearterialization. Am. J. Surg., *123*:715, 1972.
2. Bates, H. R., Jr.: Carcinoid tumors of the rectum—a statistical review. Dis. Colon Rectum, *9*:90, 1966.
3. Bernier, J. J., et al.: Diarrhea associated with medullary carcinoma of the thyroid. Gut., *10*:980, 1969.
4. Berry, E. M., Maunder, C., and Wilson, M.: Carcinoid myopathy and treatment with cyproheptadine (Periactin). Gut., *15*:34, 1974.

5. Bivens, C. H., Marecek, R. L., and Feldman, J. M.: Peyronie's disease—a presenting complaint of the carcinoid syndrome. N. Engl. J. Med., *289*:844, 1973.
6. Costello, C.: Carcinoid tumor metastases. Prospective study of twenty-two patients. Am. J. Surg., *130*:756, 1975.
7. Dabek, J. T.: Bronchial carcinoid tumour with acromegaly in two patients. J. Clin. Endocrinol. Metab., *38*:329, 1974.
8. Davis, Z., Moertel, C. G., and McIlrath, D. C.: The malignant carcinoid syndrome. Surg. Gynecol. Obstet., *137*:637, 1973.
9. Deftos, L. J., et al.: Simultaneous ectopic production of parathyroid hormone and calcitonin. Metabolism, *25*:543, 1976.
10. Engelman, K., Lovenberg, W., and Sjoerdsma, A.: Inhibition of serotonin synthesis by para-chlorophenylalanine in patients with the carcinoid syndrome. N. Engl. J. Med., *277*:1103, 1967.
11. Erspamer, V., and Asero, B.: Identification of enteramine, the specific hormone of the enterochromaffin cell system, as 5-hydroxytryptamine. Nature, *169*:800, 1952.
12. Feldman, J. M., et al.: Growth hormone and prolactin secretion in the carcinoid syndrome. Am. J. Med. Sci., *269*:333, 1975.
13. Friesen, S. R., Hermreck, A. S., and Mantz, F. A., Jr.: Glucagon, gastrin and carcinoid tumors of the duodenum, pancreas and stomach: Polypeptide "apudomas" of the foregut. Am. J. Surg., *127*:90, 1974.
14. Godwin, J. D. II.: Carcinoid tumors. An analysis of 2837 cases. Cancer, *36*:560, 1975.
15. Goldman, N. C., Hood, I. and Singleton, G. T.: Carcinoid of the larynx. Arch. Otolaryngol., *90*:90, 1969.
16. Gonzalez-Licea, A., Hartmann, W. H., and Yardley, J. H.: Medullary carcinoma of the thyroid. Ultrastructural evidence of its origin from the parafollicular cell and possible relation to carcinoid tumors. J. Clin. Pathol., *49*:512, 1968.
17. Gossett, A., and Masson, P.: Tumeurs endocrines de l'appendice. Presse Med., *22*:237, 1914.
18. Grahame-Smith, D. G.: The carcinoid syndrome. Am. J. Cardiol., *21*:376, 1968.
19. Gray, T. K., Biebedorf, F. A., and Fordtran, J. S.: Thyrocalcitonin and the jejunal absorption of calcium, water and electrolytes in normal subjects. J. Clin. Invest., *52*:3084, 1973.
20. Honey, M., and Paneth, M.: Carcinoid heart disease: successful tricuspid valve replacement. Thorax, *30*:464, 1975.
21. Hübschmann, P.: Sur le carcinome primitif de l'appendice vermiculaire. Rev. Med. Suisse Romande, *30*:317, 1910.
22. Hughes, J. P., et al.: Carcinoid tumor of the thymus gland: report of a case. Thorax, *30*:470, 1975.
23. Isler, P., and Hedinger, C.: Metastasierendes Duenndarm-carcinoid mit schweren vorwiegend das rechte Herz betreffenden Klappenfehlern und Pulmonalstenose-ein eigenartiger Symptomenkomplex? Schweiz. med. Wochenschr., *83*:4, 1953.
24. Jaffc, B. M.: Prostaglandins E and F in endocrine diarrheagenic syndromes. Ann. Surg., *184*:516, 1976.
25. Kaplan, E. L., Jaffe, B. M., and Peskin, G. W.: A new provocative test for the diagnosis of the carcinoid syndrome. Am. J. Surg., *123*:173, 1972.
26. Kaplan, E. L., et al.: Humoral similarities of carcinoid tumors and medullary carcinomas of the thyroid. Surgery, *74*:21, 1973.
27. Kulchitsky, N.: Zur Frage über den Bau des Darmkanals. Arch. f. mikroskop. Anat. Bd. *49*:1897.
28. Lembeck, F.: 5-Hydroxytryptamine in carcinoid tumors. Nature, *172*:910, 1953.
29. Levine, R. J.: Serotonin and the carcinoid syndrome; histamine and mastocytosis. *In* Bondy, P. K., and Rosenberg, L. E. (eds.): Duncan's Diseases of Metabolism. Genetics and Metab-

olism. ed. 7, pp. 1651-1666. Philadelphia, W. B. Saunders, 1974.

30. Levine, R. J., and Sjoerdsma, A.: Pressor amines and the carcinoid flush. Ann. Intern. Med., *58*:818, 1963.
31. Lubarsch, O.: Über den primären Krebs des Ileum nebst Bemerkungen über das gleichzeitige Vorkommen von Krebs und Tuberculose. Virchows Arch., *111*:281, 1888.
32. McDermott, W. V., Jr., and Hensle, T. W.: Metastatic carcinoid to the liver treated by hepatic dearterialization. Ann. Surg., *180*:305, 1974.
33. Mason, D. T., and Melmon, K. L.: New understanding of the mechanism of the carcinoid flush. Ann. Intern. Med., *65*:1334, 1966.
34. Melmon, K. L., Sjoerdsma, A., and Mason, D. T.: Distinctive clinical and therapeutic aspects of the syndrome associated with bronchial carcinoid tumors. Am. J. Med., *39*:568, 1965.
35. Mengel, C. E., and Shaffer, R. D.: The carcinoid syndrome, *In* Holland, J. F., and Frei, C. E. (eds.): Cancer Medicine. Chap. 24. Philadelphia, Lea & Febiger.
36. Moertel, C. G. Dockerty, M. B., and Judd, F. S.: Carcinoid tumors of the vermiform appendix. Cancer, *21*:270, 1968.
37. Moertel, C. G., et al.: Life history of the carcinoid tumor of the small intestine. Cancer, *14*:901, 1961.
38. Oates, J. A., and Sjoerdsma, A.: A unique syndrome associated with secretion of 5-hydroxytryptophan by metastatic gastric carcinoids. Am. J. Med., *32*:333, 1962.
39. Oates, J. A., Melmon, K., Sjoerdsma, A., et al.: Release of a kinin peptide in the carcinoid syndrome. Lancet, *1*:514, 1964.
40. Oberndorfer, S.: Ergebnisse der allgemeinen Pathologie und Pathologischen Anatomie des Menschen und der Tiere, *13*:527, 1909.
41. Olurin, E. O., et al.: Cushing's syndrome and bronchial carcinoid tumor. Cancer, *31*:1514, 1973.
42. Orloff, M.: Carcinoid tumors of the rectum. Cancer, *28*:175, 1971.
43. Pearse, A. G. E.: Cytochemical and ultrastructural characteristics of cells producing polypeptide hormones and their relevance to gut hormones. *In* Chey, W. Y., and Brooks, F. P. (eds.): Endocrinology of the Gut. pp. 24-34. Thorofare, N.J., Charles B. Slack, Inc., 1974.
44. Pearse, A. G. E., and Polak, J. M.: Neural crest origin of the endocrine polypeptide (APUD) cells of the gastrointestinal tract and pancreas. Gut, *12*:783, 1971.
45. Pearse, A. G. E., Polak, J. M., and Heath, C. M.: Polypeptide hormone production by "carcinoid" apudomas and their relevant cytochemistry Virchows Arch., *16*:95, 1974.
46. Pernow, B., and Waldenstrom, J.: Paroxysmal flushing and other symptoms caused by 5-hydroxytryptamine and histamine in patients with malignant tumors. Lancet, *2*:951, 1954.
47. Peskin, G. W., and Kaplan, E. L.: The surgery of carcinoid tumors. Surg. Clin. North Am., *49*:137, 1969.
48. Plonk, J. W., and Feldman, J. M.: Carcinoid arthropathy. Arch. Intern. Med., *134*:651, 1974.
49. Rapport, M. M., Green, A. A., and Page, I. H.: Partial purification of the vasoconstrictor in beef serum, J. Biol. Chem., *174*:735, 1948.
50. Robboy, S. J., Norris, H. J., and Scully, R. E.: Insular carcinoid primary in the ovary. A clinicopathologic analysis or 48 cases. Cancer, *36*:404, 1975.
51. Roberts, W. C., and Sjoerdsma, A.: The cardiac disease associated with the carcinoid syndrome (carcinoid heart disease). Am. J. Med., *36*:5, 1964.
52. Robertson, J. I. S., Peart, W. S., and Andrews, T. M.: The mechanism of facial flushes in the carcinoid syndrome. Q. J. Med., *31*:103, 1962.
53. Rosato, F. E., and Rosato, E. F.: Carcinoid tumors of the large bowel. Cancer, *20*:353, 1970.
54. Rosenbaum, F. F., Santer, D. G., and Claudon, D. B.: Essential telangiectasia, pulmonary stenosis and neo-

plastic liver disease, a possible new clinical syndrome. J. Lab. Clin. Med., *42*:941, 1953.
55. Rosenberg, J. C.: Carcinoid and other amine producing tumors. Prog. Clin. Cancer, *2*:297, 1966.
56. Samaan, N. A., et al.: Hyperparathyroidism and carcinoid tumor. Ann. Intern. Med., *82*:205, 1975.
57. Sylora, H. O., et al.: Primary carcinoid tumor of the urethra. J. Urol., *114*:150, 1975.
58. Thorson, A. H., Biörck, G., Bjorkman, G., and Waldenstrom, J.: Malignant carcinoid of the small intestine with metastasis to the liver, valvular disease of the right side of the heart, peripheral vasomotor symptoms, bronchoconstriction and an unusual type of cyanosis. A clinical and pathologic syndrome. Am. Heart J., *47*:795, 1954.
59. Vaidya, A. B., Wustrack, K. W., and Levine, R. J.: Failure of epinephrine to provoke flushing in patients with systemic mastocytosis. Ann. Intern. Med., *74*:711, 1971.
60. Vane, J. R.: The release and fate of vasoactive hormones in the circulation. Br. J. Pharmacol., *35*:204, 1969.
61. Weichert, R. F., III, et al.: Carcinoid-islet cell tumors of the duodenum. Report of twenty-one cases. Am. J. Surg., *121*:195, 1971.
62. Wilson, H., Cheek, R. C., Sherman, R. T., and Storer, E. H..: Carcinoid tumors. Curr. Probl. Surg., *7*:1, 1970.
63. Yalla, S. V., et al.: Primary argentaffinoma of the testis: A case report and survey of the literature. J. Urol., *111*:50, 1974.

Selected Reading

Friesen, S. R., Hermreck, A. S., and Mantz, F. A., Jr.: Glucagon, gastrin and carcinoid tumors of the duodenum, pancreas and stomach: polypeptide "apudomas" of the foregut. Am. J. Surg., *127*:90, 1974.
(A presentation of various clinical pictures of foregut carcinoid-apudomas.)

Grahame-Smith, D. G.: The carcinoid syndrome. Am. J. Cardiol., *21*:376, 1968.
(A comprehensive discussion of the manifestations of the carcinoid syndrome.)

Levine, R. J.: Serotonin and the carcinoid syndrome; histamine and mastocytosis. *In* Bondy, P. K., and Rosenberg, L. E. (eds.): Duncan's Diseases of Metabolism. Genetics and Metabolism. pp. 1651-1666. Philadelphia, W. B. Saunders, 1974.
(A vital review of carcinoid syndrome, its pharmacology and treatment.)

Weichert, R. F. III, et al.: Carcinoid-islet cell tumors of the duodenum. Report of twenty-one cases. Am. J. Surg., *121*:195, 1971.
(The above paper discusses the multiple combinations of amine and peptide secretions associated with some foregut carcinoid-islet cell tumors in a clear and comprehensive manner.)

Wilson, H., Cheek, R. C., Sherman, R. T., and Storer, E. H.: Carcinoid tumors. Curr. Probl. Surg., *7*:1, 1970.
(An extensive survey, with emphasis on the malignant potential of the various carcinoid tumors.)

EDITORIAL COMMENTARY

The enterochromaffin (EC) cells are almost ubiquitous in that they are present in the mucosa of the entire gastrointestinal tract and presumably in other sites as well because of the observations of carcinoid (EC cell) tumors in other neuroendocrine organs. These cells assume their rightful place in the APUD system because they synthesize, store and secrete amines, notably serotonin (5-HT), and those of the small intestine (not stomach or colon) also secrete motilin, a 22-amino acid peptide. Tumors of these cells, depending on their location, also elaborate other humoral products which characterize not only the site of the tumor but also the type of carcinoid syndrome observed clinically. The classical (typical) carcinoid syndrome occurs in some of those patients in whom the primary tumor is in the midgut (usually ileum) with metastases present in the liver; in such situations, 5-HT emanates chiefly from metastases in the liver, thus bypassing hepatic metabolism so that high levels of serotonin, subs. P, motilin and kallikrein-induced bradykinin produce a biologic effect on blood vessels, heart, gastrointestinal tract and lungs. On the other hand, the characterization of variants of the carcinoid (atypical) syndrome which result from EC tumors of the foregut, including the bronchi and lungs, consists of the more prolonged and brighter skin flush, facial edema, lacrimation and even hypotension. These symptoms may be due to the elaboration of histamine, in addition to the liberation of 5-hydroxytryptophan (5-HTP); the latter substance, rather than 5-HT, is usually liberated because of the absence of the enzyme 5-HTP decarboxylase. Furthermore, the greatest distinction of foregut carcinoid tumor lies in the associated elaboration of other peptides such as corticotropin, insulin, gastrin, glucagon, calcitonin, vasoactive intestinal peptide and parathyrinlike peptides. These peptides then modify the clinical picture of the atypical syndrome by masking it with their own specific biologic effects. Because of the peptide capabilities, the morphologic criteria for the diagnosis of carcinoid tumor, particularly of the foregut, should be extended to include its functional characteristics, potential or actual (i.e., carcinoid-gastrinoma, etc.). The bronchial variant differs from the syndromes of other origins in two other aspects: The endocardial complications are left-sided rather than of the right heart, and glucocorticoids have an ameliorating effect on the syndrome.

Interestingly, carcinoid tumors at any site are frequently multiple and may also be associated with other endocrine tumors and even other nonendocrine carcinomas. When the parathyroid glands are involved by association all of them are usually hyperplastic, as is similar to their involvement in the multiple endocrine adenopathy (MEA) syndromes. Another infrequently observed aspect of the carcinoid syndrome is the pellagralike malnutrition in patients, because of the diversion of tryptophan from its role in protein and niacin synthesis.

As in other endocrinopathies, refinements in diagnosis of the carcinoid syndrome include not only specific analyses of the circulating hormones and their metabolic products, but also the development of stimulation (and suppression) tests. The calcium stimulation test to elucidate the syndrome and the peaked blood serotonin level is such an example. This confirmatory maneuver is much safer than the epinephrine provocation test which if used at all should be done with much caution and regard for safety of the patient, particularly in the patient with heart disease. *S.R.F.*

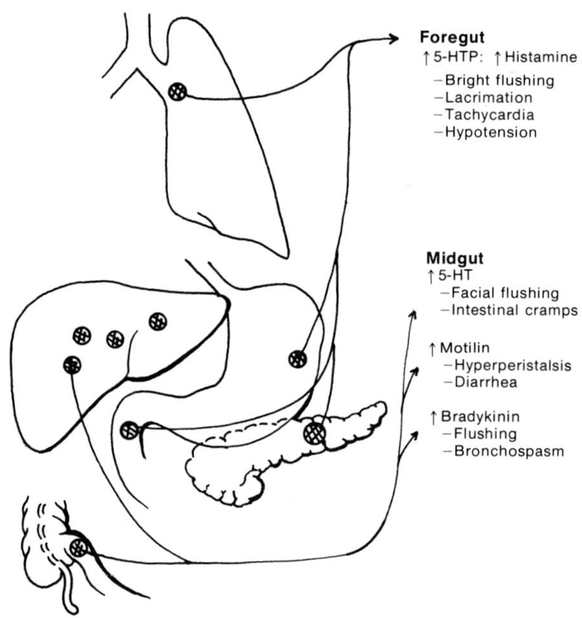

Fig. 11-12. Pathophysiology of the carcinoid syndromes (5-HT, 5-HTP, motilin-secreting tumors, of EC cells).

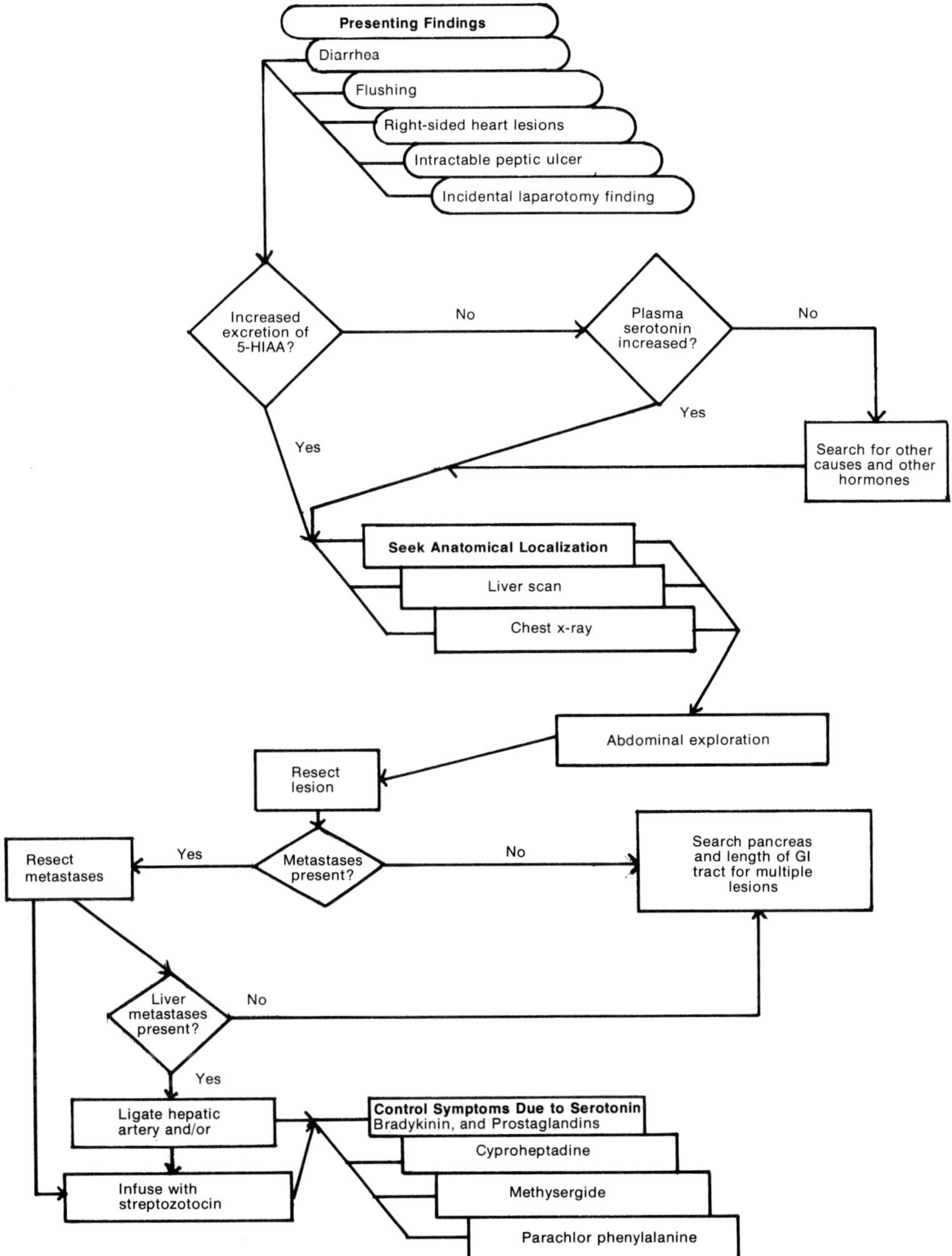

Fig. 11-13. Management flowchart of the carcinoid syndromes.

PART 2
Polypeptides

12

The Hypoglycemic Syndrome: Endogenous Hyperinsulinism

Timothy S. Harrison, M.D.

The brain has an absolute requirement for glucose as an energy substrate, and consequently it is hardly surprising that the symptoms of hypoglycemia are predominantly of central nervous system origin. Deprived of their cerebral energy source by dangerously low glucose levels in the circulating blood, hypoglycemic patients are often unable to think coherently, are forgetful and frequently indulge in bizarre and uncharacteristic behavior for which they usually have no memory. Hypoglycemic patients may have seizures of one sort or another, and still others may have obvious motor system uncoordination with garbled dysarthric speech, stumbling and coarse intentional movements prominent among their problems. A few of these hypoglycemic patients have been found in mental hospitals to which they have been committed because of their bizarre behavior. Discovery of their hypoglycemia has been delayed only because it has not been suspected.

These impairments of the mind are most striking after fasting and characteristically are relieved by eating. If the blood glucose falls rapidly hypoglycemia excites the release of epinephrine, and the patient will exhibit classical signs of epinephrine release: tachycardia, apprehension, sweating and nervousness. If the blood glucose falls over a period of hours rather than minutes, the central nervous system symptoms already mentioned will predominate.

The brain can be damaged irreversibly by profound hypoglycemia if the hypoglycemia is too prolonged. In adult patients objective signs of neurologic impairment (e.g., memory defect, extensor plantar responses and abnormal electroencephalographic changes) tend to be transient, and one can hope for long-term improvement in these patients as time passes. Permanent neurologic damage from extended, profound hypoglycemia is fortunately rare in the adult patient with insulin-secreting tumors. Although there are insufficient data available to make a definitive statement one gets the impression from a handful of cases that permanent brain damage and impaired mental development are more likely to be seen in infants and children who have had prolonged and often repeated exposure to profound hypoglycemia.

CASE STUDIES

Patient 1: A 42-yr.-old father of three, a responsible public school administrator in a midwestern town of 50,000 became a source of embarrassment and deep concern to his wife and family. A competent and respected official, he had taken to driving off by himself just before dinner or breakfast. There was no consistent pattern or plan to his bizarre behavior; when found by police or others he was usually incoherent, disoriented with unintelligible, thick, garbled speech and was incapable of explaining either his predicament or who he was.

Dinner or breakfast would follow these excursions and after eating, his recovery was rapid and complete and he was able to go on to work. He had absolutely no memory for these bizarre happenings and disbelieved that they had occurred.

Repeated blood alcohol tests were negative. After a year and a half of these episodes, a blood glucose level was determined during an attack and found to be dangerously low, 40 mg./100 ml.

Eventual pathologic diagnosis: Solitary pancreatic beta islet cell adenoma.

Patient 2: A 12-yr.-old girl, the daughter of a physician, had been doing excellent schoolwork but became a persistent and unusual behavior problem. In the hour before the noon lunch period her attention would wander and she would respond inappropriately or not at all to questions. After the noon recess her customarily fine performance resumed.

After a year and a half of such behavior she was placed in a special section of the school for children with behavioral problems. Of further concern now were grand mal seizures which came once or twice a week and always in the late morning session of school. The seizures lasted 10 to 20 minutes.

Two years after the beginning of her problems a blood glucose level was drawn just after a seizure—the report was returned to her father—36 mg./100 ml.

Eventual pathologic diagnosis: Nesidioblastosis of the pancreatic islets.

Patient 3: A 36-yr.-old congenitally blind woman had, with considerable resourcefulness, organized her life effectively after an unsuccessful marriage to a blind classmate terminated in divorce. During her marital difficulties she began to drink heavily but managed to stop.

Accomplished with braille she was employed part time as an accountant. In addition she played the cello and was active through a surprisingly wide range of intellectual interests.

Her behavior changed. She became querulous and combative in the morning and often difficult to arouse. With time the situation became worse and her admission to a mental hospital was planned.

A fasting glucose of 41 mg./100 ml. led to a pancreatic exploration for an islet cell tumor but none was found. Her hypoglycemia worsened, she became semicomatose and was referred for further treatment with a blood glucose of 32 mg./100 ml. At a second operation an islet cell adenoma was removed; 7 days postoperatively her fasting blood glucose was 40 mg./100 ml.

Eventual pathologic diagnosis: Pancreatic beta-cell adenomatosis, macroscopic and microscopic.

CLINICAL FEATURES AND DIFFERENTIAL DIAGNOSIS OF HYPOGLYCEMIA

In endocrinology there are really no conditions of exaggerated hormonal release that mimic hypoglycemia. However, in clinical medicine there are many types of disorders that produce hypoglycemia, and it is essential for the physician seeing such patients to have an organized view of the diagnostic possibilities that hypoglycemia might represent.[2,5]

There may be organic hypoglycemias (i.e., those recognized as being due to a distinct anatomic lesion). Prominent among these hypoglycemias are the various pancreatic beta islet cell lesions producing autonomous hyperinsulinism. These will be dealt with in depth later.

There are nonpancreatic tumors associated with hypoglycemia. Pleural mesotheliomas, soft-tissue sarcomas and carcinoid tumors are among the more common. Adrenal cortical carcinoma, hepatocellular carcinoma and gastrointestinal tract carcinomas all may be associated with hypoglycemia. The carcinoid tumors may produce insulin itself whereas the mesenchymal tumors mentioned produce some other compound, perhaps a somatomedin, which lowers the blood glucose level.

Diffuse liver disease, anterior pituitary hypofunction and adrenocortical insufficiency for any reason (i.e., primary adrenocortical failure), hypothalamic-pituitary dysfunction or specific enzymatic defects of glucocorticoid biosynthesis all may have hypoglycemia as their initial manifestation.

There are a group of specific enzyme defects of the liver: the so-called glycogen storage diseases (glucose-6-phosphatase deficiency, phosphorylase deficiency, amylo-1, 6-glucosidase deficiency) all of which limit seriously the quantity of hepatic glycogen that is available for breakdown into glucose and hence may first appear as hypoglycemia.

Other hepatic enzyme defects, for example, hereditary fructose intolerance (fructose-1-phosphate aldolase deficiency), galactosemia (deficiency of galactose-1-phosphate uridyl transferase), aglycogenesis (glycogen synthetase deficiency) and familial fructose and galactose intolerance all may initially become apparent as hypoglycemia.

Functional hypoglycemias (i.e., that is those patients with hypoglycemia for which there is no persistently recognizable anatomic cause) include reactive hypoglycemias; hypoglycemias associated with diabetes, rapid glucose absorption following gastrectomy, alcohol and poor nutrition, and glucagon deficiency; the hypoglycemias of the newborn and of childhood. Erythroblastosis fetalis and infantile gigantism may have hypoglycemia associated with them.

Finally one needs to be aware of patients who take insulin, or oral hypoglycemic agents or other drugs that may cause hypoglycemia.

If this list of differential diagnostic possibilities seems formidable and intimidating at first glance: it remains so after continued familiarity with it. Nevertheless, it is essential to recognize that hypoglycemia is not a disease but a sign that something has gone wrong in the complex series of biochemical reactions that customarily regulate blood glucose within carefully protected physiologic levels.

As noted (p. 153), many of the hypoglycemic disorders may be associated with fasting hypoglycemia. This presents a significant problem when one wishes to establish whether or not islet cell lesions of the pancreas are present which require surgical control.

It was thought that the occurrence of central nervous system symptoms brought on by overnight fasting, a fasting blood glucose of less than 50 mg./100 ml., and relief of the central nervous system symptoms by glucose ingestion specifically indicated the presence of beta islet cell pathology. This triad of findings was set forward most vigorously by the late Allen O. Whipple and is known today as Whipple's triad. There is still a tendency for physicians to ascribe diagnostic precision and specificity to the demonstration of Whipple's triad. This is an unacceptably dangerous oversimplification in that there are, as we have just pointed out, many other causes of fasting hypoglycemia and there are as well, more than a few instances of insulin-secreting tumors in which overnight fasting does not produce hypoglycemia of less than 50 mg. glucose/100 ml. blood. It is no more correct to suggest that Whipple's triad categorically denotes the presence of pancreatic beta islet cell pathology than it is to imply that all patients with episodic hypertension have a pheo-,chromocytoma.

Classification of Spontaneous Hypoglycemia

I. Organic hypoglycemia*—recognizable anatomical lesion
  A. Pancreatic islet cell disease with hyperinsulinism
    1. Adenoma, single or multiple
    2. Microadenomatosis, with or without macroscopic islet adenomas
    3. Carcinoma, with metastases
    4. Adenoma(s) or carcinoma, associated with adenomas of other endocrine glands al multiple endocrine adenomatosis)
    5. Hyperplasia (very rare in adults) in infancy and childhood
      (a) Hyperplasia
      (b) Nesidioblastosis
      (c) Adenoma
  B. Nonpancreatic tumors associated with hypoglycemia
  C. Anterior pituitary hypofunction
  D. Adrenocortical hypofunction
  E. Acquired extensive liver disease.
  F. Severe congestive heart failure
  G. Severe renal insufficiency in noninsulin-dependent diabetic patient
II. Hypoglycemia due to identified specific hepatic enzyme defects (infancy and childhood)
  A. Glycogen storage diseases* (deficiency of glucose-6-phosphatase or amylo-1, 6-glucosidase, or phosphorylase)
  B. Fructose-1, 6-diphosphatase deficiency*
  C. Hereditary fructose intolerance (deficiency of fructose-1-phosphate aldolase)
  D. Galactosemia (deficiency of galactose-1-phosphate uridyl transferase)
  E. Aglycogenesis* (deficiency of glycogen synthase)
  F. Familial fructose and galactose intolerance (specific enzyme defect undetermined)
III. Functional hypoglycemia—no recognizable, or no persistent, anatomical lesion
  A. Reactive functional hypoglycemia
  B. Reactive hypoglycemia secondary to mild diabetes
  C. Alimentary hyperinsulinism
  D. Alcohol and poor nutrition*
  E. Deficiency of glucagon*
  F. Transient hypoglycemia in the newborn of low birth weight*
  G. Transient postnatal hypoglycemia in an infant of a diabetic mother*
  H. "Idiopathic hypoglycemia" of infancy and childhood*
    1. Ketogenic hypoglycemia (childhood)
    2. Leucine-sensitive type
    3. Leucine-insensitive type
    4. Others
  I. Erythroblastosis fetalis, transient*
  J. Infantile gigantism with visceromegaly, microcephaly, macroglossia and omphalocele* (hyperplasia of pancreatic islet cells has been reported in some patients classified under G, H, I, and J)
  K. "Insulin autoimmune syndrome" (no previous insulin administration) and hyperinsulinemia
IV. Hypoglycemia due to exogenous causes
  A. Iatrogenic } insulin or sulfonylurea compounds*
  B. Factitious }
  C. Other drugs that may cause hypoglycemia

*Fasting hypoglycemia

(Fajans, S. S., Floyd, J. C., Jr., and Vij, S. K.: Differential diagnosis of hypoglycemia. p. 459. *In* Kryston, L. J., Shaw, R. A., and Schwager, E. [eds.]: Endocrinology and Diabetes. New York, Grune & Stratton, 1975. By permission. See also Fajans, S. S., and Floyd, J. C., Jr., N. Engl. J. Med., *294*:766, 1976)

Fortunately, there are now diagnostic measures available for hyperfunctioning pancreatic beta islet cell lesions that have brought clarity and precision to this situation which had been dangerously confused before such measures became available.

MODERN LABORATORY DIAGNOSIS

Autonomous Hyperinsulinism

In the era preceding the measurement of immunoreactive insulin, the diagnosis of hyperfunctioning islet cell tumors was an uncertain one at best. As mentioned previously the demonstration of Whipple's triad will include a large variety of conditions unrelated to endogenous hyperinsulinism and therefore Whipple's triad is not specific for islet cell lesions. Early in their experience with islet cell tumors, Whipple and Frantz reviewed the published experiences with insulin-secreting tumors and found that in 44 percent of the patients explored for hypoglycemia no islet cell pathology was found.[12] As time went by the error rate for successful diagnosis was probably somewhat decreased, but the successful diagnosis of hyperfunctioning beta islet cell lesions still did not achieve the precision for which one would hope.

The ability to measure insulin levels accurately in the circulating blood has improved dramatically the diagnostic precision for hyperfunctioning beta islet cell lesions. It is now a rare occurrence not to be able to demonstrate pathologic changes in beta cells of the pancreatic islets in all patients undergoing exploration for endogenous hyperinsulinism. At the heart of this diagnostic precision is the demonstration of fasting immunoreactive plasma insulin levels that are inappropriately elevated when related to the concomitant level of blood glucose. In physiologic circumstances glucose is a potent stimulus for the release of pancreatic insulin. In the situation of pathologic islet cells, insulin is released independently from any stimulation by glucose, and furthermore insulin's release is not inhibited by a deficiency of circulating glucose. Hence, with hyperfunctioning beta islet cell lesions a situation develops in which insulin levels tend to be at the upper limit of normal or obviously elevated, and the glucose content of the same blood sample is inappropriately low.

This combination of findings is called autonomous hyperinsulinism which is meant to convey the fact that insulin release is occurring independently of the usual controlling factor of blood glucose levels. There are other stimuli which could function physiologically for insulin release but, relative to glucose, their regulatory role on insulin release is less well understood and felt to be less important in physiologic conditions. Among such stimuli are the pancreatic islet alpha cell peptide hormone, glucagon and certain amino acids (e.g., leucine and arginine) which on infusion in man, can stimulate increased plasma-insulin levels presumably by releasing pancreatic insulin, although interference with insulin binding or inhibition of insulin breakdown are theoretically possible explanations for their action. The role of glucagon and amino acids in the physiologic control of insulin release is not known, and whether or not these amino acids play any part in stimulating insulin release from pathologically abnormal islet cells is even less clear.

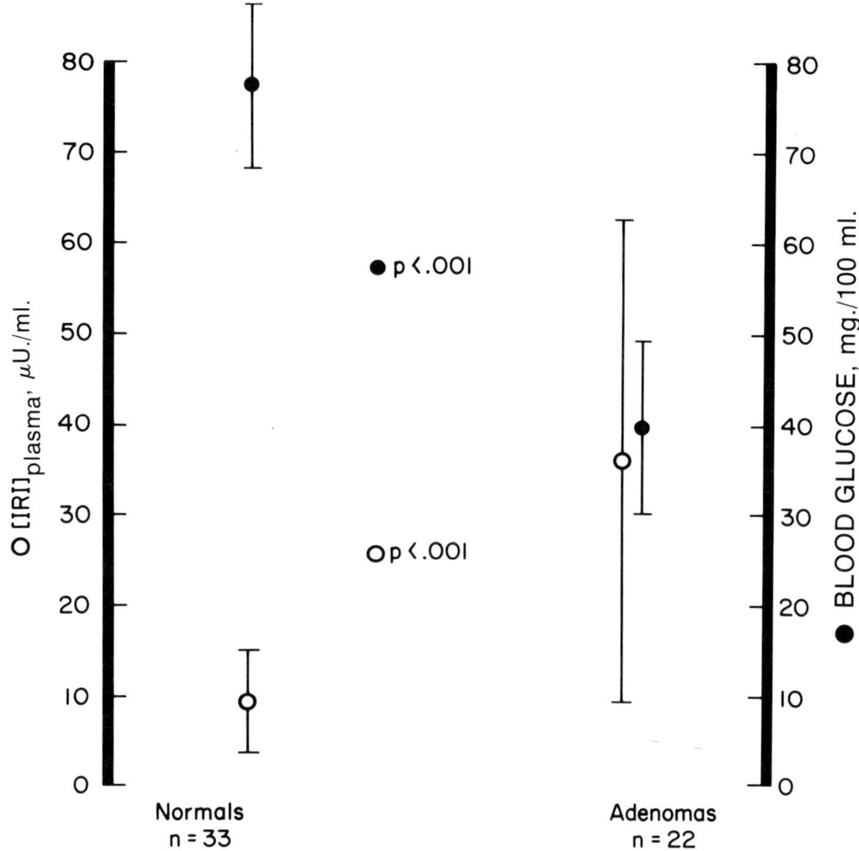

Fig. 12-1. Plasma insulin μU./ml. and blood glucose mg./100 ml., relationships after overnight fasting in normal subjects and in 22 subjects with solitary β islet cell adenomas. Both plasma insulin and blood glucose show highly significant differences between the two groups. (Harrison, T. S., Hyperinsulinism and its surgical management: *In* Hardy, J. D. [ed.]: Rhoad's Surgery, Principles and Practice. ed. 5, Chap. 35. Philadelphia, J. B. Lippincott, 1977)

Fasting Immunoreactive Insulin/Glucose Ratios

To avoid the effect of exogeneous glucose stimulation on their distortions of concomitant insulin and glucose levels, patients suspected of islet-cell tumors are studied generally after fasting for at least 12 hours. The fasting immunoreactive insulin (IRI)/glucose relationships in these patients are most easily portrayed by calculating the ratio of circulating insulin μU./ml. to blood glucose mg./100 ml. Such an IRI/glucose ratio could, in normal conditions of fasting, be insulin 14 μU./ml. and glucose 80 mg./100 ml. a ratio of 0.175. If the same insulin level 14 μU./ml. were found in fasting blood sample whose glucose content was 40 mg./100 ml. the IRI/glucose ratio would become 0.35 well into the range in which autonomously functioning pancreatic beta islet-cell lesions have been found. In 43 patients under our care all were proven at surgery to have islet-cell pathology and in them the fasting IRI-glucose ratios exceeded 0.3.[5]*

*Fajans, S. S., and Floyd, J. C., Jr.: Unpublished data.

In a few patients suspected of autonomous hyperinsulism, overnight fasting may be insufficient to demonstrate an abnormal elevation of the IRI/glucose ratio. The most convenient thing to do in this circumstance is to extend the fasting period for as long as 72 hours if necessary. In patients with islet cell pathology it would be most unusual not to demonstrate increased IRI/glucose ratios after a 72-hour fast. If the diagnosis of autonomous hyperinsulinism is not confirmed after one period of study, it is often wise to study the patient again, several months later. In this way trends may become apparent in the IRI/glucose ratio that make the diagnosis of autonomous hyperinsulinism more apparent.

Some groups have objected to IRI/glucose ratios because they depend on the assumption that at zero insulin levels a blood glucose of 30 mg./100 ml. should still persist: a situation which is felt to be physiologically untenable. These objections are more theoretical than real but have led others to develop "amended" IRI/glucose ratios in which a correction is introduced to overcome this objection. In fact amended ratios do not offer any advantage or any increased diagnostic precision when compared to the conventionally expressed IRI/glucose ratio already discussed. The suggestion that plasma insulin levels be used by themselves as an absolute criterion for the diagnosis of hyperfunctioning islet cell lesions has been made[11] but seems to be a dangerous oversimplification in that some patients with high normal plasma insulin values will have their lesions overlooked by this approach.

If a fasting IRI/glucose ratio has been ambiguous or negative on repeated study and one wishes to further substantiate normal pancreatic beta islet cell function, a variety of other tests are available. Of these the simplest is to measure proinsulin which is the precursor of insulin. Proinsulin is a large peptide with a molecular weight of about 9,000. Its amino acid sequence is known and antibodies have been raised to it. Levels of proinsulin are elevated in patients with endogenous hyperinsulinism from demonstrated beta islet cell lesions. It is still too early and experience with it too limited to know whether or not determination of proinsulin will be as helpful in the diagnosis of beta cell lesions as the determination of IRI/glucose plasma levels has been.

When proinsulin is cleaved to form insulin, the remaining C-peptide fragment can also be measured by specific radioimmunoassay. Human C-peptide has 31 amino acid residues the sequence of which is now known. C-peptide levels are increased in autonomous hyperinsulinism, but it is still too early in the collected experience with C-peptide assay to know whether it will improve further the precision for the diagnosis of pancreatic beta islet cell lesions.[8] Furthermore, whether or not there are lesions which can be picked up by either proinsulin levels or C-peptide levels having been overlooked by fasting IRI/glucose ratios cannot be stated yet. Experience should give better answers to these questions than we now have.

Pharmacologic Stimulation of Insulin Release

A variety of other tests are available which are helpful in securing or excluding the diagnosis of hyperfunctioning beta cell lesions. The more widely used of these involves stimulation of insulin release. However, taken at their best the stimulation tests are less precise and less persistently accurate diagnostic aids than the measurement of fasting IRI/glucose ratios mentioned previously. The best known and most widely used of the stimulation tests is the tolbutamide test: 1 g. sodium tolbutamide is dissolved in 20 ml. distilled water and injected intravenously over a 22-minute period. Blood samples are taken every 5 minutes for the first 15 minutes, every 15 minutes for the first hour and every 30 minutes in the second and third hours of the test. The tolbutamide test was designed by Fajans before the measurement of immunoreactive insulin was available and blood glucose depression was the only response that could be followed.[4] However, if a patient starts the test with a low fasting glucose, 50 mg./100 ml., blood glucose depression cannot be a dependable measurement in that situation. Now that measurement of immunoreactive insulin has been added to the tolbutamide test the usefulness of the tolbutamide test in the diagnosis of beta cell lesions has increased.[5,10] The accuracy of the tolbutamide test in patients with proven islet cell lesions is about 86 percent when they have been compared to the response seen in nonobese controls.[6] Obese subjects will increase their plasma insulin with tolbutamide, but in them there is no concomitant decrease in circulating glucose levels. IRI/glucose ratios 120 and 180 minutes after tolbutamide have recently been suggested as the most useful samples for diagnostic precision in this test.[10]

The leucine test is another stimulating test in which 200 mg./kg. of the amino acid leucine is infused over a 30-minute period and blood samples taken 30, 60, and 90 minutes later; 79 percent of adult subjects with proven islet cell pathology showed plasma insulin responses greater than 95 percent (2 SD) of those seen in normal nonobese controls.[6] In children the leucine test will not differentiate between idiopathic hypoglycemia and insulin-secreting tumors. Also in patients who have been taking oral hypoglycemic agents, such as the sulfonylurea drugs, the IRI and blood sugar response will be greatly enhanced.

The third test stimulating insulin release which is sometimes helpful in confirming the diagnosis of insulinoma is the injection of 1 mg. of glucagon intravenously. At 5, 10, 15, 30, 40, and 60 minutes after glucagon significant plasma insulin increases, compared to normal nonobese controls, occurred in 69 percent of subjects with proven islet cell pathology in whom the test was used.[5]

With all of these stimulating tests it is well to remember that obese subjects may exhibit an exaggerated rise in plasma insulin but that their hyperinsulinism is not accompanied by decreased blood glucose.

In patients who have been suspected of self-administration of insulin it is essential to establish that this indeed is the fact. Fortunately, these patients develop antibodies to either beef or pork insulin which can be demonstrated in their circulating blood. This can be most helpful in establishing this diagnosis of factitious hyperinsulinism.

Subselective Angiography

Once the diagnosis of autonomous hyperinsulinism is established, it is important to know as much as possible about the precise pathology involved. About 75 percent of the lesions responsible for endogenous hyperinsulinism are solitary adenomas. In recent years considerable effort has been expended on demonstrating solitary adenomas by selective and subselective arteriography. The success rate in the hands of expert angiographers is roughly 44 percent.[1] Others have reported success rates as high as 70 percent but the actual numbers of cases involved are not great, and the difference between such experiences is neither great nor important. When lesions are less than 1 cm. in diameter, the failure rate of angiographic demonstration increases and with increasing sophistication in diagnosis we can expect to diagnose more lesions of this small size.

Thus, it should be clear that failure to demonstrate a pancreatic lesion by subselective angiography should never be taken as evidence against the diagnosis of autonomous hyperinsulinism.

Beside negative arteriography in patients who nevertheless harbor hyperfunctioning beta islet cell lesions, there is another even more subtle trap which subselective arteriography will sometimes create. We explored two patients with well-defined autonomous hyperinsulinism in whom the typical angiographic blush of an insulinoma was clear. One of the patients had been explored previously, and no lesions could be palpated in the pancreas. In each of these two patients an adenoma was found and removed without trouble because the arteriographic localization had been accurate. Postoperatively it was clear within 2 weeks in both patients that there was persistent hyperinsulinism. At reexploration in both patients a generous segment of pancreas, about 80 percent, was removed and it was clear on microscopic examination of permanent histologic sections of the resected pancreas that their beta cell lesion was pancreatic adenomatosis distributed throughout the entire gland. Both patients have done well since their 80 percent resection, but one still requires diazoxide therapy to control milder hyperinsulinism experienced preoperatively. Islet cell adenomatosis will be discussed in more depth but for the moment it is worth emphasizing that simply because a solitary pancreatic lesion is angiographically visible is no assurance that it is not part of the larger problem of pancreatic beta islet cell adenomatosis.

A final point can be made concerning the usefulness of subselective abdominal arteriography in patients with hyperinsulinism. In patients whose hyperinsulinism is more pronounced than usual, the possibility of hyperfunctioning malignant islet cell tumor should be considered. If the hepatic metastases in these patients can be demonstrated arteriographically, it is wise to do so since percutaneous liver biopsy may then provide histologic confirmation of the diagnosis. Such patients can therefore be spared laparotomy which would otherwise be required to make a definite tissue diagnosis in this situation.

MANAGEMENT

GENERAL PREOPERATIVE CARE

Only a few remarks need be made to emphasize other preoperative measures unique to patients with hyperinsulinism. As noted, before, the brain and nervous system in general can be irreversibly damaged by persistent profound hypoglycemia in hyperinsulinemic patients. A properly functioning intravenous line, careful and frequent assessment of the patient's mental status, and frequent monitoring of blood glucose levels are all important. In urgent conditions 20 percent or even 50 percent glucose can be infused in small quantities to reverse profound hypoglycemia.

Ideally one wishes to have a patient reach the operating room with a blood glucose level of at least 50 mg./100 ml. Excessive hypoglycemia should be avoided when the patient is under anesthesia, just as it should be in the diagnostic and preoperative period.

INTRAOPERATIVE CARE

Solitary Islet Cell Adenomas

The surgeon exploring a patient with endogenous hyperinsulinism needs to have a sensitive awareness of the variations in islet cell pathology that may confront him.

The most common lesion, about 80 percent of cases, will be a solitary beta cell adenoma; 85 percent of the solitary adenomas are palpable, and when this is the case it is usually a simple matter to locate the lesion and tease it from the surrounding pancreas. If the adenoma is located in the distal two-thirds (body or tail) of the pancreas, one can remove that portion of the pancreas with no great difficulty rather than teasing the lesion out. Occasionally, solitary adenomas may be surprisingly inaccessible. The uncinate process is one such location that should always be inspected with care. On one occasion we found it necessary to divide the neck of the pancreas to gain access to a solitary adenoma sequestered in the head of the pancreas posterior to the common duct in the mid-portion of the vertical axis of the gland. The distal 80 percent of the pancreas was removed in this patient and this handled the situation gracefully.

The 15 percent of solitary adenomas that cannot be palpated may present real problems. Subselective angiography is a considerable help with these patients, and enabled us to locate and successfully remove three lesions other surgeons had not been able to find. In two other patients angiography did not reveal nonpalpable lesions; one was removed in a blind 85 percent distal pancreatic resection and in the other blind distal pancreatectomy failed to produce a lesion. This latter patient is now in her 70's and has been managed smoothly for 8 years with diazoxide treatment. Both her insulin and proinsulin levels have remained elevated with fasting, and there is no reason to doubt the diagnosis. Her lesion is probably deep in the pancreatic head or in an ectopic location but she does not wish further surgery, and there is no reason to suggest reexploration to her at this time.

Ectopically located pancreatic tissue should be sought at the operation if a lesion cannot be felt within the pancreas itself. The most common location for ectopic pancreas is just underneath the mucosa of the duodenum and some have advocated a small duodenotomy and insertion of a finger onto the mucosal surface of the duodenum to sensitively rule out this possibility.

Some authors have suggested that primary total pancreatectomy or resection of the pancreatic head with a pancreaticoduodenectomy is wise if a nonpalpable adenoma cannot be found. There are three arguments against this approach: (1) It is no more likely to produce a hidden lesion than is a blind distal pancreatectomy; (2) the mortality and morbidity of pancreaticoduodenectomy is higher than that for distal pancreatic resection; and (3) the patient may be suffering from diffuse islet cell disease and would respond to 85 percent distal pancreatic resection.

Considerable interest has been given to monitoring intraoperative blood glucose levels as an aid to deciding whether or not hyperfunctioning islet cell tissue has been totally removed. This so-called hyperglycemic rebound has been described by many and has been felt to represent a response to the sudden decrease in circulating insulin associated with excision of a solitary adenoma. Actually, the blood glucose of all patients tends to rise during surgery and in five operations in four patients operated on by us, in whom residual islet cell disease was left in place, the intraoperative glucose levels climbed at the same rate after partial pancreatic resection as that seen in 16 patients whose solitary adenomas had been successfully removed.[7]

The probable reason for this rise in intraoperative blood glucose is that other hormones are released by the excitement of surgery and general anesthesia, and some of these will cause an increase in blood glucose. Blood glucose should never be regarded as solely reflecting insulin release. Prominent among such hormones that serve to elevate blood glucose are epinephrine, glucagon, growth hormone and cortisol. If the blood glucose is persistently low after blind pancreatic resection for an insulin-secreting tumor, this is legitimate cause for concern and has in fact led to the successful removal of a lesion which had been overlooked. However, the recorded experiences with excision of insulinomas suggest that persistently low blood glucose intraoperatively is a rare occurrence.

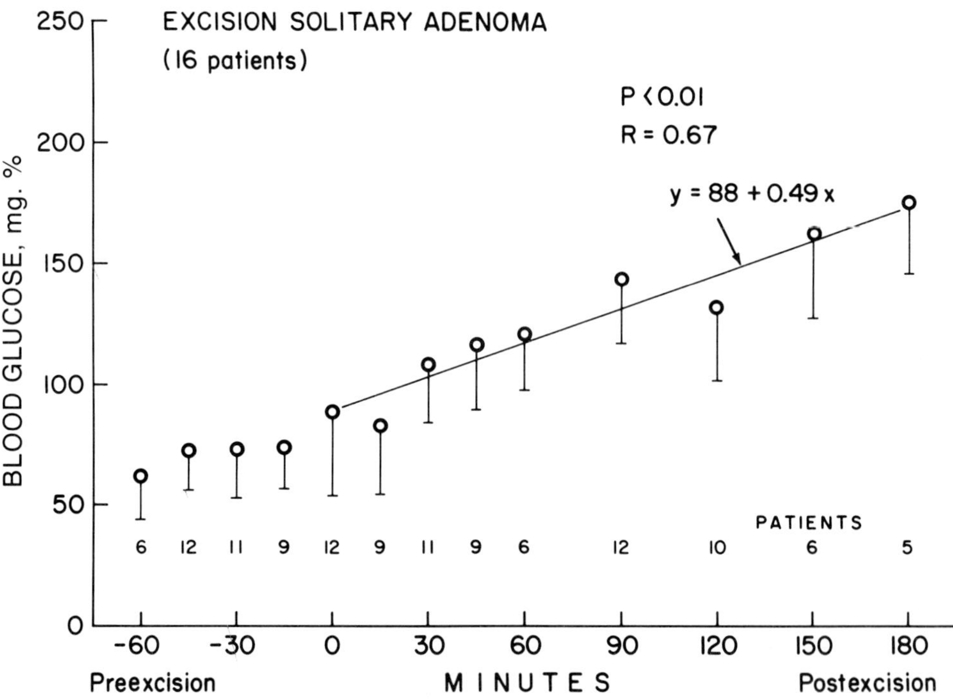

Fig. 12-2. Shown is the rate of mean blood glucose measurements after excision of solitary β cell adenomas at time 0. The ideal curve has been fitted mathematically to the depicted means by the method of least squares. The rate of glucose increment is 29 mg./100 ml. per hour. (Harrison, T. S., et al.: Ann. Surg., *178*:485, 1973[7])

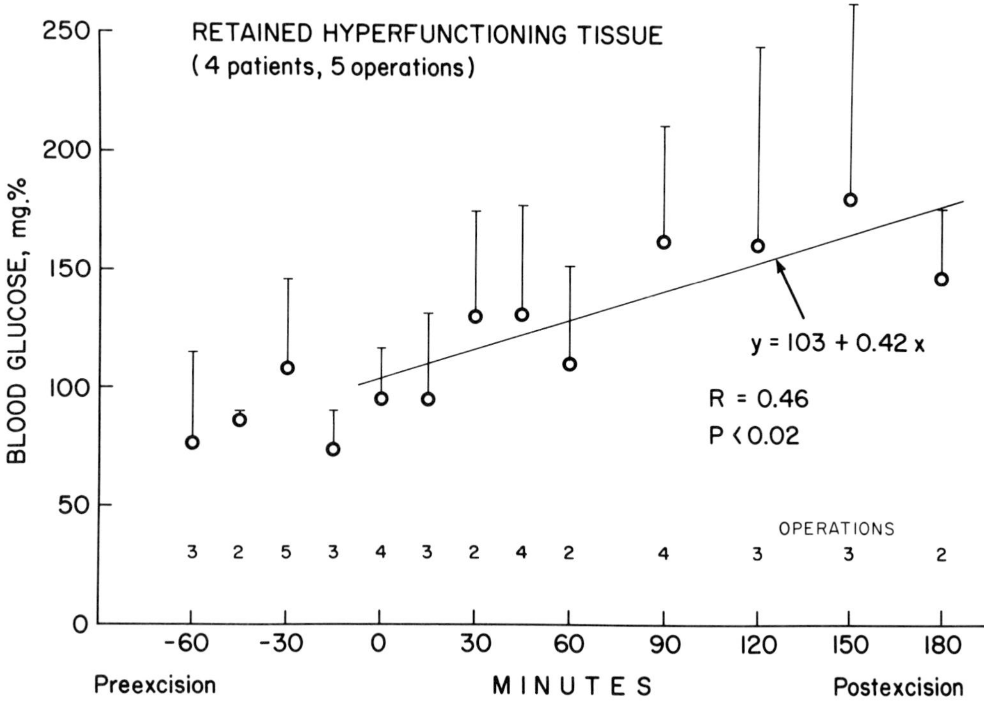

Fig. 12-3. The rate of mean blood glucose increment after resection of pancreatic tissue is shown for five operations on four patients who were known to have retained hyperfunctioning beta islet cell tissue. The glucose increment after time 0 is 24 mg./100 ml. per hour. This does not vary significantly from the curve shown in Fig. 12-2 up to the 180 minutes shown. There are no significant group differences at any of the comparable time points shown here and in Fig. 12-4. (Harrison, T. S., et al.: Ann. Surg., *178*:485, 1973[7])

Pancreatic Beta Cell Adenomatosis

Roughly 10 to 15 percent of patients with autonomous hyperinsulinism will have diffuse islet cell disease rather than a solitary adenoma. The most common of such lesions in the adult is islet cell adenomatosis. These lesions of adenomatosis may be macroscopically visible, and many more can be seen by microscopy of the pancreas. One will also see some normal islets in association with this lesion, since not all of the islets are affected with the changes of adenomatosis. The important thing for the surgeon to remember is that the disease is a diffuse process extending throughout the pancreas and excision of one or two visible or palpable adenomas will do nothing to reverse the hyperinsulinism. In five such patients, all adults, 85 percent distal pancreatic resection has brought the patients into a situation in which they respond to diazoxide therapy easily or, as was true in two patients into a condition in which only judicious dietary regulation was required.[7]

It is odd that islet cell adenomatosis has not received more emphasis over the years. Originally described by Frantz in 1944,[6] awareness of the lesion almost disappeared from view for almost 30 years. In the meantime accounts of patients with multiple adenomas, six, seven, or even eight lesions appeared

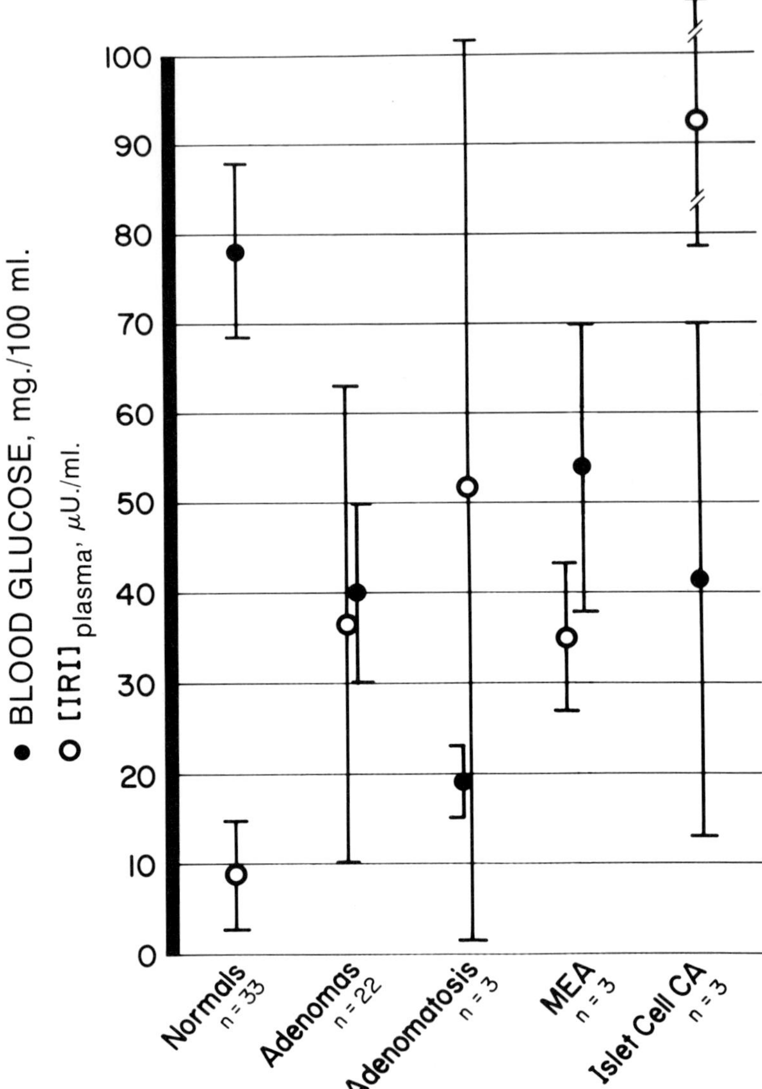

Fig. 12-4. Altered glucose, immunoreactive–insulin relationships are shown for each major category of pathology responsible for autonomous hyperinsulinism in the adult. The normals and adenomas are the same data as shown in Fig. 12-3. Of special interest are the high insulin values in the three patients with sporadic islet cell carcinoma; all three had extensive metastatic disease. (From unpublished data of Fajans, S. S., and Floyd, J. C., Jr.; and Horowitz, D. L., et al.[9])

frequently. In retrospect these multiple adenoma patients have probably been patients whose visible adenomas were part of the larger picture of diffuse adenomatosis in which both microscopically and macroscopically visible lesions are present. The obvious danger in regarding the macroscopic lesions as the only disease present is that such patients are in danger of being undertreated with too limited pancreatic resections being performed at their primary operation. Roughly 10 percent of adult patients with autonomous hyperinsulinism ultimately prove to have beta islet-cell adenomatosis.[7]

There has been a tendency to consider islet cell adenomatosis as part of the multiple endocrine adenomatosis-1 (MEA-I) syndrome. It is sometimes true that in MEA-I patients the pancreatic lesion is islet cell adenomatosis. However, many more instances of beta cell adenomatosis have appeared sporadically with no association to an MEA-I kindred.

Obviously frozen section microscopy of resected pancreatic tissue, if accurate, would be a great advantage in patients with hyperinsulinism in whom no solitary adenoma has been found. However, unless the examination is done by a pathologist highly skilled in pancreatic islet cell pathology serious errors are apt to be made. One can therefore make a good case for generous pancreatic resection, up to 85 percent if no lesion is found and examination of permanent histologic sections of this section by several groups of pathologists recognized for thier unusual competence in islet cell disease. In the adult patients at least, reexploration is not necessary, since 85 percent resection brings them into the range of medical control of their disease.

Multiple Endocrine Adenomatosis-I

Autonomous hyperinsulinism is a frequent occurrence in the MEA-I patients. The pathologic beta islet cell lesion may vary greatly within one affected kindred. Solitary adenoma, adenomatosis, multicentric islet cell carcinoma with regional lymph node metastases all may be the responsible lesion. With two exceptions no unique considerations need be applied to the MEA-I patients. The first exception is that the islet cell carcinoma associated with MEA-I tends to be a notoriously indolent and slow-growing neoplasm. Thus resection of 50 percent of the pancreas with en bloc removal of involved peripancreatic lymph nodes and local resection of a second primary in the pancreatic head will give long-term resolution of the hyperinsulinism, as was the case with one of our patients.

The second emphasis in MEA-I is that excision of two adenomas has reversed the autonomous hyperinsulinism in one of our MEA-I patients. Whether or not this remission is permanent, only extended follow-up will make clear. To date the patient has enjoyed 6 asymptomatic years, and there is little question that this fairly conservative surgical approach was worthwhile in her. It should be reemphasized that we have not seen two adenomas as the only lesions in any setting other than MEA-I.

Sporadic Beta Islet Cell Carcinoma

Beta islet cell carcinoma occurring with no recognized familial or genetic predisposition is most commonly seen in adult patients. This neoplasm is an aggressive one and frequently these patients will have demonstrable evidence of metastatic disease before their exploration is carried out. Their hyperinsulinism tends to be marked and their insulin levels much higher than those seen in patients with other forms of islet cell disease.

If the diagnosis can be suspected preoperatively on the basis of angiographic demonstration of metastases or radionuclide scanning defects of the liver, one can sometimes obtain tumor tissue by a percutaneous Silverman needle biopsy. If that is the case there is no reason to explore the patient, since a cure is clearly not possible.

When islet cell carcinoma patients are explored, there is hardly ever an instance in which the disease is confined to the pancreas. If gross tumor is confined to the pancreas, as radical a pancreatic resection as possible should be carried out en bloc with neighboring fat and involved lymph nodes. It is unlikely that the neoplasm can be cured.

If the patient has obvious involvement of regional lymph nodes and the liver, the most accessible tumor should be biopsied to confirm the diagnosis. If the primary lesion is small and mobile it can be resected, but seldom if ever will this appreciably slow down the progress of the tumor.

Patients with sporadic metastatic islet cell carcinoma which has metastasized tend to run a rapid and progressively downhill course. There are drug regimens which can be used to blunt their hyperinsulinism, and these will be discussed.

Hypoglycemias of Infancy and Childhood

In infants and children the occurrence of hypoglycemia associated with autonomous hyperinsulinism carries with it some particularly difficult problems.

The pathology varies. Solitary adenomas may be seen, but there is a higher likelihood of diffuse islet cell involvement being present than is the case in adult patients.

Nesidioblastosis. This seemingly cumbersome term originated by Laidlaw[9] from the Greek nesidion, meaning islet, has been championed by Vance, et al. for its current meaning.[12] In current usage nesidioblastosis refers to a characteristic diffuse islet cell lesion. If seen in the adult at all it is exceedingly rare but occasionally appears as part of the MEA-I syndrome. In children the lesion can occur sporadically as well as in MEA-I and in some of these patients 85 percent pancreatic resection has been successful. This is not invariably the case and more patients have been undertreated by 85 percent resection in MEA-I. If a diagnosis of nesidioblastosis is secure, and permanent section diagnosis is mandatory here, we believe that all but 5 percent of pancreatic tissue (i.e., all but a small rim of pancreatic head cradled in the duodenal sweep) should be resected. This is usually not hard to accomplish in the infant or child.

The pathologic appearance of nesidioblastosis is striking. Ribbons or sheets of islet cells parallel the pancreatic ducts and discrete islets are not seen. The lesion has been thought by some to represent a differentiation arrest of pancreatic islets.

Beta Islet Cell Hyperplasia. In infants and children as well, virulent hyperinsulinism may be encountered associated with diffuse islet cell hyperplasia. In these patients every islet scrutinized has abnormal beta cells and particular attention must be paid by the pathologists to the cellular characteristics of the beta cells which can show bizarre nuclear shapes and sizes.

Medical management of these children tends to be unsuccessful. Although enthusiasm has been expressed for 85 percent pancreatectomy in this situation, such has not been our experience. We have had to reoperate on two infants in whom 85 percent pancreatectomy reversed the hyperinsulinism for only 6 months. Again if one has a secure pathologic diagnosis, 95 percent pancreatectomy can be recommended as the surgical treatment of choice for this fortunately rare condition.

Not all of these infants with hyperinsulinism can be understood adequately by our conventional thinking on altered IRI/glucose relationships in autonomous hyperinsulinism. In one of our patients, a boy of 3 months, insulin levels were not elevated even in the presence of profound hypoglycemia. It is quite possible that heretofore unrecognized hypoglycemic mechanisms are operating in this patient. The disease of islet cell hyperplasia remains a difficult one to treat and even more difficult to understand properly.

NONOPERATIVE MANAGEMENT

Postoperative Considerations

When their hyperinsulinism has been successfully reversed, insulinoma patients are dramatically improved. Their central nervous system symptoms are gone, and they are able to resume normal lives without difficulty and in particular are capable of living with no restrictions on their diet or general activity. Some patients recognize that they are able to "think better," and that many subtle improvements occur in the vigor and confidence with which they approach their affairs. When IRI/glucose ratios are studied in these patients several months postoperatively, normal fasting and stimulated insulin-glucose relationships are found.*

For the hyperinsulinemic patient with irresectable tumor or irresectable diffuse islet cell disease and for those few patients deemed too old for surgical exploration there are a variety of measures available. For the most part these act by partially inhibiting the release of insulin from the abnormal beta cells.

Diet

The main function of dietary management in hyperinsulinism is to minimize the occurrence of dangerous hypoglycemia. Judicious spacing of food intake is advisable; in particular a snack at night before retiring may help avoid early morning hypoglycemia.

Some patients with hyperinsulinism find they do well on a relatively high protein intake. This has added appeal in that total carbohydrate and fat intake can be decreased and also daily total calories. If patients with hyperinsulinism are permitted to eat with no regulation or restraint they tend to become obese.

Drugs Inhibiting Insulin Release

Diazoxide. The most commonly used drug for the management of hyperinsulinism is diazoxide. For maximal effectiveness the drug is given with trichlormethiazide. The dose of diazoxide is usually between 300 to 800 mg. daily in patients with hyperinsulinism.

Diazoxide inhibits insulin release by a direct action on beta cells and also by stimulating epinephrine release, which itself further inhibits insulin release. There are unfortunate side effects of diazoxide the most prominent being fluid retention, gastrointestinal irritation, hypertrichosis and agranulocytosis.

---

*Fajans, S. S., and Floyd, J. C., Jr.: Unpublished data.

However diazoxide is tolerated comfortably by most patients and has been a great help in managing many insulinoma patients preoperatively. In addition diazoxide has been used to manage patients with islet cell adenomas whose lesions could not be found and who did not wish further surgery. As mentioned previously one such patient of ours has been managed with ease for 8 years and has been able to live normally while doing so.

There are many patients who do not respond successfully to diazoxide, or having initially responded to the drug later become refractory to its action. For these patients other drug regimens must be found.

Corticosteroids. Cortisone acetate, 100 to 200 mg. per day, often is helpful in raising the blood glucose of patients with hypoglycemia. Frequently the drug is used in conjunction with other agents and potentiates their effectiveness. Long-term use of cortisone is not without adverse side effects which are well known.

Streptozotocin. In recent years the drug streptozotocin has been used to increase blood glucose in patients with metastatic islet cell carcinoma. The drug is toxic and unfavorable side effects can be serious (e.g., hepatitis and progressive azotemia being the most serious reactions seen).

There are a few patients who do not respond effectively to streptozotocin, even when the drug is used in concert with cortisone or other agents.

Alloxan. Alloxan was first recognized as being capable of inhibiting insulin release by its diabetogenic action in dogs. It is toxic to the islet cells and carries with it too much toxicity to be recommended for use in humans.

Diphenylhydantoin. This anticonvulsant drug does have a recently discovered capability of raising blood glucose in a few patients with insulinoma. It is worth trying in patients refractory to other agents, but there are many patients who do not respond effectively to the drug. In hypoglycemia patients with seizure activity, the anticonvulsant actions of diphenylhydantoin should not delude one into assuming that the patient's hyperinsulinism has been successfully treated.

Somatostatin. Somatostatin, a naturally occurring peptide widely distributed in the body, inhibits the release of growth hormone.

Somatostatin also has been used effectively to reverse successfully hyperinsulinism in metastatic islet cell carcinoma.[3] Although available only for investigational use the agent, if it can be made commercially available, promises to be tremendously helpful in patients with inoperable insulin-secreting tissue. It is a natural product, and one can hope for little or no toxicity with its long-term use.

Other Measures Inhibiting Insulin Release

Radiotherapy. Palliation of patients with massive insulin-secreting tumors has been reported with x-ray therapy. It has not achieved widespread usefulness however and should be attempted only when other measures have failed.

Anti-tumor Agents. 5-Fluorouracil, nitrogen mustards and related agents have met with little success in metastatic islet cell carcinoma. The toxicity of the agents has tended to be more prominent than the relief of hypoglycemia.

CONCLUSION

Hypoglycemia should never be regarded as a specific disease entity by itself but rather as an indication that something has gone wrong in one or another of the mechanisms that physiologically regulate blood glucose levels with great sensitivity and precision.

Among the causes of hypoglycemia are pancreatic beta islet cell lesions with which is associated the release of insulin autonomous of the controlling influence of circulating levels of blood glucose. These pancreatic beta islet cell lesions can now be diagnosed with precision and should be treated surgically only when the diagnosis is securely made by well-defined laboratory criteria.

Surgical treatment carries with it a low mortality and morbidity and a strong likelihood of successfully reversing the hyperinsulinism.

REFERENCES

1. Bookstein, J. J., and Oberman, H. A.: Appraisal of selective angiography in localizing islet cell tumors of the pancreas. Radiology, *86*:682, 1966.
2. Conn, J. W., and Pek, S.: On spontaneous hypoglycemia, scope monograph. Kalamazoo, The Upjohn Co., 1970.
3. Curnow, R. T., Carey, R. M., Taylor, A., Johanson, A., and Murad, F.: Somatostatin inhibition of insulin and gastrin hypersecretion in pancreatic islet cell carcinoma. N. Engl. J. Med., *292*:1385, 1975.
4. Fajans, S. S., and Conn, J. W.: An intravenous tolbutamide test as an adjunct in the diagnosis of functioning pancreatic islet cell adenomas. J. Lab. Clin. Med., *54*:811, 1959.
5. Fajans, S. S., Floyd, J. C., Jr., and Vij, S. K.: Differential diagnosis of spontaneous hypoglycemia. *In* Kryston, L. J., and Shaw, R. A., (eds.): Endocrinology and Diabetes. pp. 453-472. New York, Grune & Stratton, 1975.
6. Frantz, V. K.: Adenomatosis of islet cells with hyperinsulinism. Ann. Surg., *119*:824, 1944.
7. Harrison, T. S., Child, C. G. III, Fry, W. J., Floyd, J. C., Jr., and Fajans, S. S.: Current surgical management of functioning islet cell tumors of the pancreas. Ann. Surg., *178*:485, 1973.
8. Horwitz, D. L., Kuzuya, H., and Rubinstein, A. H.: Circulating serum C-peptide: diagnostic implications. N. Engl. J. Med., *295*:207, 1976.
9. Laidlaw, G. F.: Nesidioblastoma, the islet tumor of the pancreas. Am. J. Pathol., *14*:125, 1938.
10. Service, F. J., Dale, A. J. D., Elveback, L. R., and Jiang, N.-S.: Insulinoma: clinical and diagnostic features of 60 consecutive cases. Mayo Clin. Proc., *51*:417, 1976.
11. Vance, J. E., et al.: Familial nesidioblastosis as the predominant manifestation of multiple endocrine adenomatosis. Am. J. Med., *52*:211, 1972.
12. Whipple, A. O., and Frantz, V. K.: Adenoma of islet cells with hyperinsulinism. Ann. Surg., *101*:1299, 1935.

EDITORIAL COMMENTARY

The clinical picture associated with hypoglycemia and relative hyperinsulinism is accountable primarily to the cerebral glucopenia which points up the continual need of the brain for glucose; additional symptoms associated with the sudden and rapid reduction in glucose levels similar to those observed after insulin overdosage are due to the compensatory elaboration of catecholamines which is stimulated by the hypoglycemia. The net effect of the excess catecholamines is ostensibly to attempt to correct the hypoglycemia by increasing the blood sugar level by means of their glycogenolytic effect on the target liver cells. This compensatory phenomenon is an example of a homeostatic mechanism in which the catecholamines seem to protect the human organism against a crisis.

Historically, the entity of tumor-induced hypoglycemia with hyperinsulinism was not recognized clinically until after the introduction of insulin for the treatment of diabetes mellitus, when the clinical similarity of iatrogenic exogenous insulin overdosage and the organic hypoglycemic attacks were noted.

It is important to understand the mechanism of the development of a relative hyperinsulinism at the time of hypoglycemia in order to arrive at an accurate diagnosis.

The physiologic action of insulin in carbohydrate metabolism can be considered to be anabolic in the sense that it causes conversion of glucose to glycogen in the liver and promotes the uptake of amino acids for protein synthesis, thus storing energy and reducing excess levels of circulating glucose in the blood. Normally insulin release is regulated by the glucose concentration of the blood perfusing the islets; an increase of glucose in the beta cells stimulates insulin release and vice versa.

Normally, during fasting, glucose is utilized by the brain and erythrocytes and during physical activity, by other tissues, and the resulting decrease in glucose concentration is accompanied by a concomitant decrease in insulin release until the circulating level of insulin is undetectable. Thus the insulin effect of converting glucose to glycogen in the liver is minimal or absent. In patients with an insulinoma, however, this capacity for hypoglycemia to inhibit insulin release is absent (in the insulinoma cells). The result is that there is a relatively high or inappropriate level of plasma insulin for that blood glucose level. Furthermore, the autonomous secretion of insulin from insulinomas continues to convert glucose to glycogen in the liver. These mechanisms during fasting, and particularly during physical activity when glucose is utilized acutely, thus exaggerate the hypoglycemia so that cerebral glucopenia ensues. Therefore, it is believed that it is not necessarily an "overproduction" of insulin, but rather an inappropriate secretory level of insulin during fasting hypoglycemia that accounts for the diminished release of glucose by the target cells in the liver.

Insulinomas release both insulin and proinsulin into the blood. These substances are measurable as immunoreactive insulin (IRI), but elevated levels of proinsulin, as determined by special radioimmunoassay (RIA) techniques, are more likely to be observed in patients with malignancies in either entopic or ectopic sites. A somatomedin is believed to be the hypoglycemic agent elaborated from ectopically located hypoglycemia-producing tumors, such as mesotheliomas. Such tumors can be confirmed by bioassay for insulinlike activity, but usually not by RIA.

Islet cell adenomatosis or hyperplasia occurs as the cause of organic hypoglycemia with about 10 percent incidence and when recognized by the surgeon and surgical pathologist, requires a subtotal distal pancreatectomy. In the absence of any discernable islet-cell pathology at the time of surgical exploration, a controversy exists as to whether a "blind" distal resection is indicated. If the hyperinsulinism is suppressible by diazoxide, as determined by prior testing, that form of medical therapy may be preferable to resection while waiting for further developments in the follow-up of the patient.

It is quite possible that in the future there may be a satisfactory nonoperative method of control of the hypoglycemic syndrome or of the endogenous hyperinsulinism by means of administration of somatostatin which inhibits the release of insulin. This relatively new polypeptide has been called "omniostatin" because of its inhibitory effect on the release of growth hormone, insulin, gastrin, glucagon, CCK and TSH. The tumor, of course, would likely not be controlled by such methods, and surgical and chemotherapeutic treatment will still be required for neoplasias. *S.R.F.*

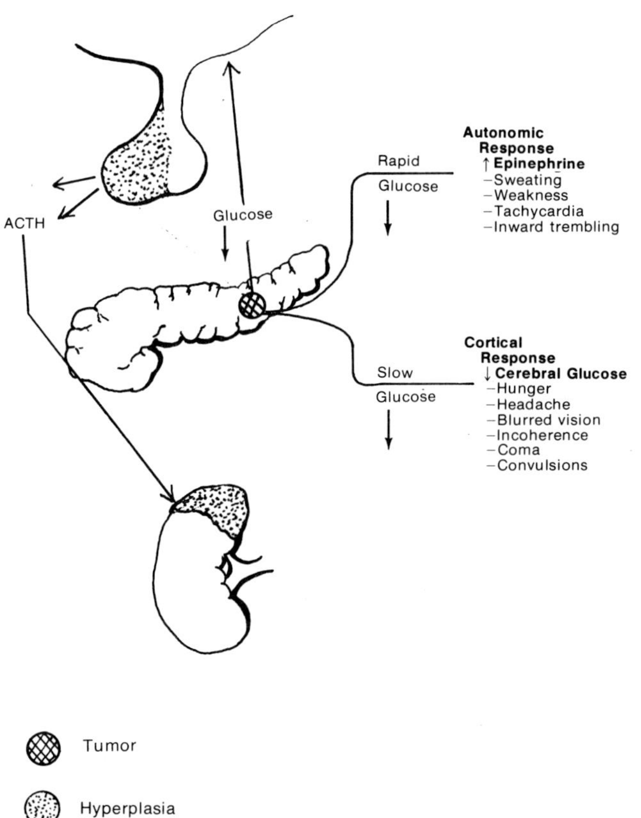

Fig. 12-5. Pathophysiology of the hypoglycemic syndrome.

(See overleaf for flowchart.)

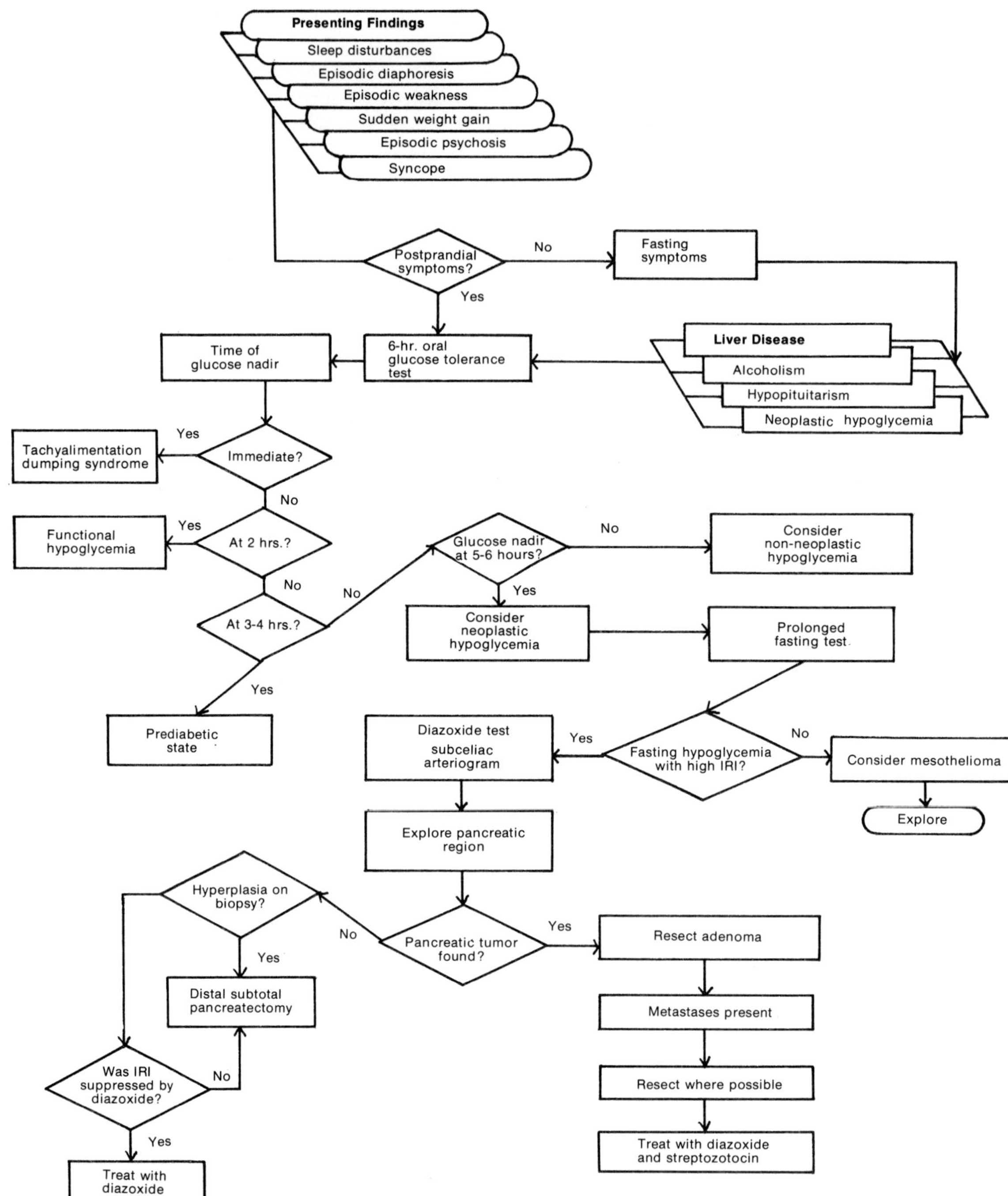

Fig. 12-6. Management flowchart of the hypoglycemic syndrome.

13

The Hyperglycemic, Cutaneous Syndrome: Pancreatic Glucagonoma

Christopher Mallinson, M.B., F.R.C.P., and Stephen R. Bloom, M.A., M.B., M.R.C.P.

Pancreatic glucagon was first identified and named in 1923 by J. R. Murlin,[24] a remarkable physiologist who was among several early workers to suggest that the hyperglycemic effect of Banting's and Best's pancreatic extract was not necessarily the result of contamination with epinephrine and could be the result of the activity of a specific hormone. Since then much has been published concerning the structure, properties, function and cellular origin of pancreatic glucagon.[14,27] Clinical medicine has few uses for this potent hormone but academic medicine has found it the subject of much research as a possible factor in the pathogenesis of diabetes mellitus and diabetic ketoacidosis.[52] During the 50 years since its discovery many workers have attempted to identify glucagon-secreting islet cell tumors. Several patients, half of whom had diabetes mellitus, have been described with a tumor consisting apparently of A_2 cells.[2,7,17,20,23,38,40,42,63] These early cases are impossible to validate now, since the staining methods used to identify tumors were nonspecific and the few studies of glucagonlike activity in tumor and plasma had used nonspecific and insensitive bioassay methods. However, in 1966 McGavran and his colleagues ushered in a new era in this field by their model report of the first convincing case of a patient with an A cell tumor containing glucagon and high plasma glucagon levels.[31] Glucagon was measured by Dr. Roger Unger with a sensitive and specific radioimmunoassay (RIA) supported by a bioassay technique. The patient's carbohydrate metabolism and glucagon levels suggested that the glucagon in the plasma originated from the tumor. However, even this classical description did not lead to the discovery of further cases. Six years elapsed before the combined efforts of dermatologists, physicians and radioimmunoassayists defined a striking and quite unexpected cutaneous syndrome accompanied by glossitis, anemia, weight loss, variable diabetes hyperglucagonemia and hypoaminoacidemia as a specific syndrome accompanying benign or malignant glucagon-containing tumors of the pancreas.[34] Since the original description of this syndrome in London several papers have been recognized from the previous records and 20 or more new patients have been diagnosed. In addition to patients with this cutaneous syndrome a smaller number of glucagonomas have been reported during the investigation of patients with diabetes mellitus, multiple endocrine neoplasia and pancreatic endocrine tumors containing more than one type of endocrine cell. None of these patients has had a rash, glossitis or anemia.

HISTORY

Although historic accounts are by definition anecdotal and hence unfashionable, the following is an account of the haphazard events which led to an understanding and classification of the clinical syndromes of glucagonomas. The first relevant reference in this subject is the description in 1942 by Becker[1] and his colleagues, from Rothman's celebrated school of dermatology in Chicago, of a patient with a malignant islet cell tumor of the pancreas, cell type unspecified, with a striking and unusual migrating erythematous rash, glossitis, stomatitis, diabetes mellitus, anemia, weight loss, severe depression and venous thrombosis. A similar syndrome was described by Gössner and Korting in 1960:[17] an extract of the tumor contained a hyperglycemic substance, possibly glucagon. The rash however was named pemphigus foliaceus, probably incorrectly since acantholysis, a diagnostic criterion of this condition, was absent. In McGavran's classic description[31] mention was also made, almost in passing, of a dermatitis, which was nevertheless severe enough to require 60 mg. of prednisolone daily, and normocytic, normochromic anemia. McGavran was not aware of the foregoing dermatologic descriptions and two subsequent dermatologic papers in 1967[9] and 1968[4] confirming Becker's original description made no reference to McGavran's paper or to glucagonomas. None of these workers knew of a penetrating paper published 10 years before in Russian in which V. C. Zhdanov[64] described a patient with what is clearly the same epidermal lesion and anemia, in whom a malignant islet cell tumor consisting of A_2 cells was identified by the histochemical reactions available. The author suggested that the diabetes at least was the result of hypersecretion of glucagon from the tumor. This author made no reference to Becker's paper. From all this we can conclude quite certainly that if English-speaking dermatologists and endocrinologists had been familiar with each other's literature not only in English but in German, Italian and Russian, and Russian pathologists had read American journals of dermatology, the whole problem of glucagonomas could have been clarified 20 years before it was. Nevertheless, Zhdanov's paper had no effect on the course of events; no further accounts have been published in Russian, and the paper was not cited in the English literature until 1976,[44] 4 years after things had come to a head in 1972. In 1971 Dr. Darrell Wilkinson demonstrated a patient with what seemed to be an unusual form of psoriasis to the Dermatological Section of The Royal Society of Medicine of London.[59] This Society still requires patients to be presented in person, and Dr. Church was present and recalling his former patient predicted firmly in discussion that this patient too would prove to have a pancreatic cancer. At a later meeting of the Section this striking piece of acumen was rewarded; it was reported that the patient did indeed have a carcinoma of the pancreas with hepatic metastases. A further case was recalled by Dr. N. R. Rowell in discussion.[60] As a direct result two further patients with the same rash, anemia and diabetes were recognized in Bristol and Plymouth by members of the Section. The patient in Bristol underwent laparotomy, after some misgivings on the part of the surgeon, and was found to have, apparently, only chronic pancreatitis. This suggested that the cutaneous syndrome might be specific simply for pancreatic disease rather than for tumor. The patient in Plymouth was referred to one of the authors for pancreatic secretion tests since the local surgical team were reluctant to operate for what seemed to be uncontrollable eczema in an uncontrollable diabetic. Fortunately, in one sense, thc tumor was in the head of the pancreas and the pancreatic secretion tests in consequence were positive.[51] What is more, the author in question had previously cared for a similar patient with a long history of migrating dermatitis, diabetes, anemia and depression, who was shown at autopsy to have an unsuspected islet cell adenoma in the tail of the pancreas. On the strength of this double confirmation the patient underwent laparotomy in Plymouth while her rash was at its worst and she required 60 units of insulin daily. A tumor was found which was removed with at least two-thirds of the pancreas. The rash abated within hours and disappeared within the week; for the first time in months, the anemia resolved, the patient gained weight without insulin and by the end of a few weeks required only modest dietary restriction to control asymptomatic diabetes. There has been no recurrence in 4 years. The tumor consisted of islet cells and contained glucagon. The plasma sent to one of us by Dr. Lightman, the house surgeon on the case, contained 20 times the normal concentration of pancreatic glucagon [24] before operation and was normal afterward (Fig. 13-1). Plasma sent by the other author to Dr. Brian Cox of the Department of Medicine at Guy's Hospital showed very reduced levels of all amino acids, for the most part lower than had previously been seen in his laboratory.[34] The authors then obtained plasma from Dr. Wilkinson's surviving patient and from two further patients diagnosed by Dr. A. P. Warin and Dr. Peter Borrie. All three patients had very high concentrations of plasma glucagon and low levels of amino acids. The last two patients were investigated in some detail and showed hyperinsulinemia, an exaggerated response to arginine, and an abnormal rise of glucagon after oral glucose,[32] findings which have all been confirmed subsequently. Shortly after this the patient in Bristol died and at autopsy a small islet cell adenoma was found in the tail of the pancreas obscured by changes of pancreatitis. The members of the British Dermatological Association were circularized and as a result three more cases, all dead, were discovered. Thus, studies of the first series of nine patients with what was felt to be a glucagonoma syndrome were published in 1974.[34] Dr. Wilkinson defined and named the rash necrolytic migratory erythema (NME) in what is the classic dermatologic description.[61] Within months two patients from the United States had been reported, one personally* and one in the full publicity of a clinicopathological conference at the Massachusetts General Hospital.[15] During the last 2 years 20 more cases have been reported or have been referred to us.[5,13,22,25,49,55,57] The clinical features of the original description have been confirmed,[15,21,44] and the majority of the tumors have been in the body and tail of the gland but comparatively few have been resectable. In addition it is clear that young men and women suffer from this syndrome and not only postmenopausal women, who composed eight of the nine patients in the first series.[35] The comparatively high incidence of severe depression* and significant venous thrombosis has been confirmed.[21] Most of the advances in understanding these tumors has been in their secretory responses; very little is known of the pathogenesis of the rash, the anemia, the mental changes or the thrombotic tendency.

---

*Hanifin, J.: Personal communication, 1975.

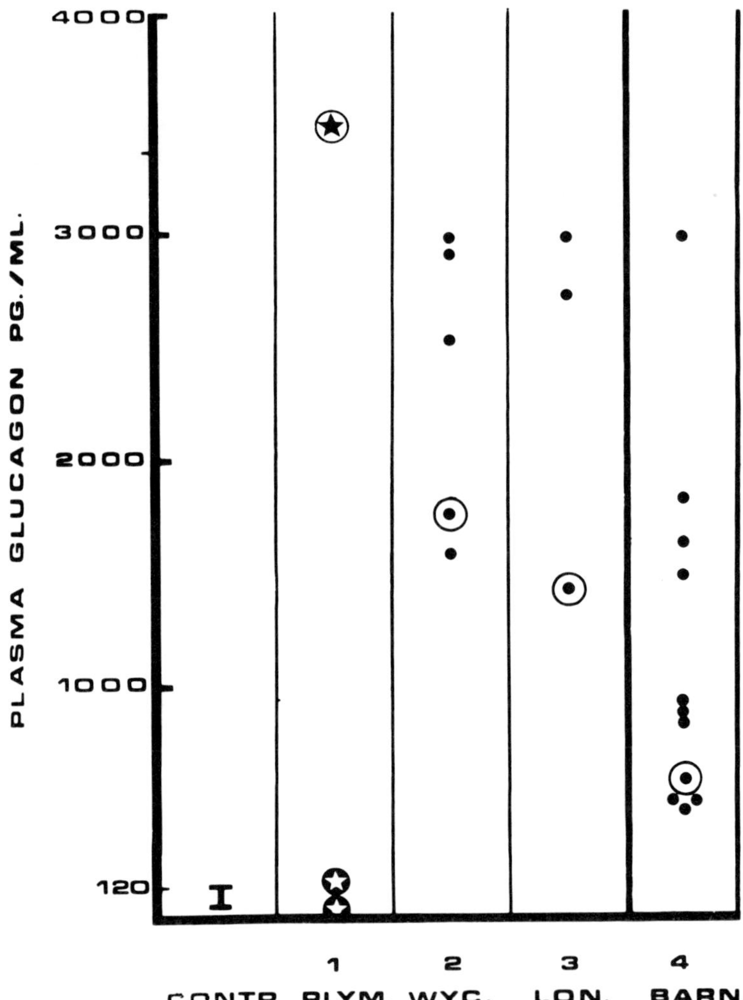

Fig. 13-1. Plasma levels of glucagon in control subjects (contr.) and in four patients with glucagonoma (1-4), being patients 1, 2, 3 and 4. (NB: *not* S.I. Units). In patient 1 the open circle is the preoperative level, the low dark circles are postoperative levels. (Mallinson, C., et al.: Lancet, *2*:1, 1974[35])

A smaller number of patients with glucagonomas have neither the rash nor the other features described with it apart from diabetes mellitus which is usually severe.[16,28,30,45] In patients with and without the rash, plasma levels of glucagon are extremely high and in a high proportion of patients abnormal forms of circulating glucagon are found.[13,45,55,57] Another recent development has been the discovery of a large number of cells containing pancreatic polypeptide in and around the glucagonomas of patients with NME.[46] So far, no patient without NME has been so studied. Glucagonomas are also found in the third type of patient, those with pluriglandular syndromes,[3,7,11,12,38,40,45,46,48,56] in whom the effect of glucagon appears to be mild and in one case at least plasma glucagon was normal.

The rash of the glucagonoma syndrome and its accompanying anemia were completely unexpected and are still unexplained. The recognition of this syndrome has led to the diagnosis of many more cases, to a measure of successful treatment of them, and to a number of advances in the understanding of glucagon, glucagonomas and endocrine tumors in general.

CLASSIFICATION

Not all glucagonomas are accompanied by NME, and not all of them produce one hormone only. In order to avoid confusion in discussion the following tentative classification is suggested. In a subject so new such a classification is likely to be revised later.

1. **Glucagonomas With the Cutaneous Syndrome.** The cutaneous syndrome consists of necrolytic migratory erythema (NME), glossitis, anemia, weight loss, diabetes mellitus, severe depression and venous thrombosis, not all of which are invariably present.

2. **Glucagonomas Without the Cutaneous Syndrome.** These are the patients reported with hyperglucagonemia, diabetes mellitus and unresectable malignant glucagonomas.[16,25,27,45,50,53] This class may prove to have a subdivision of single or multiple adenomata in association with unremarkable diabetes mellitus.[30]

3. **Glucagonomas in Patients With Pluriglandular Syndromes.** Several patients with pluriglandular syndromes show evidence of A_2 cell hyperplasia, adenomatosis, adenomas or carcinomas.[3,7,11,12,38,40,48,56] Plasma glucagon levels are not raised, diabetes is mild or absent, no rash, anemia, glossitis, etc., are seen, and the clinical picture is usually dominated by the activity of one or more of the other endocrine tumors.

CLINICAL FEATURES

The majority of patients diagnosed in life with glucagonomas have been attending a dermatology clinic and often a diabetic clinic as well; most of them have attended months or years before the diagnosis which is even now commonly made only after a tumor has been detected.[32] The second type of glucagonoma has no specific features and is usually only diagnosed by clinical vigilance after a pancreatic tumor or its metastases have appeared in a patient with diabetes. The third type of glucagonoma has no obvious clinical effect and is usually diagnosed during thorough investigation of a pluriglandular syndrome.

Glucagonoma Syndrome With NME

The Skin Rash. The most detailed descriptions of the rash are by Wilkinson,[61] Sweet[51] and Pedersen.[44] The rash is characterized by its distribution, by superficial epidermal destruction with attendant erythema, by a tendency to migrate and by highly specific histologic features.

Distribution. In all descriptions so far the rash has invariably involved the lower abdomen and the perineum (Fig. 13-2). The perioral skin and the lower limbs, in particular the feet, are also commonly involved and may be the first areas affected. The upper limbs are less commonly affected and the upper

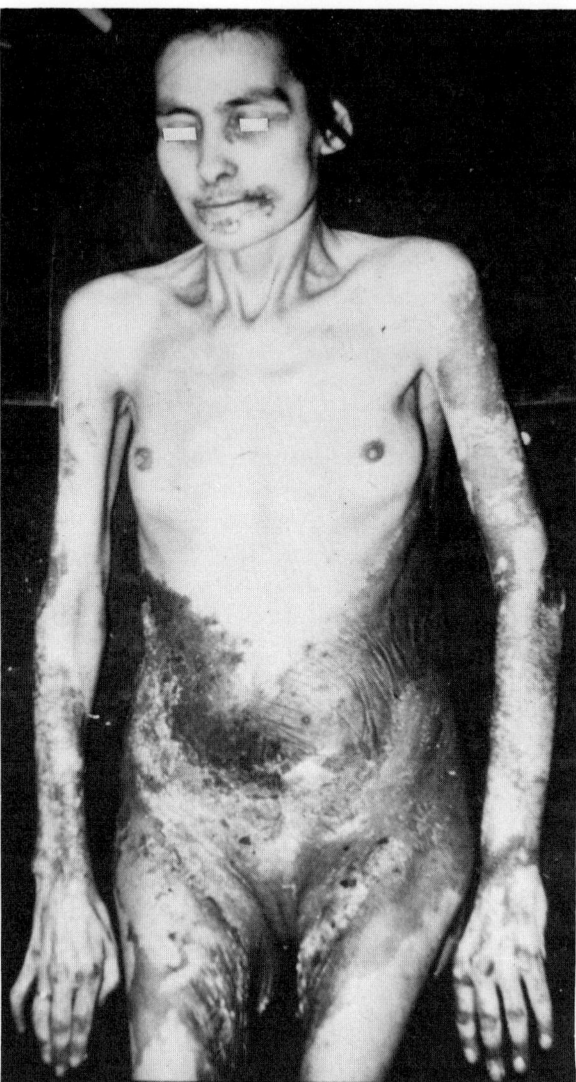

Fig. 13-2. Distribution of the rash. The lower abdomen, perineum, legs, are most affected and the perioral skin and arms less so. The edge is marginate. The darker areas over the right lower abdomen are hyperpigmented healed skin. The patient died within months of a malignant glucagonoma. (Courtesy Dr. N. R. Rowell, Leeds)

abdomen and the thorax rarely so. Most patients have angular cheilitis and glossitis with striking vermilion discoloration of the tongue. Oral ulceration has not been reported.

Appearance and Migration. In its early stages the rash is highly characteristic but may be confusingly altered if the lesions become secondarily infected.[61] The earliest abnormality is a slightly raised reddened edematous patch (Fig. 13-3*A*) which spreads within 2 or 3 days. At this stage the superficial layers of the epidermis can be rubbed off leaving a raw surface exposed to infection. The skin of the perineum and the feet is commonly rubbed raw by clothes and shoes, whereas affected areas of the face, hands and legs may not weep but do show superficial blistering followed by crusting. The edge of the lesion tends to spread, whereas the older central portion heals even when the damage has been severe. The healed skin often shows brown pigmentation which marks areas previously affected. Apparently normal skin is abnormally fragile,[51] and the sites of election of NME may be partly determined by the rubbing they receive. As the rash spreads it may take on a marginate and geographic appearance with an erythematous edge and a less affected or healed center (Fig. 13-3*B*). In this case the whole process passes through a cycle of 7 to 14 days. In some cases however the course is more indolent; the centers of the lesions do not heal, particularly if they are infected, and migration is less striking or absent. The appearance of the earliest lesion is very similar to a moderately severe scald with a reddened skin covered by a very superficial layer of dead epithelium. The whole rash is most commonly confused with atypical forms of psoriasis,[59] pemphigus[17] or eczema.[51] It bears some resemblance to acrodermatitis enteropathica seen in children which is now recognized as being the result of zinc deficiency. It has also been suggested that the lesion resembles iatrogenic zinc deficiency seen in adults. So far, this has caused marked alopecia and lesions in the face and scrotum and to this extent is different from NME. No histologic material is on record.

Histology. The earlier reports of the histology of these lesions were confusing until Wilkinson demonstrated that it is essential to biopsy the edge of the fresh lesion to avoid the confusing appearance of secondary infection.[60,61] When this precaution has been followed, the histologic changes are remarkably consistent and appear to be specific.[5,15,44] In Figure 13-4 a biopsy from a new lesion is contrasted with one from skin from a healthy patient. In NME the dermis is normal as is staining in the lower levels of the epidermis. There is an abrupt

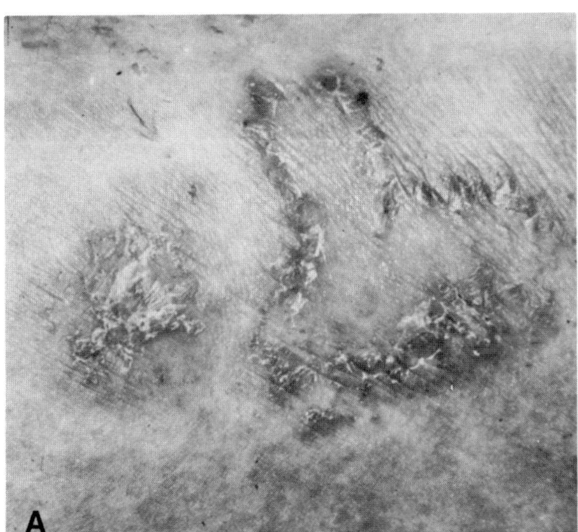

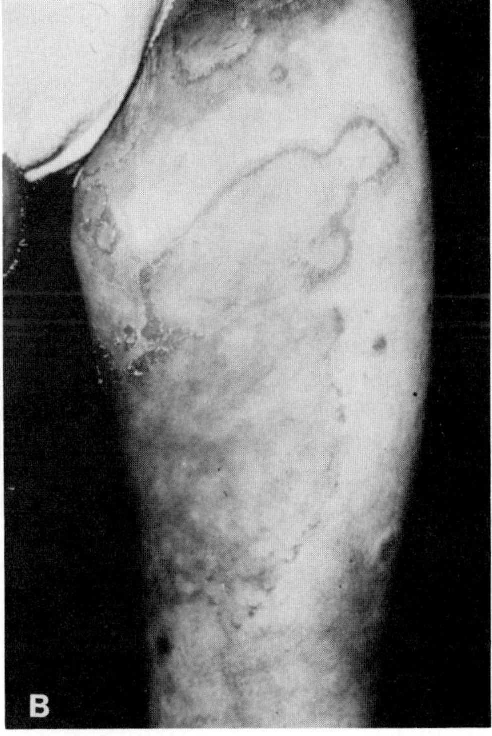

Fig. 13-3. *(A)* Two early patches of NME. The smaller lesion seen on the left is 1 day old, the one on the right resembled it exactly 3 days before. Spreading of the edge occurs with necrolysis of the epidermis in the center. *(B)* Extensive NME on the inner thigh; erythematous margin which is spreading with healed skin in center of affected patch.

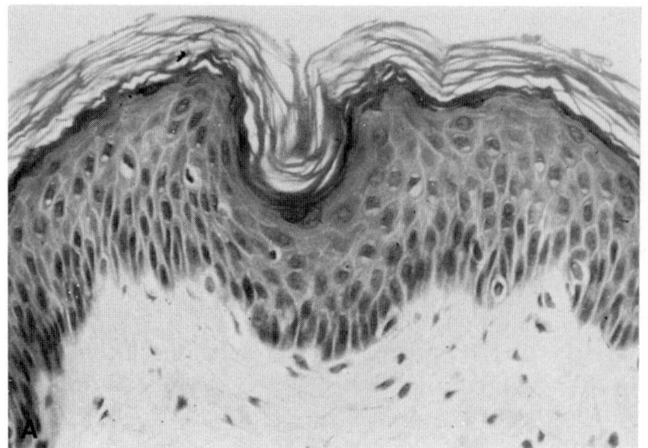

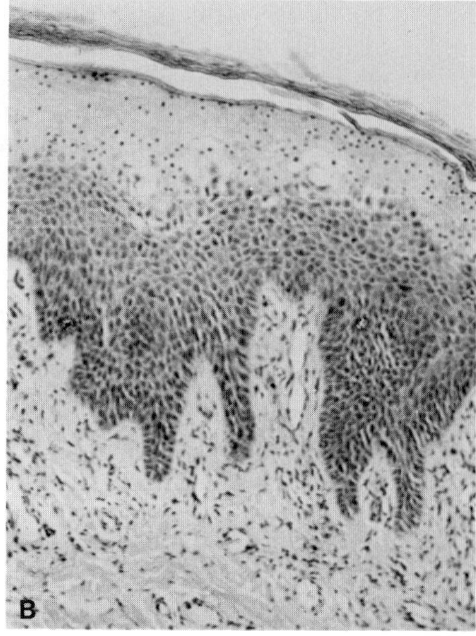

Fig. 13-4. *(A)* Histologic appearance (H & E stain) of biopsy of normal skin. The epidermis stains darkly and evenly from bottom to top and the layers of keratin are regular and adherent to the uppermost layer of epidermis. *(B)* Histologic appearance of NME. The dermis and lower layers of epidermis are normal. The upper half of the epidermis is necrotic and shows lysis; the keratin is spreading to form a superficial vesicle.

transition of staining characteristics in the upper half of the epidermis which shows necrosis and lysis (necrolysis). The dead layer of upper epidermis tends to separate from the viable layer below with the formation of superficial vesicles or bullae.

Whereas there are wide variations in quality and degree of this picture, it appears to be specific to patients with glucagonomas. However, occasional patients have been referred to us with many or all the features of this rash, who appear to have no pancreatic tumor and no hyperglucagonemia. This anomaly is unlikely to be solved until there is some knowledge as to the fundamental cause of the rash which is almost completely lacking. Indirect immunofluorescent studies have failed to reveal any evidence of an immune basis to the rash,[37,44] and there is no histologic evidence of any vascular abnormality. It seems possible that the lesion is the result of an abnormality of keratinization, or to activation of lysosomal enzymes in the middle layers of the epidermis; these two generalizations however are so broad as to have the same degree of truth and helpfulness as astrology.

Diabetes. All but one of the patients reported have been found to have an abnormal glucose tolerance test at some point in their history. This may precede or succeed the rash by a varying interval which can be many months or years. The diabetes is often a mild degree as judged by blood glucose levels and satisfactory control with oral hypoglycemic agents or diet alone. Certain patients have required insulin, a few in high doses, but brittle diabetes is unusual. In one patient on insulin some endogenous insulin secretion probably persisted and certainly was evident after the tumor had been resected and carbohydrate intolerance almost disappeared.[29] No systemic complications of diabetes such as retinopathy, neuropathy or nephropathy have been reported and the prevalence of arterial disease is unremarkable. Only one patient has had a family history of diabetes mellitus and that the only one with ketoacidosis. As is discussed below it seems probable that the diabetes in many of these patients is the result of high levels of biologically active circulating glucagon. Reduction of these levels is commonly followed by an improvement in glucose tolerance, unless the treatment used has affected B cell function as well as is the case with streptozotocin. What is also striking in these patients is that the very high levels of plasma glucagon are commonly associated with mild diabetes and so far almost never with ketoacidosis. Most of the patients have hyperinsulinemia, usually of less striking degree than the raised glucagon levels, and this seems to offset the hyperglycemic effect of the glucagon surprisingly well if glucagon were indeed a major causative factor of diabetes. The modest elevations of glucagon seen in patients with primary diabetes mellitus who have far greater degrees of carbohydrate intolerance are in sharp contrast to patients with glucagonomas.

All degrees of diabetes are seen in patients with glucagonomas. The diagnosis must not be excluded on the finding of a normal glucose tolerance test, since this may develop late in the disease.[51]

Anemia. In all but the exceptional patient some degree of normocytic, normochromic anemia has been reported during relapses of the rash.[35] This has been present in patients with small but actively secreting adenomas, but it is more severe in patients with advanced carcinomas and hepatic metastases. In the patients in whom data are available, it is clear that in remissions of the skin rash the hemoglobin tends to rise, often to normal levels.[35] In patients with NME in whom anemia has been absent the degree of activity of the skin rash at the time the hemoglobin was measured has not been recorded. The cause of this anemia is obscure; in a very few patients serum iron has been low and iron-binding protein desaturated, and courses of oral or parenteral iron have been effective in raising the hemoglobin slightly but not to normal levels. Marrow examinations have been carried out in well over half of the reported cases and showed no abnormality in erythropoiesis or iron stores. In two earlier cases ring sideroblasts were seen in the bone marrow but no features of sideroblastic anemia were recorded. Radioiron studies reported by McGavran suggested an increased turnover of iron but normal red cell turnover and intestinal iron absorption. This is the only detailed investigation into the anemia so far recorded. In one of our patients studied as the rash reappeared following a quiescent phase the levels of plasma glucagon and amino acids did not significantly alter but the hemoglobin fell from 12.4 g. to 9.6 g./100 ml. within 48 hours without evidence of hemolysis or blood loss.[32] There was a slight fall in albumin at the same time from 3.6 g. to 3.0 g./100 ml. suggesting that hemodilution could have been responsible for the fall in hemoglobin concentration.

Venous Thrombosis. Significant venous thrombosis has been reported in approximately 30 percent of patients,[35,44] with several cases of pulmonary embolus. There has been no report of thrombophlebitis migrans, a well-recognized complication of tumors of the body of the pancreas. There is no obvious correlation between the incidence of deep vein thrombosis in these patients and the severity of emaciation or the degree of malignancy of the tumors. In a personal series of 60 patients with adenocarcinoma of the exocrine pancreas, deep vein thrombosis and pulmonary embolus as complications were not seen at all. Standard laboratory prothrombin time estimations have been invariably normal (except in those patients treated with anticoagulants) and platelet counts have not been abnormally high. No systematic investigation of coagulation has been reported.

Weight Loss and Depression. Weight loss, varying from 2 to 20 kg., has been the rule in these patients and depression has been notable in about one-third. Not surprisingly loss has been greatest in patients with malignant disease, but even in patients with solitary adenomas emaciation and depression have sometimes been striking. Both conditions tend to reverse during remissions of the skin rash and have invariably done so after successful resection of tumors. The two features are discussed together because they may share the same causes in patients who have malignant disease, hypersecretion of glucagon (a catabolic hormone), diabetes mellitus, painful glossitis, an ugly skin rash and long periods in hospital undergoing observation or investigations which are unpleasant in themselves and may expose the patient to weeks away from home, being offered unpalatable food in disturbing surroundings. Nevertheless, it is tempting to think that both features are in some degree specific to glucagonomas, since all these factors, with the exception of hyperglucagonemia, operate in other groups of patients who do not show such a marked degree of weight loss or depression.

Glucagonoma Syndrome Without NME[16,25,27,45,50,53]

There are absolutely no specific clinical pointers to patients with single glucagonomas without NME apart from the consistent finding of severe diabetes mellitus and, eventually, the findings of a malignant pancreatic tumor. Although, as will be discussed later, these patients appear to have the same degree and type of hyperglucagonemia as patients with NME no rash, anemia, venous thrombosis or unusually severe depression are seen. All these features of course may take some time to develop in patients with NME and this second class of glucagonoma may simply represent an early form or a forme fruste of the first. So far no tumor has been resectable, and so the relationship of the tumor to the diabetes is uncertain. The minority and speculative view of one author is that these are patients with a primary diabetic diathesis, hence with reduced or absent endogenous insulin secretion in whom hyperglucagonemia cannot be offset by hyperinsulinemia. This may account for the severity of the diabetes and it is possible that hypersecretion of both hormones is in some way necessary for NME to develop.

Lomsky et al.[30] reported a series of 336 consecutive autopsies on diabetic patients in which three had shown A_2 cell adenomas. No evidence of a causal connection between the tumors and the diabetes was given and the findings have not been followed up. However, if such tumors are so frequent, are functioning glucagonomas and the cause of the diabetes they would presumably be the commonest form of endocrine tumor.

Glucagonomas in the Pluriglandular Syndromes[3,7,11,12,38,40,46,48,56]

The pluriglandular syndromes have been described in detail elsewhere in this book. From these accounts it will be clear that whereas glucagonomas have occasionally been described in cases of pluriglandular syndrome, no case of NME or its associated clinical features has been described. The mild diabetes found in some of these patients may be related to glucagon secretion or to the effect of a pancreatic tumor in a patient with a stressful disease. Diagnosis has only been made by meticulous investigation of patients in whom it is well-recognized that a galaxy of unsuspected endocrine tumors may be present.

Miscellaneous Findings

A number of apparently miscellaneous clinical findings have been recorded in patients with glucagonoma syndromes of all sorts. A number of patients have experienced episodic diarrhea, others have had constipation. One patient appeared to have adult celiac disease responding to a gluten-free diet,[35] which had no effect on the skin rash or anemia. Several patients have had barium studies of the small intestine which showed "coarse mucosal folds" but jejunal biopsies have been reported on as normal.[35] A recent case showed very large jejunal villi, similar to those found in the only reported case of enteroglucagonoma. This finding calls for quantitative evaluation of the available jejunal biopsies from other cases. The known physiologic and pharmacologic effects of glucagon have led to a number of other laboratory investigations: blood urea, electrolytes, calcium, magnesium, phosphate, alkaline phosphatase, acid phosphatase, bilirubin, "liver transaminases," cardiac-specific enzymes, creatinine, creatine and plasma levels of many hormones including parathormone. The latter has only been measured in one patient and was normal, the others have been repeated many times in many patients and have also been normal. In relapses of the skin rash there is commonly a slight fall in plasma albumin which is asymptomatic, accompanied by a comparable fall in calcium but no more. Many estimations of urinary VMA and 5-HIAA levels have been normal.

THE TUMORS

Glucagonomas share several characteristics with other islet cell tumors in regard to their site, light microscopic appearance, electron microscopic characteristics[5,27,31,35] and in their association with cells containing human pancreatic polypeptide.[46] They are distinguished from other pancreatic endocrine tumors by containing significant amounts of glucagon,[5,12,13,15,21,24,31,35,49,55,57] showing indirect immunofluorescent reactions for pancreatic glucagon alone[35] (apart from HPP) and in certain rather nonspecific histologic and cytochemical properties.[19]

Site

The majority of pancreatic endocrine tumors are found in the tail, body, neck and superior part of the head of the pancreas. These are the derivatives of the embryonic dorsal lobe of the pancreas which in all vertebrates bear all or most of the islet cell tissue. This distribution is in striking contrast to tumors of the exocrine pancreas which are more commonly present in the head.

Light Microscopy

The most detailed accounts of the light microscopic characteristics of these tumors are given by McGavran[31] and Leichter.[27] The tumors consist of cells of varying size, the most characteristic being cylindrical with a slightly enlarged nucleus and extremely few mitotic figures. Cells are arranged in a variety of more or less differentiated patterns, from a trabeculated and glandular arrangement of normal islets to haphazard "medullary" masses, with a variety of rosettes and follicular patterns between. Many tumors contain several patterns. The cells are supported by a variable quantity of delicate connective tissue and are usually highly vascular if they are malignant, and much less so if well-differentiated adenomata. Apart from these features which can be made out on standard hematoxylin and eosin stains there are a number of cytochemical reactions[19,43] formerly used to discriminate between islet cells of different type, and now largely superseded, in classical practice at least, because they are not entirely specific in normal tissue and even less so in tumors.

Electron Microscopy (EM)

Normal human A_2 cells have characteristically dense round secretory granules approximately 400 mp. in diameter, hence smaller than B-cell granules. An agranular limiting membrane surrounds the granules with a narrow gap between it and the core. Cells containing similar granules have been identified in glucagonomas, but other cells with granules of other sizes and shapes are usually also found. Thus EM is helpful in confirming that tumor cells are of endocrine type, but less so in defining the secretion contained.

Indirect Immunofluorescent Methods

This technique is both sensitive and highly specific in identifying individual endocrine polypeptides within cells.[25,43,54] Thus, the entire series of endocrine polypeptides can be tested for in one sample of tissue, and the endocrine content of any given tissue, normal or not, can be verified in a direct and convincing fashion. This method has confirmed that glucagonomas associated with NME are single cell tumors containing only glucagon, and that the hyperinsulinemia seen in these patients is not accompanied by insulinoma or B-cell hyperplasia.[35] It is also by this method that the cells containing HPP have been identified in and around pancreatic endocrine tumors and their metastases.[46]

It was by indirect immunofluorescence that direct confirmation was possible in one patient with overt clinical Cushing's syndrome found to have a tumor containing several endocrine polypeptides including glucagon.[3] In patients with multiple endocrine neoplasia indirect immunofluorescence again provides direct confirmation of cell content. This is an important part of the investigation since the spectrum of hypersecretion in such patients may be due to the presence of autonomously secreting tumor, to secondary hyperplasia, or simply to a pharmacologic response of normal cells to complicated endocrine discord.

Tumor Glucagon Content

Other types of pancreatic endocrine tumor and exocrine carcinomas contain little or no detectable glucagon. Glucagonomas themselves contain a variable amount of glucagon,[35] often surprisingly little, which may reflect a state of low storage and high secretion, or the care with which tissue was preserved. The highest concentration of glucagon in a tumor yet reported was in a patient with almost normal plasma glucagon levels and hence little evidence of hypersecretion. Thus, a concentration of glucagon only in the range of that found in normal pancreas is not unusual in true glucagonomas; the point is that any such level in any other sort of tumor would be quite unexpected in the absence of some A_2-cell content in the tumor.

A glucagonoma is diagnosed on the finding of islet cell morphology under the light microscope, preferably electron microscopic confirmation of endocrine granules in the cells, a significant concentration of pancreatic glucagon in the tumor extract and, probably most important, the demonstration of glucagon in the tumor cells by indirect immunofluorescence. Hyperglucagonemia and hypoaminoacidemia suggest that the tumor is secreting abnormally actively.

SECRETORY ACTIVITY

Patients with glucagonomas show variable but high basal levels of glucagon accompanied by a lesser degree of hyperinsulinemia. Both can be increased, or more rarely decreased, by various modifiers of normal glucagon secretion.[5,13,24,27,32,45,49,55,56,57] In common with many other endocrine tumors both anomalous and exaggerated responses to such modifying agents are seen. Moreover, agents which would not normally be expected to have any effect on glucagon secretion, such as streptozotocin[13,49,55] and diphenylhydantoin,[24] appear to reduce glucagon secretion. Whereas these tumors may or may not synthesize glucagon at an abnormal rate, it is certain that most of them release glucagon in an abnormal way in a pattern which is just beginning to become apparent. There is now evidence that certain glucagons which are either normally retained with A_2 cells or are not found at all are present in the circulation of glucagonoma patients. Thus, both abnormally large[13,45,55,57] and small[55] molecules showing glucagon immunoreactivity are detectable in the plasma of patients with glucagonoma.

Basal Levels

Basal levels of plasma glucagon in patients with glucagonoma are usually grossly elevated apart from those with pluriglandular syndromes. Levels do however vary widely from 500 to 6,000 pMol./ml. within and between patients (normal 10 to 120 pMol./ml.). There is also marked variability from minute to minute, accounting for the erratic baseline measurements in certain studies.

Plasma levels of endogenous insulin are often raised; this is attributed to the insulin-releasing effect of glucagon[32] and probably accounts for the mildness of the carbohydrate intolerance in most of these patients. Fasting blood glucose levels are commonly slightly high.

Glucose Tolerance

Without exception so far the blood glucose levels in oral glucose tolerance tests have been in the diabetic range. The abnormality is often mild even in the presence of very high levels of plasma glucagon. This suggests that glucagon is not a potent diabetogenic hormone, or one which can contribute greatly to the production of diabetic ketoacidosis. In most patients *oral* glucose has produced an anomalous and marked rise in plasma glucagon[5,13,24,27,32,49,55,56,57] (Fig. 13-5) in contrast to normal subjects who show a slight depression of glucagon levels. This rise does not seem to be due simply to an anomalous response to a

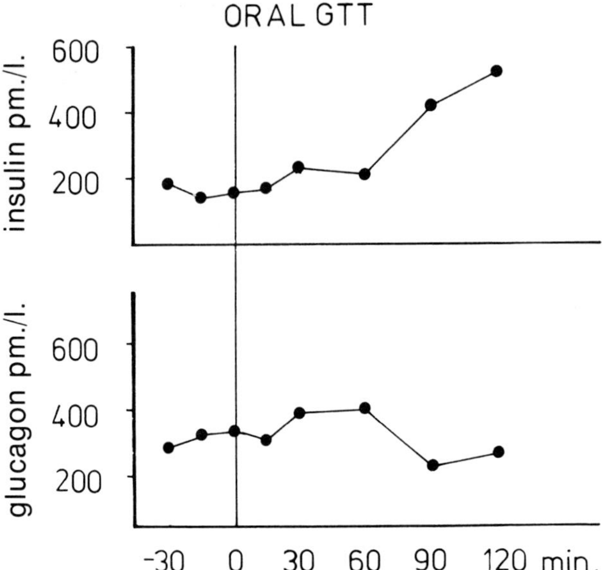

Fig. 13-5. Results of an oral glucose load on plasma glucagon and insulin in a patient with glucagonoma. The rise in glucagon is less striking than in some patients but is nevertheless quite distinct from the depression seen in normal subjects after oral glucose. Note the high basal levels of insulin.

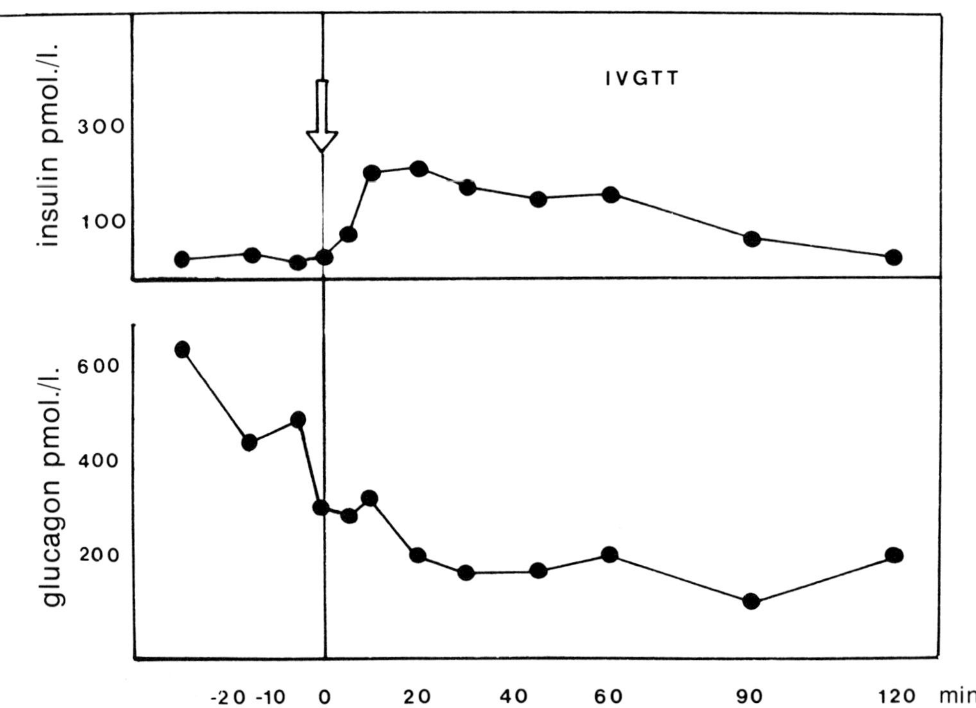

Fig. 13-6. Effect of an intravenous glucose load on plasma glucagon and insulin levels in a patient with a glucagonoma. Note the increase in insulin and depression of glucagon, which is in contrast to the rise in glucagon with oral glucose.

rise of blood glucose levels since raised blood glucose caused by *intravenous* glucose in the same patients causes depression of plasma glucagon levels or, in some, no change at all[5,13,24,49,55,57] (Fig. 13-6). This dissociation of effect of oral and intravenous glucose suggests that the oral load activates a gastrointestinal factor which is either itself abnormal, is abnormally released, or excites an abnormal response in tumor cells: it also overrides the inhibitory effect of a rise in blood glucose.

Tolbutamide

Intravenous tolbutamide normally stimulates the secretion of insulin and depresses glucagon and of course lowers blood glucose. In contrast glucagonoma patients show a brisk rise in plasma glucagon following intravenous tolbutamide,[5,13,24,49,55,57] a slower rise in insulin and an unremarkable and slow fall in blood glucose (Fig. 13-7). The rise in glucagon appears to be a direct effect of tolbutamide not mediated by changes in blood glucose or insulin. This again suggests that some abnormal mode of release of glucagon is operating either by the direct effect of tolbutamide on the cells, or by the activation of some unusual glucagon-releasing mechanism. The effect of oral tolbutamide is unknown.

Arginine

Normally intravenous arginine (or alanine) stimulates glucagon and insulin release from islet cells, whereas the blood glucose is slightly elevated. Glucagonoma patients respond to intravenous arginine by a dramatic increase in plasma glucagon, in absolute and relative terms far greater than normal, and a less marked increase in insulin levels.[5,13,24,28,33,49,55,57] Blood glucose may rise slightly but commonly stays unchanged. In one patient with extremely high basal levels of glucagon, no increase was seen with arginine although there was a slight increase in insulin secretion. Possibly that tumor was different from others, or was already secreting to capacity.[32]

Alpha-Adrenergic Blockade

Plasma glucagon usually rises during alpha-adrenergic stimulation with, for example, intravenous epinephrine. Leichter[27] found that in a patient with glucagonoma without a rash short-term alpha-adrenergic blockade reduced the stimulatory effect on glucagon levels of epinephrine and, incidentally, arginine. In the long term however these drugs were associated with a steady rise in basal glucagon and insulin levels and a slight improvement in glucose tolerance.

ABNORMAL CIRCULATING GLUCAGONS

Recent work has shown that human plasma glucagon immunoreactivity normally consists of several molecules of different size, as indicated by different mobility in filtration systems, but with identical immunoreactivity, suggesting that they have a common terminal peptide.[54] In the plasma of fasting man 55 percent or so of glucagon immunoreactivity is accounted for by a glucagon of high molecular weight (approximately 160,000), known as big plasma glucagon (BPG), or big plasma glucagon immunoreactivity (BPGI), or again, the interference factor. This material however is only readily detected by assays based on

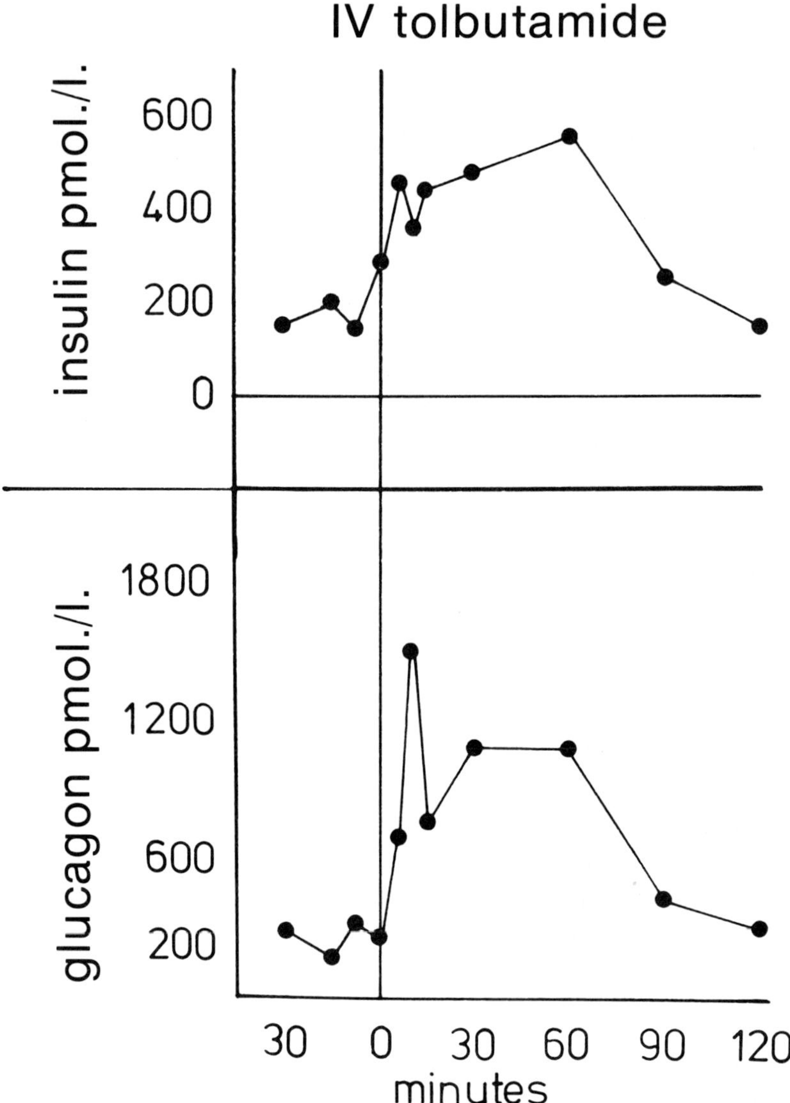

Fig. 13-7. Brisk rise of plasma glucagon (and insulin) with intravenous tolbutamide (1 g. in 1 min.). Normal subjects show a fall in glucagon.

Dr. Unger's 30K antisera. The antisera used for glucagon assay by the authors does not detect this material and consequently gives rather lower basal readings. Thirty-five percent of glucagon is so called "true" glucagon with molecular weight of 3,500 daltons. A third component, large glucagon immunoreactivity (LGI) of molecular weight 9,000 daltons, is found in pancreatic extracts and may be a precursor or storage form of glucagon—a proglucagon analogous to proinsulin.[39] A glucagon of this molecular weight is found only in very low concentration plasma but is consistently found in higher concentrations in patients with renal failure. In patients with glucagonomas it may be a major plasma glucagon component[45,49] (Fig. 13-8). There are also accounts of other forms of glucagon immunoreactivity in the circulation. In one family the presence of a glucagon of 10 to 20,000 daltons showed dominant inheritance.[41] In a second family containing one member with a glucagonoma, 85 percent of circulating glucagon immunoreactivity was in the large form in the relatives; in the patient 70 percent of the glucagon was true glucagon and 30 percent large.[5] Patients with glucagonomas, whether with NME or not, have been consistently found to have raised total plasma glucagon immunoreactivity and in the majority of these patients the increase is due to true glucagon.[5,13,55,57] Small or substantial amounts of large glucagon were found in basal conditions in plasma samples from both types of patients[45] and these two glucagons were found in one patient whether she was in remission from the rash or not.[8] Following stimulation or suppression of glucagon secretion by arginine or glucose, Weir and his colleagues[58] found the major changes in glucagon immunoreactivity to be in the true glucagon fraction, with a less-marked change in large glucagon and an uncertain change in big glucagon. In one glucagonoma patient a very small amount of glucagon with molecular weight of 2,000 daltons was found together with elevated levels of true and large glucagon.[55]

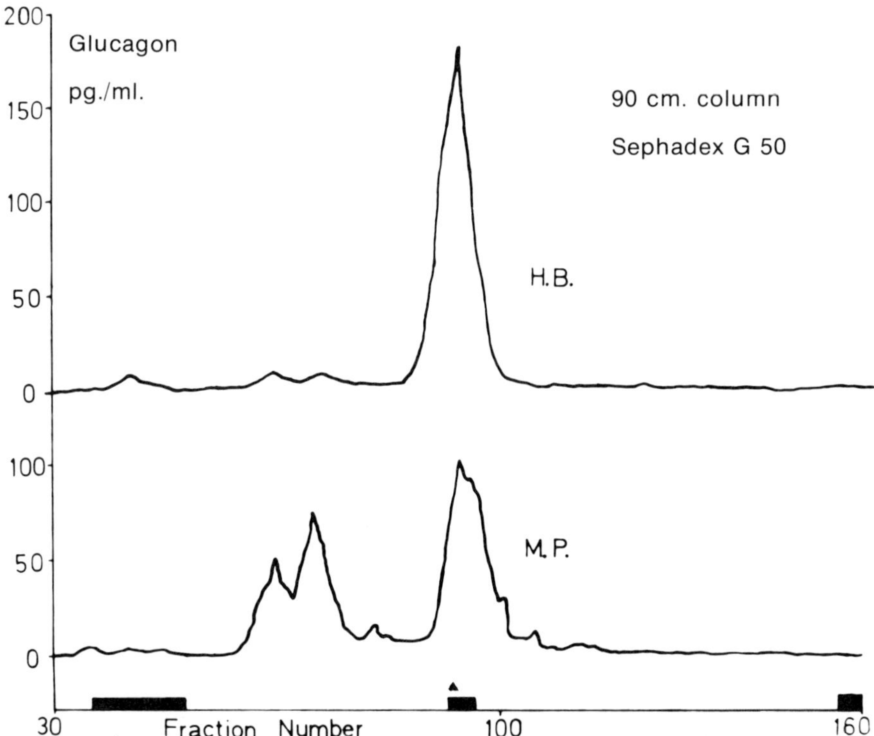

Fig. 13-8. Plasma glucagon immunoreactivity in two patients. The upper tracing shows a single peak in the gel filtrate corresponding to "true" glucagon of molecular weight 3,500 daltons. The lower trace is from a different patient and shows an earlier peak of glucagon immunoreactivity demonstrating a slower moving molecule of higher molecular weight—9,000 daltons.

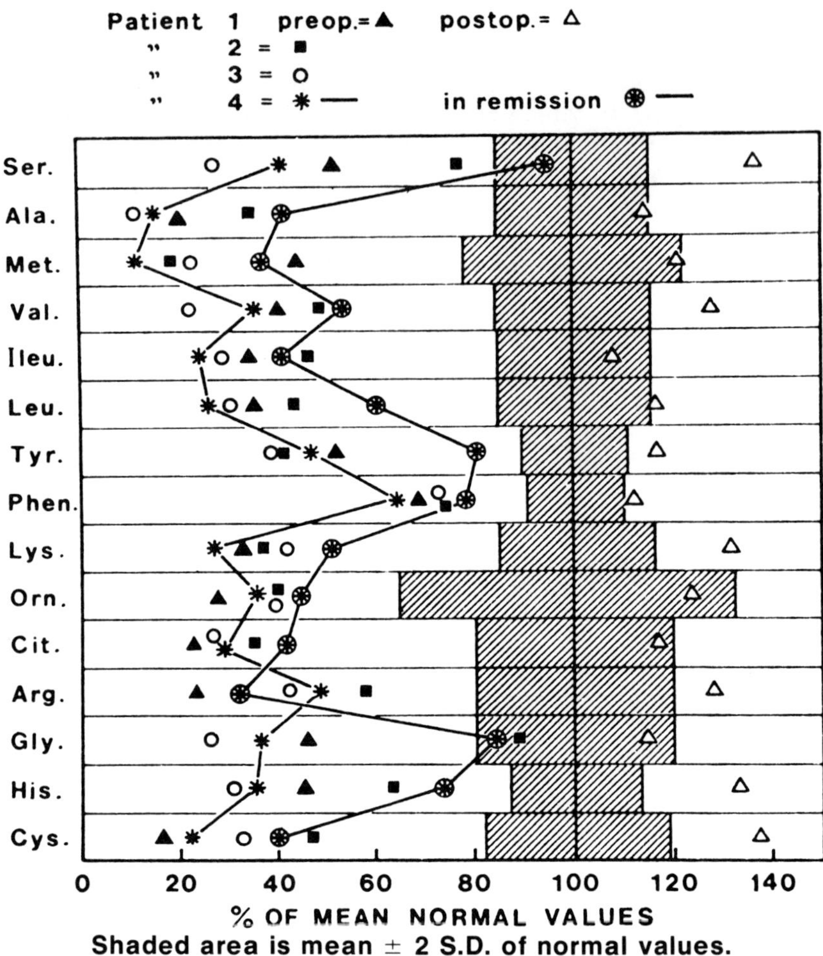

Fig. 13-9. The fasting plasma amino acid level in patients 1 to 4. The open triangles are levels seen in the patient 1 month after curative resection when plasma glucagon was normal and no clinical abnormalities remained. (Mallinson, C., et al.: Lancet, *2*:1, 1974[35])

The precise identity of the plasma LGI in these patients remains unproven. In Weir's phrase there is persuasive evidence of a precursor of glucagon in A cells which is probably also a polypeptide of 9,000 daltons.[39,58] Moreover, higher levels of LGI were found in veins draining two glucagonomas than in peripheral blood. This suggests that this size of glucagon is in fact secreted from the tumors rather than being a product of extracellular aggregation. The secretion of hormone precursors by endocrine tumors has a precedent in the case of insulinomas which may secrete proinsulin in preference to true insulin.[47] The abnormal release of a glucagon precursor is obviously of great importance to the fundamental understanding of the functioning of these tumor cells, the implication that further understanding may provide insight into the origins of tumors and the possibilities of specific therapy. In addition, estimation of abnormal plasma glucagons is of some diagnostic help, and the serial measurements of abnormal glucagons may give additional information as to the effectiveness or otherwise of antisecretory treatment.

When Dr. Recant first wrote to us concerning her finding of a large glucagon in the plasma of a patient who had a glucagonoma but no rash, we all speculated that the cutaneous syndrome might depend upon a critical proportion of some abnormal glucagon. However, increasing data suggest that there is no consistent pattern of abnormal glucagons in patients with or without NME. The finding that one family secreted large glucagon preferentially apart from the member who had a glucagonoma[5] is fascinating but will be difficult to interpret until the cause of the hyperglucagonemia and the metabolic activity of each glucagon is known.

The Biologic Activity of Plasma Glucagon

The normal "true" plasma glucagon has the same biologic activity, immunoreactivity and molecular weight as crystalline porcine glucagon used in clinical practice. The suspicion exists, reinforced by the finding of glucagons of

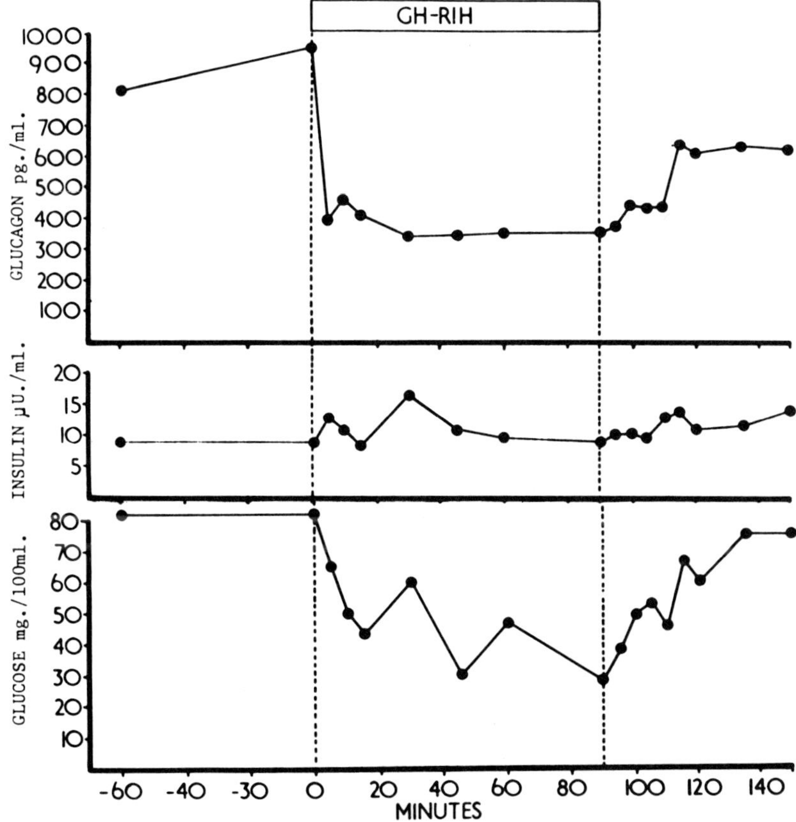

Fig. 13-10. The effect of somatostatin in one patient with glucagonoma. Plasma glucagon fell but insulin did not. Blood glucose fell and the patient experienced hypoglycemic symptoms. The glucagon was presumably biologically active in the maintenance of normal and on occasion high blood levels.

abnormal size, that glucagonomas secrete a form of hormone which is antigenically similar to "true" glucagon but of different biologic activity. Only McGavran has attempted to test this possibility formally[31] and found that the plasma glucagon immunoreactivity in his patient corresponded to its being an active "normal" glucagon. Other evidence also suggests, in a less quantitative way, that the plasma glucagon in these patients is active even though biologic assays are lacking. Many of the patients are hyperglycemic with raised plasma insulins as are normal subjects injected with glucagon. The global reduction in plasma amino acids (Fig. 13-9) is seen in no other condition apart from iatrogenic hyperglucagonemia.[36] Two attempts have been reported to measure circulating cyclic AMP.[33,45*] In one the levels were raised, in the other only marginally so. There are two vivid clinical demonstrations that the plasma glucagon is actively responsible for hyperglycemia and hypoaminoacidemia. One is the much-quoted result of complete removal of a tumor in one diabetic patient who promptly stopped requiring 60 units of insulin daily and whose amino acid pattern is shown in Figure 13-9. The other was the patient who received intravenous somatostatin (a potent inhibitor of endocrine secretion). The results are shown in Figure 13-10. Plasma glucagon fell promptly after somatostatin, and with it the blood sugar and the patient became clinically hypoglycemic. The plasma insulin remained unchanged for some unknown reason. This suggests that both hormones were present in an active form; before somatostatin they were in equilibrium in their effect on blood glucose. The reduction in glucagon but not insulin resulted in hypoglycemia which is strong evidence that the glucagon was present in its biologically active, hyperglycemic form.

DIAGNOSIS

The diagnostic workup of some of the earlier patients with glucagonoma was highly complex, partly because the investigators were floundering. However, one of the attractions of clinical work in this field is that a diagnostic flow chart can be organized in a critical manner and, however many ancillary investigations are carried out, the confirmation of the diagnosis proceeds in a few orderly steps. The exigencies of clinical life usually dictate that some of the steps are a little out of time. The individual moves are:

1. *Clinical suspicion*
   a. Suggestive clinical picture
   b. High (very) plasma glucagon
2. *Localization of tumor*
   a. Isotope scan of pancreas and liver
   b. Computerized axial tomography (when available)
   c. Selective angiography
3. *Action*
   a. Biopsy accessible metastasis
   b. Laparotomy—complete removal
   c. Laparotomy—palliative resection; tissue for diagnosis
4. *Confirmation of diagnosis*
   a. Light microscopy

b. Indirect immunofluorescence
c. Tumor glucagon content
5. *Serial postoperative follow-ups*
a. Clinical picture
b. Plasma glucagons
c. Carbohydrate tolerance
d. Metabolic responses
e. Repeat localization procedures if recurrence occurs

Plasma Glucagon Levels

All cases reported to date have consistently had very high concentrations of fasting plasma glucagons in the first sample taken. Although, as shown in Figure 13-1, the absolute levels vary, no levels have fallen anywhere near the upper limit seen in normal subjects or in conditions associated with high plasma glucagon such as trauma, burns and diabetic ketoacidosis. It is probably not essential to insist on a fasting sample, although they are traditional. Recent work suggests that effective cytotoxic drugs and diphenylhydantoin, significantly lower glucagon levels and so could cause confusion. A more common cause of error is that plasma samples are not satisfactorily prepared, glucagon decays and the result is artificially low. Appendix A indicates the most satisfactory method of preserving plasma. Although the finding of an abnormal form of glucagon in the circulation is highly suggestive that a tumor is present, so far the reliability of this as a diagnostic procedure has not been established and is not widely available. The absence of abnormal glucagons in no way excludes the diagnosis.

Metabolic Studies

The response to various factors modifying pancreatic glucagon secretion have now been widely reported in patients with glucagonomas. Although a general pattern of response is now emerging, which is discussed in a foregoing section, this is not sufficiently consistent to give more than supporting weight to the diagnosis of glucagonoma. *Nevertheless,* at this state of knowledge every patient with glucagonoma provides important new information, and detailed metabolic studies before, during and after operation when possible are mandatory in every patient.

Localization of a Tumor

Following the clinical diagnosis and the finding of even only a single very raised plasma glucagon level the next step is to initiate a search for a tumor. The search is usually begun before the glucagon levels have returned since they may take a week or two.

Isotope scanning is quick, safe and well tolerated. It has been the most widely practiced diagnostic technique and is the most successful in detecting hepatic metastases. Occasionally confusing results can be obtained; one patient had what seemed to be clear-cut hepatic metastases on an initial scan which disappeared on subsequent scans but were eventually confirmed at laparotomy.[33] Isotopic scanning has been far less successful in detecting primary pancreatic tumors. A more promising technique, still not widely available outside the

United States, is computerized axial tomography (CAT, better known as EMI scanning). This is by current accounts accurate in localizing primary pancreatic tumors; the only report known to us was highly convincing and also showed, accurately, that the tumor had a liquified center.[33] EMI scanning also provides a noninvasive technique for measuring the effect of treatment on unresectable tumors.

Endoscopic retrograde cholangiopancreatography (ERCP) has been little used in this context, and in at least one patient has been highly misleading since it revealed the changes of chronic pancreatitis clearly but missed the tumor in the tail.[35]

Angiography. Selective celiac and superior mesenteric arteriography has been carried out in the majority of patients reported from the United States and has proved the most reliable way of detecting the primary tumor so far. The majority of tumors so diagnosed have been vascular and highly malignant and commonly show a pathologic circulation. Adenomata have been more elusive, since they are less vascular, and simply show up by vessel displacement. In the tail of the pancreas where the principal vessels are small and inconstant, such changes are subtle and in at least one case have been undetectable. Fortunately this did not deter the clinicians and an adenoma was successfully removed.* Thus a positive result from arteriography can give valuable diagnostic information as to the presence of a primary tumor, of its size, vascularity and possible resectability and also the existence of metastases. *A negative angiogram does not exclude the diagnosis.*

Percutaneous Transhepatic Portal Venography. This is a promising technique whereby the pancreatic vessels can be visualized by retrograde injection of contrast and samples of portal blood obtained at one procedure. The value of differential portal/systemic plasma glucagon levels could be of particular value in patients with small tumors or A_2-cell hyperplasia. This method has proved useful in the diagnosis of insulinomas and is equally applicable to glucagonomas.

Biopsy of Accessible Tumor

Occasionally needle biopsy of superficial metastasis has confirmed the diagnosis. In spite of such confirmation laparotomy is usually still strongly indicated, but the operation can be planned in detail to obtain the fullest information.

Laparotomy

Laparotomy is strongly indicated in all patients with glucagonoma who are fit to undergo it. Patients with single adenomata are little safer than those with carcinomas and should be operated on with reasonable speed. Patients with malignant tumors and metastases may have a resectable primary, the removal of which makes the remaining metastases more amenable to chemotherapy. It is usually only by laparotomy that adequate tissue diagnosis can be obtained and an accurate assessment of the extent of the tumor made. Both pieces of information materially assist in selecting and evaluating the most appropriate treatment.

---

*Higgins, G. W.: Personal communication, 1977.

It cannot be emphasized too strongly that laparotomy should be approached only after careful consultation with the relevant laboratory colleagues. Techniques for preserving tissue are highly specialized and essential if the fullest possible information is to be obtained. None of them involves the operating surgeon in a moment of extra time, and usually the laboratory will send the relevant staff to the theater to carry out the necessary procedures on any tissue removed. No assumptions can be made about these patients, except that each one is slightly different and sometimes greatly so from the others.

Postoperative Follow-up

In patients with NME a complete resection of the tumor is followed by a striking improvement. However, a careful investigation of the patient in the immediate and postoperative period is necessary, since only in this way can unsuspected residual tumor be detected and treated and persisting diabetes mellitus or anemia be treated. It is preferable to follow the patient at intervals for years since the tumors are slow growing and recurrence can be delayed. Apart from this, valuable information concerning the fundamental responses of the patients previously harboring such tumors is likely to be essential to our understanding of the pathogenesis of these unusual lesions, justifying repetition of several metabolic investigations.

TREATMENT

Without doubt the most satisfactory treatment for glucagonomas associated with symptoms is complete surgical resection.[5,20,29,35] In 1974 the impression was that approximately half the patients with NME had resectable tumors,[35] whether benign or malignant. Since then however only two or three patients of the 20 or so reported have had removable tumors, and the incidence of malignant lesions with metastases is obviously higher than suspected. Two patients died unexpectedly after resection, one during the operation, of a massive pulmonary embolus,[33] the other within 3 days of operation at which all tumor was removed.[24] The other patients with NME in whom a single lesion has been resected have shown a dramatic clinical improvement within days. The rash has spontaneously improved as has the anemia, weight loss and depression. Glucose tolerance has usually improved in spite of the removal of a large portion of the normal pancreas, although a degree of chemical diabetes commonly persists.[29,35] In one patient insulin treatment is still needed, but this is the only patient who had a family history of diabetes (and indeed hyperglucagonemia) and showed ketoacidosis associated with NME; he may therefore have had a primary diabetic diathesis.[5] In one patient a palliative resection of a primary tumor was performed in the presence of small hepatic metastases.[49] This approach is justifiable on current evidence; it seems reasonable to reduce the mass of a tumor which appears to produce its effects more by secretory than mitotic activity. In this patient the skin was quiescent before operation and provided no indication of the resection's effect, but plasma glucagon levels fell postoperatively to near normal levels and the initially mild carbohydrate intolerance was little altered.

Anti-tumor Chemotherapy

The majority of patients with unresectable malignant tumors have received some form of chemotherapy. The drug most commonly used has been streptozotocin which is known to inhibit the secretion and growth of insulinomas and to inhibit insulin secretion from normal B cells. Whereas there is no evidence that the drug inhibits glucagon secretion from normal A_2 cells, initial reports of its use in tumors which secreted glucagon, among other hormones, showed a reduction in glucagon levels, (albeit measured by rather nonspecific methods). At least three reports since 1974 suggest that streptozotocin causes a significant improvement in plasma glucagon, NME and patient well-being.[13,49,55] Carbohydrate tolerance has been variably affected, not surprisingly in view of the effect of the drug on pancreatic B cells. In another patient the rash was strikingly improved as were plasma glucagon levels but severe depression was not.* The most evidently successful course of streptozotocin described by Danforth[13] was 1.5 g./square meter body surface per day for 6 weeks. In this patient and in one of ours plasma glucagon levels did not fall completely for 4 weeks. 5-Fluorouracil and DTIC (di-amino triazeno imidazole carboxamide) have been used, rather empirically, because they are believed to be effective against gastrointestinal tumors.[55] DTIC was effective in improving NME and this was accompanied by a fall in true and large glucagon in our patient.[55] The effectiveness of these drugs on tumor is not documented. The tumors are extremely slow growing and these agents which simply effect cell growth are inherently difficult to evaluate in addition to the difficulty of measuring deep-seated tumors.

Specifically Antisecretory Treatment

As discussed in the foregoing section the secretion of glucagon from these tumors can be modified, if in sometimes unexpected ways. Both oral glucose and intravenous tolbutamide, which suppress normal glucagon secretion, backfire in the presence of tumors by increasing glucagon secretion. Intravenous glucose usually reduces the glucagon levels in these patients but does not offer a promising therapeutic approach. Likewise, whereas alpha-adrenergic blocking drugs reduce glucagon secretion stimulated by alpha-adrenergic drugs, their long-term effect was therapeutically unpromising, since they increased plasma glucagon progressively.

A very interesting observation by Kramer[24] which may have some therapeutic application was that a short trial course of diphenylhydantoin (DPH), 1 g. daily for 5 days, reduced basal levels of plasma glucagon from a range of 2,600 to 4,000 pg./L to 2,000 pg./L. The drug was used because it is known to inhibit insulin secretion, rather in the same way that streptozotocin has been tried in glucagonomas. Moreover, in this patient DPH damped the stimulating effect of arginine on plasma glucagon but on the other hand reduced the inhibitory effect of intravenous glucose. This particular form of treatment perhaps in lower and more prolonged dosage may prove to be complimentary to other more toxic chemotherapy. Anything which allows the dose of streptozotocin or DTIC to be reduced is worth investigating.

---

*Hanifin, J.: Personal communication, 1975.

Treatment of NME

Apart from anti-tumor treatment NME has been treated directly itself in many ways. Topical antiseptic and antifungal agents and antibiotics have been used for proven superinfection. Systemic tetracycline and corticosteroids have also been used. One patient underwent a prolonged remission while taking methotrexate and again on corticosteroids and relapsed promptly on stopping each.

These treatments have been of doubtful value; assessment is difficult because NME improves spontaneously in many patients. A transient but definite improvement seen in two patients given diiodohydroxyquin (diiodohydroxyquinoline) was interesting;[35] this was formerly the specific treatment for acrodermatitis enteropathica of children which is slightly like NME, and is due to zinc deficiency. The possible connection in NME and zinc metabolism is so far tenuous, but any unexpected result in such puzzling conditions is worth noting. Treatment with zinc supplements or with amino acids has not been attempted.

SUMMARY

1. Glucagonomas are present in three clinical forms:
   a. With a characteristic skin rash, anemia, diabetes, weight loss, severe depression and venous thrombosis
   b. With severe diabetes
   c. In the presence of pluriglandular syndromes
2. The most common form of clinically significant glucagonoma is the first of these types.
3. Raised levels of plasma glucagon have been found in all patients where glucagonomas appear to exert a clinical effect. Hypoaminoacidemia has also been present.
4. Plasma glucagon is present not only as "true" glucagon but as large glucagon and possibly other forms as well.
5. Nevertheless, a significant proportion of circulating glucagon appears to be biologically active.
6. Plasma insulin is also increased in those patients with the capacity for endogenous insulin secretion.
7. The tumors, benign or malignant islet cell tumors, have variable electron microscopic features, but show indirect immunofluorescence of glucagon-containing cells and contain significant amounts of pancreatic glucagon.
8. Diagnosis is currently usually too late for effective surgical treatment. The diagnostic criteria are a raised plasma glucagon, evidence of a primary pancreatic tumor with or without secondaries by scanning or angiography, and tissue confirmation by biopsy or laparotomy.
9. An energetic metabolic investigation of all aspects of glucagon response is to be encouraged in each patient and can be used after successful resection or during palliative chemotherapy to follow progress.
10. The most satisfactory treatment is complete surgical resection; failing this several forms of chemotherapy are worth trying, notably streptozotocin, DTIC and possibly DPH.
11. It is for the future to reveal the origin of these tumors, the nature of the

abnormal gastrointestinal glucagon-releasing mechanism, the full range and explanation of the glucagon-releasing abnormalities of the cells, the basis of the rash and anemia, etc., in NME, and more specific and less toxic chemotherapy to be used until earlier diagnosis makes resection more commonly possible.

REFERENCES

1. Becker, S. W., Kahn, D., and Rothman, S.: Cutaneous manifestations of internal malignant tumours. Arch. Dermatol. Syph., *45*:1069, 1942.
2. Behrendt, W.: Ein Beitrag zur Pathologie des A-zellkarzinoms. Zentral. bl. Pathologie und Pathologische Anat., *104*:199, 1962.
3. Belchetz, P. E., et al.: ACTH, glucagon and gastrin production by a pancreatic islet cell carcinoma and its treatment. Clin. Endocrinol., *2*:307, 1973.
4. Bianchi, C., Macor, M., and Zar, E.: Dermatosi paraneoplastica in carcinoma di tipo endocrino del pancreas. Riv. Pinato. Patol. Oncol., *33*:319, 1968.
5. Boden, G., and Owen, O. E.: Familial hyperglucagonaemia: an autosomal dominant disorder. N. Engl. J. Med., *296*:534, 1977.
6. Boden, G., Owen, O. E., Rezvani, I., Elfenbein, B. I., and Quickel, K. E.: An islet cell carcinoma containing glucagon and insulin. Diabetes, *26*:128, 1977.
7. Broder, L. E., and Carter, S. K.: Pancreatic islet cell carcinoma. Ann. Intern. Med., *79*:101, 1973.
8. Bryant, M.: Unpublished observations, 1976.
9. Church, R. E., and Crane, W. A.: A cutaneous syndrome associated with an islet-cell carcinoma of the pancreas. Br. J. Dermatol., *79*:284, 1967.
10. Coons, A. H., Leduc, E. H., and Connolly, J. M.: Studies on antibody production I. A method for the histochemical demonstration of specific antibody and its application to a study of the hyperimmune rabbit. J. Exp. Med., *102*:49, 1955.
11. Croisier, J. C., Lehy, T., and Zeitoun, P.: A_2-cell pancreatic microadenomas in a case of multiple endocrine adenomatosis. Cancer, *28*:707, 1971.
12. Croughs, R. J. M., Hulsmans, H. A., Israel, D. E., Hackena, W. H. L., and Schopman, W.: Glucagonoma as a part of the polyglandular syndrome. Am. J. Med., *52*:690, 1972.
13. Danforth, D. N., et al.: Elevated plasma proglucagon-like component with a glucagon-secreting tumour. Effect of streptozotocin. N. Engl. J. Med., *295*:242, 1976.
14. Foa, P. P.: *In* Lefebvre, P. J., and Unger, R. H., (eds.): Glucagon. Oxford and New York, Pergamon Press, 1972.
15. Freedberg, I. M., and Galdabini, J. J.: Dermatitis, weight loss and filling defects in the liver. Case records of the Massachusetts General Hospital. N. Engl. J. Med., *292*:1117, 1975.
16. Friesen, S. R., Hermreck, A. S., and Mantz, F. A.: Glucagon, gastrin and carcinoid tumours of the duodenum, pancreas and stomach: polypeptide "apudomas" of thc foregut. Am. J. Surg., *127*:90, 1973.
17. Gössner, W., and Korting, G. W.: Metastasierendes inzellenkarzinom vom A zelltyp bei einem fall von pemphigus foliaceous mit diabetes renalis. Dtsch. Med. Wochenschr., *85*:434, 1960.
18. Greider, M. H., Bencosme, J. A., and Lechago, J.: The human pancreatic islet cells and their tumours. I. The normal pancreatic islet. Lab. Invest., *22*:344, 1970.
19. Hellman, B., and Hellerström, C.: The specificity of the argyrophil reaction in the islet of Langerhans in man. Acta Endocrinol., *36*:22, 1961.
20. Hess, W.: Ueber ein endokrin inaktives Carcinom der Langerhansschen Inseln. Schweiz. Med. Wochenschr., *76*:802, 1946.
21. Holst, J. J., Jonsson, J., Pedersen, N. B.,

and Thomsen, K.: The glucagonoma syndrome. Ugeskr Laeger., *137*:2631, 1975.

22. Kay, R. G., and Tasman-Jones, C.: Acute zinc deficiency in man during intravenous alimentation. Aust. N. Z. J. Surg., *45*:325, 1974.
23. Kimball, C. P., and Murlin, J. R.: Aqueous extracts of pancreas. III. Some precipitation reactions of insulin. J. Biol. Chem., *58*:337, 1923.
24. Kramer, S., Machina, T., and Marcus, J.: Metabolic studies in the malignant glucagonoma syndrome. Diabetes, *25*:370, 1976.
25. Larsson, L. I., Sundler, F., Grimelius, L., Hakanson, R., and Holst, J.: Immunohistochemical demonstration of glucagon in an A_2 cell carcinoma. Experientia, *29*:698, 1973.
26. Lefebvre, P. J., and Unger, R. H., (eds.): Glucagon. Oxford and New York, Pergamon Press, 1972.
27. Leighter, S. B., Pagkiara, A. S. Greider, M. H., Pohl, S., and Kipnis, D. M.: Uncontrolled diabetes mellitus and hyperglucagonaemia associated with an islet cell carcinoma. Am. J. Med., *58*:285, 1975.
28. Levin, M. E.: Endocrine tumors of the pancreas. Med. Clin. North Am., *52*:295, 1968.
29. Lightman, S. L., and Bloom, S. R.: Cure of insulin-dependent diabetes mellitus by removal of a glucagonoma. Br. Med. J., *1*:367, 1974.
30. Lomsky, R., Langer, F., and Vortel, V.: Demonstration of glucagon in islet cell adenomas of the pancreas by immunofluorescent technique. Am. J. Clin. Pathol., *51*:245, 1967.
31. McGavran, M. H., et al.: A glucagon secreting alpha-cell carcinoma of the pancreas. N. Engl. J. Med., *274*:1408, 1966.
32. Mallinson, C. N., Cox, B., and Bloom, S. R.: Plasma levels of aminoacids and glucagon in patients with pancreatic glucagonomas. Gut, *15*:340, 1974.
33. Mallinson, C. N., Gent, A. E., and Bloom, S. R.: Unpublished observations, 1977.
34. Mallinson, C. N., Salmon, P. R., Barrowman, J., and Bloom, S. R.: The association of a specific skin lesion with islet-cell tumours of the pancreas. Gut, *14*:827, 1973.
35. Mallinson, C. N., Bloom, S. R., Warin, A. P., Salmon, P. R., and Cox, B.: A glucagonoma syndrome. Lancet, *2*:1, 1974.
36. Marless, E. B., Aoki, T. T., Unger, R. H., Soeldner, J. S., and Cahill, G. F.: Effects of glucagon in fasting man. J. Clin. Invest., *49*:2256, 1970.
37. Mortimer, C. H., et al.: Effects of growth hormone release inhibitory hormone on circulating glucagon, insulin and growth hormone in usual, diabetic, acromegalie and hypopituitary patients. Lancet, *1*:697, 1974.
38. Murray-Lyon, I. M., Eddleston, A. L. W. F., and Williams, R.: Treatment of multiple-hormone-producing malignant islet-cell tumour with streptozotocin. Lancet, *2*:895, 1968.
39. Noe, B. D., Bauer, G. E., Steffes, M. W., Sutherland, D. E. R., and Najavian, J. S.: Glucagon biosynthesis in human pancreatic islets: preliminary evidence for a biosynthetic intermediate. Hor. Metab. Res., *7*:314, 1975.
40. O'Neal, L. W., Kipnis, D. M., Luse, S. A., Lacy, P. E., and Jarrett, L.: Secretion of various endocrine substances by ACTH-secreting tumours—gastrin, melanotropin, norepinephrine, serotonin, parathormone, vasopressin glucagon. Cancer, *21*:1219, 1968.
41. Palmer, J. P., Werner, L., Benson, J. W., and Ensinck, J. W.: Dominant inheritance of large molecular weight immunoreactive glucagon. Diabetes, *25* [Suppl. *1*]:326, 1976.
42. Patellani, E.: Chirurgia, *10*:351, 1955.
43. Pearse, A. G. E., and Polak, J. M.: Endocrine tumours of neural crest origin: neurolophomas, apudomas and the A.P.U.D. concept. Med. Biol., *52*:3, 1974.
44. Pedersen, N. B., Jonsson, L., and Holst, J. J.: Necrolytic migratory erythema and glucagon cell tumour of the pancreas: the glucagonoma syndrome. Acta Derm. Venereol., *56*:391, 1976.
45. Perrino, P. P., Lavine, R. L., Bhathena,

S. J., Burns, W. A., and Recant, L.: Big glucagon in glucagonoma. Clin. Res., *37*:446A, 1975.
46. Polak, J. M., et al.: Pancreatic polypeptide in insulinomas, gastrinomas, vipomas and glucagonomas. Lancet, *1*:328, 1976.
47. Rubenstein, A. H., et al.: Circulating proinsulin in patients with islet cell tumours. Diabetes: Proc. Eighth Cong. Internat. Diabetes Fed., Brussells, July 15-20, 1973. Edited by Malaisse, W. J., and Pirat, J. Excerpta Medica; Amsterdam (I.C.S. No. 132) pp. 736-756.
48. Schein, P. P., De Lellis, R. A., Kahn, C. R., Gordon, P., and Draft, A. R.: Islet cell tumours: current concepts and management. Ann. Intern. Med., *79*:239, 1973.
49. Soler, N. G., Oatis, G. D., Malins, J. M., Cassar, J., and Bloom, S. R.: Glucagonoma syndrome in a young man. Proc. R. Soc. Med., *69*:429, 1976.
50. Sturner, W. Q.: Sudden death from noninsulin secreting islet cell tumour of the pancreas ("glucagonoma"). Human Pathol., *3*:113, 1972.
51. Sweet, R. D.: A dermatosis specifically associated with a tumour of pancreatic alpha cells. Br. J. Dermatol., *90*:301, 1974.
52. Unger, R. H., and Orci, L.: The essential role of glucagon in the pathogenesis of diabetes mellitus. Lancet, *1*:14, 1975.
53. Unger, R. H., Eisentraut, A. M., and Lochner, J. R.: Glucagon producing tumours of the islets of Langerhans. J. Clin. Invest., *42*:987, 1963.
54. Valverdi, I., Villaneuva, M. L., Lozano, I., and Marco, J.: Presence of glucagon immunoreactivity in the globin fraction of human plasma (big plasma glucagon). J. Clin. Endocrinol. Metab., *39*:1090, 1974.
55. Valverde, I., Lemon, H. M., Kessinger, A., and Unger, R. H.: Distribution of plasma glucagon immunoreactivity in a patient with suspected glucagonoma. J. Clin. Endocrinol., *42*:792, 1976.
56. Vance, J. E., Stoll, R. W., Kitabchi, A. E., Williams, R. H., and Wood, F. C.: Nesidioblastosis in familial endocrine adenomatosis. JAMA, *207*:1979, 1969.
57. Weir, G. C., Horton, E., Aoki, T. T., and Slovik, D. M.: Increased large glucagon immunoreactivity in the glucagonoma syndrome. Diabetes, *25*:326, 1976.
58. Weir, G. C., et al.: Secretion by glucagonomas of a possible glucagon precursor. J. Clin. Invest., *59*:325, 1976.
59. Wilkinson, D. S.: Pustular psoriasis with features of necrolysis. Proc. R. Soc. Med., *63*:892, 1970.
60. ——: Necrolytic migratory erythema with pancreatic carcinoma. Proc. R. Soc. Med., *64*:1196, 1971.
61. ——: Necrolytic migratory erythema with carcinoma of the pancreas. Trans. St. Johns Hosp. Dermatol. Soc., *59*:244, 1973.
62. Wise, J. K., Hendler, R., and Felig, P.: Influence of glucocorticoids on glucagon secretion and plasma aminoacid concentrations in man. J. Clin. Invest., *52*:2774, 1973.
63. Yoshinaga, T., Okuno, G., Shinji, Y., Tsujii, T., and Nismikawa, M.: Pancreatic A-cell tumour associated with severe diabetes mellitus. Diabetes, *15*:709, 1966.
64. Zhdanov, V. C.: Diabetes and malignancy of islet cells in pancreas (Russian title translated). Arch. Pathol. (Moskva), *92*:306, 1956.

Special Reading

Ganda, O. P., et al.: "Somatostatinoma." A somatostatin-containing tumor of the endocrine pancreas. N. Engl. J. Med., *296*:963, 1977.

Larsson, L. I., et al.: Pancreatic somatostatinoma. Clinical features and physiological implications. Lancet, *1*:666, 1977.

APPENDIX 13-A

All known gastrointestinal polypeptides are stable in plasma at −20° C providing *Trasylol has been added.* Add 0.2 ml. of freshly opened Trasylol (20,000 μ/ml.) to a standard lithium heparin tube as used for plasma electrolytes. Make up to 10 ml. with freshly drawn blood. Spin down, separate plasma and store at −20° C within 5 minutes. The critical point is to get the blood into Trasylol, after that a 5- to 10-minute interval at room temperature is less likely to affect glucagon levels.

Trasylol should be fresh. A number of tubes can be made up with 0.2 ml. Trasylol in each, stored at −20° C and used as needed.

APPENDIX 13-B

Tumor tissue should be divided into four wedges.

1. A standard wedge is put into routine fixative for clinical microscopy.
2. As large a wedge as can be spared is dried and put into a sealed polyethylene bag and put immediately into dry ice or stored at −20° C for glucagon extraction.
3. A wedge is dried and put into a watertight polyethylene bag and kept on ordinary ice for indirect immunofluorescence. The technicians may prefer to process the material in the operating theater. **In any event they must be warned that tissue is expected and told as soon as it is available.** Tissue is unsuitable which is wet, fixed, or frozen.
4. Ten or 20 very small cubes of tissue are cut with a razor blade into 1 *millimeter* cubes and placed into fixative provided by the electron microscopist.

EDITORIAL COMMENTARY

Little is known of the biologic significance of pancreatic glucagon or how increased pancreatic elaboration of this polypeptide in its several molecular forms produces the clinical syndrome(s) ascribed to it. The most characteristic and unique feature of the classic form of the syndrome is that of the skin rash, a necrotizing, migrating erythema, the severity of which seems to correlate with the level of glucagon in the plasma. Also typical but much less dramatic, is the diabetes-like hyperglycemia observed in these patients; this is an unfortunate distraction leading the unwary clinician to a diagnosis of diabetes mellitus instead of pancreatic islet cell tumor. The hyperglycemia with its associated carbohydrate intolerance is usually not severe in these patients with pancreatic glucagonomas owing to the unexpected accompanying hyperinsulinemia due to the insulin-releasing effect of glucagon; this is an important diagnostic feature. Moreover, the systemic complications of diabetes mellitus rarely are seen with the hyperglycemia of hypersecreting glucagonomas. Confirmatory diagnostic procedures which differentiate this hypersecretory state from diabetes mellitus or from tumors of the exocrine pancreas include the radioimmunoassay of highly elevated levels of glucagon, the stimulatory effects of oral glucose, tolbutamide and arginine on plasma glucagon concentration, the inhibitory effect of intravenous glucose administration, and the failure of intravenously administered exogenous glucagon (1 mg.) to further elevate blood glucose levels in the already hyperglucagonemic state. Immunofluorescent and ultrastructural studies confirm the endocrine cell origin and humoral capability of the tumors.

The tumor, of alpha islet cell origin, may also be diagnosed histologically as a carcinoid (EC cell) tumor of the pancreas or as an ectopic tumor of the lung, liver or kidney. When islet cell hyperplasia is the pathologic entity, usually in families, it has been implicated in the process of nesidioblastosis with associated hypergastrinism, hyperinsulinism and hyperparathyroidism.

Abnormalities of pancreatic glucagon release have been implicated in several conditions, including diabetes mellitus, hyperparathyroidism with and without associated chronic pancreatitis, hypocalcemia with thyrocalcitonin release, nonhypoglycemic "black-out spells," and in association with polyhormonal and pluriglandular endocrinopathies. One patient with an enteroglucagonoma has been described, as noted in this chapter.

The catabolic nature of the hormone is clinically evident in the weight loss, mental depression, intestinal atonia, anemia, and tachycardia, as well as the glycogenolysis and the hypoaminoacidemia observed in these patients. (These actions are the antithesis of the anabolic action of insulin.) These catabolic features are more related to the physiologic and pharmacologic actions of the hormone than to the nature of the tumor or to the extent of its neoplasia; such debilitating and wasting signs may be present in patients with benign but hyperfunctioning tumors or islet cell hyperplasia. Unfortunately, however, the diagnosis is rarely made before metastases from malignancies occur.

Early diagnosis and surgical excision thus are presently hopeful attainments in the management of pancreatic (or intestinal) glucagonomas; chemotherapy with streptozotocin or diphenylhydantoin appears to be of value but the possible use of the polypeptide, somatostatin, as an inhibitor of hormone release holds real promise of benefit, as has already been demonstrated by the authors of this chapter, in reducing circulating glucagon and glucose in a patient with a glucagonoma.

Mallinson, by personal communication, more recently describes a patient with severe necrotizing migratory erythema and persistently elevated plasma glucagon levels with a proven glucagonoma who was treated first with oral zinc sulphate (600 mg. daily). Within 1 week the skin lesions improved and in 4 weeks they disappeared. The cutaneous lesions reappeared on ceasing zinc treatment and then once again cleared on restarting treatment. During treatment with zinc the plasma glucagon levels did not alter. Long-acting somatostatin given subcutaneously by injection controlled plasma glucagon levels.

Of new interest is that the actions of somatostatin have also recently been observed clinically in two reported patients by Larsson, et al. and by Ganda, et al. In these patients the D cell islet tumor produced SST-like immunoreactivity and bioactivity. Extracts of the tumor were potent in inhibiting insulin and glucagon secretion from isolated perfused porcine pancreas. Clinical abnormalities included hypochlorhydria, steatorrhea and diabetic glucose tolerance. In one study the tumor cells in tissue culture released somatostatin.

It appears that the pancreatic islet cell hormones, including insulin, glucagon, somatostatin and perhaps the humoral marker, pancreatic polypeptide, are inextricably interrelated in their metabolic effects and in their mutual control of each other. *S.R.F.*

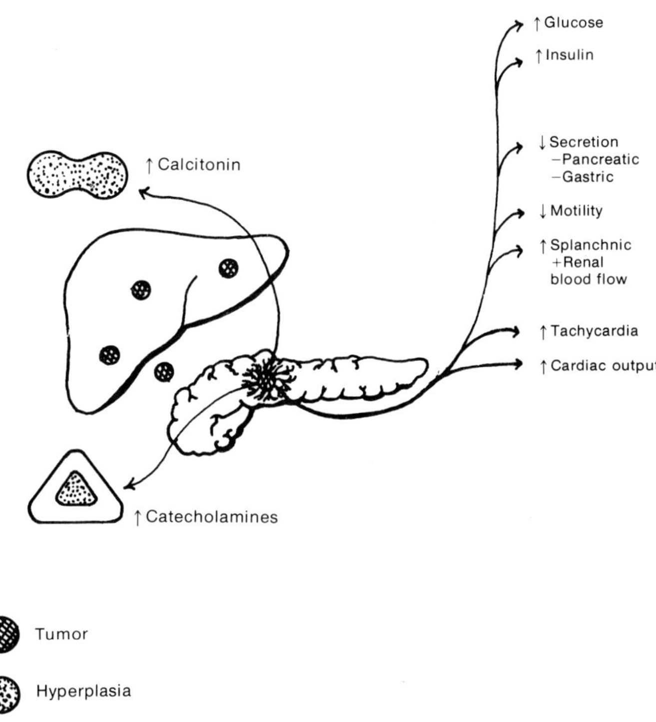

Fig. 13-11. Pathophysiology of the hyperglycemic syndrome (glucagon-secreting tumor of alpha cells).

(See overleaf for flowchart)

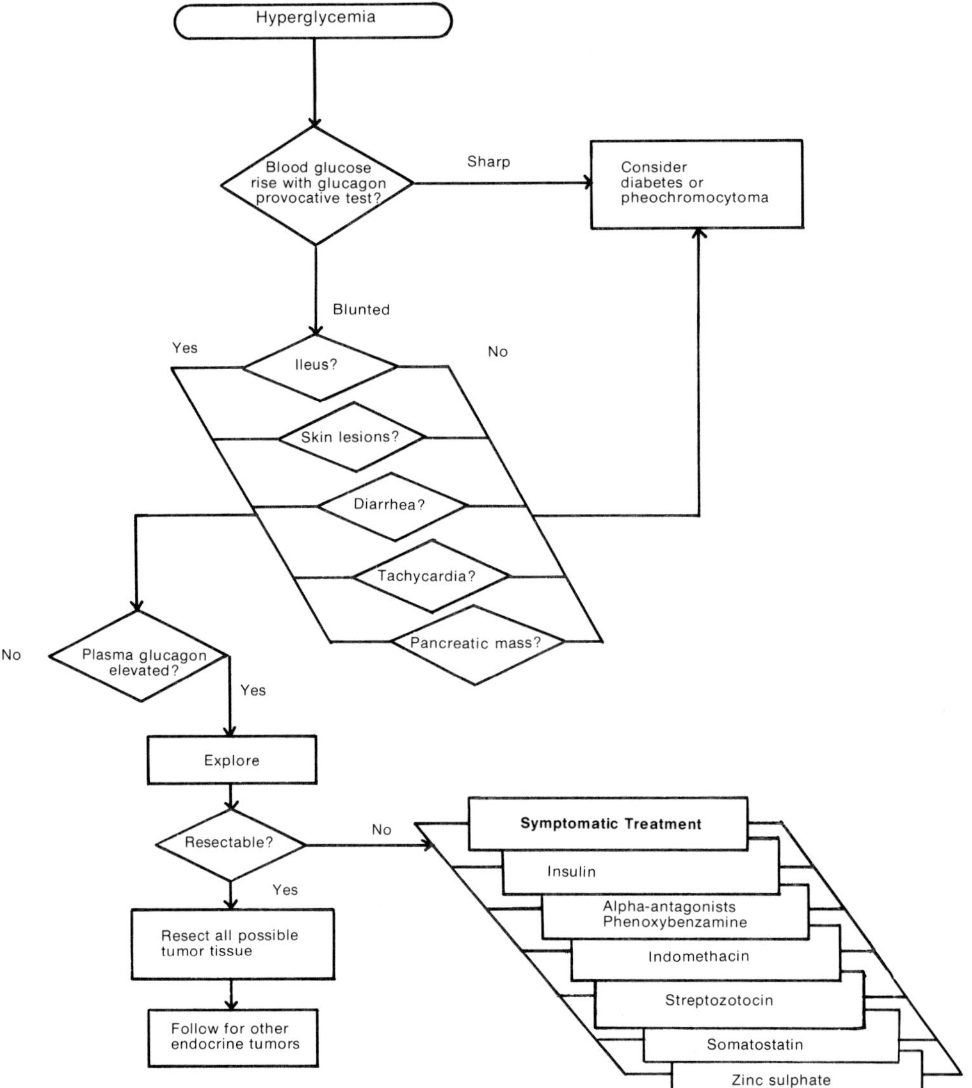

Fig. 13-12. Management flowchart of the hyperglycemic syndrome.

14

The Ulcerogenic (Zollinger-Ellison) Syndrome

Robert M. Zollinger, M.D.

CLINICAL FEATURES

Over the years an occasional patient was encountered who had severe and recurrent peptic ulceration, despite having undergone the most heroic medical or radical surgical procedures. In 1955, two such patients were reported. Both required complete removal of all acid-secreting surface by total gastrectomy in order to control excessive gastric hypersecretion.[15] A non-insulin-producing islet cell tumor of the pancreas was found in both patients. It was suggested that these islet cell tumors were producing a potent gastric secretagogue which stimulated the stomach to produce a tremendous volume of gastric juice rich in hydrochloric acid. Until this time, it had been assumed that islet cell tumors produced only excessive amounts of insulin or were nonfunctioning. Both of the original patients had severe ulceration in the jejunum just beyond the ligament of Treitz, and one had had a severe diarrhea.

An ulcerogenic islet cell tumor syndrome was evolved as a triad, consistent with the original triad of Whipple associated with an insulin-producing adenoma. The diagnostic features of the islet cell ulcerogenic syndrome consisted of a fulminating ulcer diathesis; excessive gastric hypersecretion; and the presence of a non-beta islet cell tumor. Within 5 years, Gregory, et al. had proved that the tumors as well as their metastases did produce the potent gastric secretagogue gastrin, in amounts approximately 35 times greater than that extracted from an equal weight of porcine antrum.[4] Within several years a sufficient number of cases were reported to document the syndrome as a clinical entity.[14]

It is true that these cases are very unusual and at the same time very mischievous and capricious in making their presence known. All tumors must start small with a limited hormonal output, producing symptoms which cannot be separated from those of the usual duodenal ulcer clinical history. These carcinoidlike tumors grow very slowly, tend to be multiple, and have a malignant potential to metastasize to local lymph nodes or liver in two-thirds to three-fourths of all patients.[16] Some patients have digestive complaints consistent with duodenal ulcer, whereas others complain of only a severe diarrhea which may have existed for years.

The diagnosis should be suspected in patients who have severe ulcer symptoms in their early teens, or who develop their initial ulcer symptoms late in life. The diagnosis is most likely to be considered in patients who develop recurrent ulceration after a customary surgical procedure for ulcer. This is especially true if the recurrent ulceration develops immediately following surgery and the patient is obviously producing large volumes of gastric juice with high acid values. The tumor should also be suspected when a complication of ulcer occurs in a woman shortly after delivery when the protective phenomenon of the hormones of pregnancy are no longer present. Persistent diarrhea is not an uncommon finding in approximately one-third of the patients. The presence of digestive complaints associated with hypercalcemia should raise the question not only of a parathyroid adenoma, but also the presence of a pancreatic gastrinoma. The suspicion that one endocrine tumor exists should alert the physician to look for others, since the finding of multiple endocrine adenomata in a single patient is not uncommon.

Although it is rare, the clinician must constantly be aware of the potential of the gastrin-producing islet cell tumor to produce variable gastrointestinal complaints which are too often overlooked until serious life-threatening complications develop.

PREOPERATIVE MANAGEMENT

When an ulcerogenic tumor (gastrinoma) is suspected from the patient's history, it is currently possible to either cinch or rule out the diagnosis in a relatively short time. The roentgenologist suspects a gastrinoma when large folds and evidence of an excess of fluid are observed in an unobstructed stomach.[2] Duodenal or gastric ulceration may be absent or multiple ulcerations may be present in unusual locations such as the second or third portion of the duodenum. The duodenum is enlarged and the mucosal folds tend to be edematous and may have a cobblestone appearance due to hyperplasia of Brunner's glands. Deformity of the first portion of the duodenum may be caused by an ulcer or the presence of an aberrant islet cell tumor in the submucosa. Ulceration beyond the ligament of Treitz is present in approximately one-fifth of the patients and should be considered pathognomonic of the disease.

The gastric analysis may provide an early clue to the diagnosis if the output of gastric juice from an unobstructed stomach equals or exceeds 100 ml. per hour. Twelve-hour overnight volumes of gastric juice may approximate 3 or more liters. The persistent hypergastrinemia results in hypertrophy of the gastric mucosa with a persistent maximal stimulation of the gastric glands. The basal acid output (BAO) tends to exceed 15 mEq. per hour. As a result of the continuous stimulation of the gastric glands the ratio of the BAO is 0.6 or more of the maximal acid output. Many times the first clue to the missed diagnosis results from the finding of hypersecretion with high acid values in the immediate postoperative period following a customary operation for duodenal ulcer. The diagnostic significance of the gastric analysis has been altered in recent years by the development of the gastrin immunoassay by McGuigan.[6]

The normal fasting gastrin level varies among laboratories but levels of more than 200 pg./ml. suggest the diagnosis of a gastrinoma in the presence of gastric hypersecretion. Gastrin levels may be elevated over 100,000 pg./ml. in the presence of extensive tumor involvement, including hepatic metastases. However, fasting gastrin levels do not always provide an accurate picture of the extent of the tumor involvement. Accordingly, provocative infusion studies have been used to mobilize the gastrin from the tumorous tissue.[7] Calcium gluceptate, 15 mg./kg. of body weight over a 4-hour period with performance of gastrin and calcium determinations every hour demonstrates a doubling of the fasting gastrin level by the fourth hour in more than 80 percent of the cases. This test is especially valuable when elevation in the fasting gastrin levels is only borderline.[7]

Magnesium sulfate, 1.6 mEq./kg. of body weight over a 4-hour period may also be used in the presence of cardiac disorders or hypercalcemia from hyperparathyroidism, since the magnesium lowers rather than elevates the serum calcium levels.[11] Jorpes secretin, 1 to 3 clinical U/kg. of body weight, is preferred by many, since it produces a prompt response in the gastrin levels within 30 to 60 minutes with little alteration in the serum calcium levels.[5]

Although the gastrin levels may be elevated in the presence of a postoperative retained antrum, the secretin infusion will lower the gastrin level; in marked contrast, it exerts a simulation effect in the presence of a gastrinoma. The gastrin levels may be elevated in some patients having antral biopsy proof of G cell hyperplasia associated with gastric hypersecretion. However, no further elevation occurs during the provocative infusion studies. This is an important differential diagnostic point. Hypergastrinemia not associated with gastric hypersecretion may also occur in the presence of pernicious anemia, atrophic gastritis, renal failure and carcinoma of the body of the stomach.

Approximately one-fourth of the patients with gastrinoma will have chemical evidence of hyperparathyroidism in elevated serum calcium levels. The excess serum calcium tends to act as a constant stimulus for hypergastrinemia. Parathyrin levels should be obtained to support the diagnosis of primary hyperparathyroidism. When the parathyrin, calcium, and fasting gastrin levels are elevated, it is highly probable that the patient harbors a parathyroid as well as a non-beta islet cell tumor.[13] The decision for the type of initial surgical treatment should depend upon the endocrine glands which seem to be producing the greater threat to the patient. Temporary improvement in the patient's gastrointestinal complaints accompanied by a fall in serum gastrin levels may follow the removal of a parathyroid adenoma.

A general endocrine survey should be made to assess possible adrenal and pituitary involvement. As the gastrin immunoassay becomes more widely available and its determination made routinely in all patients with digestive complaints, it well may be that gastrinoma will be recognized far more frequently and certainly much earlier than in the past.

Sufficient time should be taken to coordinate the several laboratory findings with the clinical history unless emergency surgery is indicated because of a catastrophic complication, such as a free perforation or massive hemorrhage. Intensive antacid therapy may need to be combined with constant gastric suction to lessen the effectiveness of the massive gastric hypersecretion. Those patients with severe diarrhea are relieved by continuous gastric suction. However, the fluid and electrolyte losses may be so great as to require heroic replacement around the clock with frequent determinations of body weights.

Roentgen therapy is ineffective in controlling the gastric hypersecretion. A histamine H_2-receptor antagonist such as Cimetidine is effective in suppressing acid secretion and controlling symptoms.[10] Such a drug may also be useful in controlling the severe gastric hypersecretion in patients having recurrent symptoms following less than total gastrectomy. This therapy should also be considered in those patients who either refuse total gastrectomy or who are at least temporarily very poor risks. Such therapy provides only palliation and does not alter the rate of growth of the original tumor or its metastases. An aggressive approach including total gastrectomy ensures the best long-term overall survival.

CHOICE OF OPERATION

The choice of operation depends upon the severity of the patient's symptoms and general condition, as well as the documented evidence supporting the diagnosis. The patient, regardless how young or how old, as well as the family, should be informed of the probability of total gastrectomy and possible partial pancreatectomy, as well as splenectomy. Special consideration must be given to the replacement of the excessive losses of fluids and electrolytes from constant gastric suction as well as diarrhea. The patient's weight should be frequently monitored, blood volume restored, and assurance made that all electrolytes are in order early on the day of operation. Constant gastric suction must be maintained and may on rare occasions be useful in avoiding a total gastrectomy by showing a dramatic decrease in the volume output of gastric juice following vagotomy and local excision of an obvious tumor.

A midline incision extending from over the xiphoid down to or beyond the left side of the umbilicus is made. When previous incisions are present, the one nearest the midline may be selected. Whenever the xiphoid is prominent or unduly long, it is removed and active bleeding on each side controlled by a suture ligation. This tends to provide an improved exposure of the esophagogastric junction.

In an abdominal cavity not previously operated upon the increased vascularity of the stomach is quite apparent. Because of the thickened mucosa the stomach feels spongy upon palpation. Evidence of an enlarged duodenum is usually present. Single or multiple metastatic nodules may be apparent in the liver. Evidence of an ulcer in the jejunum just beyond the ligament of Treitz should be considered pathognomonic of an ulcerogenic tumor. Enlarged lymph nodes about the pancreas or in the region of the gastrohepatic ligament are excised for a frozen section examination for islet cell metastases as the rest of the pancreas is searched for tumor. The head of the pancreas is mobilized by the Kocher maneuver and the greater omentum completely separated from the transverse colon to permit a clear exposure of the body and tail of the pancreas.

A tumor may be palpated in the submucosa of the first portion of the duodenum in 10 percent of these patients. If thorough exploration of the head of the pancreas as well as the mobilized body and tail fails to reveal a second tumor, some surgeons prefer to excise the duodenal tumor following with vagotomy, pyloroplasty, or antrectomy. In approximately one-half of the patients so managed, gastrin-producing metastases or tumor will remain and recurrence will take place. Blind resection of the left side of the pancreas searching for evidence of tumor is unnecessary if the preoperative provocative infusion studies show high gastrin levels which equal or exceed three or four times the elevated fasting gastrin level.

Total gastrectomy provides the best outlook for the patient, even in the presence of gross and extensive involvement of the regional lymph nodes or liver (Fig. 14-1). Contrary to established surgical principles, it is desirable to leave

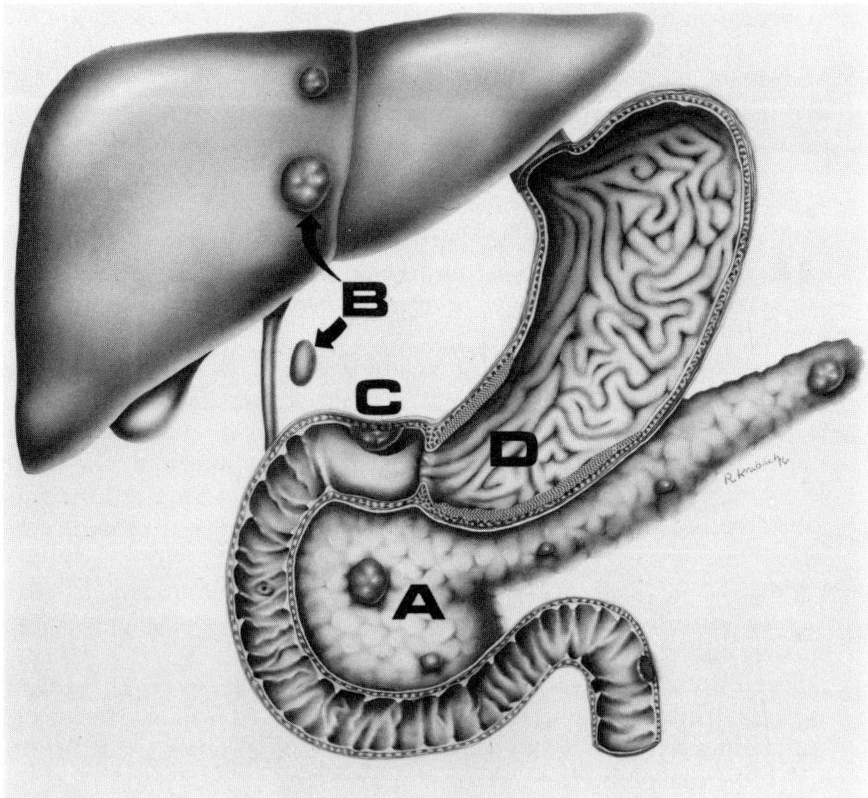

Fig. 14-1. The multicentric locations of the gastrin-producing islet cell tumors (A) and (C) and the frequency of functioning metastases (B) support the removal of the acid-secreting surface by total gastrectomy. Hyperplasia of antral G cells (D) is a possible cause of hypergastrinemia.

tumor behind and remove all of the acid-secreting surface of the stomach by total gastrectomy rather than perform a radical pancreatic resection such as a Whipple procedure. Friesen has suggested that removal of the end-organ by total gastrectomy may inhibit the further growth and development of the metastases.[3] Total gastrectomy is advisable in the teenager or even younger children, as well as in the elderly, as insurance against an almost certain morbidity and mortality expectancy. Total gastrectomy does not prevent normal growth and development in the very young.[12] There may be a temptation to remove a solitary islet cell tumor from the pancreas without following through the total gastrectomy. This approach has special appeal if the output of gastric juice, from the inlying nasogastric suction tube, which has been steady and voluminous, dramatically falls following excision of the tumor. The author has had only one successful case with a 9-year survival following excision only of a solitary tumor.

Fewer postoperative complications occur if splenectomy as well as hemipancreatectomy is avoided. The duodenum is divided and the stump closed and inverted. Following division of the short gastrosplenic vessels and double ligation of the left gastric artery, the region of the esophagus is exposed. This may prove quite challenging because of adhesions from a previous vagotomy, free perforation, or gastric resection. The left lobe of the liver should be mobilized and rotated upward and toward the midline. The vagus nerves are divided and great care is taken to avoid fraying the nonperitonealized muscles of the esophagus. After modest traction is exerted on the esophagus, it is anchored in three or four places to the margins of the hiatus to prevent retraction. A vascular type of noncrushing clamp is applied to the esophagus well above the stomach. A few interrupted sutures are placed to encircle the esophageal wall adjacent to the clamp front and back, to prevent fraying and insure a good protruding cuff of esophageal mucosa for subsequent esophagojejunal anastomosis.

A Roux-en-Y anastomosis functions well and lessens the incidence of regurgitation esophagitis. To insure a sizable stoma and minimize postoperative stenosis, an Ewald tube as well as a Levin tube are passed down the esophagus and into the jejunum before completion of the anterior row of sutures in the esophagojejunal anastomosis. The larger tube is then removed and the Levin tube directed around into the closed duodenal stump to provide constant aspiration of the duodenal contents. Solitary metastastic tumors of the liver may be excised as well as any enlarged lymph nodes obviously filled with tumor. The construction of pouches from the jejunum does not appear to improve the postoperative nutrition of the patient.[1]

Some prefer to resect only the antrum of the stomach in the presence of hypergastrinemia which is not altered following a provocative calcium infusion, but accompanied by biopsy and immunofluorescence evidence of an antral G cell hyperplasia in the absence of an islet cell tumor.[9] Further long-term observations are essential in evaluating this suspected uncommon cause of gastric hypersecretion.

Drainage is not used unless a procedure has been carried out on the pancreas which might lead to a leakage of pancreatic juice.

POSTOPERATIVE CARE

Although the ulcerogenic tumor patients may have had one or more previous gastric procedures and currently may have a variety of serious complications, they do surprisingly well following total gastrectomy. The blood volume is restored, body weight observed daily and the fluid and electrolyte levels carefully monitored. Amylase determinations are made the night of operation and daily therafter until normal levels are attained. The nasal Levin tube directed into the area of the closed duodenal stump is maintained on constant gastric suction until bowel action has returned.

The assistance of a dietitian is sought early to reassure the patient and family that normal eating habits will eventually be possible. The caloric intake is slowly increased with six small feedings a day. In a few weeks the patient's diet should be liberalized and the quantities of food gradually increased. The patient must be taught to be weight-conscious. Until a satisfactory postoperative weight is attained, the patient should refrain from smoking as well as an excessive intake of either hot or cold drinks. These patients sustain a better nutritional status than patients having a total gastrectomy for carcinoma of the stomach.

The patients must be indoctrinated with the firm concept that B_{12}-injections on a monthly basis are mandatory. During the first postoperative year a complete blood count is indicated at regular 3-to-6 month intervals. Approximately two-thirds of the patients will eventually sustain an ideal weight. Better long-term results are attained if the patients are admitted to the hospital on a yearly basis after the first year. Some may have weight loss because of stenosis of the esophagojejunal anastomosis. This can usually be corrected by careful dilatation, but surgical correction will be occasionally required. The enlargement of the esophagojejunal stenosis is probably more easily accomplished through the chest. Some develop digestive complaints which can be traced to cholelithiasis. Carcinoma of the colon was found in one patient more than 5 years after total gastrectomy.

The serum calcium level deserves regular evaluation since hyperparathyroidism may persist or develop, owing to the presence of the second endocrine tumor. Occasionally an anemia will be found which requires whole blood replacement followed by iron supplementation. Fasting serum gastrin levels should be monitored every 6 months, and every year a provocative infusion study should be performed. Fasting serum gastrin levels may be misleadingly low in comparison to levels obtained by a provocative infusion study.[8] Experience indicates that the fasting gastrin levels remain persistently elevated in almost all patients after operation. This is consistent with multicentric involvement of the islets of Langerhans and the high incidence of malignancy (66-75%) and suggests the adage "once a tumor, always a tumor."

Once a year a calcium infusion of calcium gluceptate, 15 mg./kg. of body weight, is given over a 4-hour period. Fasting gastrin and calcium levels are made every hour up to and including the fifth hour. Magnesium sulfate, 1.6 mEq./kg. of body weight can be given over a 4-hour period. The gastrin level tends to elevate despite a lowering of the serum calcium levels. The patient may be uncomfortable with the latter infusion. One to three clinical units of Jorpes secretin/kg. of body weight is well tolerated and produces a prompt elevation of the serum gastrin within 30 to 60 minutes with minimal alterations in the serum calcium levels. In cardiac patients or in those patients with elevated serum calcium levels associated with hyperparathyroidism, further elevations in the serum calcium levels should be avoided. Under these circumstances a secretin or magnesium sulfate infusion should be used instead of calcium. In approximately 85 percent of the postoperative patients, the fasting serum gastrin will be doubled following the infusion of calcium. The presence of persistent high serum gastrin levels is not associated with diarrhea as might be anticipated. Perhaps the persistent hypergastrinemia plays a role in stimulating the appetite and ensuring an improved postoperative nutrition.

When either the fasting or the provocative infusion gastrin level exceeds 1,000 pg./ml., a hepatic angiogram should be considered in a search for hepatic metastases. The angiogram may be positive in approximately one-half of such patients, although the patient may be symptom-free.

A persistent and interesting finding is the tendency for the fractionization of the alkaline phosphatase to show an elevation of the bone isoenzyme. The liver isoenzyme may also be elevated in some patients with hepatic metastasis. The presence of skeletal metastases is rare but multiple osteoblastic metastases have been reported by Pederson, et al.[8] Pain was completely controlled by radiation therapy. Smart has also observed a patient with gastrinoma and skeletal metastases.*

Chemotherapy should be considered when diffuse metastases to other structures including the liver are found at the time of surgery. Furthermore, a mounting gastrin level, especially if the level reaches 1,000 and if the hepatic angiogram is positive, is an indication for possible chemotherapy.[16] A variety of drugs have been used including streptozotocin alone or in combination with Tubercidin and 5-fluorouracil.[16] These carcinoid tumors grow so slowly and their behavior is so erratic that evidence of serious metastatic involvement may not be apparent more than 5 years following total gastrectomy. Patients may tolerate numerous metastases to their liver without clinical evidence of serious difficulty for several years.

SUMMARY

Sufficient time has elapsed since this syndrome was introduced in 1955 to appraise more accurately the growth habits of these tumors. Friesen has proposed the interesting observation that removal of the end-organ stomach may in fact stop the growth of the metastases from these tumors. Certainly it is difficult to explain how one of the original two patients has continued to do well and work every day, 22 years after total gastrectomy as well as removal of several lymph nodes containing metastatic islet cell tumor. The long-term survival studies suggest that more and more of these patients are getting into difficulty. It seems appropriate to suspect that from two-thirds to three-fourths have a tumor with a malignant potential.[16] Although the rate of growth may be slow and variable like other carcinoidlike tumors, it can become unexpectedly active. However uncertain the future of these patients may be, it is clear that the average length of survival has been greatly extended as a result of following the principle, in most cases, of removing all acid-secreting surface as soon as the diagnosis has been firmly established. Chemotherapy may further extend their survival if it is given before massive hepatic involvement has occurred. The gastrinoma has served as a tremendous stimulus for the study and better understanding of the polypeptides associated with the gastrointestinal tract.

REFERENCES

1. Bradley, E. L. III, et al.: Nutritional consequences of total gastrectomy. Ann. Surg., *182*:415, 1975.
2. Christoforidis, A. J., and Nelson, S. W.: Radiological manifestations of ulcerogenic tumors of the pancreas, the Zollinger-Ellison syndrome. JAMA, *198*:511, 1966.
3. Friesen, S. R.: Effect of total gastrectomy on the Zollinger-Ellison tumor: observations by second-look procedures. Surgery, *62*:609, 1967.
4. Gregory, R. A., and Tracy, H. J.: The constitution and properties of two gastrins extracted from hog antral mucosa. Gut, *5*:103, 1964.
5. Isenberg, J. I., et al.: Unusual effect of secretin on serum gastrin, serum calcium and gastrin acid secretion on a patient with suspected Zollinger-Ellison syndrome. Gastroenterology, *62*:626, 1972.
6. McGuigan, J. E., and Trudeau, W. L.: Studies with antibodies to gastrin:

*Smart, C. R.: Personal communication.

radioimmunoassay in human serum and physiological studies. Gastroenterology, *58*:139, 1970.
7. Passaro, E., Jr., et al.: Newer studies in the Zollinger-Ellison syndrome. Am. J. Surg., *120*:138, 1970.
8. Pederson, R. T., et al.: Osteoblastic bone metastasis in Zollinger-Ellison syndrome. Radiology, *118*:63, 1976.
9. Polak, J. M., and Stagg, B., and Pearse, A. G. E.: Two types of Zollinger-Ellison syndrome: immunofluorescent, cytochemical and ultrastructural studies of the antral and pancreatic gastrin cells in different clinical states. Gut, *13*:501, 1972.
10. Richardson, C. T., and Walsh, J. H.: The value of histamine H_2-receptor antagonist in the management of patients with the Zollinger-Ellison syndrome. N. Engl. J. Med., *294*:3, 144, 1976.
11. Thompson, J. C., et al.: Zollinger-Ellison syndrome: natural history and experience with diagnosis and treatment. Surg. Gynecol. Obstet., *140*:5, 1975.
12. Wilson, S. D., and Ellison, E. H.: Total gastric resection in children with the Zollinger-Ellison syndrome. Arch Surg., *91*:165, 1965.
13. Wilson, S. D., et al.: Does hyperparathyroidism cause hypergastrinemia? Surgery, *80*:231, 1976.
14. Zollinger, R. M., and Coleman, D.: The Influences of Pancreatic Tumors of the Stomach. 50th Annual Beaumont Lectures. Springfield, (Ill.), Charles C Thomas, 1974.
15. Zollinger, R. M., and Ellison, E. H.: Primary peptic ulcerations of the jejunum associated with islet cell tumors of the pancreas. Ann. Surg., *142*:709, 1955.
16. Zollinger, R. M., et al.: Observations on the postoperative tumor growth behavior of certain islet cell tumors. Ann. Surg., *184*:4, 525, 1976.

EDITORIAL COMMENTARY

The report in 1955 of the surprising observations by Zollinger and Ellison that a humoral agent from non-insulin-secreting pancreatic islet tumors was associated with marked gastric acid hypersecretion and recurrent ulceration was a remarkable impetus to all phases of endocrine research. It was the first suggestion that a gastrinlike substance might emanate from a source other than the gastric antrum. These clinical observations preceded the biochemical identification of gastrin as a polypeptide in the antral mucosa by Gregory and Tracy,[4] and their confirmation of this gastrinlike agent in primary and metastatic ulcerogenic tumors. The determination of the composition of the polypeptide and the synthesis of the active portion of it led to immunofluorescent identification of the G cell of the antrum by McGuigan in 1968, which was 13 years after the clinical report of the ulcerogenic syndrome and 63 years after Edkins postulated an antral secretagogue.

For many years it had been assumed that the delta cell (D cell) of the islets in the pancreas was the APUD cell capable of secreting gastrin. Not all cytologists agreed with this; currently it appears that a "gastrin cell," as observed by immunofluorescence, is present in the islets of the *fetal* pancreas (not in the adult pancreas). This recent finding suggests that a primitive APUD cell in the fetal islets undergoes normal repression, only to be derepressed later upon neoplastic instigation. Therefore, the gastrin which has been found in high concentrations in ulcerogenic tumors probably emanates from reactivated primitive APUD cells which are totipotential and capable of secreting variations of the gastrin molecules, as well as other polypeptides and amines which produce other islet-producing syndromes.

The migration of APUD cells from the neural crest and from the embryonic neurodectodermal "placodes" to many locations in the entire foregut accounts for the various sites for gastrin-secreting tumors that are seen clinically. Thus, at the time of operation such tumors may not be found within the pancreas, but in adjacent areas and in the duodenum and even in parathyroid tumors. The phenomenon of totipotentiality of the APUD cells also may account for the high incidence of multiplicity of gastrin-secreting tumors in some patients, the associated islet cell hyperplasia, the neoplastic proclivity and finally, the not infrequent association of pancreatic gastrinomas with other endocrine adenopathies seen in MEA-I. Incidentally, it has now been shown that the D cell of the pancreas is associated with somatostatin-secreting capability.

The frequency with which multiple foci or metastases are found in patients with ulcerogenic syndrome lends support to the necessity of end-organ excision, by total gastrectomy, as advocated by Zollinger and others. This operation effectively eliminates the fatal consequences of severe ulceration due to continuing gastrin-stimulated acid hypersecretion, leading to apparent good health, but may also provide the milieu for the infrequent but definite objective regression of the tumor and metastases which have occasionally been observed. The latter circumstances are conjectured to be due, possibly, to interruption of abnormal feedback phenomena perhaps involving secretin; or of course they may be "spontaneous" regressions. Whatever the mechanism, there are rather frequent observations of patients who survive an exceedingly long time without tumor after total gastrectomy and in whom only metastatic deposits have been removed for diagnostic confirmation without a primary tumor having been observed or removed. Long-term follow-up is important in any case, not only for detection of possible recurrent or persistent gastrinoma, but also for the recognition of other endocrine tumors. The possible use of histamine-2 blockers of gastrin receptor activity will most likely eliminate the acid hypersecretion as does total gastrectomy, but such treatment may not affect tumor growth if the absence of the stomach or "gastric factor" is of any theoretical importance.

The occasional location of an "isolated" gastrinoma such as in the duodenum is easily overlooked, but should be searched for and removed; however, successful long-term amelioration of the syndrome by local excision only of that tumor has been exceedingly infrequent, so that it is generally advised that total gastrectomy be added to the surgical treatment. Furthermore, total gastrectomy is safer in most instances than pancreaticoduodenectomy (Whipple's procedure) for such lesions. Multiple duodenal gastrinomas have been observed and removed, some of which have the histologic appearance of carcinoid tumors; these nodules are not to be confused with nodular hyperplasia of Brunner's glands of the first portion of the duodenum which is sometimes seen radiologically as a diagnostic feature of the Zollinger-Ellison syndrome. Such hyperplasia, together with parietal cell hyperplasia (gastric hyperrugation radiologically) may be evidence of the trophic capability of gastrin.

The question of gastrin cell hyperplasia of the antral mucosa without a pancreatic component as a cause of the Zollinger-Ellison syndrome has been raised. Disregarding the fact that such a circumstance is incompatible with the classic definition of the Zollinger-Ellison syndrome, there are patients who have clinical findings highly suggestive of the syndrome, including elevation of the serum gastrin; if it were not for the elevated serum gastrin in these patients, they could be considered to have severe duodenal ulcer disease, in which case the serum gastrin concentration and G cell popluation of the antrum would be normal. Usually in such unusual situations the elevated fasting serum gastrin concentration is in a range between 400 and 800 pg./ml. In such cases further diagnostic steps can be carried out to help elucidate the diagnosis. Antral mucosal biopsy obtained by flexible gastroscopy, with tissue fixed in glutaraldehyde and stained by toluidine blue dye, as if in preparation for electron microscopy, may in these instances reveal antral G cell hyperplasia, a finding not observed in pancreatic islet-induced ulcerogenic syndrome. Furthermore, provocative tests using calcium, magnesium and secretin stimulation are important in determining whether the gastrinemia has a tumor as its source; the fasting elevated serum gastrin concentration is not elevated further when the source is the antral mucosa; but it is significantly increased if the islets are the source. It is reasonable, in view of these findings, to consider that the clinical picture which is compatible with the syndrome, but which originates in the antrum with G cell hyperplasia and with no further elevation of serum gastrin on provocative testing, represents an intermediate stage between duodenal ulcer disease and pancreatic-induced Zollinger-Ellison syndrome; for this situation vagotomy and antrectomy have been shown to suffice completely as appropriate treatment. As is pointed out in this chapter, the first clue to an overlooked ulcerogenic tumor after operations for duodenal ulcer is the observation of continued gastric acid hypersecretion in the postoperative gastric aspirate; this possible circumstance should be kept in mind routinely.

Another syndrome, which may be confused with the ulcerogenic syndrome has been described by Wilson, in which there is cholecystokinin elaboration from islet cell hyperplasia. The diarrhea and gastric acid hypersecretion, however, is associated with normal serum gastrin levels, and secretin infusion decreases gastric acidity and serum gastrin values. *S.R.F.*

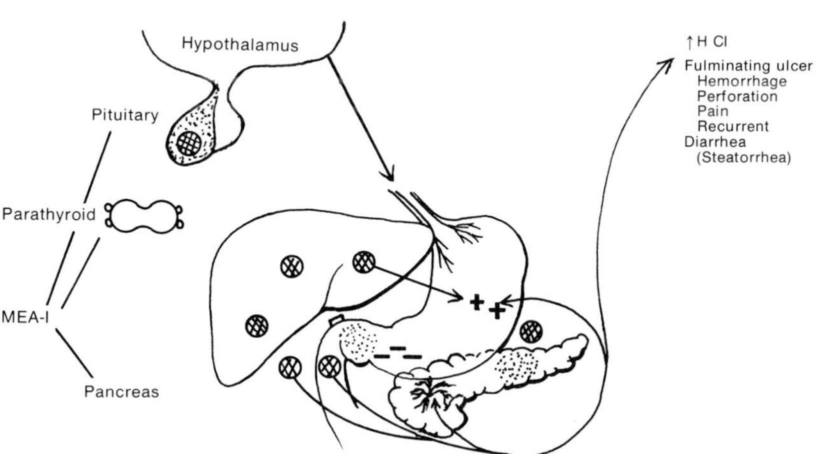

 Tumor

 Hyperplasia

Fig. 14-2. Pathophysiology of the ulcerogenic syndrome.

(See overleaf for flowchart)

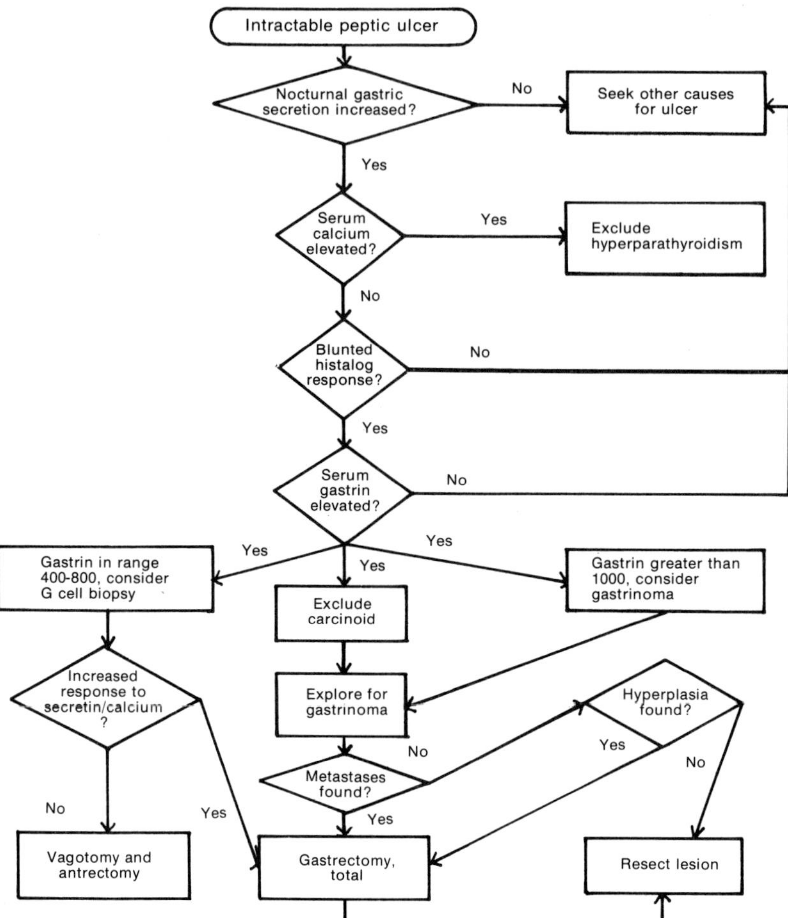

Fig. 14-3. Management flowchart of the ulcerogenic syndrome.

15

The Diarrheogenic Syndrome: Verner-Morrison, WDHA Syndrome

Bernard M. Jaffe, M.D.

When Priest and Alexander[72] first reported the association of diarrhea and non-beta islet cell tumors, it was thought that this symptom complex was a variant of the Zollinger-Ellison syndrome. The "diarrheogenic syndrome" was defined and characterized as a separate entity by Verner and Morrison[99] who recognized the prominent role of hypokalemia and the conspicuous absence of gastric hypersecretion and peptic ulceration. Several investigators, including Murray, et al.,[65] Espiner and Beavan,[21] and Hindle and associates,[38] noted the association with achlorhydria despite normal gastric parietal cells. On the basis of these observations, they suggested that the diarrheogenic hormone secreted by the islet cell tumors must also be a potent inhibitor of gastric acid secretion. A number of designations have been proposed for the syndrome, each emphasizing specific clinical attributes. Because of the etiologic role of the pancreas and the similarities with cholera, Matsumoto and colleagues[58] suggested that the syndrome be called "pancreatic cholera." Marks and associates[56] coined the acronym WDHA syndrome, representing watery diarrhea, hypokalemia, achlorhydria. Since most patients with the syndrome have hypochlorhydria (rather than achlorhydria), Verner and Morrison[100] have recently suggested the modification, WDHH. In this chapter, the designations diarrheogenic syndrome, WDHA/WDHH syndrome, Verner-Morrison syndrome, and pancreatic cholera will all be used interchangeably.

The diarrheogenic syndrome is an extremely rare clinical entity, accounting for only a miniscule percent of cases of chronic, unexplained diarrhea. To date, approximately 85 well-documented cases have been described. Since the pathophysiology of the complex is still poorly understood and no single responsible humeral mediator has been clearly identified, it is extremely difficult to make the diagnosis with assurance. Furthermore, the complexity and severity of the electrolyte disturbances, as well as the relatively limited experience with surgical and postsurgical therapy contribute to making this a very challenging clinical problem. Advances in the pathophysiology of the syndrome have been summarized by Rambaud and colleagues,[75] and its clinical features have been recently reviewed by Verner and Morrison.[101] This chapter will attempt to derive a logical and systematic approach to the diagnosis and management of the diarrheogenic syndrome.

CHARACTERISTICS OF THE DIARRHEOGENIC SYNDROME

Clinical Features and Electrolyte Abnormalities

The diarrheogenic syndrome is most often a disease afflicting middle-aged females. At the time of diagnosis the patients have averaged 47 years of age,[100] however, their ages have ranged from 5 to 72 years. Two-thirds (65%) of the patients reported have been female.

Watery diarrhea has uniformly been the presenting complaint. Initially the diarrhea has been reported as intermittent in approximately half the patients with alternating symptomatic episodes and quiescent periods during which time the stools are few in number and semisolid in consistency. As the syndrome progresses, the symptomatic episodes increase in frequency and eventually coalesce, resulting in constant unremitting diarrhea. In general, when the WDHA syndrome has been caused by malignant tumors, the diarrhea has been constant from the outset.

During the active phases of the syndrome, the diarrhea is profuse, averaging 4.6 liters per day, (range 3-10).[100] The diarrhea has the appearance of weak tea and is extremely rich in electrolytes, particularly potassium (200-400 mEq. per day) and bicarbonate. The fecal loss of electrolytes is responsible for the biochemical abnormalities which makes the syndrome so difficult to manage. These anomalies will be described below.

Most patients with the WDHA syndrome have described 10 to 15 motions per day. Since, as will be described below, this is almost purely a secretory diarrhea in which hypermotility plays no significant role in the pathogenesis, patients have reported remarkably few symptoms and crampy abdominal pain is unusual. However, once the patients become hypokalemic, they develop symptoms of potassium deficiency per se, including muscular weakness, lethargy, nausea, vomiting and crampy abdominal pain; these symptoms can be alleviated by potassium administration.

Despite the extraordinary diarrhea, malabsorption and steatorrhea are uncommon and of relatively minor importance. Normal fecal fat excretion was reported in 19 of 22 patients studied by Matuchansky.[73] Minimal steatorrhea has been reported in only four patients.[30,63,68,88] Abnormal Schilling and D-xylose tests as well as small bowel biopsies have been described in only one patient each.[73]

The characteristics of the diarrhea can explain a number of the electrolyte abnormalities. Fecal excretion of potassium and bicarbonate result in profound hypokalemia and acidosis. Serum K^+ levels have averaged 2.1 mg./100 ml. at the time of hospitalization for diagnosis and arterial pHs of 7.1 are common. Dehydration has been a major problem and most patients have had a significant element of prerenal azotemia. Three patients have had congestive heart failure secondary to hypokalemia-induced myocardial damage[14,54] and several uremic deaths have been ascribed to hypokalemic vascular tubular nephropathy.[76] The electrolyte depletion and dehydration have been extremely severe and have been directly responsible for the deaths of seven patients (almost 10% of the cases reported).[34,57,68,72,96,99]

Characteristic abnormalities in gastric acid secretion have been described in patients with the Verner-Morrison syndrome. In contrast to the Zollinger-

Ellison syndrome (see Chap. 14), peptic ulcer disease and gastric hypersecretion are distinctly uncommon. Only two patients have had peptic ulceration; one developed a superficial gastric ulcer while taking adrenal corticosteroids[72] and we have treated one normochlorhydric patient who had a coexisting duodenal ulcer. Furthermore, hyposecretion of gastric acid and pepsin have been rather consistent. In their review of the WDHA syndrome, Verner and Morrison[100] have reported that 59 percent of the patients tested had basal achlorhydria and half of them had no secretory response to injection of histamine. Among a compilation of 54 patients[98,100] only 14 had histamine-fast achlorhydria, whereas another 16 had hypochlorhydria. A number of mechanisms have been proposed to explain the gastric hyposecretion. Although hypokalemia has been shown to suppress gastric acid secretion,[18] depletion of this electrolyte alone cannot explain the observed hypochlorhydria; a number of patients have been described in whom gastric hyposecretion persisted after correction of the hypokalemia. The most likely etiology is tumor secretion of a gastric inhibitor. The evidence for this suggestion includes:

1. Gastric biopsies have invariably revealed normal parietal cells even in achlorhydric patients.
2. Gastric hyposecretion of pepsin and intrinsic factor has been corrected by resection of diarrheogenic tumors.[3]
3. Following resection of islet cell tumors, 8 of 13 patients studied both pre- and postoperatively developed rebound gastric hypersecretion; several of these patients developed duodenal ulcer disease, one of whom required vagotomy for control.

The nature of the gastric inhibitor is still uncertain but the potential candidates will be discussed below.

Although flushing is an uncommon symptom, having been described in only 14 patients, it is quite characteristic.[65,90,94] Patients have reported episodic erythema associated with urticaria and some induration affecting primarily the face and upper trunk. The etiology of the abnormality is unknown. Despite the resemblance to the carcinoid-induced flush, only two patients have had elevated circulating levels of serotonin or daily urinary excretion rates of 5 hydroxyindole acetic acid.[29,85]

In addition to acidosis, hypokalemia, and azotemia, hypercalcemia and hyperglycemia have also been noted in patients with the WDHA syndrome.

Hypercalcemia has been reported in 18 of 37 collected patients,[100] and we have observed the abnormality in every patient we have treated. Balance studies have revealed that patients with diarrheogenic tumors are in negative calcium balance and have suggested that the calcium originates from the bone.[47] Although the mechanism of hypercalcemia is still uncertain, it appears to be induced by the iselt cell tumor rather than by abnormalities in the parathyroid glands. Serum phosphorus levels have generally been normal and parathyroidectomy has been uniformly unsuccessful in lowering serum calcium.[10,72,99] In contrast, resection of islet cell adenomas has corrected the hypercalcemia in a number of patients.[10,13,21,30,54,56,65] Tetany, thought to be due to hypomagnesemia, has been reported in four hypercalcemic patients,[10,94,99] This unusual abnormality is particularly dangerous, since it is worsened by potassium administration during attempts to correct the associated hypokalemia.

Glucose intolerance has been described in half the patients with the Verner-Morrison syndrome (17/32 collected patients). Although hypokalemia has been shown to raise serum glucose levels, the hyperglycemia observed is almost certainly due to a diabetogenic effect of the secreted hormone. In support of this suggestion, in one patient, operative manipulation of an islet cell tumor resulted in pronounced hyperglycemia[21] and, as a general rule, resection of diarrheogenic tumors has normalized glucose tolerance tests.[13,36,103]

Pathophysiology

Understanding the pathophysiology of the WDHA syndrome is critical to evaluating and managing the associated clinical, and more specifically, the electrolyte abnormalities. Accordingly, the pathophysiology of the syndrome, as recently characterized by Rambaud and associates,[75] is described in this section.

The gastric secretory abnormalities have been alluded to on page 216. Briefly, basal hyposecretion of gastric acid and pepsin are characteristic. Although 30 percent of patients have histamine-fast achlorhydria,[100] most patients have relatively normal gastric secretory responses to pentapeptide and histamine. Basal gastric hypersecretion has rarely been detected on individual determinations; although very unusual, hypersecretion does not necessarily rule out the WDHA syndrome and may be explained by elevations in serum gastrin (noted in 4 of 17 patients[41]) and in urinary gastric secretagogue activity.[75]

Abnormalities in the biliary tract have been emphasized particularly by Zollinger and colleagues.[104] They have described gallbladders containing bile with increased concentrations of chloride and bicarbonate and low levels of bile acids (including cholic, chemodeoxycholic and deoxycholic acids). Although this observation has been confirmed by several investigators,[58,75,103] the humeral mediator of this phenomenon is still in question. The rate of hepatic bile flow has been shown to be slightly elevated whereas basal and secretin-stimulated rates of pancreatic secretion have generally been normal.[28,40,56,67,75]

Despite their consistency, these abnormalities in upper gastrointestinal function do not seem to play a significant role in the pathogenesis of the syndrome. The volume and composition of the fluid arriving at the ligament of Treitz is normal.[75] This feature explains an important diagnostic characteristic of the WDHA syndrome, that the diarrhea is not affected by nasogastric suction.

The small intestine is the site of the major abnormalities. Despite normal absorption of leucine and glucose, Rambaud and colleagues[74] have demonstrated that these two nutrients fail to stimulate normal jejunal absorption of water and electrolytes. In addition, there is active secretion throughout the entire length of the intestine. As a result, the total volume of fluid leaving the distal ileum is approximately 10 times normal. Within the jejunum, the luminal concentrations of potassium and especially bicarbonate have been shown to be increased; the latter abnormality results in abolition of the normal bicarbonate gradient from the proximal to distal small bowel. The composite effect of these small intestinal abnormalities is the luminal loss of vast quantities of water and electrolytes, an effect which has been reproduced by the injection of at least one tumor extract.[27]

In contrast to the small intestine, the colon has been shown to function normally in this syndrome. Although the colon reabsorbs the great majority of the water, sodium, chloride and bicarbonate which enters the cecum, the volume of fluid and mass of electrolytes far exceeds the finite absorptive capability of the large bowel.[19] Colonic (but not intestinal) reabsorption has been shown to be responsive to aldosterone[77]; patients with the diarrheogenic syndrome have a significant component of secondary hyperaldosteronism[12,75] which has been documented by elevations in serum aldosterone as well as in the urinary excretion of aldosterone metabolites. As a consequence of the hyperaldosteronism, potassium is exchanged for sodium in the colon. The result of this aldosterone-mediated effect is, therefore, colonic absorption of sodium and secretion of potassium.

By considering the pathophysiology, the electrolyte abnormalities seen clinically can readily be ascribed to specific alterations in intestinal function. Dehydration and acidosis are due to small intestinal losses of water and bicarbonate, whereas hypokalemia is due to colonic secretion of potassium ion.

Humoral Mediators

Despite extensive studies performed by a number of laboratories, no one hormone has been implicated in the etiology of the WDHA syndrome. As will be discussed later, on page 222, the lack of a single humoral mediator considerably complicates the establishment of the diagnosis. In this section, possible mediators will be discussed and the evidence implicating them will be presented. This information is relevant to the interpretation of hormone profiles in patients with the diarrheogenic syndrome.

A number of suggested mediators have been largely ruled out, including a combination of gastrin and glucagon[4] and serotonin. Although glucagon inhibits gastric acid secretion and causes hyperglycemia, it is a potent inhibitor of pancreatic exocrine function and hypocalcemic agent and its proposed intestinal secretory activity in vivo is, at best, equivocal. Similarly, gastrin stimulates intestinal secretion but its spectrum of biologic actions is incompatible with the symptoms of the WDHA syndrome; gastrin causes hypoglycemia, hypocalcemia and hyperchlorhydria.

Although recent studies have demonstrated that serotonin inhibits intestinal absorption of water and electrolytes,[45] the predominant diarrheogenic action of the amine is caused by increased intestinal tone and motility[35]; this is manifested clinically by shortened intestinal transit time and, to a lesser degree, by steatorrhea, features that are notably absent in patients with pancreatic cholera.

Thus, despite the fact that occasional elevations of serum levels of gastrin and glucagon[14,41] and of urinary excretion of 5-HIAA[12,14,21] have been reported, in the overwhelming majority of patients, these determinations have been normal.

Zollinger and his associates have proposed that secretin is responsible for the diarrheogenic syndrome. The initial evidence for this possibility was based on the observation of secretinlike effects on the biliary tract and gallbladder.[104] Extracts of some (but not all) diarrheogenic tumors have stimulated pancreatic volume and bicarbonate secretion and Tompkins and colleagues[97] have demonstrated that these extracts possessed secretinlike choleretic activity. Wormsley has reported that secretin caused diarrhea in man.[102] Thus, secretin possesses an appropriate spectrum of activities, including intestinal secretion,[39,61,97] inhibition of gastric acid secretion[33] and hypercalcemia. In specific patients, positive bio-[3,15,85] and radioimmunoassays[48,85] have been reported. However, there are also a number of negative factors. Secretin stimulates rather than inhibits gastric pepsin secretion. The great majority of patients with the diarrheogenic syndrome have had both normal basal pancreatic exocrine function and secretory responses to exogenous secretin.[14,28,40,56,75] Finally, most patients have had normal circulating secretin levels.[41]

Currently, the three potential mediators which are receiving the majority of attention are vasoactive intestinal polypeptide (VIP), human pancreatic polypeptide (HPP) and prostaglandin E_2 (PGE_2). As will be discussed below, measurements of these agents are particularly important in the diagnostic workup, and they are available in specific centers in the United States and abroad.

VIP is a peptide which shares a number of structural similarities with secretin and glucagon.[82] It is synthesized by specific cells both in the intestinal tract, particularly the ileum and colon,[70] and in the peripheral and central nervous systems[83]; its presumed role is as a neurotransmitter substance.[11] The spectrum of its biologic activities (at least as determined by the administration of exogenous VIP) coincides perfectly with the clinical features of the WDHA syndrome[55,80]; infusion of VIP results in intestinal secretion and diarrhea, peripheral vasodilation, hypercalcemia, hyperglycemia (due to glycogenolysis), inhibition of gastric secretion and motility, augmentation of bile flow, and minimal stimulation of pancreatic bicarbonate secretion. Bloom and associates[9] first reported elevated VIP levels in the plasma and tumors from patients with the diarrheogenic syndrome. A number of case reports rapidly verified this observation.[22,31,75,85,89,91,95] Two relatively large series have evaluated the role of VIP in the WDHA syndrome, those of Said and Faloona[81] and of Bloom and Polak.[7] In the former series, elevated levels of VIP were described in the 26/28 plasma samples and 13/13 diarrheogenic tumor extracts. Plasma VIP levels were high in patients with pancreatic islet cell tumors as well as those with ectopic (lung and adrenal) lesions and pancreatic islet cell hyperplasia. VIP levels seemed to correlate well with activity of the disease, falling rapidly after resection of tumors as well as after steroid- and streptozotocin-induced alleviation of diarrhea; however, VIP levels remained elevated in three patients subjected to subtotal pancreatectomy for islet cell hyperplasia. Bloom and Polak[7] similarly reported elevated plasma VIP levels (200-2000 pg./ml.; normal 20 pg./ml.) in 17 patients; VIP concentrations in 10 diarrheogenic tumors ranged from 1 to 100 μg./g. In contrast to the above series,[81] patients with islet cell hyperplasia had normal plasma levels of VIP. Based on this distinction, Bloom and Polak classified patients with islet hyperplasia as "pseudo-Verner-Morrison syndrome."[8] Despite these observations, there are several pieces of evidence that disprove the fact that VIP is the sole humoral mediator of the diarrheogenic syndrome:

1. According to the data of Gardner and colleagues (personal communication), the concentrations of VIP achieved are not high enough to produce diarrhea.
2. Since the intestinal effects of VIP are mediated by cyclic AMP,[86] the normal intestinal concentrations of cyclic AMP noted rules VIP out as the sole mediator.

3. Elevated levels of VIP have been reported in patients with a glucagonoma[52] and surreptitious laxative and diuretic abuse,[49] implying a lack of specificity.
4. A number of patients with pancreatic cholera have had normal plasma levels of VIP.[7,20,41,49,52]

Recently, Polak and her associates reported that half of the pancreatic endocrine tumors examined contained large amounts of HPP.[71] HPP is a member of the homologous family of pancreatic peptides produced by specific endocrine cells both within the islets and throughout the exocrine tissue[5,50,51]; patients who have undergone total pancreatectomy have immeasurably low levels of this peptide.[1] Although HPP is released following a normal meal[1,2,87] and after insulin-induction of hypoglycemia,[2] the physiologic role of this hormone is still unknown. There is no evidence that infusion of HPP reproduces the symptoms of the WDHA syndrome and consequently, this peptide cannot currently be implicated in the pathogenesis of the diarrheogenic syndrome. HPP is released by infusions of a number of gastrointestinal hormones.[69] However, the frequency of elevation of plasma levels of HPP makes it a useful tumor marker.

The activities of prostaglandin E (PGE) includes all those associated with the symptoms of the diarrheogenic syndrome; this agent can cause secretory diarrhea,[17,59,60] flushing associated with vasodilitation,[66] hypercalcemia,[25] hypochlorhydria[78] and hyperglycemia.[79] Although occasional elevations of bioassayable and radioimmunoassayable PGE have previously been reported in patients with the WDHA syndrome,[84,85] we have carefully evaluated the etiologic role of this mediator.[41] Among 23 patients with the diarrheogenic syndrome, 10 had elevated levels of PGE (5 of whom had normal plasma levels of VIP). PGE levels averaged 1,000 pg./ml. for the total group (of 23 patients) compared to control levels of 250 pg./ml. Two patients were particularly interesting. The first, who had normal levels of VIP, had significantly elevated plasma concentrations of PGE before resection of a pancreatic islet cell carcinoma (9,939 pg./ml.) and 8 months later, prior to extirpation of a solitary metastasis from the left lobe of the liver (1,063 pg./ml.); following each of these procedures, PGE levels returned to normal and the diarrhea abated. The second patient, a hyperprostaglandinemic 63-year-old woman, had a remarkable response to indomethacin, a potent inhibitor of prostaglandin biosynthesis. Within 24 hours after initiation of indomethacin therapy (25 mg. t.i.d.), daily stool volume fell from 3 to 4 liters of watery diarrhea to one or two semiformed or formed bowel movements. With this therapy, plasma PGE levels were profoundly lowered. Although this is the only known patient who had such a dramatic response to indomethacin, the data support the contention that PGE was involved in mediating the diarrheogenic response in this woman. (She has been asymptomatic without drugs since the resection of a pancreatic adenoma.) Despite the bulk of this evidence, 13 of our 23 patients, and several others reported, had normal levels of PGE, making it quite unlikely that PGE is the sole mediator of the diarrheogenic syndrome.

In summary, the current impression is that the WDHA syndrome is not a uniform clinical entity caused by a single, well-defined humoral mediator. A more realistic concept is that it is a heterogeneous composite of secretory diarrheogenic states whose pathogenesis involves several interrelated hormones. This concept is consistent with the possibility that diarrheogenic tumors are APUDomas (see Chap. 2).

PREOPERATIVE EVALUATION

Management of Electrolyte Abnormalities

At the time of hospitalization a primary problem facing the physician is correction of the electrolyte abnormalities. The specific deficits and their etiologies have already been described. It is difficult to put the severity of the dehydration and electrolyte depletion in perspective, but it is appropriate to emphasize that nearly 10 percent of the patients with diarrheogenic tumors died during attempts to manage these problems. It is not within the scope of this chapter to provide a detailed description of a management plan. However, a few suggestions may be in order:

1. Since virtually all the patients have had diarrhea and tolerated the dehydration and electrolyte deficit for several years, it is inappropriate, even dangerous, to attempt to rapidly correct the deficiencies. A useful example of the potential problems relates to the correction of hypokalemia. Most patients have lost 200 to 400 mEq. of K^+ per day over prolonged periods of time. Adequate replacement would therefore necessitate infusion of *many* thousand milliequivalents of K^+. Potassium replacement should be performed slowly in order to allow for equilibration of extra- and intracellular potassium and evaluation of true potassium requirements. A reasonable suggestion might be 100 mEq. per day above the measured daily losses.

2. During the course of electrolyte management, patients continue to excrete huge amounts of fluid and electrolytes. These continuing losses must be taken into consideration when planning replacement therapy. Careful measurements of the volumes and composition of dietary intake and fecal and urinary output are critical and must be quantitated daily. Despite the fact that fasting does not significantly alter the stool volume, electrolyte replacement is usually more effective if the patient is not permitted to eat or drink anything but measured small volumes of water.

3. The combination of hypokalemia and hyperchloremic acidosis is quite unusual. Massive transfusion of KCl must therefore be avoided and potassium should be administered with other anions, including sulfate, phosphate and bicarbonate. In hypercalcemic patients, potassium repletion may precipitate hypomagnesemic tetany; in order to avoid this complication, small doses of magnesium sulfate should be utilized. Finally, the massive diarrhea may cause deficiencies of trace metals, a problem which can be prevented readily by infusion of small amounts of plasma.

4. Since it may be difficult to distinguish the signs and symptoms of the WDHA syndrome from those of the related electrolyte abnormalities, the full diagnostic workup is best postponed until after the correction of the deficiencies.

Diagnosis

The diagnostic workup can be divided into two distinct phases, establishing the diagnosis of the WDHA syndrome and attempting to localize the tumor. The first three divisions of this section are devoted to the diagnosis of pancreatic cholera; the final division will discuss the value of diagnostic modalities designed to localize tumors.

Differential Diagnosis. A number of chronic diarrheal states may mimic the diarrheogenic syndrome.

Villous adenomas of the rectosigmoid colon may cause diarrhea and hypokalemia. In this clinical entity (in contrast to WDHA), the stool characteristically contains large amounts of mucus. The humoral mediator of the hypokalemia has never been identified. Nonetheless, this colonic lesion can readily be identified by sigmoidoscopy and barium enema and should cause no major difficulty in differential diagnosis.

Surreptitious abuse of laxatives and diuretics can be extremely difficult to distinguish from the WDHA syndrome. One complicating factor is that VIP levels are frequently reported as elevated under these conditions. Specific chromatographic and spectrophotometric tests have been developed to measure each of the commonly used laxatives and diuretics. Fecal excretion of phenophthalein (a component of most commercially available laxatives) is suggested if the stool develops a red color after alkalinization with 0.1N NaOH; positive identification of this drug depends on spectrophotometric proof that peak absorption occurs at a wavelength of 525 nm. (and coincides with a phenophthalein standard).[49] Since most clinical laboratories are capable of detecting phenophthalein in the stool, this determination should be performed routinely in patients with symptoms suggestive of pancreatic cholera. Although thorough investigation may reveal illicit drug use, nasogastric intubation and suction is an effective way of preventing surreptitious drug abuse.

In its florid form with extensive intestinal involvement, celiac disease causes profuse diarrhea. It is not uncommon for such patients to have more than 10 stools per day and to develop acidosis and hypokalemia. The similarity with pancreatic cholera is accentuated by the fact that patients with celiac disease have intestinal secretion of water and electrolytes.[24] Despite these similarities, this enteropathy should be distinguished readily from the WDHA syndrome. In celiac disease, malabsorption is a major characteristic and thus, the stools are usually oily and foul smelling. Abnormalities in the D-xylose tolerance tests are usual. As a result of poor nutrition, patients complain of severe weight loss, weakness, lassitude and fatigue. Since the diarrhea is due to the osmotic effects of malabsorbed foodstuffs (protein, fat, and carbohydrate) and to hydroxyfatty acids synthesized by bacteria from unabsorbed lipid precursors, it can be ameliorated by nasogastric suction. Histologic abnormalities on small bowel biopsy, clinical responsiveness to a gluten-free diet, hypocalcemia associated with osteomalacia, and iron- and folic acid-deficiency anemias are characteristics of celiac sprue that further serve to distinguish this clinical entity from pancreatic cholera.

Other endocrine diarrheogenic syndromes should be reasonably easily distinguished. Patients with the Zollinger-Ellison syndrome have massive gastric hypersecretion as the result of which they may develop metabolic alkalosis. Other metabolic abnormalities include hypocalcemia and hypoglycemia, effects which are induced by circulating gastrin. In addition, Z-E patients routinely have malabsorption and steatorrhea. Crosby capsule biopsies reveal evidence of acid-induced damage to the small intestinal mucosa. Gastrin levels may not necessarily be diagnostic, since elevated gastrin levels (in the Z-E range) have been reported in several patients with the WDHA syndrome.

As described in Chapter 11, the diarrhea associated with the carcinoid

Table 15-1. Differential Diagnosis of the WDHA Syndrome

Differential Diagnosis	*Diagnostic Procedure*	*Hormone Analysis*
Villous adenoma	Barium enema Sigmoidoscopy (colonoscopy)	
Drug abuse	Stool examination for phenophthalein	
Celiac disease	Fecal fat quantitation D-xylose tolerance test Crosby capsule biopsy	
Zollinger-Ellison syndrome	Basal and histamine-stimulated gastric secretion	Gastrin
Carcinoid syndrome	Intestinal transit time Liver scan	Serotonin Urinary 5-HIAA
Medullary carcinoma of thyroid	Thyroid scan, T_3, T_4	Calcitonin
Parasitic and infectious diseases	Stool culture Ova and parasites	
Inflammatory bowel disease	Upper GI and small bowel roentgenographic study	
WDHA syndrome	Superior mesenteric angiography Intravenous pyelogram Chest x-ray with necessary laminograms CAT scan of the retroperitoneum	VIP PGE_2 HPP Secretin

syndrome is caused by elevated peripheral blood levels of serotonin.[44,62] Serotonin-induced diarrhea is associated with increased motility and shortened intestinal transit time,[35] characteristics that serve to distinguish this clinical entity from the Verner-Morrison syndrome. Additional differential criteria include bronchoconstriction, steatorrhea and weight loss. Increased urinary excretion of 5-HIAA has been described in patients with the diarrheogenic syndrome as well as in those with carcinoid tumors.

Medullary carcinoma of the thyroid (MCT) causes diarrhea in one-third the afflicted patients and as described in Chapter 18, this symptom is commonly the presenting complaint.[37] Diarrhea associated with MCT has a significant secretory component, and thyrocalcitonin has been shown to cause jejunal secretion of water and electrolytes.[32] However, elevated calcitonin levels are not absolutely diagnostic of MCT, since they have also been reported in patients with pancreatic cholera.[75,85] Elevated levels of PGE have also been reported in both syndromes.[41,42] Although patients with medullary thyroid cancer have shortened intestinal transit times,[6,37] the major distinguishing characteristic is the presence of a palpable thyroid nodule which is "cold" on radioactive scan. Thorough clinical and isotopic evaluation of the thyroid should be performed routinely in the evaluation of patients suspected of having pancreatic cholera.

Parasitic, infectious and inflammatory bowel diseases are unlikely to cause any difficulty in differential diagnosis, but stool examinations for ova and parasites, stool cultures and radiographic examination of the small bowel should be included in the diagnostic workups.

The differential diagnosis of the WDHA syndrome and the appropriate diagnostic modalities are summarized in Table 15-1. This composite list of procedures constitutes a thorough diagnostic workup.

Hormone Analysis. The appropriate hormone analyses are listed in Table 15-1. Although not all of these determinations are routinely performed in all hospitals, the analyses can usually be obtained, either commercially or from the specific laboratories in which the techniques were developed. Despite the sophistication applied to these hormone analyses, none of these measurements is absolutely diagnostic of the WDHA syndrome. Accordingly, abnormalities in hormone levels must be considered in light of the entire diagnostic workup and should never be interpreted as indications for diagnostic laparotomy.

Intestinal Perfusion. Intestinal perfusion is currently the most specific modality available for documenting intestinal secretion and confirming (or excluding) the diagnosis of pancreatic cholera. In a recent article, Krejs and his associates[49] reported that all three patients with the WDHA syndrome studied had objective evidence of jejunal secretion, whereas this was not observed in patients with other diagnoses. Although the technique, recently described in detail,[49] is demanding and is not suitable for routine screening by most physicians, pertinent information about its performance is included.

Perfusion studies were performed in fasting patients receiving intravenous electrolyte solutions.[49] The small intestine was intubated using triple-lumen polyvinyl tubes.[16,23] Jejunal perfusions were performed when the infusion hole was located at the ligament of Treitz (90 cm.); the corresponding length for the midileal studies was 200 cm. from the teeth. Infusions, bubbled with 5 percent CO_2 and 95 percent O_2 to a pCO_2 of 40 mm. Hg. and containing polyethylene glycol as a recovery marker, were performed for 60 minutes (after a 45-minute equilibration period) at a constant rate of 11 ml. per minute. Aspirates from the 30-cm. long test segment were sampled and analyzed. The composition of the test perfusion solutions and the ranges of normal values are included in Table 15-2.

Table 15-2. Normal Ranges of Water and Electrolyte Movement Data During Intestinal Perfusion[49]

	Water (ml. per hour/30 cm.)	*Sodium (mEq. per hour/30 cm.)*	*Potassium (mEq. per hour/30 cm.)*	*Chloride (mEq. per hour/30 cm.)*	*Bicarbonate (mEq. per hour/30 cm.)*
Jejunal Perfusion					
1. Plasmalike[1]	−15 to −115	−3.0 to −14.6	0 to 0.8	+2.3 to −11.3	−1.3 to −8.1
2. Mannitol[2]	—	+1.0 to +12.6	—	—	—
3. Glucose[3]	—	−2.1 to −20.6	—	—	—
Ileal Perfusion					
1. Plasmalike[4]	−8 to −128	−0.9 to −18.1	+0.6 to −1.0	−1.1 to −16.7	+1.3 to −3.0
2. Mannitol-low salt[5]	+20 to −48	+1.1 to −4.1	—	−1.3 to −8.1	—

Test Solutions

1. Plasmalike	NaCl 105mM;	$NaHCO_3$ 30mM;	KCl 5mM
2. Mannitol	NaCl 105mM;	KCl 5mM;	mannitol 65mM
3. Glucose	NaCl 105mM;	KCl 5mM;	glucose 65mM
4. Plasmalike	NaCl 105mM;	$NaHCO_3$ 35mM;	KCl 5mM
5. Mannitol-low salt	NaCl 50mM;	KCl 5mM;	mannitol 160mM

Other Workup. As described below (Treatment) 70 percent of the patients with the WDHA syndrome have pancreatic tumors. Ectopic diarrheogenic tumors (10%) have been reported in the retroperitoneum and the adrenal glands as well as in the lungs. Thus, diagnostic studies aimed at localizing the sites of diarrheogenic tumors must focus on these areas. Suggested studies are listed in Table 15-1. Although occasional successes have been reported,[30,54,91,99,104] in general, superior mesenteric angiography has been disappointing and frequently has failed to visualize even large tumors. Selenomethionine (^{75}Se) scanning of the pancreas has so consistently failed to visualize lesions that it is no longer warranted. CAT scanning of the retroperitoneum holds particular promise, but not enough experience has been accumulated to evaluate the effectiveness of this new modality in localizing pancreatic tumors; in a recent personal case, a CAT scan failed to identify a diarrheogenic tumor (5 x 7 cm.) in the tail of the pancreas. Having established the diagnosis of the WDHA syndrome on the basis of clinical and chemical parameters, assuming there is no evidence of a pulmonary neoplasm, the definitive diagnostic modality is exploratory laparotomy.

Preparation for Operation

After rehydration and correction of the electrolyte deficiencies and establishing the diagnosis of the diarrheogenic syndrome, the patient should be prepared for laparotomy. If at all possible, it is suggested that the diarrhea should be controlled with medication for several days prior to operation. As will be discussed below, steroids (e.g., prednisone 30 mg. per day) have usually been successful in alleviating the diarrhea in these patients. We have also recently aborted profuse diarrhea in one patient with pancreatic cholera using indomethacin in a dose of 25 mg. t.i.d. Since these drugs are effective within 48 hours, if at all, short trial courses of prednisone and indomethacin are warranted in the preoperative period.

TREATMENT

Pathology and Location of Tumors

In a recent review of 55 patients with pancreatic cholera,[101] 43 had pancreatic non-beta islet cell tumors (78%), 23 of which were benign adenomas. All 20 patients with malignant lesions had metastases at the time of diagnosis. However, this is a skewed statistic, since it is quite difficult for the pathologist to establish a diagnosis of malignancy on the basis of histologic criteria alone. As described above (p. 219) there is still considerable conflict as to the cells of origin of the tumors and their humoral products. In addition to those with pancreatic tumors, 11 of the 55 reported patients (20%) had islet cell hyperplasia. This diagnosis is quite difficult to interpret, since no firm histologic criteria have been established. The diagnosis of islet hyperplasia cannot be made accurately on frozen section and requires intensive examination of pancreatic tissue by pathologists with specific interest and experience in islet abnormalities.

Fausa and associates[22] first reported a patient in whom the WDHA syndrome was cured following resection of a retroperitoneal ganglioneuroma. Similar patients were reported by Swift and colleagues[95] and Said and Faloona.[81] It is difficult to establish the frequency with which retroperitoneal neoplasms cause the WDHA syndrome. Pediatricians have seen a number of infants and children with neuroblastomas and diarrhea but the possibility that they have pancreatic cholera or a closely-related variant has not seriously been entertained until recently. In addition to retroperitoneal ectopic lesions, Said and Faloona[81] have recently reported that 5 of 30 patients studied had bronchogenic (diarrheogenic) carcinomas. Overall, approximately 10 percent of cases of the WDHA syndrome have been caused by diarrheogenic tumors arising from extrapancreatic sites.

Surgical Therapy

Resection of diarrheogenic tumors provides the only effective means for cure or long-lasting remission. In a collected series,[101] all patients with benign islet cell tumors were cured of their symptoms by resection of the adenomas. Pancreatic adenomas have usually not been very difficult to locate at surgery, since 80 percent have been in the body and tail, most have been large (>3 cm.), and only very rarely have more than one adenoma been recognized.[3] In several patients with malignant lesions, palliative resections have provided temporary remissions and relief of symptoms. If total resection is impossible, the surgeon can offer maximal palliation by resecting as much gross tumor as is possible.

Surgical management of pancreatic islet cell hyperplasia is more difficult. If a tumor cannot be located, subtotal pancreatotomy (just to the left of the superior mesenteric vessels) is the procedure of choice. Frozen section evaluation of the number and size of islet cells is unreliable and thus, islet hyperplasia cannot be diagnosed intraoperatively. Furthermore, 8 of 11 reported patients treated by partial pancreatectomy were cured of their symptoms.[10,36,40,53,92,104] However, subtotal pancreatectomy should not be considered a universally successful therapeutic modality; several patients have required completion pancreatectomy to control the symptoms of pancreatic cholera.[101]

When effective, surgical resection provides virtually immediate relief of symptoms. Postoperative electrolyte management has not been difficult and when intestinal propulsive function returns, bowel movements have been normal. During the immediate postoperative period, antacids should be administered in order to avoid the potential problems with rebound gastric hypersecretion.

Chemotherapy

In patients with unresectable and/or metastatic diarrheogenic tumors, attention must be directed both to the alleviation of symptoms and to chemotherapeutic control of tumor growth.

Adrenal corticosteroids were effective in controlling the diarrhea in 7 of 12 treated patients.[13,38,46,48,58,72,89,93] Our experience has confirmed this observation, and steroids have proven to be a valuable adjunct in the management of the diarrhea associated with pancreatic cholera. We have also noted dramatic control of diarrhea in one hyperprostaglandinemic female using indomethacin; since this is the first patient in whom indomethacin-mediated inhibition of prostaglandin biosynthesis has been clinically useful, it is difficult to estimate how frequently this response might be anticipated.

Neither radiation therapy nor 5-fluorouracil has consistently been effective in controlling the growth of malignant diarrheogenic tumors.[12,64] Recently, Kahn and colleagues[43] have reported that intra-arterial administration of streptozotocin produced dramatic remissions in two patients. This observation was confirmed by Gagel and associates[26] who also noted that previously elevated plasma levels of VIP returned to the normal range after four courses of this chemotherapeutic agent. The addition of this agent to our armamentarium adds substantially to the prospects of control of diarrheogenic tumor growth.

CONCLUSIONS

Our knowledge about the diarrheogenic syndrome has rapidly progressed. We have recently come to understand its pathophysiology and thus, can more effectively manage the complicated electrolyte problems. Substantial clinical experience has recently been accumulated and our approach to the diagnosis and management of this disorder has become considerably more enlightened. However, there are still a number of important unresolved problems particularly relating to the nature of the humoral mediator(s). It seems quite likely that with continued research and clinical observation, many of these questions will be answered within a short period of time.

REFERENCES

1. Adrian, T. E., Bloom, S. R., Bryant, M. G., Polak, J. M., Heitz, Ph., and Barnes, A. J.: Distribution and release of human pancreatic polypeptide. Gut, *17*:940, 1976.
2. Adrian, T. E., Besterman, H. S., Cooke, T. J., Bloom, S. R., Barnes, A. J., Russell, R. C. G., and Faber, R. G.: Mechanism of pancreatic polypeptide release in man. Lancet, *1*:161, 1977.
3. Andersson, H., Dotevall, G., Fagerberg, G., Raotoma, H., Walan, A., and Zederfeldt, B.: Pancreatic tumor with diarrhea, hypokalemia, and hypochlorhydria. Acta Chir. Scand., *138*:102, 1972.
4. Barbezat, G. O., and Grossman, M. I.: Cholera-like diarrhea induced by glucagon plus gastrin, Lancet, *1*:1026, 1971.
5. Bergstrom, B. H., Loo, S., Hirsch, H. J., Schutzengel, D., and Gabbay, K. H.: Ultrastructural localization of pancreatic polypeptide in human pancreas. J. Clin. Endocrinol. Metab., *44*:795, 1977.
6. Bernier, J. J., Rambaud, J. C., Cattan, D., and Prost, A.: Diarrhea associated with medullary carcinoma of the thyroid. Gut, *10*:980, 1969.
7. Bloom, S. R., and Polak, J. M.: The role of VIP in pancreatic cholera. *In* Thompson, J. C. (ed.): Gastrointestinal Hormones. pp. 635-642. Austin, University of Texas Press, 1975.
8. ——: VIP measurement in distinguishing Verner-Morrison syndrome and pseduo Verner-Morrison syndrome. Clin. Endocrinol., *5* [Suppl.]:2235, 1976.
9. Bloom, S. R., Polak, J. M., and Pearse, A. G. E.: Vasoactive intestinal peptide and watery diarrhea syndrome. Lancet, *2*:1053, 1968.
10. Brown, C. H., and Crile, G., Jr.: Pancreatic adenoma with intractable diarrhea, hypokalemia, and hypercalcemia. JAMA, *190*:30, 1963.
11. Bryant, M. G., Polak, J. M., Modlin, I., Bloom, S. R., Albuquerque, R. H., and Pearse, A. G. E.: Possible dual role for vasoactive intestinal peptide as gastrointestinal hormone and neurotransmitter substance. Lancet, *1*:991, 1976.

12. Cerda, J. J., Raffensberger, E. C., and Rawnsley, H. M.: Cholera-like syndrome and pancreatic islet cell tumors. Med. Clin. North Am., *54*:567, 1970.
13. Chears, W. C., Jr., Thompson, J. E., Hutcheson, J. B., and Patterson, C. O.: Pancreatic islet cell tumor with severe diarrhea. Am. J. Med., *29*:529, 1960.
14. Classen, M., Gail, K., Breining, H., and Demling, L.: Verner-Morrison syndrome. Dtsch. Med. Wochenschr., *97*:277, 1972.
15. Cleator, J. G. M., Thomson, C. G., Sircus, W., and Coombes, M.: Bioassay evidence of abnormal secretin-like and gastrin-like activity in tumour and blood in cases of "choleraic diarrhoea." Gut, *11*:206, 1970.
16. Cooper, H., Levitan, R., Fordtran, J. S., and Ingelfinger, F. J.: A method for studying absorption of water and solute from the human small intestine. Gastroentorology, *50*:1, 1966.
17. Coupar, I. M., and McColl, I.: Stimulation of water and sodium secretion and inhibition of glucose absorption from the rat jejunum during intra-arterial infusions of prostaglandins. Gut, *16*:759, 1975.
18. DeMuro, P., Rownski, P., Calaresu, I., and Fragui, A.: The importance of potassium in the mechanism of gastric hydrochloric acid secretion. Acta Med. Scand., *170*:403, 1961.
19. Devroede, G. J., and Phillips, S. J.: Studies of the perfusion technique for colonic absorption. Gastroenterology, *56*:92, 1969.
20. Ebeid, A. M., Murray, P., Hirsch, H., Wesdorp, R. I. C., and Fischer, J. E.: Radioimmunoassay of vasoactive intestinal peptide. J. Surg. Res., *20*:355, 1976.
21. Espiner, E. A., and Beaven, D. W.: Nonspecific islet-cell tumor of the pancreas with diarrhea. Q. J. Med., *31*:447, 1962.
22. Fausa, O., Fretheim, B., Elgjo, K., Semb, L. S., and Gjone, E.: Intractable watery diarrhoea, hypokalaemia, and achlorhydria associated with non-pancreatic retroperitoneal neurogenous tumour containing vasoactive intestinal peptide (VIP). Scan. J. Gastroenterology, *8*:713, 1973.
23. Fordtran, J. S., Rector, F. C., and Carter, N. W.: The mechanisms of sodium absorption in the human small intestine. J. Clin. Invest., *47*:884, 1968.
24. Fordtran, J. S., Rector, F. C., Locklear, T. W., and Ewton, M. F.: Water and solute movement in the small intestine of patients with sprue. J. Clin. Invest., *46*:287, 1967.
25. Franklin, R. B., and Tashjian, A. H., Jr.: Intravenous infusion of prostaglandin E_1 raises plasma calcium concentration in the rat. Endocrinology, *97*:240, 1975.
26. Gagel, R. F., Costanza, M. E., DeLellis, R. A., Norton, R. A., Bloom, S. R., Miller, H. H., Ucci, A., and Nathanson, L.: Streptozotocin-treated Verner-Morrison syndrome. Arch. Intern. Med., *136*:1429, 1976.
27. Gardner, J. D., and Cerda, J. J.: In vitro inhibition of intestinal fluid and electrolyte transfer by a non-beta islet cell tumor. Proc. Soc. Exp. Biol. Med., *123*:361, 1966.
28. Gjone, E., Fretheim, B., Nordoy, A., Jacobsen, C. D., and Elgjo, K.: Intractable watery diarrhea, hypokalemia and achlorhydria associated with pancreatic tumors containing gastric secretory inhibitory. Scand. J. Gastroenterol., *5*:401, 1970.
29. Gloor, V. F., Pletscher, A., and Hardmeier, T.: Metastasierendes. Inselzelladenom des Pancreas mit 5-Hydroxytryptamin und Insulinproduktion. Schweiz Med. Wochenschr., *94*:1476, 1964.
30. Goulon, M., Mercier, J. N., Reilly, J., and LaPorte, A.: Carcinome Langerhansien Responsable d'Hypersecretion Gastrique Acid, de Diarrhee Chronique, d'Hypokaliemie Severe avec Paralysies et d'Hypoglycemie. Sem. Hop. Paris, *36*:812, 1960.
31. Graham, D. Y., Johnson, C. D., Bentlif, P. S., and Kelsey, J. R., Jr.:

Islet cell carcinoma, pancreatic cholera, and vasoactive intestinal peptide. Ann. Intern. Med., *83*:782, 1975.

32. Gray, T. K., Bieberdorf, F. A., and Fordtran, J. S.: Thyrocalcitonin and the jejunal absorption of calcium, water and electrolytes in normal subjects. J. Clin. Invest., *52*:3084, 1973.
33. Greenlee, H. B., Longhi, E. H., Guerrero, J. D., Nelson, T. S., El-Bedri, A. L., and Dragstedt, L. R.: Inhibitory effect of pancreatic secretin on gastric secretion. Am. J. Physiol., *190*:396, 1957.
34. Gutch, C. F., and Kisner, P.: Islet cell tumor, diarrhea, and hypotassemia. Nebr. Med. J., *47*:119, 1962.
35. Haverback, B. J., and Davidson, J. D.: Serotonin and the gastrointestinal tract. Gastroenterology, *35*:570, 1958.
36. Hess, W.: Dearrhoen mit Hypokaliamie, Pradiabetes und Subacitat: Ein Neues Syndrom bei Uberfunktion des Inselapparetes. Helv. Chim. Acta, *35*:87, 1968.
37. Hill, C. S., Ibanez, M. L., Samaan, N., et al.: Medullary (solid) carcinoma of the thyroid gland: an analysis of the M. D. Anderson Hospital experience with patients with the tumor, its special features and its histogenesis. Medicine, *52*:141, 1973.
38. Hindle, B., McBrien, D. J., and Cramer, B.: Watery diarrhea and an islet cell tumor, Gut, *5*:359, 1964.
39. Hubel, K. A.: Effects of secretin and glucagon in intestinal transport of ions and water in the rat. Proc. Soc. Exp. Biol. Med., *139*:656, 1972.
40. Jacobs, W. H., Halperin, P., and Mantz, F. A.: Watery diarrhea and hypokalemia due to non-beta islet cell hyperplasia of the pancreas. Am. J. Gastroenterol., *15*:333, 1972.
41. Jaffe, B. M., and Condon, S.: Prostaglandins E and F in endocrine diarrheagenic syndromes. Ann. Surg., *184*:516, 1976.
42. Jaffe, B. M., Behrman, H. R., and Parker, C. W.: Radioimmunoassay measurement of prostaglandins E, A, and F in human plasma. J. Clin. Invest., *52*:398, 1973.
43. Kahn, C. R., Lev, A. G., Gardner, J. D., Miller, J. V., Gorden, P., and Schein, P. S.: Pancreatic cholera: beneficial effects of treatment with streptozotocin. N. Engl. J. Med., *292*:941, 1975.
44. Kaplan, E. L., Jaffe, B. M., and Peskin, G.: A new provocative test for the diagnosis of the carcinoid syndrome. Am. J. Surg., *123*:173, 1972.
45. Kisloff, B., and Moore, E. W.: Effect of serotonin on water and electrolyte transport in the in vivo rabbit small intestine. Gastroenterology, *71*: 1033, 1976.
46. Knappe, V. G., Fleming, F., Stobbe, H., and Wendt, T.: Pankreasinselzelladenom mit der Trias Diarrhoe, Hypokaliamie, und Hyperglykamie. Dtsch. Med. Wochenschr., *91*:1224, 1966.
47. Kofstad, J., Froyshov, I., Gjone, E., and Blix, S.: Pancreatic tumor with intractable watery diarrhea, hypokalemia and hypercalcemia. Electrolyte balance studies. Scand. J. Gastroenterol., *2*:246, 1967.
48. Kraft, A. R., Tompkins, R. K., and Zollinger, R. M.: Recognition and management of the diarrheal syndrome caused by non-beta islet cell tumors of the pancreas. Am. J. Surg., *119*:163, 1970.
49. Krejs, G. J., Walsh, J. H., Morawski, S. G., and Fordtran, J. S.: Intestinal perfusion studies and plasma VIP concentrations in patients with pancreatic cholera syndrome and surreptitious ingestion of laxatives and diuretics. Am. J. Dig. Dis., *22*:280, 1977.
50. Larsson, L.-I., Sundler, F., and Hakanson, R.: Immunohistochemical localization of human pancreatic polypeptide (HPP) to a population of islet cells. Cell Tiss. Res., *156*:167, 1975.
51. Larsson, L.-I., Sundler, F., and Hakanson, R.: Pancreatic polypeptide—a postulated new hormone: identification of its storage site by light and

electron microscopic immunocytochemistry. Diabetologia, *12*:211, 1976.

52. Larsson, L.-I., Schwartz, T., Lundquist, G., Chance, R. E., Sundler, F., Rehfeld, J. F., Grimelius, L., Fahrenkrug, J., Schaffalitzky de Muckadell, O., and Moon, N.: Occurrence of human pancreatic polypeptide in pancreatic endocrine tumors. Am. J. Pathol., *85*:675, 1976.
53. Leger, L., Bertola, J., and Riberi, A. M.: Hyperplasia Adenomatuse del Pancrease Endocrino y Dolores. Prensa Med. Argent., *49*:1715, 1962.
54. Lopes, V. M., Reis, D. D., and Cunha, A. B.: Islet cell adenoma of the pancreas with reversible watery diarrhea and hypokalemia. Am. J. Gastroenterol., *53*:17, 1970.
55. Makhlouf, G. M., and Said, S. I.: The effect of vasoactive intestinal peptide (VIP) on digestive and hormonal function. *In* Thompson, J. C. (ed.): Gastrointestinal hormones. pp. 599-610. Austin, University of Texas Press, 1975.
56. Marks, I. N., Bank, S., and Louw, J. H.: Islet cell tumor of the pancreas with reversible watery diarrhea and achlorhydria. Gastroenterology, *52*:695, 1967.
57. Martini, G. A., Strohmeyer, G., Haug, P., and Gusek, W.: Inselzelladenom des Pankreas mit Urtikarielleum Exanthem Durchfallen, Sowiekalium ant Eiweissverlust uber den Darm. Dtsch. Med. Wochenschr., *89*:313, 1964.
58. Matsumoto, K. K., Peter, J. B., Schultze, R. G., Hakim, A. A., and Franck, P. T.: Watery diarrhea and hypokalemia associated with pancreatic islet cell adenoma. Gastroenterology, *50*:231, 1966.
59. Matuchansky, C., and Bernier, J. J.: Effect of prostaglandin E_1 on glucose, water and electrolyte absorption in the human jejunum. Gastroenterology, *64*:1111, 1973.
60. Matuchansky, C., Mary, J.-Y., and Bernier, J.-J.: Further studies on prostaglandin E_1-induced jejunal secretion of water and electrolytes in man with special reference to the influence of ethacrynic acid, furosemide, and aspirin. Gastroenterology, *71*:274, 1976.
61. Mekhjian, H., King, D., Sanzenbacher, L., and Zollinger, R.: Glucagon (Gl) and secretin (Se) inhibit, water and electrolyte transport in the human jejunum. Gastroenterology, *62*:782, 1972.
62. Misiewicz, J. J., Waller, S. L., and Eisner, M.: Motor responses of human gastrointestinal tract to 5-hydroxytryptamine in vivo and in vitro. Gut, *7*:208, 1966.
63. Moldawer, P. M., Nardi, G. L., and Raker, J. W.: Concomitance of multiple adenomas of the parathyroids and pancreatic islets with tumor of the pituitary: a syndrome with familial incidence. Am. J. Med. Sci., *222*:190, 1954.
64. Moore, F. T., Nadler, H., Radefeld, D. A., and Zollinger, R. M.: Prolonged remission of diarrhea due to non-beta islet cell tumor of the pancreas by radiotherapy. Am. J. Surg., *115*:845, 1968.
65. Murray, J. S., Paton, R. R., and Pope, C. E. II: Pancreatic tumor associated with flushing and diarrhea. N. Engl. J. Med., *264*:436, 1961.
66. Nakano, J., and McCurdy, J. R.: Cardiovascular effects of prostaglandin E_1. J. Pharmacol. Exp. Ther., *156*:538, 1967.
67. Pabst, K., Kummerle, F., Hennekenser, H. H., and Mappes, G.: Beitrag zum Krankheitsbild des Verner-Morrison Syndroms. Dtsch. Med. Wochenschr. *94*:9, 1969.
68. Parkins, R. A.: Severe watery diarrhea and potassium depletion associated with an islet-cell tumor of the pancreas. Br. Med. J., *2*:356, 1961.
69. Pearse, A. G. E., Polak, J. M., and Bloom, S. R.: The newer gut hormones. Gastroenterology, *72*:746, 1977.
70. Polak, J. M., Pearse, A. G. E., Garaud, J.-C., and Bloom, S. R.: Cellular localization of a vasoactive intestinal pep-

tide in the mammalian and avian gastrointestinal tract. Gut, *15*:720, 1974.

71. Polak, J. M., Adrian, T. E., Bryant, M. G., Bloom, S. R., Heitz, Ph., and Pearse, A. G. E.: Pancreatic polypeptide in insulinomas, gastrinomas, VIPomas, and glucagonomas. Lancet, *1*:328, 1976.
72. Priest, W. M., and Alexander, M. K.: Islet cell tumor of the pancreas with peptic ulceration, diarrhea and hypokalemia. Lancet, *2*:1145, 1957.
73. Rambaud, J. C., and Matuchansky, C.: Diarrhoea and digestive endocrine tumors. Clin. Gastroenterol., *3*:657, 1974.
74. Rambaud, J. C., Bitoun, A., Matuchansky, C., Modigliani, R., and Bernier, J.-J.: Etude de l'Absorption Jejunale et Ileale de l'Eau et des Electrolytes dans un Cas de Syndrome de Verner-Morrison; Effet du Glucose. Biol. Gastroenterol. (Paris), *5*:627c, 1972.
75. Rambaud, J. C., Modigliani, R., Matuchansky, C., Bloom, S., Said, S., Pessayre, D., and Bernier, J.-J.: Pancreatic cholera. Gastroenterology, *69*:110, 1975.
76. Relman, A. S., and Schwartz, W. B.: The nephropathy of potassium depletion: a clinical and pathological entity. N. Engl. J. Med., *255*:195, 1956.
77. Ricour, C., Millot, M., and Balsan, S.: Sodium conservation after total or subtotal colonic resection in children. Scand. J. Gastroenterol., *8*:743, 1973.
78. Robert, A., Nezamis, J. E., and Phillips, J. P.: Inhibition of gastric secretion by prostaglandins. Am. J. Dig. Dis., *12*:1073, 1967.
79. Robertson, R. P., Gavareski, D. J., Porte, D., Jr., and Bierman, E. L.: Prostaglandin (PG) E_1: inhibition of glucose-stimulated insulin secretion in the intact dog. Clin. Res., *21*:635, 1973.
80. Said, S. I.: Vasoactive intestinal polypeptide (VIP). Current status. *In* Thompson, J. C. (ed.): Gastrointestinal Hormones, pp. 591-597. Austin, University of Texas Press, 1975.
81. Said, S. I., and Faloona, G. R.: Elevated plasma and tissue levels of vasoactive intestinal polypeptide in the watery diarrhea syndrome due to pancreatic, bronchogenic and other tumors. N. Engl. J. Med., *293*:155, 1975.
82. Said, S. I., and Mutt, V.: Isolation from porcine intestinal wall of a vasoactive octacosapeptide related to secretin and to glucagon. Eur. J. Biochem., *28*:199, 1972.
83. Said, S. I., and Rosenberg, R. N.: Vasoactive intestinal polypeptide: abundant immunoreactivity in neural cell lines and normal nervous tissue. Science, *192*:907, 1976.
84. Sandler, M., Karim, S. M. M., and Williams, E. D.: Prostaglandins in amine-peptide-secreting tumors. Lancet, *2*:1053, 1968.
85. Schmitt, M. G., Jr., Soergel, K. H., Hensley, G. T., and Chey, W. Y.: Watery diarrhea associated with pancreatic islet cell carcinoma. Gastroenterology, *69*:206, 1975.
86. Schwartz, C. J., Kimberg, D. V., Sheerin, H. E., Field, M., and Said, S. I.: Vasoactive intestinal peptide stimulation of adenylate cyclase and active electrolyte secretion in intestinal mucosa. J. Clin. Invest., *54*:536, 1974.
87. Schwartz, T. W., Stadil, F., Chance, R. E., Rehfeld, J. F., Larsson, L.-I., and Moon, N.: Pancreatic-polypeptide response to food in duodenal-ulcer patients before and after vagotomy. Lancet, *1*:1102, 1976.
88. Scudamore, H. H., McConahey, W. M., and Priestley, J. T.: Nontropical sprue and functioning islet-cell adenoma of the pancreas: report of a case. Ann. Intern. Med., *49*:909, 1958.
89. Seif, F. J., Sadowski, P., Heni, F., Fischer, R., Bloom, S. R., and Polak, J. M.: Das Vasoaktive Intestinale, Polypeptid beim Verner-Morrison Syndrome. Dtsch. Med. Wochenschr., *100*:399, 1975.
90. Shafer, W. H., McCormack, L. J., and Hoerr, S. O.: Non-beta islet cell car-

cinoma of the pancreas with flushing attacks and diarrhea. Cleve. Clin. Q., *32*:13, 1965.
91. Shield, C. F., and Haff, R. C.: The VIPoma: Further confirmation of VIP as the hormonal agent in the WDHA syndrome. Am. J. Surg., *132*:784, 1976.
92. Sircus, W., Brunt, P. W., Walker, R. J., Small, W. P., Falconer, C. W. A., and Thomson, C. G.: Two cases of pancreatic cholera with features of peptide-secreting adenomatosis of the pancreas. Gut, *11*:197, 1970.
93. Smith, R.: The Zollinger-Ellison syndrome. Ann. R. Coll. Surg., *37*:160, 1965.
94. Stoker, D. J., and Wynn, V.: Pancreatic islet cell tumor with watery diarrhea and hypokalemia. Gut, *11*:911, 1970.
95. Swift, P. G. F., Bloom, S. R., and Harris, F.: Watery diarrhea and ganglioneuroma with secretion of vasoactive intestinal peptide. Arch. Dis. Child., *50*:896, 1975.
96. Telling, M., and Smiddy, F. G.: Islet cell tumors of the pancreas with intractable diarrhoea. Gut, *2*:12, 1961.
97. Tompkins, R. K., Kraft, A. R., and Zollinger, R. M.: Secretin-like choleresis produced by a diarrheagenic non-beta islet cell tumor of the pancreas. Surgery, *66*:131, 1969.
98. Verner, J. V.: Clinical syndromes associated with non-insulin producing tumors of the pancreatic islets. *In* Demling, L., and Ottenjahn, R. (eds.): Non-Insulin Producing Tumors of the Pancreas. pp. 165-186. Stuttgart, George Thieme Verlag, 1969.
99. Verner, J. V., and Morrison, A. B.: Islet cell tumor and a syndrome of refractory watery diarrhea and hypokalemia. Am. J. Med., *25*:374, 1958.
100. ———: Non-B islet cell tumors and the syndrome of watery diarrhea, hypokalemia and hypochlorhydria. Clin. Gastroenterol., *3*:595, 1974.
101. ———: Endocrine pancreatic islet cell disease with diarrhea. Arch. Intern. Med., *133*:492, 1974.
102. Wormsley, K. G.: Response to secretin in man. Gastroenterology, *54*:197, 1968.
103. Zenker, R., Forrell, M. M., and Erpenbeck, R.: Zum Kenntnis eines Seltenen Durch ein Pankreasadenom Verursachten Krankeitsyndroms. Dtsch. Med. Wochenschr., *91*:634, 1966.
104. Zollinger, R. M., Tompkins, R. K., Amerson, J. R., Endahl, G. L., Kraft, A. R., and Moore, F. T.: Identification of the diarrheogenic hormone associated with non-beta islet-cell tumours of the pancreas. Ann. Surg., *168*:502, 1968.

EDITORIAL COMMENTARY

Even though a single polypeptide has not been incriminated conclusively as the sole mediator of the "diarrheogenic" syndrome, the specific clinical hypersecretory condition has been well documented. The findings include profuse watery diarrhea, often explosive, without steatorrhea or hyperperistalsis, resulting in hypokalemia. It is also associated with gastric achlorhydria or hypochlorhydria, hence the acronym, WDHA or WDHH syndrome of Verner and Morrison. The ensuing dehydration is often accompanied by acidosis and azotemia and there may also be flushing, hypercalcemia, hyperglycemia and tetany, the latter being due to loss of magnesium. The syndrome has been called, "pancreatic cholera," by Matsumoto and Sircus when the source of the humoral elaboration is the pancreatic islets, and because of the clinical similarity to cholera. The pathologic findings in the pancreas include benign and malignant non-beta islet cell tumors and hyperplasia, including nesidioblastosis; approximately 10 percent of the secreting tumors are in extrapancreatic sites, particularly retroperitoneal ganglioneuromas of the sympathetic neural tissue, adrenal medulla and rarely, bronchogenic carcinomas, all embryonic sites of APUD cells.

The humoral products involved in the watery diarrhea syndrome have a secretinlike action, except that pancreatic exocrine function is usually normal. The leading hormonal candidate is vasoactive intestinal peptide (VIP) which has been identified in both pancreatic and nerve tumors and which has additionally been found normally in the hypothalamus, intestine and placenta. In addition to its dual function of being a hormone and a neurotransmitter, VIP also has a stimulatory effect on mucosal cyclic AMP metabolism at its target cell, similar to that of cholera enterotoxin and prostaglandin. Pancreatic polypeptide (PP) secreted from cells dispersed throughout the pancreas has also been found in approximately half of the pancreatic tumors of this syndrome (and in other syndromes) but not from neural diarrheogenic tumors. Pancreatic polypeptide has been found to be elevated in the plasma of pancreatic cholera patients and also in patients after infusion of some gastrointestinal hormones; for these reasons it is reasonable to assume at this time that PP is a marker of pancreatic islet cell tumor activity. The finding of elevated prostaglandin E (PGE_2) elaboration in patients with the WDHH syndrome due to pancreatic tumors and subsequent decrease, together with cessation of the diarrhea, after treatment with a potent inhibitor of prostaglandin synthesis (indomethacin), substantiates its role in the syndrome. The cause of the inhibition of gastric secretion is not known, but several polypeptides have been suggested. Hypochlorhydria has been shown to be present in patients whose tumors elaborate VIP; it is reasonable to assume that histamine-fast achlorhydria may be due to GIP or to another secretinlike hormone or secretin itself. PGE_2 is a potent inhibitor of acid secretion.

The fact that parietal cells are present in the hyposecreting stomach suggests that the parietal cell receptors are either blocked or inhibited by the diarrheogenic hormone. Moreover, it has been reported that after treatment by surgical excision of the tumor or by the administration of steroids, there is a gastric hypersecretory rebound phenomenon. The overall favorable responsiveness of patients to glucocorticoids can be a positive diagnostic feature of this syndrome in approximately half of the patients.

The recent important contributions relating to the mechanisms of action in the diarrheogenic syndrome clearly show that the major biologic effects of the hormones take place in the small intestinal mucosa (midgut). Physiologic studies of jejunal and ileal mucosal secretion demonstrate a hypersecretory loss of water and electrolytes into the lumen, not found in the gastroduodenal-pancreatic or colonic areas. The stomach, of course, participates to the extent that there is gastric hyposecretion. The normal absorptive capacity of the colon is overwhelmed by the large volume reaching it and may participate to the extent that an aldosteronelike effect is present in which potassium is exchanged for sodium in the colon, which results in further losses of potassium.

The treatment of the diarrheogenic syndrome, as outlined in this chapter, is straightforward. Surgical exploration for confirmation of the diagnosis and the identification of the underlying pathologic process is usually necessary. Since approximately half of the patients have an islet cell adenoma, its excision is indicated. When hyperplasia is present as confirmed by an experienced pathologist, a distal subtotal pancreatectomy usually suffices, but may on occasion require total pancreatectomy. When metastatic malignancy is found, excision of the primary lesion plus selective intra-arterial chemotherapy with streptozotocin, an islet cell cytotoxic agent, and/or indomethacin by mouth, in patients with hyperprostaglandinemia, to inhibit prostaglandin synthesis, have been beneficial.

Available information relating to the pathogenesis of diarrheogenic syndrome suggests that several humoral products may be involved, a finding which is consistent with the APUD concept. *S.R.F.*

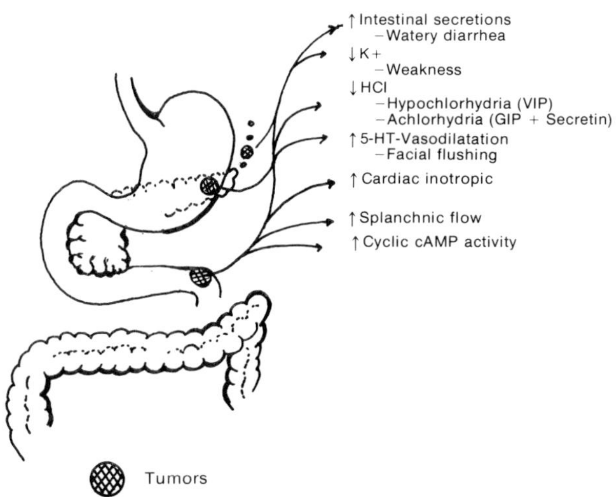

Fig. 15-1. Pathophysiology of the diarrheogenic (WDHA) syndrome (VIP-secreting tumor, or GIP, or secretin).

(See overleaf for flowchart)

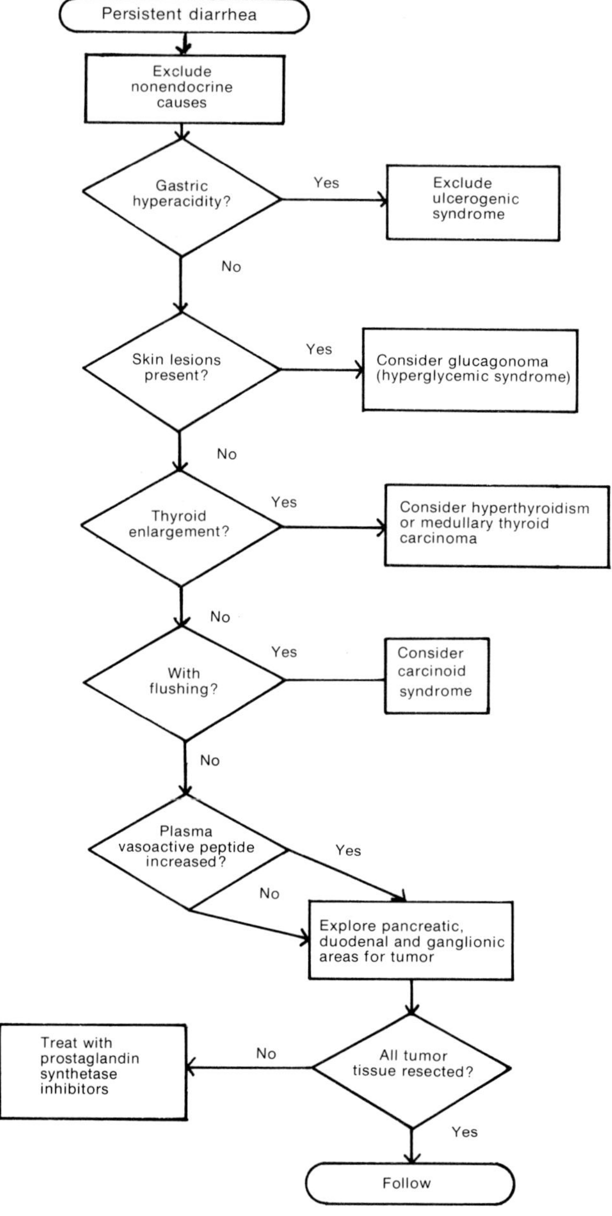

Fig. 15-2. Management flowchart of the diarrheogenic syndrome.

16

The Hypercalcemic Syndrome: Hyperparathyroidism

Orlo H. Clark, M.D., and Lawrence W. Way, M.D.

Hyperparathyroidism, once thought to be a rare disease, is now known to occur in about one of every 1,000 hospitalized patients, making it one of the most common endocrinopathies.[13] Hyperparathyroidism is unusual in children, more common in women than in men, with the peak incidence occurring between the third and fifth decades of life.[73]

Between 1926 and 1932, hyperparathyroidism was only recognized in patients who presented with osteitis fibrosa cystica.[1] In 1932, Albright noted that 80 percent of patients with osteitis fibrosa cystica had renal stones, and for the next 30 years nephrolithiasis was the principal clue to the presence of hyperparathyroidism.[28] During this period, Rogers and Keating noted an association of peptic ulcer disease with hyperparathyroidism,[90] and Cope reported an association with pancreatitis.[29] Today most patients with hyperparathyroidism are diagnosed when hypercalcemia is detected by routine screening tests.[48] When questioned carefully most of these patients relate subtle symptoms of hypercalcemia, but some of them are completely asymptomatic.

The diagnosis of hyperparathyroidism may be comparatively easy or exceedingly complex. In some cases parathyroidectomy can be performed successfully by a surgeon with no specialized training or experience other than familiarity with thyroid operations; in other cases, the operation can be tedious and frustrating, even for one who performs parathyroidectomy regularly. It is axiomatic that the surgeon be *convinced* preoperatively that the diagnosis of hyperparathyroidism is correct. Otherwise, if the initial search fails to reveal a lesion the surgeon may be tempted to conclude the exploration prematurely.

The surgeon who cares for patients with primary hyperparathyroidism must be familiar with (a) the physiology of calcium metabolism, (b) the clinical manifestations of hyperparathyroidism and associated conditions, (c) the differential diagnosis of hypercalcemia, (d) the diagnostic approach to hypercalcemia and the normocalcemic patient suspected of having hyperparathyroidism, (e) the medical and surgical treatment for hypercalcemia and hyperparathyroidism, (f) the rationale of the various operative strategies, and (g) the management of patients after parathyroidectomy.

ETIOLOGY

Primary Hyperparathyroidism

The etiology of primary hyperparathyroidism is not known with certainty, but most experts interpret the evidence to indicate that in about 90 percent of cases the disease results from neoplastic transformation of one, or occasionally more than one, parathyroid gland.[5] When hyperparathyroidism occurs in association with multiple endocrine adenomatosis, Type I (MEA-I; Wermer's syndrome), or multiple endocrine adenomatosis, Type II (MEA-II; Sipple's syndrome), the multiple neoplasms are thought to arise by a genetically determined process from a common stem cell originating from the neurocrest.[79]

In addition to causing secondary hyperparathyroidism, chronic, excessive stimulation of the parathyroid glands may be the cause of some cases of primary hyperparathyroidism. Clinical and laboratory data supporting this theory are:

1. Prolonged phosphate-rich, calcium-poor diets produce hyperparathyroidism in animals, occasionally with marked enlargement of the parathyroid glands.[59]
2. Chronic administration of glucagon lowers the serum calcium and may produce hyperparathyroidism.[76]
3. Hyperparathyroidism is common in postmenopausal women, a time of metabolic change and osteoporosis.[73]
4. In dogs, chronic administration of thiazide diuretics produces hypercalcemia, hypophosphatemia, and histologic evidence of increased parathyroid activity.[80]
5. Autonomous parathyroid hyperfunction indistinguishable from primary hyperparathyroidism eventually develops in some patients with secondary hyperparathyroidism.[34]

Nevertheless, because removal of a single adenoma cures most patients, chronic stimulation of the glands must be a relatively uncommon cause of primary hyperparathyroidism.[25]

The frequent coexistence of hyperparathyroidism with other conditions that cause hypercalcemia, such as thyrotoxicosis, sarcoidosis, Paget's disease, carcinoma, and the milk-alkali syndrome may be of etiologic as well as diagnostic importance.[84] For unknown reasons hyperparathyroidism also seems to be more common in patients with differentiated thyroid carcinomas.[64]

Secondary and Tertiary Hyperparathyroidism

Secondary hyperparathyroidism denotes chronically increased secretion of parathyroid hormone (PTH) in response to low plasma concentrations of ionized calcium. If the stimulation of PTH secretion is prolonged, as may occur in renal disease or intestinal malabsorption, chief cell hyperplasia may appear. In secondary hyperparathyroidism due to renal failure, the serum phosphorus is usually high; when secondary hyperparathyroidism is due to malabsorption, osteomalacia, or rickets, the phosphorous is usually low or normal.

Secondary hyperparathyroidism with renal osteodystrophy, a common sequela of hemodialysis, is primarily the result of phosphate retention caused by decreased renal function.[14] Other contributing factors in this condition are (a) deficient renal hydroxylation of 25-hydroxyvitamin D to the biologically active metabolite (1,25-dihydroxyvitamin D) causing impaired intestinal absorption of calcium,[72] (b) resistance of bone to the action of parathyroid hormone,[72] (c) depletion of total body magnesium,[63] and (d) defective catabolism of PTH and other effects that produce elevated serum PTH levels.[87]

Secondary hyperparathyroidism may evolve into autonomous parathyroid hyperfunction, in which case the condition is termed tertiary hyperparathyroidism.[20] For example, in some patients what was originally secondary hyperparathyroidism persists after renal transplantation has restored renal function to normal. However, in most cases of secondary hyperparathyroidism associated with renal failure, the serum calcium concentration returns to normal within 6 months after transplantation.[32]

MINERAL AND SKELETAL HOMEOSTASIS

The action of parathyroid hormone (PTH), vitamin D and its derivatives, calcitonin, and calcium and phosphate ions in extracellular fluid are metabolically interrelated. **Parathyroid hormone** is secreted in response to a fall in the serum level of ionized calcium. The major target organs for PTH action are the kidneys, the skeletal system, and to a lesser degree, the intestines. The actions of PTH are listed below.

PTH is secreted as an intact 84-amino acid polypeptide, which immediately undergoes degradation into N- and C-terminal fragments. Using specific radioimmunoassays for the N- and C-terminal fragments, it has been demonstrated that the N-terminal fragment has biologic activity,[18] but that the C-terminal fragment has none.[4]

In man **vitamin D** is converted in the liver to 25-hydroxycholecalciferol, which is hydroxylated by the kidney to 1,25-dihydroxycholecalciferol.[45] These are the biologically active derivatives of vitamin D, which increase calcium and phosphate retention and control mineralization of bone. The overall physiologic effect of vitamin D is to elevate plasma calcium and phosphate and enhance mineralization of bone. PTH is essential for the conversion of 25-hydroxycholecalciferol to 1,25-hydroxycholecalciferol.[47] Low levels of phosphate enhance the conversion and high levels inhibit it.[100] When 1,25-dihydroxycholecalciferol becomes available for clinical use, it should be able to prevent osteitis fibrosa in patients with chronic renal failure.

Calcitonin, a hormone secreted by the specialized C cells or parafollicular cells of the thyroid, acts in concert with PTH to modulate ionized calcium levels in plasma.[68] Calcitonin inhibits bone resorption, an action apparently independent of PTH.[46] Hypercalcemia increases the secretion of calcitonin and reduces the secretion of parathyroid hormone; hypocalcemia has opposite ef-

Direct Actions of Parathyroid Hormone

1. Increases plasma calcium concentration
2. Decreases plasma phosphate concentration
3. Increases tubular excretion of phosphate
4. Increases tubular resorption of calcium
5. Increases bone remodeling by increasing the number and activity of osteoclasts and osteoblasts
6. Increases bicarbonate excretion by the kidney
7. Increases the rate of conversion of 25-hydroxyvitamin D_3 to 1,25-hydroxyvitamin D_3 in the kidney
8. Activates adenylate cyclase in cells of target tissues
9. Increases gastrointestinal absorption of calcium by enhancing vitamin D synthesis

fects. Other hormones involved in regulating mineral homeostasis and skeletal remodeling are thyroxine, growth hormone, adrenal corticosteroids and estrogens.

CLINICAL MANIFESTATIONS

Most of the clinical manifestations of hyperparathyroidism are caused by hypercalcemia, but several symptoms, including those of neuromuscular dysfunction, appear to be due to other factors. The symptoms of hyperparathyroidism (see below) principally involve the renal, musculoskeletal, gastrointestinal, nervous and cardiovascular systems.

General
Polydipsia and weight loss
Renal
Colic, hematuria, back pain, polyuria
Musculoskeletal
Aches and pains, bone pains, arthritis, pathologic fractures
Gastrointestinal
Anorexia, nausea, emesis, constipation, dyspepsia, epigastric pain, upper abdominal pain radiating through to back
Neurologic
Depression, lethargy, weakness, confusion, neurosis, psychosis, insomnia, headache, apathy
Cardiovascular
Hypertension, heart block

The initial clinical manifestations that led to the diagnosis of hyperparathyroidism at the University of California, San Francisco are listed in Table 16-1.

Patients with hyperparathyroidism may develop nephrolithiasis, nephrocalcinosis, hypertension, peptic ulcer disease, pancreatitis, gout, or pseudogout. The pathogenesis of these conditions in hyperparathyroidism has not been entirely clarified. Other conditions that cause hypercalcemia, include Paget's disease, sarcoidosis, carcinoma, hyperthyroidism, and milk-alkali syndrome, and may coexist with hyperparathyroidism.

Hyperparathyroidism is also part of MEA-I[8] and MEA-II.[98] MEA-I is characterized by tumors of the parathyroid, pituitary, pancreas, adrenal cortex, and less commonly, the thyroid or ovaries. MEA-II consists of hyperparathyroidism, medullary carcinoma of the thyroid, multiple neurofibromas, gut ganglioneuromatosis and pheochromocytoma.[19]

DIAGNOSIS AND MANAGEMENT OF THE PATIENT WITH SUSPECTED HYPERPARATHYROIDISM

The approach to a patient suspected of having hyperparathyroidism varies depending upon the serum calcium concentration and the clinical manifestations of the disorder. For example, a normocalcemic ($Ca^{++} < 10.5$ mg./dl.) patient with hypercalciuria and renal colic requires a different evaluation from a patient with persistent hypercalcemia. Furthermore, the management of pa-

Table 16-1. Initial Manifestations of Hyperparathyroidism

	Percent of Patients
Hypercalcemia on screening test (routine physical exam)	40 (8)*
Renal stones	28
Symptoms of hypercalcemia (weakness, constipation, lethargy, polyuria, polydipsia)	7
Peptic ulcer disease	5
Hypertension	4
Bone disease	4
Diabetes mellitus	3
MEA-I	3
Thyroid disease	3
Pancreatitis	2
Lump in neck	1

*Eight percent of the patients were completely asymptomatic.

tients with moderate hypercalcemia differs from that of patients with severe hypercalcemia (Ca^{++}>14.5 mg./dl.).

When evaluating moderate hypercalcemia (Ca^{++} 10.5-14.5 mg./dl.) one must consider all possible causes, including artifacts (e.g., laboratory error or a tight tourniquet) and the various clinical conditions (Table 16-2). Although its prevalence seems to be increasing, hyperparathyroidism is not the most common cause of hypercalcemia.[48] In some patients the reason for the hypercalcemia is obvious, whereas in others the diagnosis may be exceedingly difficult.

Table 16-2. Causes of Hypercalcemia

Condition	*Approximate Frequency (%)*
Malignancy	35
Breast cancer	
Metastatic tumor	
PTH secreting tumor (lung, kidney, others)	
Multiple myeloma	
Acute and chronic leukemia	
Hyperparathyroidism	28
Artifact (e.g., laboratory error, dirty glassware, cork stopper, tight tourniquet)	10
Vitamin D overdose	8
Thiazide diuretics	4
Hyperthyroidism	3
Milk-alkali syndrome	3
Sarcoidosis	3
Miscellaneous	6
Immobilization	
Paget's disease	
Addison's disease	
Idiopathic hypercalcemia of infancy	
Dysproteinemias	
Vitamin A overdose	
Myxedema	
WDHA syndrome	

To diagnose hyperparathyroidism one should exclude all other causes of hypercalcemia. The history should document the duration of any symptoms possibly related to hyperparathyroidism or the conditions associated with this disease; excessive use of milk products, antacids, or baking soda; symptoms of malignant disease, such as bone pain, cough, or hemoptysis; or palpitations and nervousness suggestive of hyperthyroidism. A long history of nephrolithiasis or peptic ulcer disease suggests that hyperparathyroidism is the most likely diagnosis, whereas an acute progressive illness with weight loss suggests malignancy. A careful review of the patient's laboratory data from previous hospitalizations frequently reveals that hypercalcemia has been present for several years, suggesting hyperparathyroidism.

Laboratory Evaluation of Hypercalcemia

With few exceptions, every patient with hypercalcemia should receive the entire battery of tests listed below before one attempts to make a final diagnosis. If the diagnosis is still unclear at this point, special tests described in the text may be indicated.

Blood Tests	Creatinine and BUN
Calcium	pH
Phosphorus	Uric acid
Chloride	
Protein; albumin/globulin	X-rays
Parathyroid hormone	Chest film
Alkaline phosphatase	Abdominal plain films

Certain other tests also will be helpful in some cases such as serum magnesium, erythrocyte sedimentation rate (ESR), urinary calcium, tubular resorption of phosphate (TRP), serum and urinary protein electrophoresis, intravenous pyelogram as well as roentgenograms of the hands and skull.

Blood Tests. Hypercalcemia, the keystone to diagnosis of hyperparathyroidism, is found in most patients. In our hospital normal total calcium levels range from 8.5 to 10.5 mg./dl.; the normal range may differ slightly between laboratories. The normal concentration of plasma calcium is lower in women than in men; in women the calcium concentration rises after 30 years of age in spite of a fall in serum albumin, whereas in men the calcium concentration decreases with age.[56] Approximately 75 percent of patients with hypercalcemia and primary hyperparathyroidism have hypercalciuria (urinary calcium excretion greater than 300 mg. per day in men and 250 mg. per day in women) although urinary calcium levels may be normal or even decreased.[78,84]

Serum **parathyroid hormone** (PTH) levels are usually increased in patients with primary and ectopic hyperparathyroidism and are low or absent in other conditions causing hypercalcemia. Serum PTH levels also rise in normal subjects in response to hypocalcemia and in patients with excessive gastrointestinal or renal calcium losses; therefore, an elevated PTH level in the presence of a normal or low serum calcium does not usually indicate primary hyperparathyroidism.

In patients with parathyroid adenomas the magnitude of the increase in serum PTH and calcium usually corresponds directly with the size of the adenoma[71];

thus, patients with intermittent or minimal hypercalcemia often have normal or only slightly increased PTH levels and small adenomas. The diagnosis of primary hyperparathyroidism may be difficult in such patients. Occasionally, PTH levels are either low or undetectable even though the patient is subsequently proven to have primary hyperparathyroidism. The assumption in such cases is that the circulating form of PTH would not react with the PTH antibodies used in the PTH assay.

PTH radioimmunoassays have been developed that are specific for the N- or the C-terminal fragments of the hormone. Because the N-terminal fragment is cleared from blood more rapidly than the C-terminal fragment, assays for the N-terminal fragment are more valuable when attempting to localize an adenoma by selective venous catheterization. Assays measuring the concentration of the C-terminal fragment in peripheral serum are more sensitive to screen for hyperparathyroidism.

Patients with ectopic or pseudohyperparathyroidism due to malignant nonparathyroid tumors often have increased PTH levels.[89] The increase in PTH is usually lower than would be expected for the magnitude of the increase in serum calcium because the tumor secretes fragments of PTH that incompletely cross-react with antibodies developed against the normal N- and C-terminal fragments. To overcome the diagnostic confusion in this situation, specific antibodies have been produced against the PTH variants secreted by nonparathyroid tumors.[10]

Analysis of parathyroid hormone levels obtained during highly selective venous catheterization is useful in localizing the abnormal parathyroid gland(s) in patients who have previously had unsuccessful operations. The technique of highly selective venous catheterization consists of (a) percutaneous passage of a catheter from the right femoral vein into the internal jugular veins, (b) selective cannulation of the thyroid and other cervical and mediastinal veins, (c) injection of small amounts of water-soluble contrast media to confirm the position of the catheter tip; and (d) collection of 5-ml. samples of blood at different positions in the venous network of the anterior neck. Veins carrying blood with especially high PTH concentrations compared with the others most likely drain hyperfunctioning parathyroid tissue. Selective venous catheterization is not necessary in patients undergoing an initial exploration because an experienced surgeon can identify the adenoma(s) by visual inspection alone in 95 percent of patients. Highly selective venous catheterization is not useful in the diagnosis of hyperparathyroidism because increased PTH levels are occasionally present in thyroid veins in subjects without hyperparathyroidism.[96]

Parathyroid hormone decreases renal tubular resorption of phosphate (TRP), which produces the **hypophosphatemia** (phosphate<2.5 mg./dl.) found in about 50 percent of patients with hyperparathyroidism. Thus, 81 percent of hyperparathyroid patients on a regular diet without renal failure have a low TRP (less than 78%); the TRP is low in only 6 percent of normal subjects.[48]

$$\text{TRP (in \%)} = 100 \times 1 = \frac{\text{urinary phosphate} \times \text{serum creatinine}}{\text{urinary creatinine} \times \text{serum phosphate}}$$

Unfortunately a low TRP is occasionally seen in all other conditions that cause hypercalcemia.[40]

When hypophosphatemia is found in a patient with hypercalcemia, hyperparathyroidism is by far the most likely diagnosis. Patients with vitamin D intoxication, sarcoidosis, malignant disease without metastases, and hyperthyroidism only rarely have hypophosphatemia. In patients with breast cancer or other malignant tumors with skeletal metastasis, the serum phosphate is normal or elevated. If hypophosphatemia and hypercalcemia occur in a patient with breast cancer, concomitant parathyroid hyperfunction is the most likely explanation because breast cancers rarely secrete PTH.[40,102] Measurement of serum PTH is valuable in this situation, since the PTH is low or undetectable with hypercalcemia due to all causes other than hyperparathyroidism.

In the presence of hypercalcemia an elevated serum **chloride** concentration suggests hyperparathyroidism. PTH decreases the resorption of bicarbonate from the proximal renal tubule, leading to increased resorption of chloride and mild hyperchloremic renal tubular acidosis; in other causes of hypercalcemia the serum chloride is normal. In the absence of vomiting or renal insufficiency, serum chloride levels in hyperparathyroidism are usually above 102 mEq./L., and in 40 percent of patients they exceed 107 mEq./L.[107] The ratio of **chloride to phosphate** suggests hyperparathyroidism if it exceeds 33 in a patient with hypercalcemia.[86]

Serum protein concentrations should be measured because about 0.8 mg. of calcium is bound by 1 g. of protein and the definition of hypercalcemia must be adjusted accordingly in patients with low or high levels of serum proteins.[85] Protein electrophoresis should be performed to search for hyperglobulinemia, which is rare in hyperparathyroidism but common in mulitple myeloma and sarcoidosis.[39]

Serum **alkaline phosphatase** levels are elevated in about 20 percent of patients with primary hyperparathyroidism. The alkaline phosphatase may also be increased in Paget's disease and malignant disease. A 5′-nucleotidase or leucine aminopeptidase level (enzymes produced by the liver but not by bone) should be obtained if the alkaline phosphatase is elevated. If these tests are normal, the high alkaline phosphatase usually reflects increased bone turnover due to hyperparathyroidism.

The **hydrocortisone suppression test** (150 mg. of hydrocortisone per day for 10 days) reduces the serum calcium concentration to normal in sarcoidosis and vitamin D intoxication, [37] but only rarely in hyperparathyroidism.[48,84] The effect of cortisone on the hypercalcemia of multiple myelomatosis, carcinoma and milk-alkali syndrome is variable.[67,101] Hydrocortisone suppression is especially helpful if PTH levels cannot be obtained or if the results of the assay are equivocal.

Patients with hyperparathyroidism often are mildly acidotic and hyperuricemic. Anemia and an increased erythrocyte sedimentation rate are uncommon.[48,84] If there is a history of peptic ulcer disease and diarrhea or a family history of MEA-I, skull films and a serum gastrin level should be obtained. If there is a history of marked hypertension or a family history of MEA-II, a serum calcitonin level and urinary VMA and urinary metanephrine should be determined before parathyroid operation. Other tests indicated rarely include bone biopsy, bone densitometry, I^{125} photon absorption, urinary hydroxyproline determinations, calcium infusion tests and radioactive calcium turnover studies.

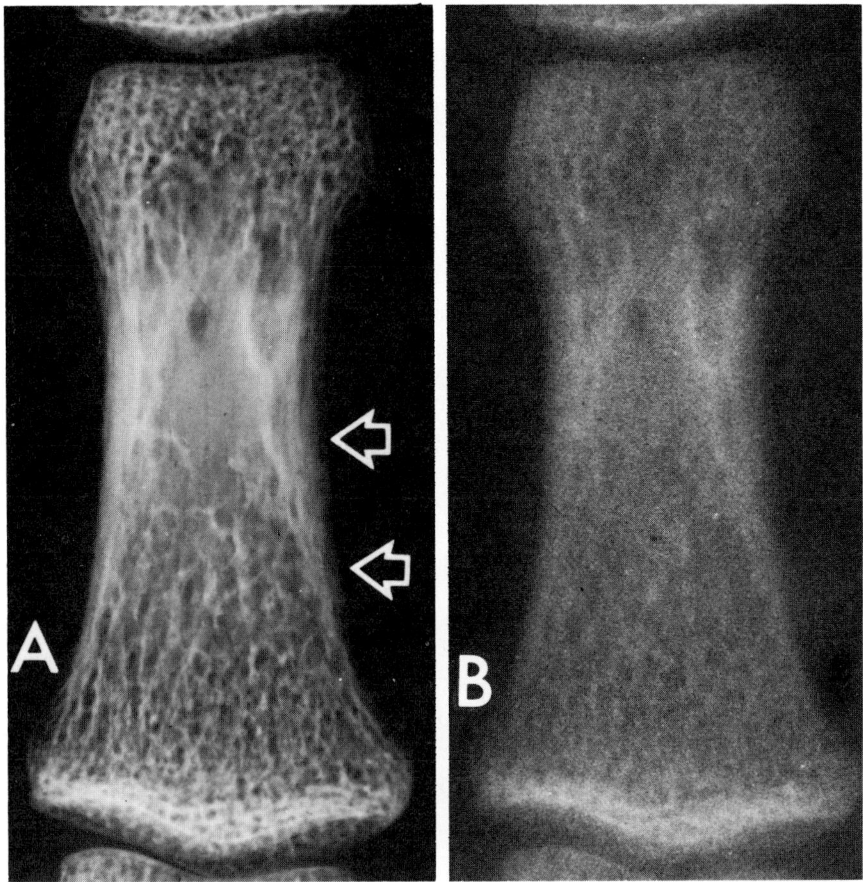

Fig. 16-1. The middle phalanx of a patient with primary hyperparathyroidism. *(A)* Diagnostic subperiosteal bone resorption *(arrows)* and intracortical tunneling can be seen along the radial aspect on the fine grain industrial film. *(B)* Findings are much less obvious on conventional film. (Roentgenographs optically magnified X 5) (Courtesy H. K. Genant)

Roentgenographic Findings

A chest roentgenogram is valuable in eliminating carcinoma of the lung as a cause of the hypercalcemia. Abdominal films revealing nephrolithiasis or nephrocalcinosis suggest chronic hypercalcemia and probable hyperparathyroidism. *Roentgenographic examination* of bone aids in the diagnosis of hyperparathyroidism, but overt skeletal changes are found in only 10 percent of patients nowadays. Roentgenographic evidence of bone changes is rare in hyperparathyroidism unless the serum alkaline phosphatase concentration is increased. The roentgenographic findings pathognomonic of hyperparathyroidism (both primary and secondary) are subperiosteal resorption of the phalanges, resorption of the distal clavicles, and bone cysts (Fig. 16-1). A ground-glass appearance of the skull with loss of definition of the tables and demineralization of the outer aspects of the clavicles are less frequent findings.

Paget's disease or malignant disease should be suspected in patients with markedly elevated serum alkaline phosphatase levels without subperiosteal resorption of bone on roentgenograms.

Differential Diagnosis

Malignancy. Hypercalcemia is a frequent complication of nonparathyroid malignant disease and most often is caused by demineralization of bone from metastases.[49] In some cases, it is due to secretion by the tumor of a PTH-like substance. Other substances such as prostaglandin E_2, metabolites of vitamin D, and various unidentified humoral factors have been implicated occasionally.[81] About 25 percent of patients with breast cancer,[35] 10 percent of patients with lung cancer,[9] and 15 percent of patients with renal cell carcinoma have hypercalcemia at some point during their disease.[104]

Findings that suggest malignancy as the cause of hypercalcemia are an illness of short duration, bone pain and tenderness; a mass lesion; an abnormality on chest x-ray or IVP; anemia; increased sedimentation rate; serum chloride levels below 102 mEq./L.; hematuria; proteinuria; an elevated alkaline phosphatase level without x-ray evidence of subperiosteal bone resorption; or a decrease in hypercalcemia following steroid treatment.[61] Hypercalcemic patients with skeletal metastases usually have high or normal serum phosphate levels.

Since parathyroid tumors may occur in patients with malignant neoplasms, it is important to note the response of serum calcium levels to removal (or other treatment) of the nonparathyroid tumor. Highly selective venous catheterization and PTH radioimmunoassay are also valuable in determining the source of the increased PTH levels in selected patients with malignancy and suspected hyperparathyroidism.[93]

Milk-Alkali Syndrome. This may complicate prolonged ingestion of large amounts of milk, calcium and absorbable antacids.[17] The usual clinical manifestations include thirst, polyuria, weakness, dyspepsia, pruritus and corneal calcification.

Laboratory tests usually reveal hypercalcemia, normal or elevated serum phosphate, mild renal failure, alkalosis, **absence of hypercalciuria** and low serum PTH levels. Renal calculi and nephrocalcinosis occasionally occur.[69] The clinical picture can mimic hyperparathyroidism, and milk-alkali syndrome may coexist with hyperparathyroidism. If calcium-containing products are discontinued the hypercalcemia will resolve, although this may take several months.

Thiazide-induced Hypercalcemia. The administration of thiazide diuretics to normal subjects produces little change or a transient increase of less than 1 mg./dl. in serum calcium levels.[41] In patients with primary hyperparathyroidism or idiopathic juvenile osteoporosis the increase may be greater.[77] Since thiazides are sometimes used to treat hypertension and to decrease renal excretion of calcium in idiopathic hypercalciuria, multiple myeloma, and Paget's disease, coexisting hyperparathyroidism may be difficult to identify if hypercalcemia develops in these patients.

If hypercalcemia appears in patients receiving thiazide diuretics, the thiazides should be discontinued. If hypercalcemia persists after several weeks another cause of hypercalcemia should be suspected. Since in humans PTH secretion is not affected by thiazides, an elevated PTH level suggests hyperparathyroidism.

Vitamin D Intoxication. Chronic excessive ingestion of vitamin D may produce hypercalcemia by increasing bone resorption and gastrointestinal absorption of calcium. The diagnosis is usually suspected because of a history of excessive vitamin D intake. The serum phosphorus level is often increased, but it may be normal or decreased. The hypercalcemia may persist for weeks to months after discontinuing vitamin D, because vitamin D is stored in the liver and released slowly.[58]

Administration of hydrocortisone is the best way of diagnosing and treating vitamin D intoxication, since serum calcium levels fall in patients with vitamin D intoxication but remain elevated in hyperparathyroid patients. Specific radioimmunoassays for vitamin D are being developed and should help to confirm the diagnosis.

Sarcoidosis. Hypercalcemia occurs in about 20 percent of patients with sarcoidosis.[70] The cause appears to be excessive absorption of calcium from the intestines (low fecal calcium levels). Differentiation from hyperparathyroidism may be very difficult. Patients with sarcoidosis may have polyuria, nephrocalcinosis, nephrolithiasis, band keratopathy and bone cysts.[84,95] Although the serum phosphorus level is usually normal or increased, it may be low; the alkaline phosphatase may be normal or increased; and sarcoidosis and hyperparathyroidism may coexist. Serum PTH levels are low[31] and hypercalcemia disappears within 1 week of treatment with cortisone. The presence of an increased gamma-globulin level, a chest x-ray revealing a diffuse fibronodular infiltrate and prominent hilar adenopathy suggest sarcoidosis. The finding of noncaseating granulomas in a lymph node or liver biopsy specimen is diagnostic.

Multiple Myeloma. About 40 percent of patients with multiple myeloma have hypercalcemia, apparently because of direct erosion of bone by the neoplasm.[11] Patients with this condition usually have bone pain, especially in the lumbar region. Typical "punched out" lesions are seen in affected bones on x-ray. Serum phosphate levels are usually normal or high, but occasionally they may be low. There may be hyperchloremia and hypercalciuria. The diagnosis of myeloma is suggested by the presence of markedly elevated serum and urine globulin levels. Confirmation results from demonstrating myeloma cells on bone marrow examination. The administration of corticosteroids lowers serum calcium in this condition by directly suppressing the tumor, thus reducing the increased turnover of bone. With steroid treatment the morphology of the marrow improves, hemoglobin levels rise, and the excretion of abnormal urinary and serum proteins falls.[11]

Hyperthyroidism. The total serum calcium concentration is elevated in 25 percent and the ionized serum calcium is elevated in about 50 percent of patients with hyperthyroidism.[16] The diagnosis usually is not difficult because symptoms of thyrotoxicosis rather than hyperparathyroidism bring the patient to the physician. However, some patients may have apathetic hyperthyroidism and others may have concomitant hyperparathyroidism. In hyperthyroid patients, hypercalcemia is produced by increased bone resorption; intestinal calcium absorption is usually low or normal, and urinary calcium is increased.[97] The heightened bone resorption may lead to hypercalciuria, hyperphosphatemia and occasionally to spontaneous fractures.

To differentiate between these two conditions one may treat the hyperthyroidism to see whether the serum calcium returns to normal; measure serum PTH levels, which are low in hyperthyroidism without associated hyperparathyroidism;[16] or determine fecal calcium excretion, which is low or normal in hyperparathyroidism and high or normal in hyperthyroidism.

Other miscellaneous causes of hypercalcemia are Paget's disease, immobilization (especially in Paget's disease, or in young patients), adrenal insufficiency, myxedema, dysproteinemias, idiopathic hypercalcemia of infancy, vitamin A intoxication, and the WDHA syndrome (intractable watery diarrhea, hypokalemia, and achlorhydria) associated with non-beta islet cell tumors of the pancreas.

ASYMPTOMATIC HYPERPARATHYROIDISM

Careful questioning of patients with hyperparathyroidism detected by screening tests reveals that many of them are not entirely asymptomatic. Purnell, Keating, and coworkers[82] at the Mayo Clinic prospectively studied 147 patients with uncomplicated or "asymptomatic hyperparathyroidism" to determine the natural history of this condition. Patients included in this prospective study had a calcium less than 11.0 mg./dl., an increased PTH level, no radiographic evidence of bone disease, normal renal function (glomerular filtration rate more than 80 ml./min.), no recent kidney stone formation and no peptic ulcer disease. No mention was made of whether these patients had hypertension, gout, polydipsia, polyuria, constipation, fatigue and psychiatric or neuromuscular problems. We think that it is more appropriate to refer to these patients as having uncomplicated hyperparathyroidism rather than asymptomatic hyperparathyroidism because the manifestations listed above usually improve after parathyroidectomy.[6]

Of the untreated patients followed by Purnell and coworkers,[83] within 5 years 20 percent developed specific indications for operation, 4 percent died and 18 percent failed to return for follow-up interviews. Unfortunately, no criteria could be identified that indicated which patients would develop renal disease, bone disease, or life-threatening hypercalcemia.

Asymptomatic patients with primary hyperparathyroidism were found by Kaplan and coworkers[55] to benefit from parathyroidectomy by improved renal function and increased bone density.

NORMOCALCEMIC HYPERCALCIURIA

Differential Diagnosis and Management

The incidence of normocalcemic hyperparathyroidism in patients with hypercalciuria and recurrent nephrolithiasis (idiopathic hypercalciuria) is not known. Patients with primary hyperparathyroidism would obviously benefit from parathyroidectomy, whereas patients with idiopathic hypercalciuria due either to hyperabsorption of calcium from the intestine (absorptive hypercalciuria)—low PTH—or to primary renal tubular calcium leak (renal hypercalciuria)—high PTH—would not. All patients thought to have normocalcemic hypercalciuria should be evaluated by obtaining at least three blood samples for calcium determinations, since hypercalcemia may be intermittent.[53] The test should be run the day the blood is drawn because the calcium level may fall with refrigeration or freezing.[26] If the proper equipment is available, the serum ionized calcium level should be measured because it may be increased in some patients with a normal total serum calcium level.[65]

When the ionized calcium and PTH levels are elevated, but the total calcium concentration is normal, normocalcemic hyperparathyroidism is present. About 60 percent of patients with hypercalciuria and renal stones have increased serum PTH levels and a normal serum calcium level.[27] It is interesting to note that about the same number of patients with hypercalciuria who were operated on by Grimelius and coworkers[50] were found to have abnormal parathyroids (22% had adenomas and 46% had hyperplasia). Postoperatively all patients with adenomas and some of the patients with hyperplasia improved. It seems likely that those with hyperplasia who benefited from operation had primary hyperplasia, and those who did not benefit had secondary hyperplasia due to renal loss of calcium. By treating patients with idiopathic hypercalciuria and increased PTH levels for several months with thiazide diuretics, which decreases urinary calcium loss, and then repeating the serum PTH level, it is possible to distinguish between idiopathic hypercalciuria and normocalcemic hyperparathyroidism.[27] In the former condition serum PTH levels become normal because thiazides correct the excessive urinary loss of calcium. In normocalcemic hyperparathyroidism, serum PTH levels remain high and serum calcium levels may rise.

The **phosphate deprivation test** is also useful in differentiating normocalcemia hyperparathyroidism from idiopathic hypercalciuria. This test involves giving for 3 days a diet normal in calories and calcium but restricted to less than 350 mg. of phosphate; aluminum hydroxide gel, 60 ml. is given 4 times daily; and serum calcium, phosphorus and protein concentrations are obtained for 4 days. Patients whose serum calcium rises above normal with phosphate deprivation or those who have persistent hypercalciuria usually have hyperparathyroidism.[75] Magnesium or vitamin D deficiency, a high phosphate diet, hypoalbuminemia, impaired renal function, or acute pancreatitis may be responsible for the presence of a normal calcium level in some patients with hyperparathyroidism, and when these conditions are corrected hypercalcemia may appear.

HYPERCALCEMIC CRISIS

Differential Diagnosis

Life-threatening hypercalcemia ($Ca^{++} > 14.5$ mg./dl.) may present acutely in patients who were previously asymptomatic or in patients with chronic disease. The symptoms include weakness, nausea and vomiting, drowsiness, stupor, coma, constipation and tachycardia. The history should record the duration of symptoms, recent medications (e.g., calcium-containing antacids, vitamin D, vitamin A, thiazide diuretics), or symptoms of bone pain or weight loss. Although only 4 percent of all patients with hyperparathyroidism have palpable parathyroid tumors, the tumor can be felt in 40 percent of those admitted in hypercalcemic crisis.[62]

The immediate objectives in managing these patients are:

1. Hydrate the patient.
2. Diurese vigorously.
3. Determine the cause of the hypercalcemia.
4. Correct electrolyte imbalance.
5. Avoid immobilization.

If the alkaline phosphatase level is elevated roentgenograms of the hands should be obtained; if subperiosteal resorption is present the patient has hyperparathyroidism and needs an urgent parathyroidectomy. If films of the hands are normal, malignancy is the most likely diagnosis. Roentgenograms of the abdomen may reveal nephrolithiasis or nephrocalcinosis suggesting hyperparathyroidism.

Management

Mild hypercalcemia can usually be treated by intravenous hydration and diuresis, whereas severe hypercalcemia (Ca^{++}>14.5 mg./dl.) requires more extreme measures. Combination of treatments can rapidly reduce the serum calcium levels to normal. Dehydration is a common complication of hypercalcemia and malignancy because of nausea and vomiting. Rehydration should be accomplished with 0.15 N saline intravenously while renal and cardiopulmonary functions are assessed. Physiologic saline (up to 2 L in 3 hours) is preferable to 5 percent dextrose solution, because sodium promotes renal excretion of calcium.[57] Isotonic sodium sulfate (1 L in 3 hours) is also effective, but it may cause hypernatremia in patients with impaired renal function.[21] Deionized water given by mouth or by nasogastric tube is also useful.

After the patient has been hydrated, renal excretion of calcium may be enhanced by giving Lasix (40 mg.) or ethacrynic acid (100 mg.) every 1 or 2 hours. Forced diuresis may drop the calcium level by 3 to 4 mg./dl. within several hours, associated with the excretion of more than 1 g. of calcium in the urine in 24 hours.[99] The effect persists only during the infusion and the calcium may return to elevated levels within hours after the infusion is stopped. Careful monitoring of body weight, electrolytes, magnesium, and plasma osmolality is necessary to avoid overhydration, underhydration, hyponatremia, hypokalemia, hypomagnesemia and hypernatremia. Thiazide diuretics should not be used because they decrease calcium excretion.

Inorganic phosphate (1,500 mg. intravenously over 6 to 8 hours) lowers the serum calcium rapidly by several mg./dl. at the end of the infusion, principally by inducing calcium deposition in bone.[42] Unfortunately, inorganic phosphate may be dangerous because it also decreases urinary excretion of calcium and evokes calcium deposition in extraskeletal sites, such as heart and kidney.[94] If phosphate is given too rapidly, severe hypocalcemia and even death may occur.

When giving oral phosphate (200 mg. daily) chronically, use the lowest dose that will keep the serum phosphate level under 5.5 mg./100 ml.[83] Several days of oral phosphate treatment are necessary before the maximal effect is achieved. Gastrointestinal intolerance may occur. Retention enemas with Fleet phosphosoda are also useful.

Adrenal corticosteroids decrease calcium absorption in vitamin D intoxication and sarcoidosis; they exert a mild calciuretic effect in all patients; and they suppress tumor activity, especially in myeloma, lymphoma and carcinoma of the breast.[84,102] Steroids are the treatment of choice for hypercalcemia accompanying vitamin D intoxication, sarcoidosis and Addison's disease. Large doses (200 mg. cortisone per day) are often needed for the treatment of hypercalcemia of malignancy. Steroids have limited value when the cause of the hypercalcemia is unknown because the response rate is only 50 percent in malignancy and is 5 to 10 percent in hyperparathyroidism.[48,61]

Parenteral **calcitonin** (0.5 to 5 MRC units/kg. per hour) decreases serum calcium levels within a few hours by inhibiting bone resorption and by increasing the renal clearance of calcium.[56] Salmon calcitonin is more potent and longer lasting than either porcine or human calcitonin. In many cases the calcitonin must be given every 3 to 8 hours to avoid escape from its effect. Calcitonin is less effective than phosphate or mithramycin in patients with hypercalcemia of malignancy, but it has fewer side effects than these other agents and can be used in the presence of impaired renal and cardiopulmonary function.[54] As yet, calcitonin has not been approved by the FDA to treat hypercalcemia.

Mithramycin (25 mg./kg. IV) directly inhibits bone resorption and lowers serum and urinary calcium.[44] It is useful when hypercalcemia does not respond to hydration and diuresis, especially in patients with malignant tumors. Important side effects are thrombocytopenia, hepatocellular necrosis, hemorrhage, azotemia, hypocalcemia and proteinuria. Hypocalcemia may occur within 48 hours and may last several days. Toxic effects are rare if only one or two doses are given.

EDTA and **sodium citrate** solutions have been used to treat hypercalcemic crises. However, because EDTA can cause hypotension and renal failure, and citrate therapy is difficult to regulate, these medications are used infrequently.[3]

Streptozotocin, a methyl-nitrosourea glucosamine antibiotic, has recently been reported to be effective for hypercalcemia associated with pancreatic islet cell carcinoma.[38]

Dialysis (either peritoneal or hemodialysis) is useful in patients with hypercalcemia and azotemia, but is only rarely needed.[56]

SURGICAL TREATMENT

In general, parathyroidectomy is indicated for all patients with primary hyperparathyroidism unless there are contraindications to operation or the diagnosis has not been firmly established. If the diagnosis is unclear the patient should be observed until a definitive diagnosis can be made.

Preoperative Preparation

The diagnosis of hyperparathyroidism should be well documented before the patient is scheduled for operation. Patients with renal insufficiency should be adequately hydrated, since renal function may temporarily deteriorate postoperatively. The EKG should be monitored in patients requiring digitalis because of synergistic effects of calcium and digitalis on the myocardium.

Most hypercalcemic patients have a shortened qT interval on EKG and some degree of heart block.[84]

Localization

Localization of parathyroid tumors is best done at operation by an experienced surgeon who is familiar with the normal and ectopic sites of the parathyroid glands. Numerous techniques have been used preoperatively in attempts to localize the adenoma, including arteriography,[60] selenomethionine and ^{131}I scanning, cine-esophagograms, thyroid lymphography, thermography and selective and highly selective venous catheterization with parathyroid hormone immunoassay.[43] The most reliable techniques are highly selective venous catheterization with parathyroid hormone immunoassay and arteriography.[43] These tests are usually indicated only in patients with persistent hyperparathyroidism after a previous unsuccessful exploration, since an experienced surgeon can locate the tumor in most patients. The success rate in finding the tumor in persistent and recurrent hyperparathyroidism is lower because tissue planes are obliterated by adhesions and in some cases the tumor is in an ectopic location.

Operative Technique

The incision is wider than for thyroidectomy but otherwise the approach is similar. In over 80 percent of cases, the parathyroid tumor is found attached to the posterior capsule of the thyroid gland, often overlying the recurrent laryngeal nerve. The parathyroid glands are usually symmetrically placed. Occasionally parathyroid tumors lie cephalad to the superior pole of the thyroid gland, along the great vessels of the neck in the tracheoesophageal area, in thymic tissue (7%), in the substance of the thyroid gland itself (1%), or in the mediastinum.[24] The operative field must be kept free of blood or the tumor may be obscured. The tumor must not be traumatized, because color is useful in distinguishing it from surrounding thyroid, thymus, lymph nodes and fat (Fig. 16-2). Two maneuvers that are helpful in finding parathyroid tumors at operation are tracing the branches of the inferior thyroid artery and gently palpating in the tracheoesophageal groove.

Although about 10 percent of patients have either more or less than four parathyroid glands,[103] the surgeon should attempt to identify four glands before removing an abnormal one. If a single, obviously enlarged parathyroid gland (adenoma) and three normal parathyroid glands are found, as occurs in 80 percent of patients, the adenoma should be removed and examined by frozen section. Obtaining a biopsy of one normal gland is optional. If two enlarged glands and two normal glands are identified, the two enlarged glands should be removed, a biopsy specimen obtained from one of the other glands and all specimens confirmed to be parathyroid tissue by frozen section. The remaining parathyroid glands should be marked with a silver clip.

In primary and secondary parathyroid hyperplasia, when all the glands are abnormal, all but one gland should be removed and the remaining gland subtotally excised (leaving about 50 mg.);[30] the remnant should be marked with a silver clip. The biopsy of the gland to be left behind should always be performed before removing the other parathyroids, so that if the remnant is not viable it can

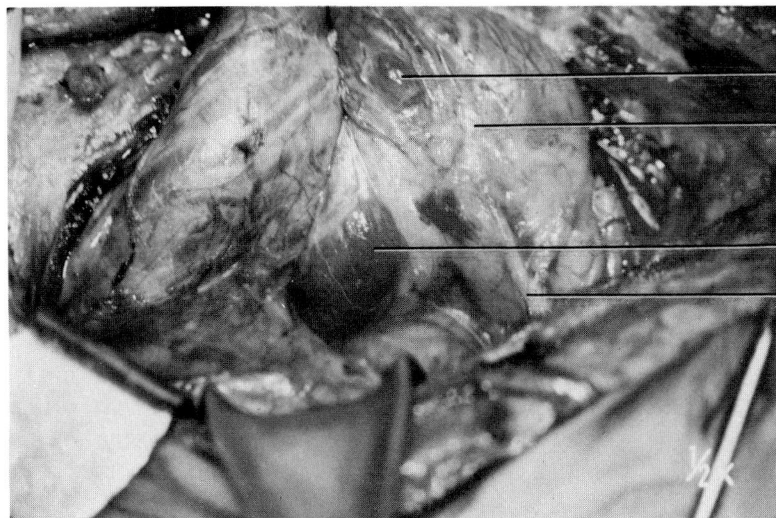

Fig. 16-2. Operative findings in a 63-year-old man with polyuria, polydypsia, weakness and severe constipation. His serum calcium was 16.1 mg./dl., phosphate 2.1 mg./dl., chloride 113 mEq./l., and parathyroid hormone 10 ng./ml. (normal less than 2.0 ng./ml.). After removal of the parathyroid adenoma, his serum calcium decreased to 9.0 mg./dl. and phosphate increased to 3.5 mg./dl.

be removed and a biopsy specimen obtained from another gland. If possible, leave the most normal-size gland that would be easy to find at a subsequent operation if recurrent or persistent hyperparathyroidism were to occur.

For primary hyperplasia, Alveryd[2] and Wells[105] and their coworkers have recently recommended total parathyroidectomy with autotransplantation into muscle of a portion of an intact or diced hyperplastic gland. Alveryd placed the transplant in the sternomastoid and Wells the muscles of the forearm. The rationale of this approach is that if hypercalcemia persists or recurs postoperatively the source of the PTH can be easily determined and, if necessary, the mass of the transplanted parathyroid tissue can be reduced by a much simpler operation than reexploration of the neck. We feel that it is premature to adopt this procedure for all patients with primary hyperplasia because most patients with this condition can be adequately managed by conventional procedures and the incidence of hypoparathyroidism following autotransplantation appears to be significant (e.g., 30-60%).[2] At present we would reserve parathyroid autotransplantation for persistent or recurrent hyperparathyroidism, where the risk of aparathyroidism following removal of the residual parathyroid tissue is significant.[22]

If exploration of the areas where the tumor is usually located is unrevealing, the thymus should be delivered from beneath the manubrium and removed and the retroesophageal area explored. Then, if less than two glands are found on one side, perform a partial thyroidectomy; if less than two glands are found on each side, perform a conservative subtotal thyroidectomy. If a thyroid nodule is present, it should be removed. The incidence of thyroid carcinoma in patients with hyperparathyroidism is about 7 percent. At the completion of the operation the surgeon should be satisfied that a parathyroid tumor is not present in the neck.

Exploration of the mediastinum by way of a sternal splitting incision is necessary in only 1 to 2 percent of cases.[48] If cervical exploration is not fruitful, or if arteriography or highly selective venous catheterization and PTH immunoassay suggest the presence of a mediastinal tumor, the patient should be allowed to recover from his initial operation and return in 6 to 8 weeks for mediastinal exploration. Median sternotomy should be performed only at the same time as the cervical exploration if the patient is in hypercalcemic crisis.

Parathyroid Biopsy

Biopsy of parathyroid glands may be indicated to determine whether the observed tissue is parathyroid, or to learn whether a parathyroid gland is normal or abnormal. Biopsy should be performed only if the remnant of the gland can be safely preserved. Biopsy is not necessary if an adenoma and three normal-size glands are identified. The biopsy technique we use is illustrated in Figure 16-3. The parathyroid gland is carefully examined and a silver clip is applied to the gland without injuring its blood supply or the surrounding fat. The clip applicator is left in place while a sliver of parathyroid is shaved off, using a new No. 15 scalpel blade. The clip applicator helps to stabilize the gland during the biopsy; the clip prevents bleeding and marks the position of the gland for future reference.

Parathyroid Pathology

Traditionally it has been taught that the best method of differentiating a parathyroid adenoma from hyperplasia is to identify a rim of normal or atrophic parathyroid tissue compressed by the tumor and to find at least one other normal-appearing parathyroid gland.[91] Although these criteria are useful in distinguishing between parathyroid adenoma and diffuse hyperplasia, they are not always reliable because the sizes of the glands vary considerably in some patients with primary chief cell hyperplasia.[12] For this reason all four parathyroid glands should be identified before any are removed. Normal parathyroid glands weigh less than 65 mg. excluding surrounding fat, and they average 5 x 3 x 1 mm. in size.[103] Roth and Gallagher[92] recently reported that normal parathyroid glands can be distinguished from hyperplastic and adenomatous glands on frozen section by the amount of intracellular fat. Histologically, both adenomas and hyperplastic glands are usually composed of chief cells, or mixed chief, water clear, and oxyphil cells with little or no fat. Less commonly only oxyphil cells are present. From the histologic pattern of a single gland, it is usually impossible to distinguish between adenoma or hyperplasia either by frozen or permanent section. Essentially the pathologist can only reliably state whether the removed tissue is parathyroid. Ultrastructural changes may be helpful in the future, but as yet reliable criteria that differentiate hyperplasia from adenoma have not been defined.

The histologic diagnosis of parathyroid carcinoma may also be difficult. The presence of fibrous trabeculae traversing the tumor, extensive capsular invasion,

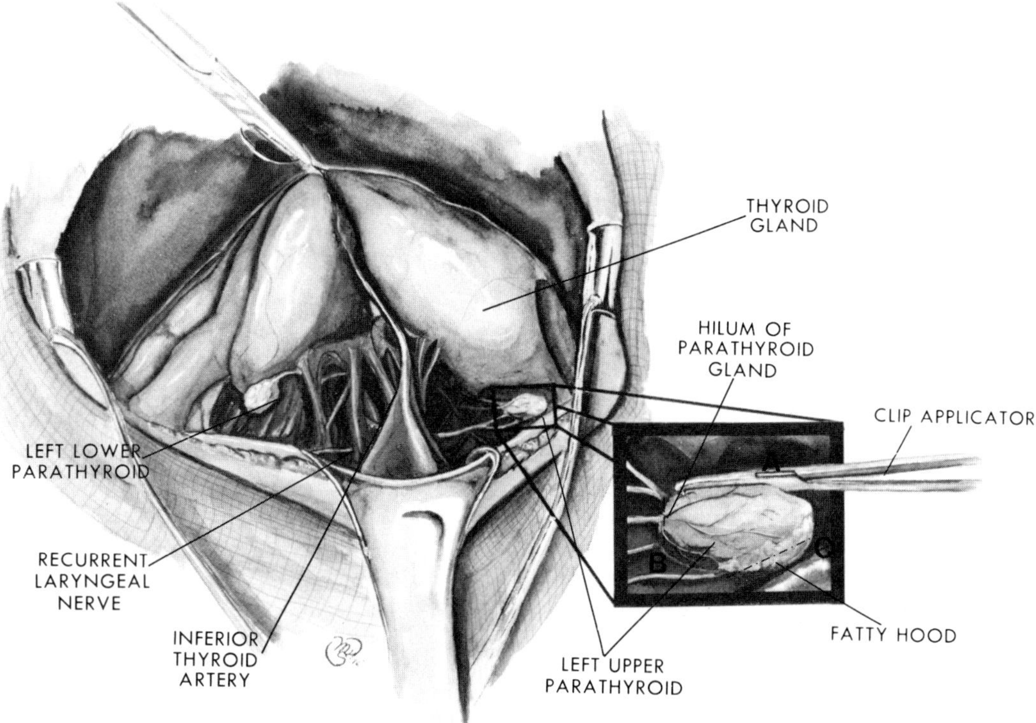

Fig. 16-3. Anatomy of the dissection performed for parathyroidectomy is viewed from the patient's left side. The insert illustrates the technique of marking a parathyroid gland with a metal clip to facilitate its identification if reoperation is required.

and mitoses suggest malignancy, but distant metastases and invasion into adjacent structures are the only pathognomonic signs. Parathyroid cancers are palpable in 50 percent of cases in contrast to benign parathyroid tumors, which can be felt in only 4 percent of cases.[52]

Postoperative Care

Following successful parathyroidectomy the serum calcium should fall to normal in 24 to 48 hours. Symptoms of hypoparathyroidism may develop in patients with severe skeletal depletion, in patients with high calcium levels preoperatively and in patients with a small parathyroid remnant. The postoperative symptoms are determined by the rate of fall and absolute serum level of ionized calcium.

The manifestations of hypocalcemia include circumoral numbness, paresthesias, muscle cramps, carpopedal spasm, anxiety and convulsions or opisthotonus. Hyperventilation and resulting respiratory alkalosis can aggravate these symptoms, whereas renal failure with acidosis may mask hypocalcemia until serum calcium levels are very low. Testing for Chvostek or Trousseau signs is useful to detect latent hypocalcemia.

Acute hypoparathyroid tetany is a medical emergency. The patient should be reassured to avoid hyperventilation and given calcium chloride (10-20 ml. of 10% solution) intravenously over 5 to 10 minutes until tetany disappears. Ten to 50 ml. of 10 percent calcium chloride may then be added to a liter of normal saline or 5-percent dextrose solution and administered at a rate that keeps the serum calcium normal. Hypomagnesemia may also cause tetany, and magnesium sulfate (10 ml. of a 25% solution) should be given by slow intravenous administration if the symptoms do not respond quickly to calcium. Once tetany has been reversed the patient can be maintained on oral calcium. Glubionate calcium (Neo-Calglucon syrup, 1-3 tablespoonsful, 3 times daily) is the best absorbed and most palatable oral preparation.

Dihydrotachysterol (Hytakerol, AT-10, 0.5 ml.) or vitamin D (25,000 to 50,000 units 3 times daily) is used for chronic therapy. Aluminum hydroxide may also be necessary to bind phosphorus in the gut and increase fecal phosphorus losses. The management of chronic hypoparathyroidism may be difficult because the difference between the controlling and intoxicating doses of vitamin D may be small.[7] Serum calcium levels should be determined frequently.

Chronic hypoparathyroidism may produce dizziness, brittle nails, alopecia, cataracts and loss of eyebrows. Important laboratory findings are hypocalcemia, hyperphosphatemia, low or absent urinary phosphate, a high tubular resorption of phosphate and undetectable serum levels of PTH. Roentgenographic studies may reveal calcification of the basal ganglia, arteries and the external ear. Hypoparathyroidism causes so much morbidity that it must be avoided if possible.

Reoperation

As emphasized previously, a thorough search for all four parathyroid glands should always be performed at the initial operation, since reexploration for persistent or recurrent hyperparathyroidism, or after a previous thyroidectomy, may present formidable problems and an increased risk of complications. Selective arteriography and highly selective venous catheterization with parathyroid hormone immunoassay are useful for tumor localization before a second exploration. Most patients with persistent hyperparathyroidism have a parathyroid tumor that can be removed through a cervical incision, making mediastinal exploration unnecessary.[48]

RESULTS OF TREATED HYPERPARATHYROIDISM

After removal of a single adenoma recurrent hyperparathyroidism develops in less than 5 percent of patients.[25,33,74] Persistent hyperparathyroidism, due to failure to remove one or more enlarged parathyroid glands, occurs in about 11 percent.[23]

In contrast, recurrent or perisistent hyperparathyroidism is found in about 33 percent of patients with MEA or familial hyperparathyroidism[25]; therefore, extra care should be taken to remove all abnormal parathyroid tissue and to mark the normal appearing glands at operation in these patients. Subtotal parathyroidectomy should be performed in MEA or FH if more than one parathyroid gland is abnormal.

When present at the time of parathyroidectomy, renal failure often progresses despite the return of normocalcemia.[15] McGeown reported that 16 percent of

104 patients died within 8 years of successful parathyroidectomy,[104] and Reinhoff found that 35 percent of patients with hyperparathyroidism died within 11 years after successful parathyroidectomy.[88] Half of these deaths were due to renal failure and the other half to hypertension and other cardiovascular complications. Early operation before renal disease develops should improve these long-term results.

When the disease is discovered early most patients benefit from parathyroidectomy.[6,84] One-third of those with hypertension become normotensive[85]; two-thirds of those with peptic ulcer disease improve[106]; two-thirds of patients with hyperuricemia become normouricemic[6]; the incidence of renal lithiasis is reduced[84]; skeletal abnormalities improve; and symptoms of hypercalcemia such as polydipsia, polyuria, constipation and neuromuscular symptoms disappear.[6]

REFERENCES

1. Albright, F., Aub, J. C., and Bauer, W.: Hyperparathyroidism: a common and polymorphic condition as illustrated by 17 cases from one clinic. JAMA, *102*:1276, 1934.
2. Alveryd, A., El-Zawahry, M. D., Herlitz, P., and Nordenstan, H.: Primary hyperplasia of the parathyroids. Acta Chir. Scand., *141*:24, 1975.
3. Amatruda, T. T., Jr.: Nonendocrine secreting tumors. *In* Bondy, P. K., and Rosenberg, L. E. (eds.): Duncan's Diseases of Metabolism. p. 1636. Philadelphia, W. B. Saunders, 1974.
4. Arnaud, C. D.: Immunochemical heterogeneity of circulating parathyroid hormone in man: sequel to an original observation by Berson and Yalow. Mt. Sinai J. Med. N.Y., *40*:422, 1973.
5. Aurbach, G. D., and Potts, J. T., Jr.: The parathyroids. Adv. Metab. Disord., *1*:45, 1964.
6. Aurbach, G. D., Mallette, L. E., Patten, B. M., Heath, D. A., Doppman, J. L., and Bilezikian, J. P.: Hyperparathyroidism: recent studies. Ann. Intern. Med., *79*:566, 1973.
7. Avioli, L. V.: The therapeutic approach to hypoparathyroidism. Am. J. Med., *57*:34, 1974.
8. Ballard, H. S., Frame, B., and Hartsock, R. J.: Familial multiple endocrine adenoma-peptic ulcer complex. Medicine, *43*:481, 1964.
9. Bender, R. A., and Hauren, H.: Hypercalcemia in bronchogenic carcinoma. Ann. Intern. Med., *80*:205, 1974.
10. Benson, R. C., Jr., Riggs, B. L., Pickard, B. M., and Arnaud, C. D.: Immunoreactive forms of circulating parathyroid hormone in primary and ectopic hyperparathyroidism. J. Clin. Invest., *54*:175, 1974.
11. Bentzel, C. J., Carbone, P. P., and Rosenberg, L.: The effect of prednisone on calcium metabolism and Ca^{47} kinetics in patients with multiple myeloma and hypercalcemia. J. Clin. Invest., *43*:2132, 1964.
12. Block, M. A., Frame, B., Jackson, C. E., Parfitt, A. M., and Horn, R. C.: Primary diffuse microscopical hyperplasia of the parathyroid glands. Arch. Surg., *111*:348, 1976.
13. Boonstra, C. E., and Jackson, C. E.: Hyperparathyroidism detected by routine serum calcium analysis. Ann. Intern. Med., *63*:468, 1965.
14. Bricker, N. S., Slatopolsky, E., Reiss, E., and Avioli, L. V.: Calcium, phosphorus and bone in renal disease and transplantation. Arch. Intern. Med., *123*:543, 1969.
15. Britton, D. C., Johnson, I. D. A., Thompson, M. H., and Fleming, L. B.: The outcome of treatment and changes in presentation of primary hyperparathyroidism. Br. J. Surg., *60*:782, 1973.
16. Burman, K. D., Monchik, J. M., Earll,

J. M., and Wartofsky, L.: Ionized and total serum calcium and parathyroid hormone in hyperthyroidism. Ann. Intern. Med., *84*:668, 1976.

17. Burnett, C. H., Commons, R. R., Albright, F., and Howard, J. E.: Hypercalcemia without hypercalciuria or hypophosphatemia, calcinosis and renal insufficiency. N. Engl. J. Med., *240*:787, 1949.
18. Canterbury, J. M., Levey, G. S., and Reiss, E.: Activation of renal cortical adenylate cyclase by circulating immunoreactive parathyroid hormone fragments. J. Clin. Invest., *52*:524, 1973.
19. Carney, J. A., Go, V. L. W., Sizemore, G. W., and Hayles, A. B.: Alimentary-tract ganglioneuromatosis. A major component of the syndrome of multiple endocrine neoplasia, type 2b. N. Engl. J. Med., *295*:1287, 1976.
20. Castleman, B., and Kibbee, B. U.: Case records of the Massachusetts General Hospital. N. Engl. J. Med., *268*:943, 1963.
21. Chakmakjian, Z. H., and Bethune, J. E.: Sodium sulfate treatment of hypercalcemia. N. Engl. J. Med., *275*:862, 1966.
22. Clark, O. H.: Letter to the editor concerning management of primary parathyroid hyperplasia. N. Engl. J. Med., *295*:1203, 1976.
23. Clark, O. H., and Goldman, L.: Prophylactic subtotal parathyroidectomy should be discouraged. *In* Varco, R. L., and Delaney, J. P. (eds.): Controversy in Surgery. Philadelphia, W. B. Saunders, 1936.
24. ——: Thyroid and Parathyroid. *In* Dunphy, J. E., and Way, L. W. (eds.): Current Surgical Diagnoses and Treatment. ed. 2, p. 254. Los Altos, California, Lange Medical Publications, 1975.
25. Clark, O. H., Hunt, T. K., and Way, L. W.: Recurrent hyperparathyroidism. Ann. Surg., *184*:391, 1976.
26. Coburn, J. W., Popovtver, M. M., Massry, S. G., and Kleeman, C. R.: The physiochemical state and renal handling of divalent ions in chronic renal failure. Arch. Intern. Med., *124*:302, 1969.
27. Coe, F. L., Canterbury, J. M., Firpo, J. J., and Reiss, E.: Evidence for secondary hyperparathyroidism in idiopathic hypercalciuria. J. Clin. Invest., *52*:134, 1973.
28. Cope, O.: The story of hyperparathyroidism at the Massachusetts General Hospital. N. Engl. J. Med., *274*:1174, 1966.
29. Cope, O., Culver, P. J., Mixter, C. G., Jr., and Nardi, G. L.: Pancreatitis, a diagnostic clue to hyperparathyroidism. Ann. Surg., *145*:857, 1957.
30. Cope, O., Keynes, W. M., Roth, S. I., and Castleman, B.: Primary chief cell hyperplasia of the parathyroid glands: a new entity with surgery of hyperparathyroidism. Ann. Surg., *148*:375, 1958.
31. Cushard, W. G., Jr., Simon, A. B., Canterbury, J. M., and Reiss, E.: Parathyroid function in sarcoidosis. N. Engl. J. Med., *286*:395, 1972.
32. David, D. S.: Calcium metabolism in renal failure. Am. J. Med., *58*:48, 1975.
33. Davies, D. R.: The surgery of primary hyperparathyroidism. Clin. Endocrinol. Metab., *3*:253, 1974.
34. Davis, D. R., Dent, C. E., and Willcox, A.: Hyperparathyroidism and steatorrhea. Br. Med. J., *2*:1133, 1956.
35. Davis, H. L., Jr., Wiseley, A. N., Ramirez, G., et al.: Hypercalcemia complicating breast cancer. Clinical features and management. Oncology, *28*:126, 1973.
36. Deftos, L. J., and Neer, R.: Medical management of hypercalcemia of malignancy. *In* Creger, W. P. (ed.): Annual Review of Medicine. p. 323. Palo Alto, California, Annual Reviews, Inc., 1974.
37. Dent, C. E., and Watson, L.: The hydrocortisone test in primary and tertiary hyperparathyroidism. Lancet, *2*:662, 1968.
38. Dewys, W. D., Stoll, R., Au, W. Y.,

and Salisnjak, M. M.: Effects of streptozotocin on an islet cell carcinoma with hypercalcemia. Am. J. Med., *55*:671, 1973.
39. Dexter, R. N., Mullinax, F., Estep, H. L., and Williams, R. C.: Monoclonal IgG gammopathy and hyperparathyroidism. Ann. Intern. Med., *77*:759, 1972.
40. Dillon, R. S.: Hormones and disorders of mineral and bone metabolism. *In* Handbook of Endocrinology. p. 273. Philadelphia, Lea and Febiger, 1973.
41. Duarte, C. G., Winnacker, J. L., Becker, K. L., and Pace, A.: Thiazide-induced hypercalcemia. N. Engl. J. Med., *284*:828, 1971.
42. Eisenberg, E.: Effect of intravenous phosphate on serum strontium and calcium. N. Engl. J. Med., *282*:889, 1970.
43. Eisenberg, H., Pallota, J., and Sherwood, L. M.: Selective arteriography, venography and various hormone assay in diagnosis and localization of parathyroid lesions. Am. J. Med., *56*:810, 1974.
44. Elias, E. G., and Evans, J. T.: Hypercalcemic crises in neoplastic diseases: management with mithramycin. Surgery, *71*:631, 1972.
45. Fraser, D. R., and Kodicek, E.: Unique biosynthesis by kidney of a biologically active vitamin D metabolite. Nature, *228*:764, 1970.
46. Friedman, J., and Raisz, L. G.: Thyrocalcitonin: inhibitor of bone resorption in tissue culture. Science, *150*:1465, 1965.
47. Garabedian, M., Holick, M. F., DeLuca, H. F., and Boyle, I. T.: Control of 25-hydroxycholecalciferol metabolism by parathyroid glands. Proc. Nat. Acad. Sci. USA., *69*:1673, 1973.
48. Goldman, L., Gordon, G. S., and Roof, B. S.: The parathyroids. Progress, problems and practice. Curr. Probl. Surg., Aug., 1971.
49. Goldsmith, R. S.: Differential diagnosis of hypercalcemia. N. Engl. J. Med., *274*:674, 1966.
50. Grimelius, L., Ejerblad, S., Johansson, H., and Werner, I.: Parathyroid adenomas and glands in normocalcemic hyperparathyroidism. Am. J. Pathol., *83*:475, 1976.
51. Hellstrom , J., Birke, G., and Edvall, C. A.: Hypertension in hyperparathyroidism. Br. J. Urol., *30*:13, 1958.
52. Holmes, E. C., Morton, D. L., and Ketcham, A. S.: Parathyroid carcinoma: a collective review. Ann. Surg., *169*:631, 1969.
53. Johnson, R. D., and Conn, J. W.: Hyperparathyroidism with a long period on normocalcemia. JAMA, *210*:2063, 1969.
54. Kammerman, S., and Canfield, R. E.: Effect of porcine calcitonin on hypercalcemia in man. J. Clin. Endocrinol. Metab., *31*:70, 1970.
55. Kaplan, R. A., Snyder, W. H., Steward, A., and Pak, C. Y. C.: Metabolic effects of parathyroidectomy in asymptomatic primary hyperparathyroidism. J. Clin. Endocrinol. Metab., *42*:415, 1976.
56. Keating, F. R., Jr., Jones, J. D., Elveback, L. R., and Randall, R. V.: The relation of age and sex to the distribution of values in healthy adults of serum calcium, inorganic phosphorus, magnesium, alkaline phosphatase, total proteins, albumin, and blood urea. J. Lab. Clin. Med., *73*:825, 1969.
57. Kleeman, C. R., Bohannan, J., Bernstein, D., Ling, S., and Maxwell, M. H.: Effect of variations in sodium intake on calcium excretion in normal humans. Proc. Soc. Exp. Biol. Med., *115*:29, 1964.
58. Krane, S. M.: Selected features of the clinical course of hypoparathyroidism. JAMA, *178*:472, 1961.
59. Krook, L.: On the etiology of "primary parathyroid hyperplasia." Rev. Can. Biol., *24*:63, 1965.
60. Kuntz, C. H., and Goldsmith, R. E.: Selective arteriography of parathyroid adenomas. Radiology, *102*:21, 1972.
61. Lafferty, F. W.: Pseudo-hyperpara-

thyroidism. Medicine, *45*:247, 1966.

62. Lemann, J., Jr., and Donatelli, . A. A.: Calcium intoxication due to primary hyperparathyroidism. Ann. Intern. Med., *60*:447, 1964.
63. Lim, P., Dong, S., and Khoo, O. T.: Intracellular magnesium depletion in chronic renal failure. N. Engl. J. Med., *280*:981, 1969.
64. Livolsi, V. A., and Feind, C. R.: Parathyroid adenoma and nonmedullary thyroid carcinoma. Cancer, *38*:1391, 1976.
65. Low, J. C., Schaaf, M., Earll, J. M., Piechocki, J. T., and Li, T. K.: Ionic calcium determination in primary hyperparathyroidism. JAMA, *223*: 152, 1973.
66. McGeown, M. G.: The results of parathyroidectomy. Urol. Int., *19*:137, 1965.
67. McGeown, M. G., and Montgomery, D. A. D.: Multiple myelomatosis stimulating hyperparathyroidism. Br. Med. J., *1*:86, 1956.
68. MacIntyre, I.: Calcitonin: an introductory review. *In* Calcitonin Proceedings of the Symposium on Thyrocalcitonin and the C Cells. London, William Heinemann, 1968.
69. McMillan, D. E.: Milk alkali syndrome: A study of the acute disorder with comments on the development of this chronic condition. Medicine, *44*:485, 1965.
70. McSwiney, R. R., and Mills, J. H.: Hypercalcemia due to sarcoidosis. Lancet, *2*:862, 1956.
71. Mallette, L. E., Bilezikian, J. P., Health, D. A., and Aurback, G. D.: Primary hyperparathyroidism: clinical and biochemical features. Medicine, *53*:127, 1974.
72. Massry, S. G., Coburn, J. W., Lee, D. B. N., Jowsey, J., and Kleeman, C. R.: Skeletal resistance to parathyroid hormone in renal failure. Ann. Intern. Med., *78*:375, 1973.
73. Muller, H.: Sex, age and hyperparathyroidism. Lancet, *1*:449, 1969.
74. ——: True recurrence of hyperparathyroidism: proposed criteria of recurrence. Br. J. Surg., *62*:556, 1975.
75. Nichols, G., Jr., and Flanagan, B.: Normocalcemia hyperparathyroidism. Trans. Assoc. Am. Physicians, *80*:314, 1967.
76. Paloyan, E.: The role of glucagon hypersecretion in the relations of pancreatitis and hyperparathyroidism. Surgery, *62*:167, 1967.
77. Parfitt, A. M.: Chlorothiazide-induced hypercalcemia in juvenile osteoporosis and hyperparathyroidism. N. Engl. J. Med., *281*:55, 1969.
78. Peacock, M., Robertson, W. G., and Nordin, B. E. C.: Relation between serum and urinary calcium with particular reference to parathyroid activity. Lancet, *1*:384, 1969.
79. Pearse, A. G. E., and Polak, J. M.: Neural crest origin of the endocrine polypeptide (APUD) cells of the gastrointestinal tract and pancreas. Gut, *12*:783, 1971.
80. Pickleman, J. R., Straus, F. H., Forland, M., and Paloyan, E.: Thiazide-induced parathyroid stimulation. Metabolism, *18*:867, 1969.
81. Powell, D., Singer, F. R., Murray, T. M., Minkin, C., and Potts, J. T.: Nonparathyroid humoral hypercalcemia in patients with neoplastic diseases. N. Engl. J. Med., *289*:176, 1973.
82. Purnell, D. C., Smith, L. H., Scholz, D. A., Elveback, L. R., and Arnaud, C. D.: Primary hyperparathyroidism: a prospective clinical study. Am. J. Med., *50*:670, 1971.
83. Purnell, D. C., Scholz, D. A., Smith, L. H., Sizemore, G. W., Black, B. M., Goldsmith, R. S., and Arnaud, C. D.: Treatment of primary hyperparathyroidism. Am. J. Med., *56*:800, 1974.
84. Pyrah, L. N., Hodgkinson, A., and Anderson, C. K.: Primary hyperparathyroidism. Br. J. Surg., *53*:16, 1966.
85. Rawson, A. J., and Sunderman, F. W.: Studies in serum electrolytes XV Calcium-binding property of serum proteins (multiple myeloma, lymphogranuloma, venereum and sarcoidosis). J. Clin. Invest., *27*:82, 1948.
86. Reeves, C. D., Palmer, F., Bacchus,

H., and Longerbeam, J. K.: Differential diagnosis of hypercalcemia by the chloride/phosphate ratio. Am. J. Surg., *130*:166, 1975.

87. Reiss, E., and Canterbury, J. M.: Blood levels of parathyroid hormone in disorders of calcium metabolism. Annu. Rev. Med., *24*:217, 1973.
88. Rienhoff, W. F., Jr.: The surgical treatment of hyperparathyroidism. Ann. Surg., *131*:917, 1950.
89. Riggs, B. L., Arnaud, C. D., Reynolds, J. C., and Smith, L. H.: Immunologic differentiation of primary hyperparathyroidism from hyperparathyroidism due to nonparathyroid cancer. J. Clin. Invest., *50*:2079, 1971.
90. Rogers, H. M., Keating, F. R., Jr., Morlock, C. G., and Barker, N. W.: Primary hypertrophy and hyperplasia of parathyroid glands associated with duodenal ulcer: report of an additional case with special reference to metabolic, gastrointestinal and vascular manifestations. Arch. Intern. Med., *79*:307, 1947.
91. Roth, S. I.: Recent advances in parathyroid gland pathology. Am. J. Med., *50*:612, 1971.
92. Roth, S. I., and Gallagher, M. J.: The rapid identification of "normal" parathyroid glands by the presence of intracellular fat. Am. J. Pathol., *84*:521, 1976.
93. Samaan, N. A., Hickey, R. C., Sethi, M. R., Yank, K. P., and Wallace, S.: Hypercalcemia in patients with known malignant disease. Surgery, *80*:382, 1976.
94. Schneeberger, E. E., and Morrison, A. B.: Increased susceptibility of magnesium-deficient rats to a phosphate-induced nephropathy. Am. J. Pathol., *50*:549, 1967.
95. Scholz, D. A., and Keating, F. R.: Renal insufficiency, renal calculi and nephrocalcinosis in sarcoidosis. Am. J. Med., *21*:75, 1956.
96. Shimkin, P. M., and Powell, D.: Parathyroid hormone levels in thyroid vein blood of patients without abnormalities of calcium. Metabolism, *78*:714, 1973.
97. Singhelakis, P., Alevizaki, C. C., and Ikkos, D. G.: Intestinal calciun absorption in hyperthyroidism. Metabolism, *23*:311, 1974.
98. Steiner, A. L., Goodman, A. D., and Powers, S. R.: Study of a kindred with pheochromocytoma, medullary thyroid carcinoma, hyperparathyroidism and Cushing's disease: multiple endocrine neoplasia, type 2. Medicine, *47*:371, 1968.
99. Suki, W. N., Yium, J. J., Von Minden, M., Saller-Herbert, C., Eknoyan, G., and Martinez-Maldonado, M.: Acute treatment of hypercalcemia with furosemide. N. Engl. J. Med., *283*:836, 1970.
100. Tanaka, Y., and DeLuca, F. H.: The control of 25-hydroxyvitamin D metabolism by inorganic phosphorus. Arch. Biochem. Biophys., *154*:566, 1973.
101. Thalassinos, N. C., and Joplin, C. F.: Failure of corticosteroid therapy to correct the hypercalcaemia of malignant disease. Lancet, *2*:537, 1970.
102. Vichayanrat, A., Auramides, A., Gardner, B., Wallach, S., and Carter, A. C.: Primary hyperparathyroidism and breast cancer. Am. J. Med., *61*:136, 1976.
103. Wang, C. A.: The anatomic basis of parathyroid surgery. Ann. Surg., *183*:271, 1976.
104. Warren, M. M., Utz, D. C., and Kelalis, P. P.: Concurrence of hypernephroma and hypercalcemia. Ann. Surg., *174*:863, 1971.
105. Wells, S. A., Ellis, G., Gunnells, C., Schneider, A. B., and Sherwood, L. M.: Parathyroid autotransplantation in primary parathyroid hyperplasia. N. Engl. J. Med., *295*:57, 1976.
106. Wilder, W. T., Frame, B., and Hambrich, W. S.: Peptic ulcer in primary hyperparathyroidism. Ann. Intern. Med., *55*:885, 1961.
107. Wills, M. R., and McGowan, G. K.: Plasma-chloride levels in hyperparathyroidism and other hypercalcemic states. Br. Med. J., *1*:1153, 1964.

EDITORIAL COMMENTARY

It is evident that the hypercalcemic syndrome is associated with a variety of organic causes, the principal ones being parathyroid tumors and hyperplasia as well as malignancies of nonparathyroid tissues. The symptomatology of the syndrome is related to the effect of elevated levels of circulating serum calcium due to PTH activity, involving the kidneys, skeletal system, gastrointestinal tract and the neuromuscular apparatus, thus accounting for the oft-quoted clinical presentations referred to as, "stones, bones, groans and moans." The apparent increasing frequency of the diagnosis of hyperparathyroidism is accountable in large measure to the more routine and automated laboratory determinations of serum calcium in the screening of patients, and this serendipitous identification of patients with hypercalcemia has led to complexities of diagnostic confirmation and a relative increase in the incidence of parathyroid hyperplasia. There are reports of additional reasons for the recent surge in the number of patients having hyperparathyroidism; these include the use of thiazide diuretics, adrenal glucocorticoids and irradiation to the head and neck during infancy and childhood. The two former medications have also been shown experimentally to produce parathyroid hyperplasia; prior radiation and differentiated thyroid neoplasms, long known to be associated in incidence with each other, are now reported to be associated also with hyperparathyroidism due to tumor or hyperplasia. This expanding incidence and changing histologic basis for hyperparathyroidism has fostered the development of at least two differing conceptual plans of surgical treatment of hyperparathyroidism of parathyroid origin (i.e., excision of isolated parathyroid adenomas or the subtotal (3½), or total removal of parathyroid tissue with and without autotransplantation).

It is still difficult to differentiate between a small parathyroid adenoma and hyperplasia (of either chief or clear cells) not only by laboratory testing, but also by surgical and histologic scrutiny. Yet the surgeon must make at least two important decisions: That the preoperative data are absolutely convincing that parathyroid pathology exists, and that the type and extent of abnormal parathyroid tissue are identified and removed at operation consistent with a methodical plan such as is described in this chapter. The use of localization techniques, particularly selective venous sampling for parathyrin concentrations, is usually reserved for the more necessary application in patients with persistent or recurrent hyperparathyroidism after an initial operation. In this regard, persistently functioning parathyroid tissue in the mediastinum can usually be removed through the cervical approach so that sternal splitting operations for mediastinal exploration are rarely necessary.

There are, of course, special clinical situations, including uncomplicated (so-called asymptomatic) hyperparathyroidism, normocalcemic hyperparathyroidism, idiopathic hypercalciuria, and the severe and dramatic hypercalcemic crises in some patients which require recognition for proper management.

S.R.F.

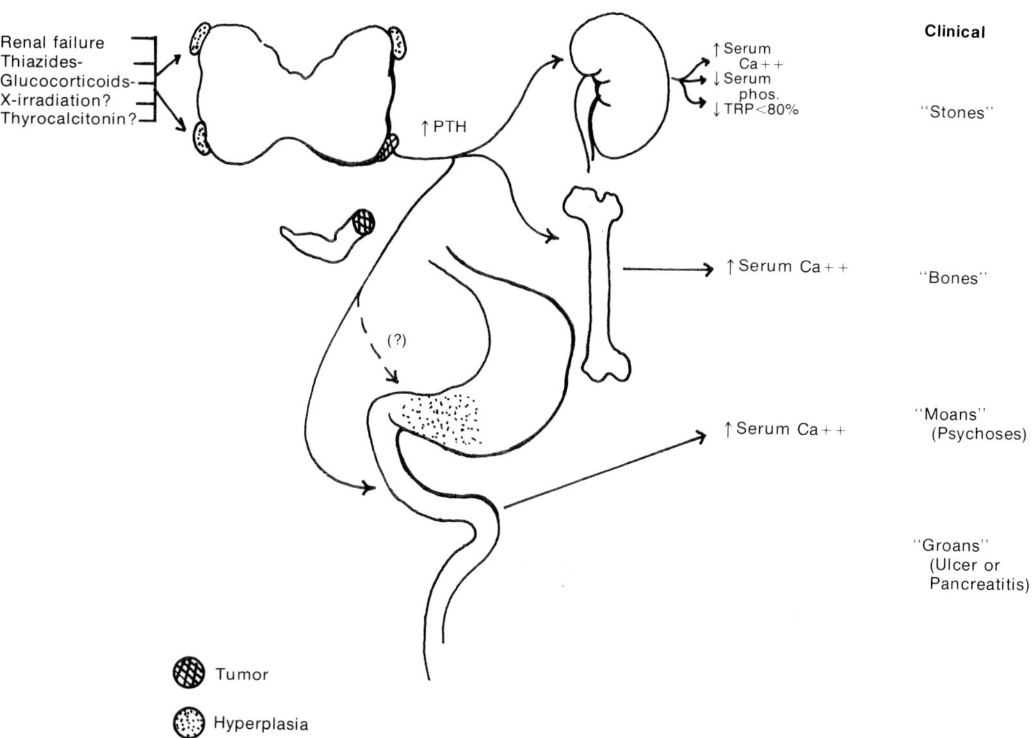

Fig. 16-4. Pathophysiology of the hypercalcemic syndrome (hyperparathyroidism).

(See overleaf for flowchart)

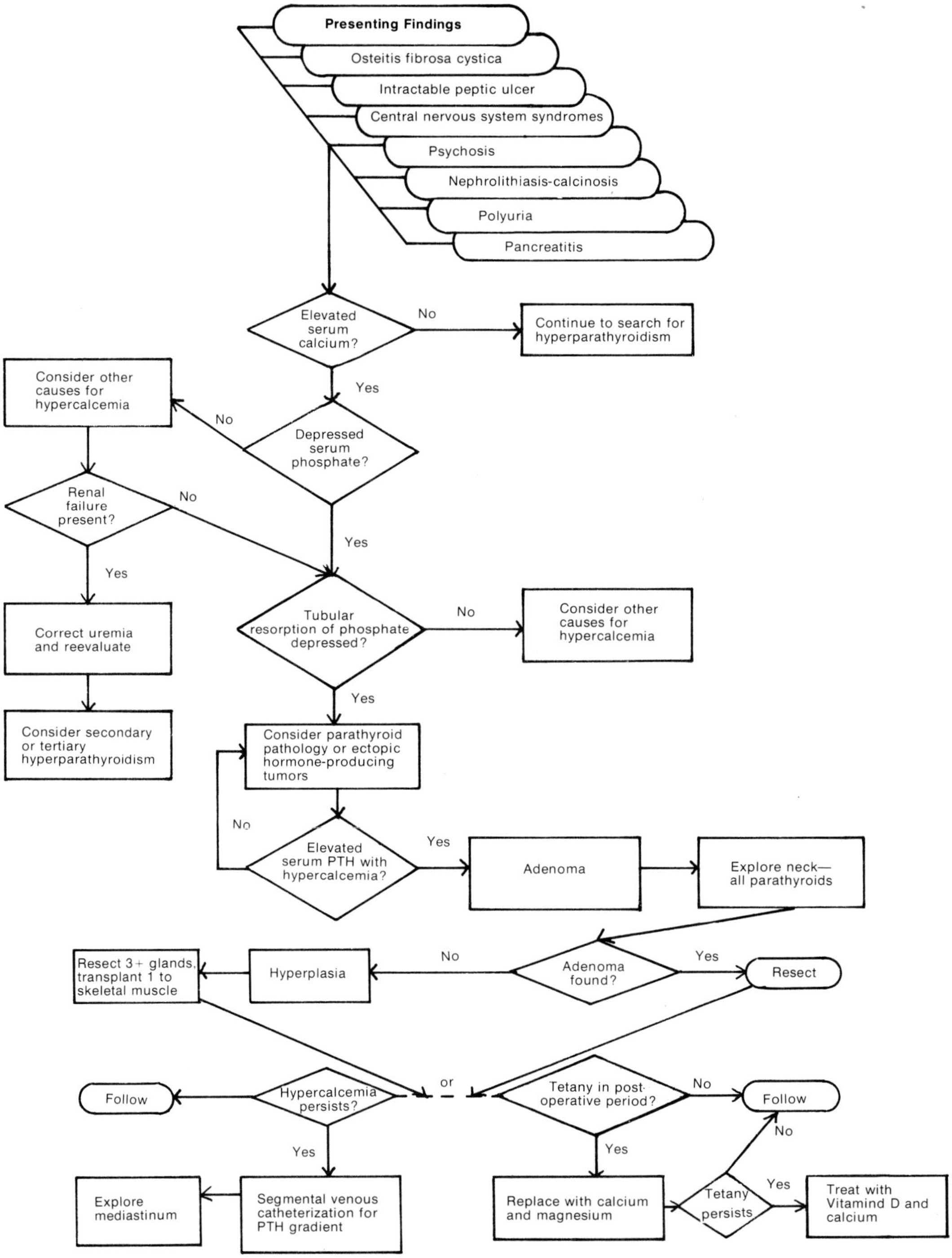

Presenting Findings
Osteitis fibrosa cystica
Intractable peptic ulcer
Central nervous system syndromes
Psychosis
Nephrolithiasis-calcinosis
Polyuria
Pancreatitis

Elevated serum calcium?
No
Continue to search for hyperparathyroidism
Yes
Consider other causes for hypercalcemia
No
Depressed serum phosphate?
Renal failure present?
No
Yes
Yes
Correct uremia and reevaluate
Consider secondary or tertiary hyperparathyroidism
Tubular resorption of phosphate depressed?
No
Consider other causes for hypercalcemia
Yes
Consider parathyroid pathology or ectopic hormone-producing tumors
No
Elevated serum PTH with hypercalcemia?
Yes
Adenoma
Explore neck—all parathyroids
Resect 3+ glands, transplant 1 to skeletal muscle
Hyperplasia
No
Adenoma found?
Yes
Resect
Follow
Hypercalcemia persists?
or
Tetany in post-operative period?
No
Follow
No
Yes
Yes
Explore mediastinum
Segmental venous catheterization for PTH gradient
Replace with calcium and magnesium
Tetany persists
Yes
Treat with Vitamind D and calcium

Fig. 16-5. Management flowchart of the hypercalcemic syndrome.

17

Wermer's Syndrome: Multiple Endocrine Adenopathy, Type I

Stuart D. Wilson, M.D.

Multiple endocrine adenopathy, Type I (MEA-I) or Wermer's syndrome are terms used to describe an inherited endocrine disorder involving pathologic changes, usually hyperfunctioning tumors, in two or more of the endocrine glands, primarily the parathyroid glands, the pancreatic islets, the pituitary gland and occasionally tumors of the adrenal and thyroid glands. Several reports of patients with coexisting endocrine tumors had been published earlier, but it was Wermer's 1954 description of a family affected with "adenomatosis of the endocrine glands" and his proposal that this syndrome was an inherited disorder that prompted investigations into such families.[24] The recent development of radioimmunoassay techniques which allow precise quantitative measurement of circulating peptide hormones secreted from endocrine glands has stimulated interest further and expanded our knowledge about this syndrome.

Genealogic studies of many affected families confirm Wermer's original hypothesis that the MEA-I syndrome is inherited and caused by an autosomal dominant gene, which has a high degree of penetrance.[2,8,11,12,14,21]

Wermer's syndrome has been used as the eponym and MEA-I as the acronym for this disorder. Wermer later used the term multiple endocrine neoplasia, Type I and the acronym MEN-I because the involved endocrine glands may present with tumors that are classified as hyperplasia or carcinoma as well as adenomas.[26] The term multiple endocrine adenopathy satisfies the latter criteria and the original and still frequently used acronym, MEA, still may be used correctly.

The MEA-I syndrome is a distinct entity from the MEA-II syndrome, another inherited endocrine disorder, in which hyperparathyroidism (HPT), medullary carcinoma of the thyroid (MCT) and pheochromocytoma are the predominant endocrine disorders. The eponym for MEA-II (a) is Sipple's syndrome.

ENDOCRINE RELATIONSHIPS IN A FAMILY WITH MEA-I

Four generations of a Milwaukee family with multiple (Fig. 17-1) endocrine adenomatosis have been traced and studied. The pedigree of this family provides insight into this inherited disorder. The father (generation-I) of seven children was known to have vomited blood and died in 1908 with "nephritis and uremia." These features suggest he may have had a gastrinoma and hyperparathyroidism. Four of his children had "stomach ulcers" and gastrointestinal bleeding; three died at an early age from intestinal hemorrhaging. In

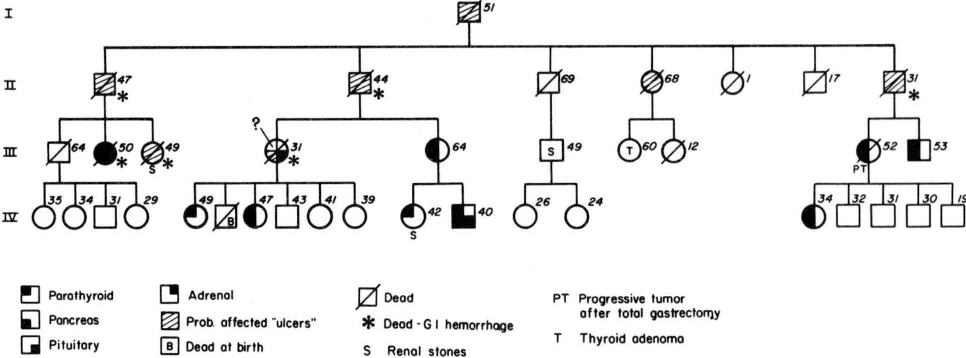

Fig. 17-1. Pedigree of family with MEA-I trait. Number adjacent to each individual is current age or age at death.

generation-III, six of the ten children had peptic ulcer disease and hyperparathyroidism has been documented in four of the six. Three of the six affected generation-III members have succumbed from ulcers and two of the remaining three had total gastrectomy. The parathyroids were not examined in the other two members who died with bleeding ulcers. Parathyroidectomy did not significantly alter the ulcer disease in any patient. The only affected member of generation-III alive beyond 60 years has had a parathyroidectomy and a total gastrectomy. Another generation-III member died as the result of progressive tumor growth (gastrinoma) several years after total gastrectomy. Four of the six generation-IV members who have lived 40 years have been studied and have hyperparathyroidism; two of these have evidence of gastrinomas. A younger member of this generation with proven hyperparathyroidism was found to have a pancreatic tumor during an abdominal procedure to remove renal calculi. Electronmicroscopy of this pancreatic islet cell tumor showed a mixture of non-beta and beta cells. However, this tumor apparently was not secreting any excessive amounts of peptide hormones. Gastrin and insulin concentrations in the blood were normal and the patient did not exhibit any signs or symptoms of hypergastrinemia or hyperinsulinism.

Some common characteristics of the MEA syndrome illustrated by this family include those listed below:

1. Hyperparathyroidism is generally present in affected family members, usually by the end of the third decade. Such patients are frequently without symptoms and the hyperparathyroidism is "mild." Unless serum calcium and parathyroid hormone are measured, the disease may go unnoticed.
2. A family history shows that members from older generations frequently succumbed from the complications of peptic ulcer disease. Methods for measuring serum calcium were not generally available at the time these people died. When an autopsy was performed, however, islet cell tumors were frequently documented and the parathyroid glands demonstrated hyperplasia.
3. The pancreatic islet cell tumors usually become clinically apparent at a later age than the parathyroid disorder. Gastrinomas are the most common of these peptide-secreting pancreatic tumors. Insulinomas are less common;

however, in some MEA-I families, insulinomas may be the predominant type of pancreatic tumor. Islet cell tumors which secrete insulin and gastrin simultaneously and tumors elaborating a diarrheogenic hormone have been reported in MEA-I family members.

4. Clinically, functioning pituitary adenomas and adrenal hyperplasia are not common; however, studies of autopsy material demonstrate that pituitary and adrenal lesions can be documented in most MEA-I patients.

Genetic Concepts and Pathogenesis

The hereditary basis of the MEA-I syndrome is proved by its familial occurrence. Approximately one-half of the offspring of an affected individual will inherit the MEA-I trait, sexes are equally affected and usually there are no skipped generations. This pattern of inheritance indicates an autosomal dominant trait. Clinical variability depends on penetrance (i.e., whether or not a family member inherits the trait) and expressivity (i.e., the degree to which the trait is expressed). The MEA-I syndrome has a high degree of penetrance which becomes more apparent when asymptomatic members of a family with the MEA-I trait are screened using radioimmunoassays that detect abnormal levels of circulating hormones. Clinical manifestations vary not only because of the different endocrine glands involved, but also because of differences in the secondary effects of the endocrine tumors. For example, a patient with hyperfunctioning parathyroid hyperplasia and a pancreatic gastrinoma may be entirely asymptomatic (penetrance of the inherited trait is proven by the findings of hypercalcemia, increased parathyroid hormone concentration, gastric hypersecretion and hypergastrinemia), whereas the affected sibling or offspring may have the same abnormal biochemical changes but also have symptomatic renal stones and peptic ulcers.

The pathogenesis of the MEA-I syndrome is still not defined. Although several hypotheses have been advanced,[9] Wermer's original hypothesis of a defect in a dominant pleiotrophic (effecting change in more than one character) autosomal gene remains attractive.[26] Pleiotropism, the genetic process which leads to involvement of a characteristic group of endocrine tissues, is compatible with Pearse's theory that the endocrine cells of the gut are cell derivatives of the neural crest and are thus both neuroectodermal and, strictly speaking, neuroendocrine.

GENERAL FEATURES

The clinical features of the MEA-I syndrome depend on the number and combinations of endocrine glands that are involved. The basic features of the syndrome are outlined in Table 17-1. These features are further detailed in the respective chapters covering the pathology of each endocrine gland. The incidence of the MEA-I syndrome is unknown but surely is more common than generally appreciated. A review in one institution of all patients admitted during a 10-year period with pituitary, parathyroid, or islet cell tumors documented five MEA-I kindreds.[28] The parathyroids, islets of Langerhans and pituitary are the primary endocrine glands involved in the MEA-I syndrome. There is frequently hyperplasia of the adrenal cortices, but the adrenal lesions usually do not cause clinical symptoms. Benign thyroid tumors have been

Table 17-1. Primary Endocrinopathies in MEA-I Syndrome

Endocrine System	*Hormone*	*Primary Biologic Action*	*Effects of Endocrine Hyperfunction*
Parathyroids			
Chief cell (usual) Oxyphil cell (occasional) Water-clear cell (rare)	Parathyrin (PTH)	↑ Serum calcium ↓ Serum phosphorus	Weakness, easy fatigability, bone pains, generalized decalcification, nephrocalcinosis and nephrolithiasis
Pancreas			
"Alpha-1" cell of pancreatic islets	Gastrin	↑ Gastric acid secretion	Gastric hypersecretion, peptic ulcer disease, diarrhea may result from excessive gastric secretions
Beta-cell of pancreatic islets	Insulin	↓ Blood sugar	Hypoglycemia (epinephrine release) Sweating Hunger Tremor Tachycardia Cerebral glucose deprivation Disorientation Incoherent speech Blurred vision Convulsions Coma
Cell type Not defined	Diarrheogenic hormone 1. Vasoactive inhibitory peptide (VIP) 2. Gastrointestinal inhibitory peptide (GIP) 3. Secretin	Stimulates water and electrolyte secretion into gut (usually associated inhibition of gastric secretion)	Watery diarrhea—frequently associated with hypokalemia and gastric hyposecretion
Pituitary			
Cell types Chromophobe Acidophilic Basophilic May be nonfunctioning or hyperfunctioning tumor(s)	1. Growth hormone (GH) 2. Prolactin (PRL) 3. Adrenocorticotrophic hormone (ACTH)	Growth of bone, cartilage and connective tissue Promotes lactation Promotes adrenocortical function	Acromegaly Galactorrhea, amenorrhea Cushing's disease

reported; however, the evidence is not convincing that they are part of the inherited syndrome. Carcinoid tumors of the jejunum, ileum or bronchi may be present, but functioning carcinoid tumors are rare. Nonendocrine tumors also have been reported. These nonendocrine lesions are subcutaneous and visceral lipomas, benign buccal mucosal tumors and multiple polyps of the colon.

HYPERPARATHYROIDISM

Clinical Features

Modern studies of families with MEA-I indicate that the parathyroid glands are involved in more than 90 percent of affected patients.[12,14,21,22] The hyperparathyroidism is often mild and the patient asymptomatic. Unless screening tests are performed, this endocrine disorder may become apparent only after the appearance of renal calculi or complications of gastric hypersecretion in the third or fourth decade. Symptoms of hyperparathyroidism in patients with the MEA-I syndrome are similar to those of the ordinary clinical forms of hyperparathyroidism except that a greater number of those with MEA-I have the "mild" form of the disease. Symptoms may be subtle and are related to the hypercalcemia. Muscle weakness, lethargy, easy fatigability, anorexia, constipation, polyuria and polydipsia are frequent complaints in symptomatic patients. Nephrocalcinosis may lead to serious impairment of renal function. Bone pains and arthralgias are related to increased bone resorption and calcium pyrophosphate deposition in the joints. The prolonged effects of parathyrin excess may cause characteristic bony changes that can be seen radiologically.

Confirmatory Laboratory Studies

The characteristic laboratory feature of hyperparathyroidism in the MEA-I syndrome is hypercalcemia. Just as in patients with the nonfamilial form of hyperparathyroidism, the serum phosphorus is usually depressed and urinary calcium excretion is increased. The differential diagnosis of hypercalcemia can be complex, but development of a radioimmunoassay to measure circulating serum parathyroid hormone (parathyrin, PTH) concentrations has been of great value. Although the measurement of parathyroid hormone by radioimmunoassay is not available in many hospitals, this test is now performed by a number of commercial laboratories. Because hyperparathyroidism generally does not require urgent surgery, it is recommended that a serum parathyroid hormone determination be obtained whenever possible to confirm the diagnosis. If an ectopic PTH-producing tumor outside the neck can be excluded, an elevated serum calcium and inappropriately elevated PTH indicates hyperfunctioning parathyroid glands. Serum parathyroid hormone should not be evaluated in terms of "normal" ranges but rather as a function of the serum calcium concentration. Using this "plot" (linear discriminate analysis), patients with even "mild" hyperparathyroidism may be discriminated from normal individuals.[18] Inappropriately elevated PTH and hypercalcemia in an MEA-I family member invariably means hyperparathyroidism and that the individual carries the MEA-I trait. A neck exploration is indicated; however, prior to operation, additional diagnostic studies as outlined in Figure 17-2 should be completed to document the status of the other endocrine glands commonly involved in the MEA-I syndrome.

Preoperative Localization Studies

Selective venous catheterization of the internal jugular veins, the smaller veins draining the area of the parathyroids and the mediastinal vessels with simultaneous collection of blood samples for measurement of parathyroid hormone concentration is a technique that has been successful in localizing parathyroid tumors preoperatively.[4,17] However, this technique is not advocated on a routine basis for hyperparathyroid patients when there has been no previous neck surgery. When hyperparathyroidism is documented in an MEA-I family member, hyperplastic changes will usually be found in more than one parathyroid gland. It is mandatory for the surgeon to identify all four glands regardless of the findings of any preoperative localization studies. Selective venous catheterization studies do have value in the patient who has had a previous unsuccessful neck exploration and in whom hypercalcemia persists. The location of a "missed-gland" as well as hyperfunctioning mediastinal tumors have been identified using this technique. (For practical reasons as well as economical, this study should be performed in referral centers.)

Selective angiography may also help to localize parathyroid lesions but potential risks mitigate against routine use. Cine-esophagrams, thermography, and selenomethionine scanning occasionally demonstrate a large parathyroid adenoma preoperatively, but these large lesions should not be missed by an experienced surgeon.[19]

Operative Management

The surgical procedure employed is a bilateral cervical exploration. A low collar incision is utilized. The platysma is divided in the line of the incision and flaps elevated superiorly to the thyroid notch and inferiorly to expose the suprasternal notch. The plane between the sternocleidomastoid muscles and the underlying strap muscles is dissected open to allow for retraction of the sternocleidomastoid muscles. The investing fascia of the neck is incised in the midline. The strap muscles are freed from the thyroid gland and divided between Bambridge clamps. The middle thyroid veins are divided and ligated bilaterally, allowing for mobilization of each thyroid lobe to expose their posterior aspects and the area of the recurrent laryngeal nerves.

Considerable controversy among surgeons exists concerning the management of the parathyroid glands in primary hyperparathyroidism. Routine excision of three parathyroid glands and a portion of the fourth in all patients has been advocated by some surgeons,[15] whereas others have shown that removal of a single adenoma is curative in more than 90 percent of hyperparathyroid patients.[19] The evidence is strong that HPT patients with a family history of parathyroid disease, gastrinomas, insulinomas and pituitary lesions usually will have hyperplasia of all four parathyroid glands.[2,21,25,28] Persistent or recurrent hypercalcemia is common when the surgeon removes only one enlarged parathyroid gland in the hyperparathyroid patient with a family history of the MEA-I syndrome.

For these reasons, identification of all four parathyroid glands is imperative in hyperparathyroid patients with the MEA-I syndrome or family history of MEA-I. After identifying all four glands, the surgeon can best assess the situation and decide on an operative strategy. When all four parathyroids are obviously enlarged and hyperplastic, three parathyroid glands and enough of the fourth gland are removed leaving only enough parathyroid tissue to provide a normal level of parathyroid hormone. Before the surgeon removes any parathyroids, he should identify all the glands and then tentatively select the gland of which a portion will be left to maintain function. The gland should be selected on the basis that a part can be left with an adequate vascular supply. Selection of an inferior gland may be advantageous because it is surgically accessible with less risk to the recurrent laryngeal nerves in the event that a secondary neck exploration is necessary because of persistent hypercalcemia. If the surgeon sees that the piece of parathyroid tissue is of questionable viability or the tissue infarcted, this remnant of parathyroid tissue is removed and one of the other parathyroid glands can be used to fashion the remnant of tissue that will be left.

On occasion, two or three glands may be very large and the remaining gland very normal in appearance and size. Removal of one-half or three-quarters of the remaining small gland may not be necessary. The important factor is to leave only enough viable tissue that approximates a normal parathyroid; however, the surgeon should biopsy the gland to confirm the impression that the tissue is indeed a parathyroid. Such biopsies are done with a small iris scissors, excising only a small 1 to 3-mm. tip of the parathyroid gland on the end away from the vascular supply.

Postoperative Management

Postoperative hypocalcemia occurs more frequently in patients with parathyroid hyperplasia who require three and a portion of a fourth gland resected than after excision of a single adenoma, which is the usual situation in nonfamilial hyperparathyroidism. There is no difference in the treatment of postoperative hypocalcemia in MEA-I patients than in those who develop hypocalcemia after single gland resection. When early postoperative symptoms of hypocalcemia such as parasthesias and perioral numbness are associated with a positive Trousseau's sign and progressively falling serum calcium, oral calcium supplements are started. Intravenous calcium is rarely needed except for overt tetany. One or two tablespoons of calcium glubionate syrup before meals and at bedtime usually prevents symptoms (each 15 ml. contains 8.4 g. calcium glubionate and 345 mg. calcium). Calcium tablets or wafers may be used in lieu of the calcium syrup preparation. During the first week, the patient is carefully monitored for signs of tetany, and serum calcium is determined daily. The oral calcium supplements may be progressively decreased as the serum calcium concentration returns to normal. If symptoms of hypocalcemia recur or the serum calcium is not maintained at near-normal concentrations as the oral calcium is decreased, oral vitamin-D is added to the oral calcium regime. The amounts of vitamin-D required to maintain a near-normal calcium varies with each individual. Usual doses of calciferol (vitamin-D_2) range from 100,000 to 400,000 units daily. The peak effect from oral vitamin-D and calcium may occur after several days to weeks. Weekly serum calcium determinations are obtained and the oral calcium supplements adjusted. After all oral calcium has been gradually discontinued, the vitamin-D may be decreased. The effect of vitamin-D may continue for several weeks. These patients should be monitored on a weekly basis for several months after calcium and vitamin-D supplements have been stopped.

PANCREATIC ISLET-CELL TUMORS

The clinical manifestations of the pancreatic islet cell tumors usually surface after signs of hyperparathyroidism have been present for a number of years. Islet cell tumors have been documented in approximately 50 percent of patients with the MEA-I syndrome; however, this may be a conservative estimate. When case reports from older generations are studied and autopsy material is available, 85 percent of those patients so studied will be found to have had pancreatic lesions.[2] When younger patients in MEA-I families are screened and the inherited trait is thought to be present because hypercalcemia and elevated parathormone concentrations are found, the incidence of functioning islet cell tumors is far less than 50 percent,[12,21,28] but the incidence increases as these patients grow older.

The pancreatic tumors may be benign adenomas or carcinomas. These lesions may be single or multiple. Islet cell hyperplasia or microadenomatosis may be the only pathology, or these changes may be associated with larger tumors. Non-beta islet cell tumors releasing excessive amounts of gastrin are the most common. Beta-cell tumors which release insulin are the second most common type of hyperfunctioning tumor. It is of interest to note that in several MEA-I families, the affected members may only develop insulinomas; however, gastrinomas predominate in most genealogies.[9,12,21,28] On occasion, the islet cell tumor may be composed of both cell types and elaborate both gastrin and insulin.[9,13,28] Pancreatic tumors secreting a diarrheogenic hormone or glucagon have been reported, but these syndromes are rare in families with the MEA-I trait.[9,28]

Gastrinoma

Clinical Features

The clinical manifestation of gastrin-secreting tumors are secondary to gastric hypersecretion.[27] Hypergastrinemia per se does not cause symptoms. Analogous to the "mild" form of hyperparathyroidism that has been documented in many MEA-I families, there appears to be a "mild" form of hypergastrinemia as well as a more severe form associated with peptic ulcer diathesis.[12,22,28] Gastric hypersecretion is the hallmark of gastrinomas and patients will usually present with pain related to peptic ulcer disease. A duodenal ulcer can be documented in most individuals. Bleeding, obstruction and perforation are complications that invariably occur; however, perhaps one in four patients experiences symptoms for more than 5 years before seeking medical help.[27] Diarrhea may be the complaint although peptic ulcer symptoms are usually associated. Indeed, the patient who presents with diarrhea and evidence of hyperparathyroidism should be considered to harbor a coexisting gastrinoma until proven otherwise.

Wermer has maintained that there are two distinct gastrinoma entities: the nonfamilial, sporadic form of the Z-E syndrome in which individuals with gastrinomas have no associated endocrine disorders, and the familial form in which individuals with gastrinomas have associated parathyroid and pituitary tumors.[26] A recent study supports this concept in that those patients with gastrinomas without associated endocrinopathies had no family history of multiple endocrinopathies, whereas those gastrinoma patients with parathyroid and pituitary tumors invariably had relatives with endocrinopathies when families were adequately screened.[12] Hypergastrinemia occurs in both forms, hence the gastrointestinal symptomatology is indistinguishable. The practical aspect of this concept is obvious; if confirmed, associated endocrine dysfunction in patients with gastrinoma means a familial disorder.

Confirmatory Laboratory Tests

Gastric Analysis. The single most important study for detecting gastrinomas is the gastric analysis. After an overnight fast, the 1-hour basal acid output (BAO) is recorded. An augmented gastric acid stimulation using subcutaneous histamine (0.04 mg./kg.) or pentagastrin (6 μg./kg.) is then done which allows calculation of the maximal acid output (MAO) and peak acid output (PAO). The latter are indirect measurements of parietal cell mass. More than 85 percent of patients harboring a gastrinoma will have a BAO>15 mEq. per hour. A BAO greater than 60 percent of the MAO is also suggestive of the diagnosis. No one secretory criterion is infallible.[28]

Serum Immunoreactive Gastrin. "Normal" values for fasting serum gastrin will vary somewhat depending on the immunoassay technique. Most laboratories report normal ranges for serum gastrin concentration from 50 to 150 pg./ml. and some up to 300 pg./ml. Patients with gastrinomas generally have gastrin concentrations greater than 500 pg./ml., most greater than 1,000 pg./ml.[10,28] Hypergastrinemia (greater than 750 pg./ml.) and basal hypersecretion (BAO greater than 15 mEq. per hr.) is diagnostic of a gastrinoma. A "mild" and frequently asymptomatic form of hypergastrinemia has been documented in several MEA-I kindreds.[12,22] These individuals usually have biochemical evidence of associated hyperparathyroidism. Gastric analysis will show gastric hypersecretion. When the serum gastrin is less than 1,000 pg./ml., and additional confimatory evidence for gastrinoma is required, a secretin provocative test is indicated.

Secretin Provocative Tests. Serum gastrin is depressed or unchanged after the intravenous infusion of secretin (two units per kg. of GIH secretin*) in patients with ordinary duodenal ulcer disease or in those conditions associated with increases in serum gastrin such as pernicious anemia, gastritis, gastric outlet obstruction, G-cell hyperplasia or the retained antral segment syndrome. Paradoxically, in patients harboring a gastrinoma, secretin infusion causes an increase in the serum gastrin.[10] The calcium infusion test and standardized test meals are other provocative tests. The secretin infusion test is safe, simple, reliable and practical for evaluating patients with the MEA-I syndrome.[12]

Gastrointestinal Roentgenograms. Characteristic roentgenographic features of

---

*Gastrointestinal Hormone Research Laboratory, Karolinoka Institute, Stockholm, Sweden.

large gastric rugal folds, peptic ulcers in atypical locations, duodenitis, jejunitis and rapid small bowel transit may be present in patients with gastrinomas; however, most will exhibit only those findings usually seen in duodenal ulcer patients. Many of the MEA-I individuals with the latent or "mild" form of hypergastrinemia have normal studies.

Gastrointestinal Endoscopy. Endoscopy may show peptic ulceration and gastric hyper-rugosity not seen on roentgenologic studies. When an ulcer is accompanied by hypergastrinemia, a gastrinoma is likely. Duodenal wall, islet-cell tumors have been reported in 5 to 10 percent of Z-E patients. An alert endoscopist may occasionally document such a tumor preoperatively.

When the diagnosis of gastrinoma is confirmed, an exploratory celiotomy is indicated in all but the "mild" forms. This latter group of asymptomatic patients presents an unresolved therapeutic dilemma, since longitudinal studies are not available. The natural history is unknown. Prior to surgery, selective celiac angiography should be performed. Although gastrinomas are less vascular than insulinomas, some reports indicate that 50 percent may be documented by angiography.[10,28] Because MEA-I individuals with gastrinomas have a greater incidence of microadenomatosis, the number of tumors visualized will be less than 50 percent. Nevertheless, an angiographic study is still indicated because it may help to locate the tumor(s) and may provide evidence for multiple or metastatic lesions (pancreas and liver) not readily apparent at operation.

Operative Management

Intraoperative management of an MEA-I patient suspected of harboring a gastrinoma is not different from that for a patient with gastrinoma (Z-E syndrome) without other endocrinopathies. Successful management depends on localizing and defining the extent of the gastrin-secreting tumor.

The abdomen is explored through a long midline incision. The body and tail of the pancreas are visualized after opening the lesser sac. Incision of the peritoneum along the superior and inferior borders of the distal pancreatic body and tail allow the surgeon to insert his fingers behind the pancreas and bimanually palpate the pancreas looking for tumors. A Kocher maneuver mobilizes the duodenum and head of the pancreas for inspection and palpation. Multiple lymph node biopsies (peripancreatic, duodenal and mesenteric nodes) are most important and should be done as the surgeon proceeds with the exploration. A concerted effort to find tumor will almost always reward the surgeon. Small, submucosal, duodenal wall tumors may be palpated. When the presence of tumor cannot be proven, resection of the tail of the pancreas may be necessary to document small tumors, microadenomatosis, or islet cell hyperplasia.

Prior to the advent of radioimmunoassay techniques to measure gastrin in peripheral blood, a tissue diagnosis was crucial before proceeding with a total gastrectomy. When gastrin concentrations are clearly elevated, gastric hypersecretion is documented (BAO>15 mEq. per hour) and the intravenous secretin test provokes the characteristic paradoxical rise in blood gastrin, total gastrectomy may be warranted even without a tissue diagnosis. Total gastrectomy, also might be justified without a tissue diagnosis, when a patient with a family history of MEA-I has these criteria and requires emergency surgery to control a complication of gastric hypersecretion (i.e., GI hemorrhage or perforation).

The tumor may be benign or malignant and even the benign lesions are frequently multiple. Experience indicates that fewer than one in four patients with gastrinoma will have a single tumor.[27] Multiple tumor sites or metastatic disease preclude complete tumor excision in most patients. The surgeon must remove all of the gastrinoma(s) or all of the stomach. Since complete removal of the gastrinoma(s) is unlikely, total gastrectomy is the recommended procedure in most situations.[6] Radical pancreaticoduodenectomy (Whipple's operation) is rarely curative. Total pancreatectomy in conjunction with total gastrectomy is not recommended. The potential added benefit of removing all of the tumor (unlikely) does not outweigh the nutritional problems of a patient without a stomach and a pancreas.

Following total gastrectomy, gastrointestinal continuity is reestablished with a Roux-en-Y, retrocolic loop of jejunum and an end-to-side esophagojejunostomy. The surgeon may be tempted to leave a small cuff or proximal gastric mucosa to facilitate the anastomosis. This step is to be condemned since even a small 1-cm. residual segment of gastric mucosa may result in recurrent ulceration and bleeding. The surgeon should have biopsy confirmation of esophageal mucosa indicating complete excision of the stomach. A jejunal pouch may be fashioned as a substitute stomach.[5] Operative mortality of total gastrectomy has been high particularly when the procedure is done as an emergency in a bleeding patient.[27] Elective total gastrectomy, however, should have less than a 5-percent mortality rate. Anastomotic leak is the most frequent operative complication of total gastrectomy. Prophylactic drainage of the esophageal anastomosis and placement of a distal feeding jejunostomy may prove lifesaving. A small leak can then be managed conservatively. The patient is fed a blenderized diet through the jejunostomy tube until radiologic studies confirm closure of the anastomotic leak. Following discharge from the hospital, close supervision and regular follow-up is mandatory. Weight loss or signs of esophageal stricture should prompt immediate hospitalization. Vitamin B_{12} injections at 1- to 3-month intervals are required for life. Oral iron, vitamins, calcium and pancreatic supplements may be necessary. Serum gastrin determinations may provide evidence of tumor progression and the possible need for chemotherapy.

Special Situation—Hyperparathyroidism and Coexisting Gastrinoma

The patient with hyperparathyroidism may present with signs or symptoms that suggest a coexisting gastrinoma. Peptic ulcer disease, gastrointestinal bleeding and diarrhea should alert the physician. Frequently, the preoperative diagnostic studies will document hypergastrinemia and gastric hypersecretion. A secretin provocative test for gastrin response will confirm the presence of a gastrinoma in most patients even when fasting gastrin concentrations are borderline.[12] The surgeon may proceed first with parathyroidectomy when the patient is not in trouble from the sequelae of gastric hypersecretion. Parathyroidectomy has been reported to decrease gastric hypersecretion in some patients; however, follow-up of successfully treated hyperparathyroid patients with evidence of coexisting gastrinoma indicates that when gastric hypersecretion and hypergastrinemia was present before parathyroidectomy, these findings usually persist after parathyroidectomy.[28,29] Gastric hypersecretion may be temporarily reduced as the result of transient hypocalcemia following parathyroidectomy, but as the calcium returns to normal levels, gastric hypersecretion recurs.

An abdominal exploration to confirm the gastrinoma follows after parathyroidectomy. The time of this interval depends on the problems the patient is experiencing from the gastric hypersecretion. When the patient has "mild" or equivocal hypergastrinemia, no symptoms or evidence of ulcer and has had no complications, a period of observation with periodic gastrin determinations and gastric analyses may be warranted. Histamine H_2-receptor antagonists may prove useful in controlling the gastric hypersecretion in these patients in the future. The physician should temper thoughts of conservatism with the knowledge that complications of gastric hypersecretion, primarily hemorrhage, have been the leading cause of death in the MEA-I syndrome.

Insulinoma

Clinical Features

The clinical manifestations of insulinomas are caused by the excessive or inappropriate release of insulin which results in hypoglycemia. The hypoglycemic episodes may result in very subtle or dramatic symptoms depending on how fast and how low blood glucose falls. Sweating, weakness, tremor, tachycardia and blurring of vision are frequent complaints which occur when the blood glucose falls rapidly, stimulating epinephrine release by the adrenal glands. A more profound lowering of the blood glucose may give rise to syncopal attacks, disorientation, bizarre behavior, convulsions or coma. Fasting or exercise may precipitate hypoglycemia episodes, and these patients often learn that drinking or eating foods with sugars will abort the attacks. Some individuals with insulinomas have been erroneously treated for neurologic or psychiatric disorders.

Confirmatory Laboratory Tests

Fasting Plasma Glucose. Plasma concentrations less than 40 mg./dl. suggest hyperinsulinism. Repeat determinations are obtained on several days. Extending the fasting period beyond the usual 12 hours may be necessary. When symptoms of hypoglycemia, an associated low plasma glucose and relief of symptoms after administration of glucose (Whipple's triad) have been demonstrated, associated increases in the serum insulin should be documented if the hypoglycemia is to be attributed to hyperinsulinism.

Simultaneous Plasma Glucose and Serum Immunoreactive Insulin (IRI) Determinations. Simultaneous determinations of plasma glucose and serum IRI allows discrimination of those patients with an insulinoma from those with noninsulin-mediated hypoglycemia. The glucose/insulin ratios provide reliable diagnostic criteria for an insulinoma.[3,20]

Intravenous Tolbutamide Test. Certain agents will stimulate the release of insulin from the beta cells. In the case of an insulinoma, excessive amounts of insulin are released. Simultaneous measurements of circulating plasma glucose and serum IRI after an injection of 1 g. of sodium tolbutamide over a 2-minute period provide additional evidence for insulinoma(s) if glucose/insulin ratios are not diagnostic. Blood samples are collected at 15- to 30-minute intervals for 3 hours. The glucose and insulin responses with calculation of a ratio allow for discrimination. A physician should monitor this test, since some patients develop marked hypoglycemia requiring glucose administration and termination of the test.

Proinsulin. A small number of patients with characteristic signs, symptoms, and pathologic findings of beta-cell tumors have been described in whom serum insulin concentrations determined by the usual radioimmunoassay techniques were not inappropriately elevated. Further studies in these patients have shown abnormally high proinsulin concentrations.[1,9,28] The physician should be aware of the potential situation of a "proinsulin-secreting" tumor. Some insulin assays will not detect the proinsulin component. When the history and findings of hyperinsulinism are characteristic, yet immunoreactive insulin concentrations are not elevated, special immunoassays that recognize proinsulin may be required.

Selective Arteriography. When the clinical and biochemical diagnoses of insulinoma have been confirmed, selective celiac arteriography should be performed before surgery. Insulinomas are generally quite vascular lesions, and not surprisingly, selective angiographic techniques have been reported to successfully localize the insulinoma(s) in 50 to 90 percent of cases.[3,9,20] However, these reports primarily concern nonfamilial cases of insulinoma. Hyperinsulinism in MEA-I families is associated with a greater incidence of multiple adenomas, microadenomatosis and diffuse islet cell hyperplasia so that the overall success rate of arteriography will be less than that reported for nonfamilial insulinomas. Small pancreatic lesions that the surgeon might easily overlook are frequently localized.

Operative Management

Insulinomas are single and benign in 80 to 90 percent of patients, so that complete tumor excision will be successful in most situations.[3,20] However, these optimistic reports may not apply directly to the MEA-I patient with an insulinoma because there is a greater tendency for multiple adenomas.[9] Exploration and localization techniques are similar to those described for gastrinomas. Simple enucleation may remove single benign lesions in the head. Multiple or single lesions in the body and tail may be removed with a distal pancreatectomy. Rarely, a large, deep-seated tumor in the head may require a pancreaticoduodenectomy (Whipple's operation). When tumor(s) cannot be found, blind distal pancreatic resection is warranted, since small occult tumors measuring less than 1.0 cm. or microadenomatosis may be present. Total pancreatectomy is not indicated as an initial procedure.

Intraoperative blood glucose monitoring may help to assure the surgeon that no additional tumors remain after excision of a primary lesion. Complete tumor removal should be followed within 30 minutes by a hyperglycemia rebound or sustained increase in blood glucose. False-positive hyperglycemic rebound can occur.

Drains should be placed leading to the site of tumor enucleation or stump of resected pancreas. Pancreatic fistulas are thus controlled. These fistulas usually stop draining in 1 to 2 weeks. Drains are not to be removed before the tenth day and may remain longer if a pancreatic fistula persists.

Postoperative Management

Postoperative hyperglycemia is common for several days following the successful removal of an insulinoma. Elevations in blood glucose may persist for longer periods when major resections are necessary. Small amounts of insulin may be required during the first several days if blood glucose exceeds 250 to 300 mg./dl.

Follow-up statistics for insulinomas limited to MEA-I patients are not available, but postoperative hyperinsulinism might be expected more often because multiple tumors and microadenomas are more common. Reoperation may be necessary when simple enucleation fails. Diazoxide is a thiazide compound that has been useful in circumstances of persistent or "mild" hyperinsulinism and in the rare situations when the patient harbors an unresectable beta-cell carcinoma with metastases. Diazoxide interferes with the release of insulin and may aid in maintaining a normoglycemic state; however, this drug has no effect on the tumor. Streptozotocin is an antibiotic with relatively greater toxicity for pancreatic beta cells. This drug has toxic side effects but may inhibit growth or cause regression of malignant insulinomas.

PITUITARY TUMORS

Clinical Features and Confirmatory Laboratory Studies

The manifestations of pituitary tumors in the MEA-I syndrome depend on the growth and size of the pituitary lesion, compression or invasion of adjacent structures and the effects of any hormones that are secreted. Modern studies of large kindreds affected with the MEA-I syndrome show that less than 30 percent of those subjects with the trait have evidence of a pituitary lesion clinically.[12,14,22,28] However, the true incidence of pituitary abnormalities is probably much greater. Ballard's 1964 review included 74 MEA-I cases reported in the literature, many of which were autopsied cases, and the incidence of pituitary tumors was 65 percent.[2]

The tumors arise from the anterior pituitary gland and are classified according to the staining characteristics of the secretory granules into chromophobe, acidophil and basophil types. More than one cell type may be found in a pituitary tumor; however, the chromophobe adenomas are the most common. Varying degrees of hypopituitarism may occur as the result of the mechanical effects of pressure on endocrine-secreting cells of the pituitary. It is unusual for the deficiencies to be complete. Studies frequently show growth hormone and gonadotrophic deficiency and, less often, ACTH and thyroid deficiency. In conjunction with such endocrine abnormalities, this type of pituitary tumor may exhibit clinical manifestations because of compression on neighboring structures. The structures most frequently affected are the optic chiasm with the resultant visual field abnormalities or compression of the cavernous sinus with secondary cranial nerve palsies and diplopia.

Pituitary tumors that secrete excessive amounts of hormone(s) may result in some dramatic syndromes including the following.

1. Growth Hormone (GH) Excess. Acromegaly is the syndrome resulting from GH excess and is manifested by excessive growth of facial and acral parts, articular problems secondary to bony and cartilaginous overgrowth, increase in connective tissue mass and cardiomegaly. Gigantism occurs when excess growth hormone production occurs before puberty.

2. Hyperprolactinemia (PRL). Modern immunoassay techniques indicate that this syndrome may be the most common hypersecreting pituitary tumor syndrome, but it is not always apparent to the physician. Prolactin promotes lactation; however, not all patients with hyperprolactinemia have galactorrhea. Galactorrhea rarely may be the presenting symptom of pituitary tumors in men. In women, nonpuerperal galactorrhea, amenorrhea and low urinary FSH are characteristic (Forbes-Albright syndrome).

3. ACTH Excess. The clinical features are caused by hypercortisolism (Cushing's syndrome) resulting from chronic adrenal stimulation. Easy bruising of the skin, osteoporosis, body fat redistributed to the face and trunk, abdominal stria, hirsutism and catabolic effects of glucocorticoids are the primary features.

4. Rare Types. Pituitary lesions that secrete excess amounts of follicle-stimulating hormone (FSH), thyrotropin (TSH), and melanocyte-stimulating hormone (MSH) have been reported but these are rare and when present are usually associated with GH-, PRL- or ACTH-secreting tumors.

Surgical and Irradiation Management

The primary methods for pituitary tumor ablation are surgery and irradiation. The choice of therapy depends on the tumor type and the expertise available at the treatment center. Pituitary tumors may be removed surgically through a transsphenoidal or transfrontal approach. The transsphenoidal approach utilizing microdissecting techniques is advantageous for small hyperfunctioning adenomas frequently found in the MEA-I syndrome. Mortality for this procedure is low and residual brain damage is rare. Supervoltage irradiation, proton-beam irradiation, and transnasal or transethmoidal implantation of radioactive seeds are the different modes of radiation management that have been used. A major disadvantage of radiation therapy is the frequent delay of weeks to several months for desired effects after therapy has begun.

ADRENAL AND MISCELLANEOUS LESIONS

Functioning adrenal tumors are not common in the MEA-I syndrome; however, adrenocortical hyperplasia has been documented in 30 to 50 percent of autopsied cases.[2,9,28] Plasma cortisol and plasma ACTH determinations should be obtained in MEA-I individuals with proven parathyroid, pancreatic, or pituitary tumors. Cushing's syndrome can be the result of a pituitary tumor-secreting ACTH or the ectopic production of an ACTH-like substance by a malignant islet cell pancreatic tumor.[7,28] Appropriate diagnostic studies should be performed to differentiate the source of excess ACTH before any surgical procedure is undertaken.

A variety of polypeptide hormones and amines may be secreted by tumors of the APUD cell series of the gut. Malignant pancreatic islet cell tumors, whether they be of the sporadic or of the familial type, have the potential for secreting one or more hormones. Potential hormones from such lesions include gastrin, insulin, ACTH, melanocyte-stimulating hormone, parathyroid hormone, glucagon, gastrointestinal inhibitory peptide and serotonin.[7,9,10,28] Pancreatic tumors that secrete ectopic or multiple hormones are usually malignant and most aggressive. The prognosis for these patients is poor.[27]

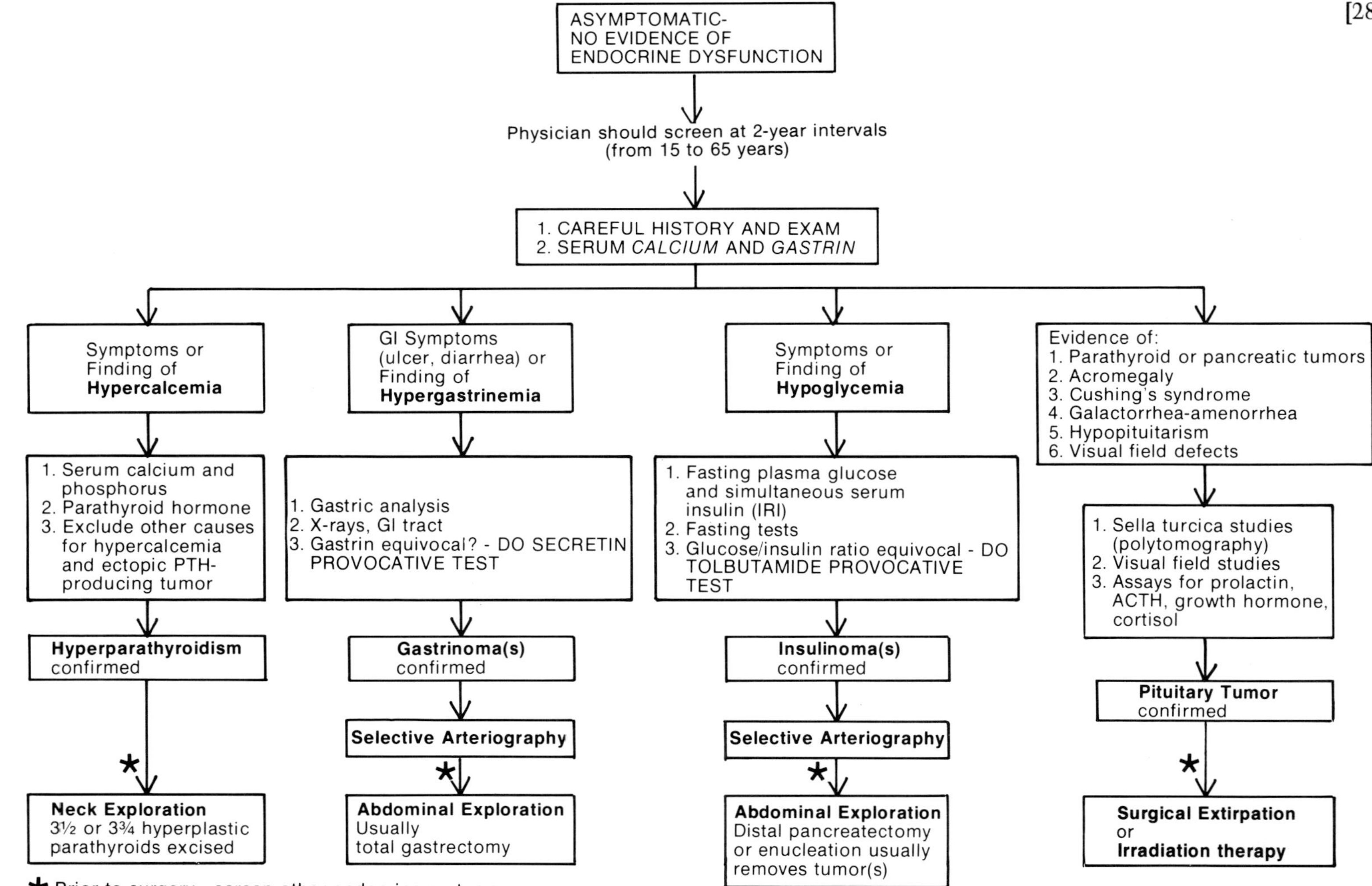

Fig. 17-2. Screening procedure for MEA-I family member.

Screening the Asymptomatic Relative

The most important diagnostic tool is a careful history (see Fig. 17-2). The usual symptomatic patient affected with the MEA-I trait presents with signs, symptoms, or sequelae of hypercalcemia or gastric hypersecretion. The family history may indicate relatives with ulcer disease, renal stones, or recognized parathyroid, pancreatic, or pituitary tumors.

From a practical point of view, screening tests for the asymptomatic relative may be kept to a minimum. In the absence of any signs or symptoms of specific endocrinopathies, a serum calcium, phosphorus and radioimmunoassay for serum gastrin concentration should single out those "asymptomatic" adult family members who have inherited the MEA-I trait. Determinations of fasting blood sugar and immunoreactive insulin are not likely to be abnormal in a family member who has been well, has no symptoms of hypoglycemia and no evidence of other endocrine disorders. If serum calcium and gastrin values are normal and there are no clinical findings indicating a pituitary disorder, pituitary screening tests are not required on a routine basis. Screening tests for pituitary tumors should be done when studies indicate parathyroid or islet-cell pathology.

FOLLOW-UP PROGRAMS

The individual with a documented endocrinopathy, and a family history of the MEA-I syndrome should be considered affected with the inherited trait. This individual must have yearly follow-up examinations for life. The natural history of patients affected with this inherited syndrome is not well defined. Longitudinal studies are not yet available. The pattern of endocrinopathies reported to date suggest that the primary endocrine organs involved, the parathyroids, islets of Langerhans and the pituitary usually will develop pathologic changes if the patient survives into the sixth and seventh decade. The tumors may not be hyperfunctioning and thus not clinically apparent.

The "recurrence rate" of hyperparathyroidism in the MEA-I syndrome is several times that reported after parathyroidectomy in the nonfamilial form of primary hyperparathyroidism. This "recurrence" may be a misnomer and "persistent" hyperparathyroidism might be a more appropriate term. This high failure rate in patients with the MEA-I syndrome is related to the frequent involvement of all four parathyroids and the surgeon's failure to adequately remove enough of the hyperfunctioning parathyroid tissue.

There have been several examples of patients with pancreatic tumors secreting one peptide-hormone who after appropriate treatment (i.e., partial pancreatectomy for insulinoma) returned several years later with symptoms of another pancreatic tumor elaborating a second and different hormone (i.e., gastrin).[7,9,28] A yearly follow-up exam is mandatory once endocrine dysfunction is documented with an awareness that hyperfunction of the other endocrine glands is likely to surface.

REFERENCES

1. Alsever, R. N., Roberts, J. P., Gerber, J. G., Mako, M. E., and Rubinstein, A. H.: Insulinoma with low circulating insulin levels: the diagnostic value of proinsulin measurements. Ann. Intern. Med., *82*:347, 1975.

2. Ballard, H. S., Frame, B., and Hartstock, R. J.: Familial multiple endocrine adenoma-peptic ulcer complex. Medicine, *43*:481, 1964.
3. Edis, A. J., et al.: Insulinoma—current diagnosis and surgical management. *In* Ravitch, M. M. (ed.): Current Problems in Surgery. Chicago, Year Book Med. Publishers, 1976.
4. Eisenberg, H., Pallotta, J., and Sherwood, L. M.: Selective arteriography, venography, and venous hormone assay in diagnosis and localization of parathyroid lesions. Am. J. Med., *56*:810, 1974.
5. Fox, P. S., Hofmann, J. W., Wilson, S. D., and DeCosse, J. J.: Surgical management of the Zollinger-Ellison syndrome. Surg. Clin. North Am., *54*:395, 1974.
6. ——: The influence of total gastrectomy on survival in malignant Zollinger-Ellison tumors. Ann. Surg., *180*:558, 1974.
7. Friesen, S. R., and McGuigan, J. E.: Ectopic apudocarcinomas and associated endocrine hyperplasias of the foregut. Ann. Surg., *182*:371, 1975.
8. Friesen, S. R., Schimke, R. N., and Pearse, A. G. E.: Genetic aspects of the Z-E syndrome: prospective studies in two kindred, antral gastrin cell hyperplasia. Ann. Surg., *176*:370, 1972.
9. Harrison, T. S., and Thompson, N. W.: Multiple endocrine adenomatosis, I and II. *In* Ravitch, M. E. (ed.): Current Problems in Surgery. Chicago, Year Book Med. Publishers, 1972.
10. Isenberg, J. I., Walsh, J. H., and Grossman, M. I.: Zollinger-Ellison syndrome. Gastroenterology, *65*:140, 1973.
11. Johnson, G. J., Summerskill, W. H. J., Anderson, V. E., and Keating, F. R.: Clinical and genetic investigation of a large kindred with multiple endocrine adenomatosis. New Engl. J. Med., *277*:1379, 1967.
12. Lamers, C. B. H. W.: Some aspects of the Zollinger-Ellison syndrome and serum gastrin. Thesis for Ph.D. in Medicine. The Netherlands, The Catholic University of Nijmegen, 1976.
13. Larsson, L. I., et al.: Mixed endocrine pancreatic tumors producing several peptide hormones. Am. J. Pathol., *79*:271, 1975.
14. Marx, S. J., et al.: Familial hyperparathyroidism, mild hypercalcemia in at least nine members of a kindred. Ann. Intern. Med., *78*:371, 1973.
15. Paloyan E., Lawrence, A. M., and Straus, F. H.: Hyperparathyroidism. New York, Grune & Stratton, 1973.
16. Pearse, A. G. E., and Polak, J. M.: Neural crest origin of the endocrine polypeptide cells of the gastrointestinal tract and pancreas. Gut, *12*:783, 1971.
17. Powell, D.: Primary hyperparathyroidism: preoperative tumor localization and differentiation between adenoma and hyperplasia. New Engl. J. Med., *286*:1169, 1972.
18. Purnell, D. C., et al.: Treatment of primary hyperparathyroidism. Am. J. Med., *56*:800, 1974.
19. Satava, R. M., Jr., Beahrs, O. H., and Scholz, D. A.: Success rate of cervical exploration for hyperparathyroidism. Arch. Surg., *110*:625, 1975.
20. Shatney, C. H., and Grage, T. B.: Diagnostic and surgical aspects of insulinoma. Am. J. Surg., *127*:174, 1974.
21. Snyder, N. III, Scurry, M. T., and Deiss, W. T., Jr.: Five families with multiple endocrine adenomatosis. Ann. Intern. Med., *76*:53, 1972.
22. Snyder, N. III, Scurry, M. T., and Hughes, W.: Hypergastrinemia in familial multiple endocrine adenomatosis. Ann. Intern. Med., *80*:231, 1974.
23. Weichert, R. F. III.: Multipotential endocrine cells and the production of polyhormonal syndromes. *In* Ballinger, W. F., and Drapanus, T., (eds.): Practice of Surgery: Current Review. vol. 1, pp. 48-63. St. Louis, C. V. Mosby, 1972.
24. Wermer, P.: Genetic aspects of adenomatosis of endocrine glands. Am. J. Med., *16*:363, 1954.
25. ——: Endocrine adenomatosis and

peptic ulcer in a large kindred. Am. J. Med., *35*:205, 1963.

26. ——: Multiple endocrine adenomatosis: multiple hormone-producing tumors, a familial syndrome. *In* Bonfils, S. (ed.): Endocrine-secreting tumors of the GI tract. Clin. Gastroenterol., *3*:671, 1974.
27. Wilson, S. D.: Ulcerogenic tumors of the pancreas: the Zollinger-Ellison syndrome. *In* Carey, L. C. (ed.): The Pancreas. pp. 295-316. St. Louis, C. V. Mosby, 1973.
28. ——: Zollinger-Ellison Tumor Registry. Milwaukee, The Medical College of Wisconsin, 1976.
29. Wilson, S. D., Singh, R. B., Kalkhoff, R. K., and Go, V. L. W.: Does hyperparathyroidism cause hypergastrinemia? Surgery, *80*:231, 1976.

EDITORIAL COMMENTARY

When two or more endocrinopathies develop in a patient, either synchronously or metachronously, there is a possibility that a genetic, hereditable clinical situation exists. This familial potentiality should be distinguishable from the sporadic and rare association of coexisting multiple but unrelated endocrine tumors. Inquiry into family history and subsequent repeated screening of the family related to the patient with multiple endocrine disorders may be the only practical means of determining the genetic etiology. The key feature of the multiple endocrinopathy syndromes is **multiplicity** of **involvement** not only of several endocrine organs in predictable combinations in multiple members of a family, but also, perhaps more important, the multiple cellular distribution and bilaterality of involvement of all glands, such as the four parathyroid glands, diffuse islet changes and bilateral adrenal hyperplasias and tumors in various combinations. This multiplicity with diffuse hyperplasia (whether or not neoplasia is also present) is precisely the distinguishing feature of multiple endocrine **adenopathy** (MEA) syndromes and is thus a more satisfactory term than is multiple endocrine neoplasia (MEN) or even adenomatosis, the original descriptive term. Semantics aside, the independent development of pathologic changes in all similar cells in several endocrine organs in a familial pattern is characteristic of a pathogenesis involving pleiotropism, as propounded by Wermer. In this mechanism the pleiotropic autosomal gene is activated by the cytoplasm of cells that are capable of interacting with it; thus, all of the chief cells (or clear cells) in all four of the parathyroid glands react identically, which explains the multiplicity and bilaterality of inherited "tumors." Furthermore, the gene is pleiotropic if it can be activated by the cytoplasm of cells in more than one organ; thus endocrine cells in different organs, though not identical, may interact with the gene if they are embryologically related, as are the cells in the APUD system. It should be noted again that the parathyroid involvement in both the MEA syndromes is explainable embryologically only because of their placodal origin in the neuroectoderm, rather than derivation strictly from the neural crest.

Another theory of the pathogenesis of multiple endocrinopathies, specifically of Type I, is proposed by Vance (1972) as familial nesidioblastosis. Parenthetically, it was Laidlaw who, as early as 1938, described insulinomas as being nesidioblastomas through a process of "islet building." Vance postulated that the inherited component consists of islet cell proliferation from which humoral hyperactivity stimulates the extrapancreatic components; for instance, chronic insulin-induced hypoglycemia leads to reactive hyperplasia of the pituitary trophic cells, with possible subsequent elaboration of polypeptides by the anterior lobe of the pituitary. This theory does not fully explain the common parathyroid abnormalities in MEA in any direct mechanism. Antral G-cell hyperplasia has been observed in patients having MEA-I[8]; Larsson has reported a case of MEA in which an antropyloric "gastrinoma" was associated with pancreatic nesidioblastosis of islets (1973). Carcinoid tumors, benign and malignant, are seen in Wermer's syndrome and are found in the bronchi, pancreas and intestines which are typical locations of the EC cells in the APUD system.

This high frequency of hyperplasia in the MEA-I syndrome leads to a number of clinical modifications of the individual sporadic syndromes. For instance, in MEA (1) a greater variability of the severity of the endocrinopathy is observed, including a gamut from asymptomatic and mild presentations to crisis manifestations, (2) suppressibility without autonomy is commonly elicited, (3) failure of angiographic demonstration of endocrine "tumors" is more frequent as a consequence of diffuse hyperplasia or microadenomatosis, (4) the surgical management usually requires total or near total excision of the endocrine organ (excision of three and a half to four parathyroid glands with and without transposition, subtotal pancreatectomy, total adrenalectomy or anterior hypophysectomy, etc.), and finally (5) treatment involving disruption of abnormal feedback mechanisms may lead to the occasional possibility of reversal of the direction of cellular changes from hyperplasia to neoplasia back to hyperplasia (regression of tumor growth).

Once having made a diagnosis of an endocrinopathy involving one of the organs which might also be suspect in a multiple endocrinopathy situation, it then becomes necessary to determine whether this is a sporadic or a familial situation; the former presentation can only be ascertained usually by the exclusion of a positive family history, a positive familial screening and a long-term follow-up for exclusion of a second subsequent endocrinopathy. When a familial association is suspect, a simple screening program of serum calcium and gastrin determinations may be carried out conveniently on an annual basis; if a genetic basis of the disease is present, asymptomatic relatives will usually become apparent and/or symptomatic by the time they reach twenty years of age. Earlier identification of suspect family members, even though asymptomatic, may be possible if, in an investigative center, antral mucosal biopsies are done which demonstrate antral G-cell hyperplasia, a possible forerunner of endocrinopathies yet to come. On the other hand, the clinical onset may be dramatic with simultaneous presentation of several components of the multiple endocrinopathy. In such instances the judicious establishment of lifesaving priorities is required; the crucial choices are usually between management of the hypercalcemic crisis and the impending jejunal ulcer perforation.

Pituitary involvement in MEA-I, probably occurs at a higher incidence than is clinically recognized; such enlargements are sometimes discovered only at the time of postmortem examination rather than by radiologic demonstration of an enlarged sella turcica. As is being learned since the more routine use of the transphenoidal surgical approach, microadenomas of the anterior pituitary lobe may be found. Furthermore, even the chromophobe tumors with apparent hypopituitarism are now being observed to be associated with increased levels of prolactin secretion because of greater availability of assays for prolactin.

Adrenocortical hyperplasia and tumors, often bilateral, with hypersecretion of glucocorticoids (Cushing's syndrome) and of aldosterone (Conn's syndrome) are occasionally observed in MEA-I; on the other hand, adrenal medullary hyperplasia and tumor, often bilateral, with hypersecretion of catechalomines, are observed in MEA-II. The cortical involvement may be due to anterior pituitary or ectopic stimulation rather than to a genetic or embryologic basis; the medullary changes are strictly genetic and embryologic, the cells being classic members of the APUD system. *S.R.F.*

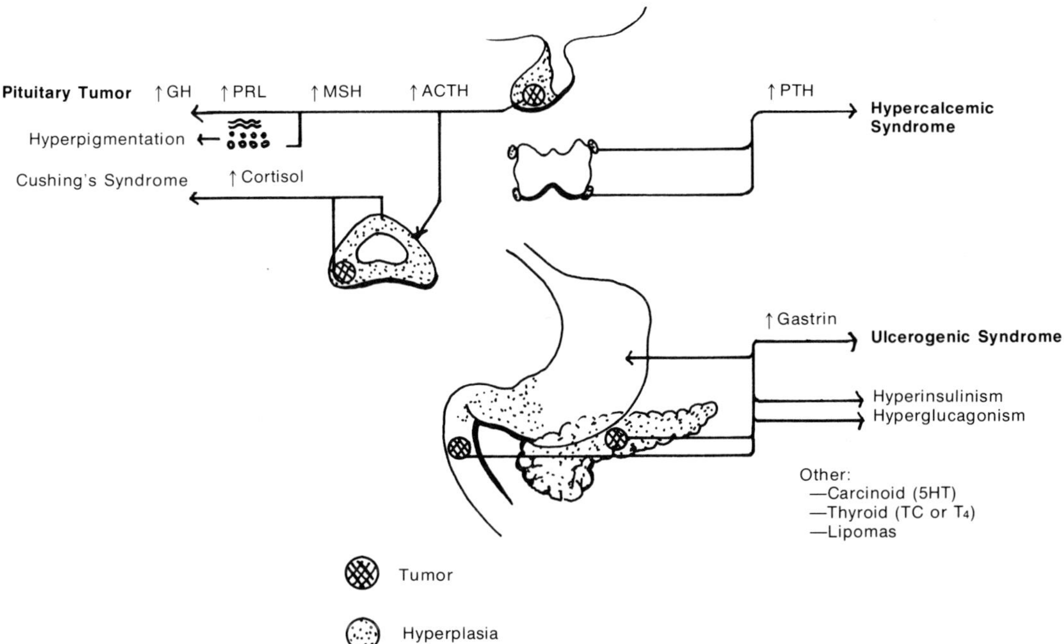

Fig. 17-3. Pathophysiology of multiple endocrine adenopathy, Type I (MEA-I) syndrome.

(See overleaf for flowchart)

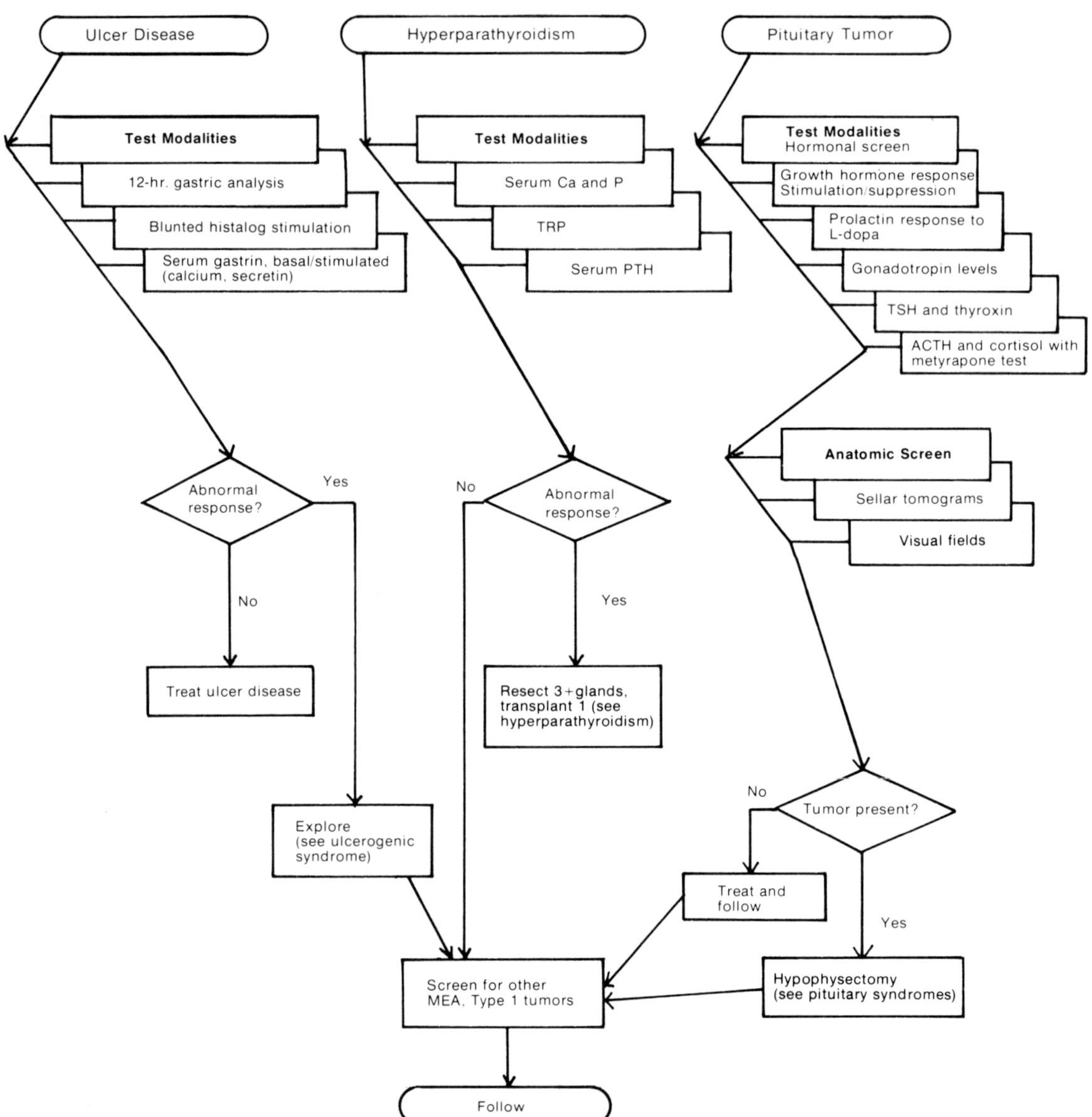

Fig. 17-4. Management flowchart of multiple endocrine adenopathy, Type I (MEA-I) syndrome.

18

Medullary Carcinoma of the Thyroid and Multiple Endocrine Neoplasia-II Syndromes*

Samuel A. Wells, Jr., M.D., and Jeffrey A. Norton, M.D.

HISTORY

In 1959, Hazard, Hawk, and Crile[3] described medullary carcinoma of the thyroid gland (MCT) as a distinct clinical and pathologic entity. In retrospect, it is surprising that the uniqueness of this malignancy was not appreciated earlier since it has rather striking histologic characteristics, being the only thyroid neoplasm demonstrating cellular argentaffin staining and amyloid production. Moreover, this neoplasm is uniquely associated with two fascinating clinical syndromes: multiple endocrine neoplasia, Type II (MEN-II) and its variant multiple endocrine neoplasia, Type IIb (MEN-IIb). In the late 1960's, several investigators reported that MCT secreted a specific hormone, thyrocalcitonin (TCT), which serves as a tumor marker for this disease. Because of the unusual histologic, endocrinologic, and clinical manifestations of this malignancy, MCT has attracted more interest than the other thyroid neoplasms even though it accounts for only 10 percent of all thyroid cancers.

Medullary carcinoma of the thyroid gland may present in one of three clinical settings. Most commonly, it occurs not as part of a syndrome, but sporadically as a solitary nodule in one lobe of the thyroid gland. Less often, patients with MCT have associated familial, clinical and pathologic findings which readily distinguish them from those having sporadic MCT.

In 1961, Sipple[11] made the observation that there was an unusual association between pheochromocytoma and thyroid cancer, and in 1965, Williams, et al.[16] and Schimke et al.[10] showed that the particular thyroid carcinoma involved was of the medullary or solid type, and that the disease complex had a definite genetic pattern, being inherited as a mendelian autosomal dominant trait. It had also been appreciated by Manning, et al.[7] that hyperparathyroidism was an integral part of this syndrome. Steiner and associates[12] termed this disease constellation of medullary carcinoma of the thyroid gland, pheochromocytoma, and hyperparathyroidism, multiple endocrine neoplasia, Type II.

MEN-IIb refers to the syndrome in which medullary carcinoma of the thyroid gland and pheochromocytoma, but usually not hyperparathyroidism, are the component parts. These patients have characteristic facies with prominent mandibles, puffy lips, and multiple mucosal neuromas involving the eyelids, lips, tongue and other mucous membranes. Additionally, they commonly have a Marfanoid habitus, pes cavus, medullated corneal nerves, and gastrointestinal

*Supported in part by National Institutes of Health contract NCI-CB-63994-39 and grant RR-30 from the General Clinical Resources Center, Program of the Division of Research Resources.

abnormalities, primarily consisting of diverticulosis and ganglioneuromatosis. Clinically, the MCT presents earliest in patients with MEN-IIb, and seems to have a more aggressive course since relatively few patients survive beyond 30 years of age. The physical appearance of the patient often suggests the diagnosis before the pheochromocytoma and MCT manifest themselves clinically. Some investigators have proposed that this disease be termed multiple endocrine neoplasia, Type III; however, it seems to clearly represent a variant of MEN-II, and the term MEN-IIb appears a more logical derivation. Although MEN-IIb can present in the same genetic pattern as MEN-II, it most commonly occurs sporadically without familial involvement (Table 18-1).

The two multiple endocrine neoplasia syndromes have provided information as to the embryologic tissue of origin of many endocrine cells and their associated tumors. The cells comprising medullary carcinoma of the thyroid gland are parafollicular cells which originate from neural crest tissue. Also, arising from neural crest tissue is the medullary portion of the adrenal gland which gives rise to pheochromocytomas. Both the MCT cells and the adrenal medullary cells have the biochemical features of a cell system designated by Pearse[9] as the APUD cell system (A=amines for the presence of amines such as serotonin and dopamine; PU=precursors to serotonin and dopamine in vitro; and D=decarboxylase for the presence of the amine synthesizing enzyme L-aromatic decarboxylase). The nature of the defect, or combination of defects, in neural crest tissue which provides for the simultaneous inheritance of MCT and pheochromocytomas remains to be defined. The presence of a parathyroid abnormality in MEN-II is less well understood, since these cells are not derived from neural crest tissue and do not have the biochemical features of APUD cells. Some investigators feel that the hyperparathyroidism is reactive to the hypocalcemic effects of high levels of thyrocalcitonin whereas others feel that the hyperparathyroidism is genetically determined and is not a secondary phenomenon.

Histologically, the medullary thyroid carcinoma arising in patients with MEN-II appears no different from the MCT occurring sporadically. However, in virtually all patients with MEN-II or MEN-IIb, the thyroid tumors are bilateral (Fig. 18-1) whereas MCT occurring sporadically seldom is. The tumor tissue almost always occupies a position in the superior-lateral part of the thyroid lobe(s); often multiple tumor foci are visible grossly. The neoplasm appears as a circumscribed whitish tan nodule, and histologically is composed of

Table 18-1. Multiple Endocrine Neoplasia, Type-II

Type II (MEN-II)	*Type IIb (MEN-IIb)*
Bilateral medullary carcinoma of the thyroid gland	Bilateral medullary carcinoma of the thyroid gland
Pheochromocytoma(s)	Pheochromocytoma(s)
Parathyroid hyperplasia	Parathyroid disease—rare
No specific phenotype	Specific phenotype
Familial inheritance as a mendelian autosomal dominant trait	Can occur in mendelian autosomal dominant pattern but more commonly is not familial
Variable rate of MCT progression, more commonly indolent	Generally MCT progresses rapidly

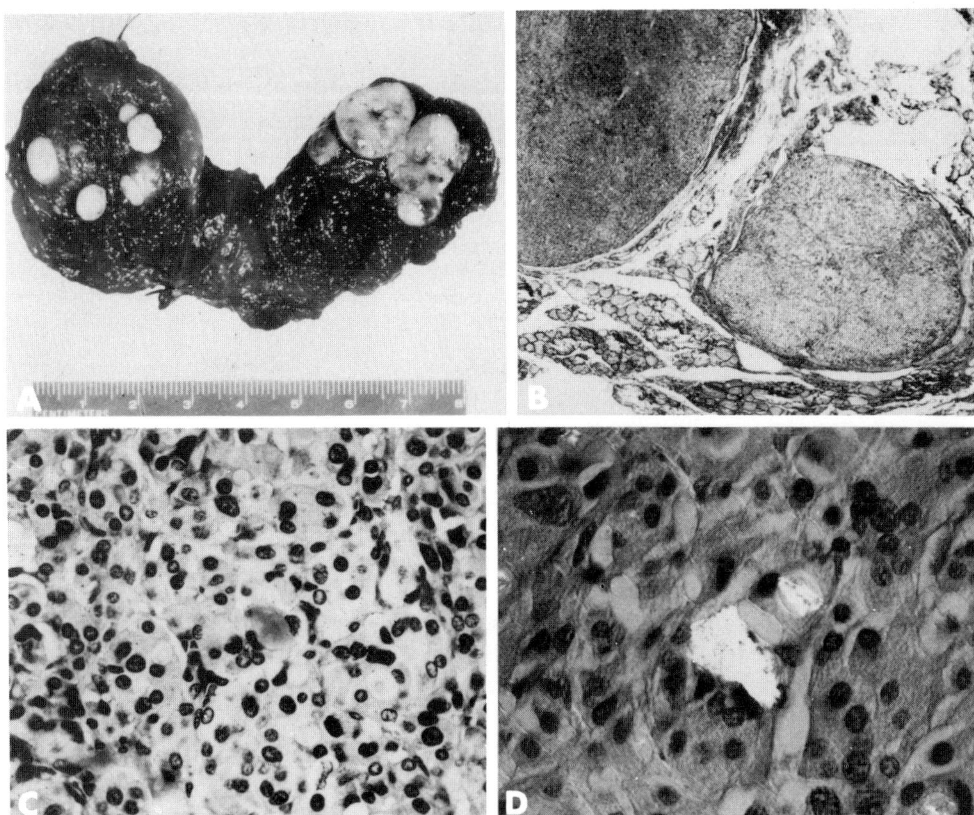

Fig. 18-1. Primary medullary carcinoma of the thyroid of the cellular type. *(A)* The thyroid gland contained multiple tumor nodules in the upper half of each lobe. *(B)* The nodules exhibited a solid growth pattern (H & E, X 10); *(C)* were composed of multiple sheets and nests of ovoid cells with hyperchromatic nuclei (H & E, X 325), and were virtually devoid of connective tissue (*B* and *C*). Small eosinophilic deposits were present in the centers of some of the nests (*C*). *(D)* In preparations stained with Congo red and examined with polarized light, these deposits exhibited the typical green birefringence of amyloid. (X 500) (Keiser, H. R., et al.: Ann. Intern. Med., *78*:571, 1973[6])

sheets or cords of round or spindle-shaped cells separated by a variable amount of amorphous stromal material. It should be noted that in older patients, MCT may be primarily composed of fibrous tissue with only a few cells present.

When MCT is stained with congo red and examined for amyloidlike material, the typical apple-green birefringence is found scattered throughout the amorphous stromal portions. Although a frequent finding, its presence is not needed to diagnose MCT since often the substance is not seen in primary or metastatic tumor foci. The amyloidlike material is supposedly composed of aggregates of a prohormone of TCT synthesized by the tumor cells.

The pheochromocytomas of MEN-II and MEN-IIb usually present in the second and third decades of life and are bilateral approximately 70 percent of the time. The lesion is seldom malignant and almost always is confined to the adrenal gland. Histologically, pheochromocytomas in MEN-II or MEN-IIb are indistinguishable from those occurring sporadically in a nonfamilial setting.

The parathyroid lesions in MEN-II consist of a pseudonodular but usually generalized multiglandular hyperplasia.

Any of the neoplasms that make up the syndrome of MEN-II or MEN-IIb may bring the patient to the physician's attention; however, the thyroid tumor is a constant feature of MEN-II or MEN-IIb, being present in virtually 100 percent of affected individuals. The presence of the other two lesions is more variable, and definitive figures are lacking; however approximately 40 percent of patients have pheochromocytomas, and in MEN-II approximately 60 percent of patients have parathyroid hyperplasia.[6]

CLINICAL PRESENTATION

Medullary carcinoma of the thyroid gland occurring sporadically affects males and females equally, and clinically there is no way to suspect that afflicted patients have MCT as opposed to any of the other thyroid tumors. The diagnosis is often not made until the resected specimen is examined histologically. Approximately 25 percent of patients will present with preceding or concurrent lymphadenopathy.

Medullary carcinomas of the thyroid gland are capable of great biosynthetic activity and are known to produce prostaglandins, serotonin, histaminase, and ACTH in addition to thyrocalcitonin. Approximately 20 patients with MCT and associated Cushing's syndrome have been reported.

Thirty percent of MCT patients, especially those with large primary lesions or with metastatic disease, develop diarrhea. The mechanism for this is unclear, however it is thought that the tumor secretes a hormonal agent(s) which causes either hypermotility of the gastrointestinal tract or increased intestinal secretion. This is suggested by the finding that frequently the diarrhea ceases in patients when the tumor is removed. Although the agent(s) causing the diarrhea is unknown, prostaglandins, serotonin, thyrocalcitonin and vasoactive intestinal polypeptide have all been proposed as the responsible substance.

It should be stated that when these paraendocrine syndromes (diarrhea and Cushing's syndrome) occur in patients with MCT, a relatively advanced disease state is indicated, and the patient is often incurable.

Many patients with MEN-II or MEN-IIb present to their physician with a history of episodic headaches, sweating, palpitations, nausea and vomiting. This should lead one to suspect the presence of pheochromocytoma(s), and the diagnosis can be confirmed by detecting elevated levels of urinary catecholamines, vanillylmandelic acid, or metanephrines. Characteristically, these patients have episodic, however, rather than sustained hypertension. The diagnosis is often difficult to make even with biochemical measurements, and provocative agents such as glucagon, tyramine and histalog occasionally will not induce a positive pressor response. In reviewing the family histories of patients with MEN-II, it is striking to see how frequently one finds young relatives who have experienced "strokes," "heart attacks," or even sudden death prior to the time that a thyroid tumor was observed. Even if the MCT is diagnosed first, it is absolutely critical that the presence of a pheochromocytoma be ruled out prior to neck exploration. Often a general anesthetic induction in an unprepared patient will provoke a hypertensive crisis which might result in severe morbidity or perhaps death.

It is unusual for patients with MEN-II to present with symptoms relative to hypercalcemia. In most patients, this is an incidental finding and there are few who actually deveolp renal stones or bone disease. As mentioned previously, the hyperparathyroidism seems to occur most often in the MEN-II syndrome, being uncommon in patients who have sporadic medullary carcinoma of the thyroid gland or MEN-IIb. It is unknown why the hyperparathyroidism occurs in MEN-II. It has been proposed that it develops secondary to the hypercalcitonemia which occurs, but if this were the case, one would expect it to develop in patients with MEN-IIb or sporadic MCT.

It should be mentioned that MCT patients rarely develop hypocalcemia even with markedly elevated plasma TCT levels and histologically normal parathyroid glands demonstrated at surgery.

PREOPERATIVE EVALUATION AND SCREENING

When the proper clinical setting for MEN-II or MEN-IIb exists, precise diagnosis depends upon familiarity with the biochemical activity of the thyroid, parathyroid and adrenal lesions. For MCT, the production of TCT by the tumor cells holds the key for diagnosis. With the advent of a radioimmunoassay technique for this hormone, Tashjian and associates[13] documented that virtually all patients with clinically detectable MCT have elevated circulating TCT levels. Most investigators feel that the upper limit of normal of TCT is 0.2 ng./ml. of plasma. Patients who present with palpable thyroid lesions caused by MCT or those who have clinically apparent metastatic disease will all have TCT levels above normal, and generally greater than 1.0 ng./ml. With extensive disease, baseline levels may exceed 1,000 ng./ml.

Therefore, patients who present with a neck mass or lateral neck lymphadenopathy may be diagnosed as having MCT by demonstrating an elevated TCT level in the plasma. It should be mentioned that minimally elevated basal levels of plasma TCT have been reported in patients with other tumors (small cell lung carcinoma, carcinoid tumors and breast carcinoma), but for practical purposes, especially in evaluating patients suspected of having either sporadic or familial MCT, elevated TCT levels are diagnostic of medullary thyroid carcinoma. The utility of the TCT assay has been demonstrated in evaluating family members in a kindred proven to have MEN-II. Screening persons in an effort to identify early stages of MCT has usually required more than determination of the TCT level in a single basal blood sample. Melvin and associates[8] showed that minimal elevations of plasma TCT can be indicative of MCT in patients who have no clinical manifestations of the neoplasm, either by palpation of the neck or by thyroid scan. Indeed, tumors no larger than 1.0 mm. can be so diagnosed. It was also found by these investigators that some patients with normal basal TCT levels had an increase to abnormal levels following calcium ion infusion (15 mg./kg. over 4 hours). Selected patients who were followed serially and had modest, but progressive increases in TCT with calcium stimulation were operated upon and found to have C-cell hyperplasia, a pathologic entity supposedly indicative of a premalignant phase of medullary carcinoma of the thyroid gland.[17]

It has been shown by other investigators that the synthetic peptide, pentagastrin is a more potent stimulus for TCT release in MCT patients that the standard

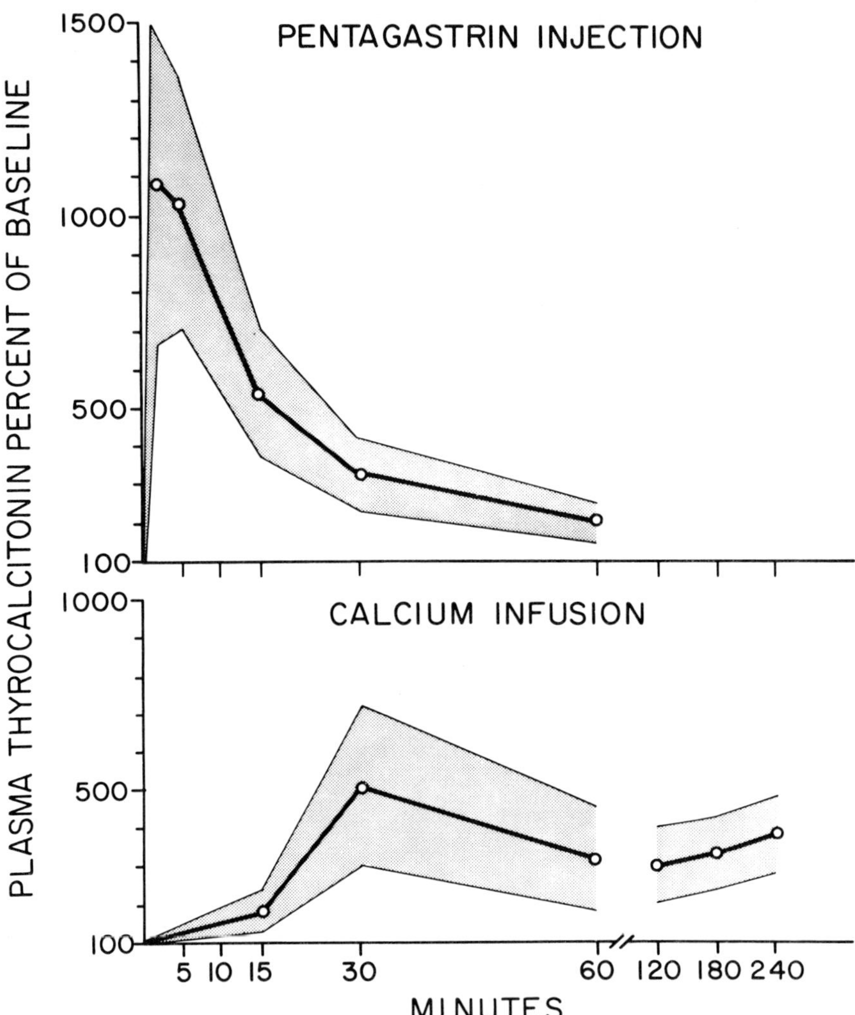

Fig. 18-2. Combined responses of seven patients with elevated baseline levels of plasma thyrocalcitonin to pentagastrin injection and calcium infusion. Responses are expressed as a percent increase in immunoreactive thyrocalcitonin above initial baseline levels. Open circles and solid lines represent the mean responses and the shaded areas indicate the range of the standard errors. (Hennessy, J. F., et al.: J. Clin. Endocrinol., *39*:491, 1974[4])

4-hour calcium infusion.[4] Following a pulse injection of pentagastrin (0.5 μg./kg.), peak TCT levels are detectable in 1 to 3 minutes, compared to 30 to 60 minutes following the beginning of a calcium ion (15 mg./kg. over 4 hours) infusion. Furthermore, peak TCT levels following pentagastrin are two to threefold higher than peak levels following calcium infusion (Fig. 18-2). Screening with pentagastrin has resulted in the detection of preclinical MCT in MEN-II patients who have no physical or radiologic evidence of MCT, and no elevation of TCT following calcium ion infusion[4,15] (Fig. 18-3). There are some side effects associated with the pentagastrin injection (flushing and epigastric

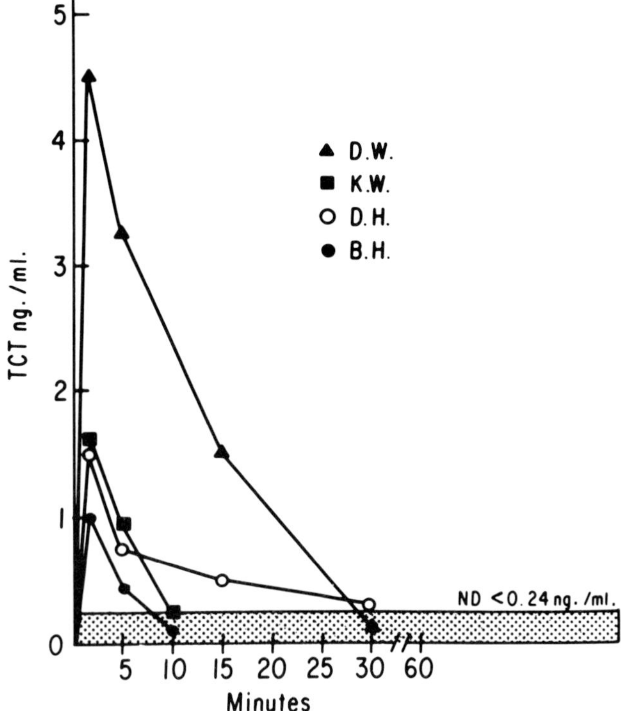

Fig. 18-3. Thyrocalcitonin response to pentagastrin stimulation in four children with a family history of MEN-II, but without elevated thyrocalcitonin levels either basally or following calcium infusion. (Wells, S. A., Jr., et al.: Ann. Surg., *182*:364, 1975[15])

pain), but these are minimal and usually last only 30 or 45 seconds. With the 4-hour calcium infusion, patients occasionally develop nausea, headache and vomiting. It has been proposed that a short bolus calcium injection (2 mg. calcium gluconate/kg. over 1 min.) would invoke a higher TCT response than pentagastrin injection. If so, this might be the test agent of choice for the early diagnosis of MCT, but adequate comparisons remain to be made. Generally, it has been the policy to operate on patients who have TCT levels greater than 1 ng./ml. following provocative stimulation with either calcium ion or pentagastrin. Occasionally patients will have undetectable basal levels of TCT, but following stimulation with pentagastrin their levels will increase to 0.3 or 0.8 ng./ml. It has been our practice in such patients to place a catheter through the femoral vein into the inferior thyroid vein and perform a pentagastrin test comparing systemic to inferior thyroid vein levels of TCT. Almost always, five to tenfold higher levels of TCT can be detected in the inferior thyroid vein effluent of MCT patients establishing the diagnosis of medullary carcinoma (Fig. 18-4). Normal patients evaluated thus far have not had inferior thyroid vein TCT levels above baseline following pentagastrin injection.[15]

Another biochemical feature of MCT is the presence of high concentrations of the enzyme histaminase in tumor tissue. Approximately 50 percent of all patients with MCT will have elevated circulating levels of this enzyme. The factors determining which patients have abnormal blood histaminase levels are not completely known; however, there is a positive correlation with the presence of metastatic disease (Fig. 18-5). Generally, patients who have abnormal levels prior to surgery, and especially those whose levels do not return to normal

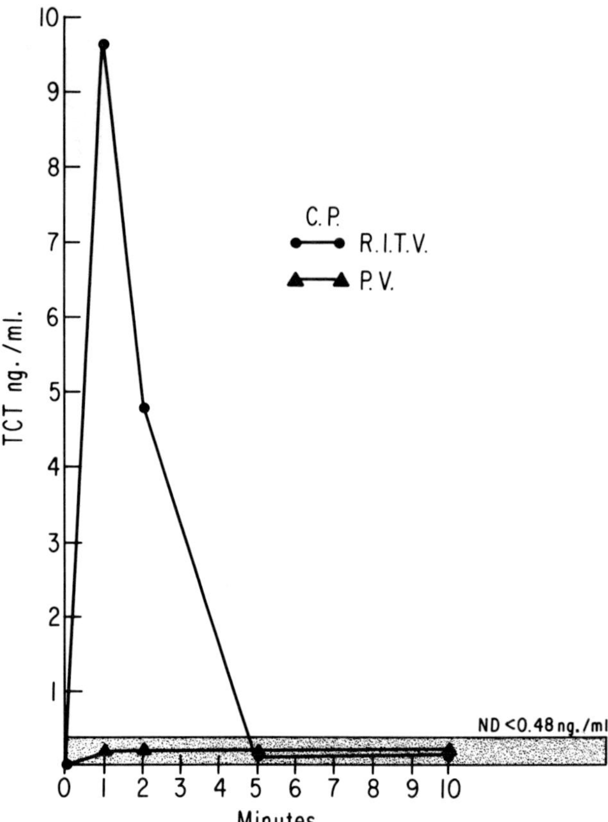

Fig. 18-4. Thyrocalcitonin response to pentagastrin stimulation in a patient C. P. in whom there was no elevated thyrocalcitonin level either basally or following calcium infusion. Note the absence of plasma thyrocalcitonin elevation in the peripheral vein (P.V.) after pentagastrin stimulation. An elevated thyrocalcitonin level is only detected in the right inferior thyroid vein (R.I.T.V.). At surgery no gross tumor was demonstrated in the patient's thyroid gland; however, C-cell hyperplasia was detected microscopically. (Wells, S. A., Jr., et al.: Ann. Surg., *182*:364, 1975[15])

postoperatively, have a high incidence of persistent disease or of subsequent recurrent disease.

The diagnosis of pheochromocytoma in patients with MEN-II or MEN-IIb depends on analysis of levels of urinary catecholamines and catecholamine metabolites. As mentioned previously preoperative determination of the presence of pheochromocytoma(s) is critical since this lesion often will not manifest itself clinically.

Intravenous pyelography with sonography or retroperitoneal air insufflation are commonly used to localize adrenal lesions. Some groups routinely use selective arteriography to localize pheochromocytomas, especially when extra-adrenal lesions are suspected.

The diagnosis of hyperparathyroidism in MEN-II depends largely on establishing the presence of an elevated blood calcium concentration on serial determinations. Any history of recurrent renal stones should, of course, make the search for hyperparathyroidism more aggressive. It has been uncommon for patients with MEN-II to have parathyroid associated bone disease.

SURGICAL MANAGEMENT

The ability to diagnose MCT in familial patients at risk allows the surgeon to diagnose and treat this malignancy in an early preclinical stage.

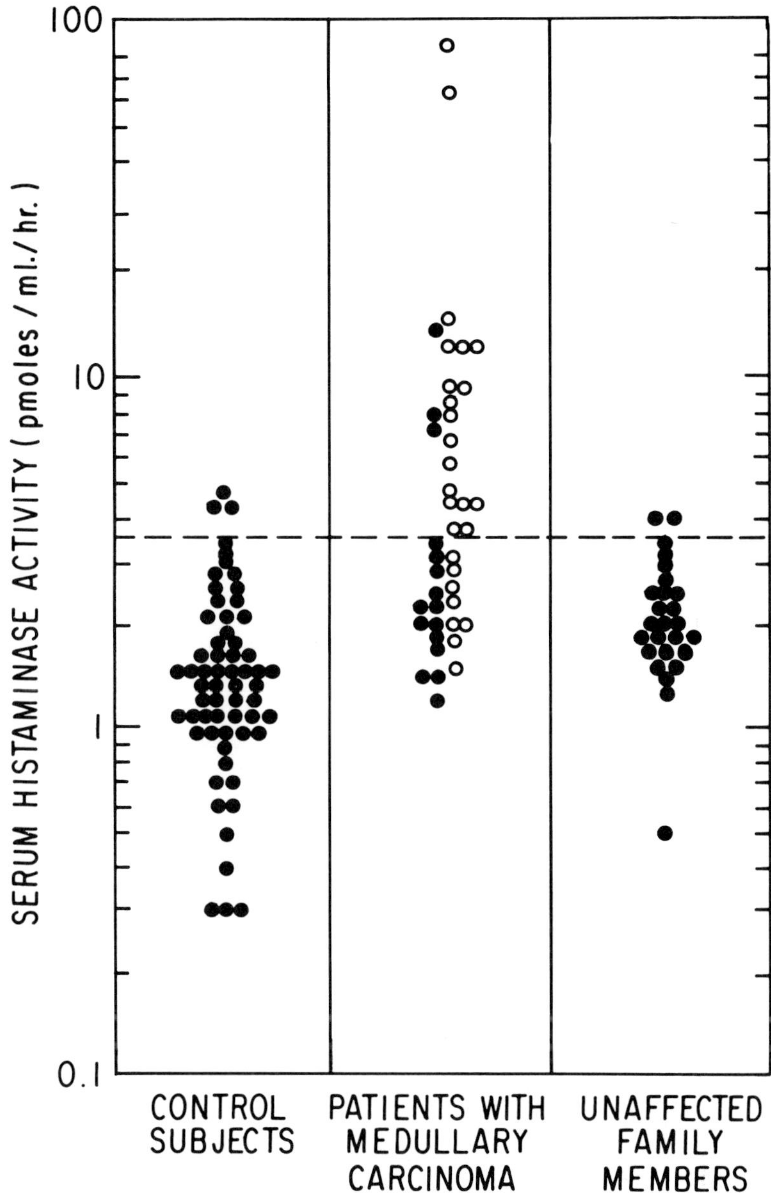

Fig. 18-5. Serum histaminase activity in 62 controls, 42 patients with medullary thyroid carcinoma and 26 relatives of patients who were clinically normal. (Baylin, S. B., Beaven, M. A., Keiser, H. R., et al.: Serum histaminase and calcitonin levels in medullary carcinoma of the thyroid gland. Lancet, *1*:456, 1972)

From previous experience with many large kindreds, investigators generally agree that the detection of an elevated blood TCT level (>1.0 ng./ml.) following provocative stimulation with either calcium or pentagastrin is virtually diagnostic of medullary carcinoma of the thyroid gland. This has been demonstrated repeatedly in patients with no palpable mass in the thyroid gland, normal thyroid scans and undetectable TCT levels in the peripheral blood even following 4-hour-calcium infusion. Should one diagnose MCT in a patient from an MEN-II kindred, it is absolutely essential that the remainder of the family members at risk be screened. It is in this situation that the pentagastrin test with TCT determination has its greatest utility. Most patients diagnosed with provocative testing have had tumors confined to the thyroid gland with no evidence of regional node metastases at the time of surgery. Testing is usually done in family members at risk beginning at 8 to 10 years of age and continuing at yearly intervals through the third decade.

As mentioned previously, should the diagnosis of pheochromocytoma(s) be made, the patient should undergo anterior abdominal exploration first with a thorough evaluation of both adrenal fossae, the organ of Zuckerkandl and the sympathetic chain. The state of adrenal medullary hyperplasia has been described in MEN-II[1] and some surgeons have advocated bilateral adrenalectomy (in the presence of unilateral gross disease) on the basis of this histologic picture. It has not been our policy to routinely biopsy a contralateral normal-size adrenal gland after resection of a unilateral pheochromocytoma. Again postoperatively patients undergoing unilateral pheochromocytoma resection should be followed carefully at 6-month or yearly intervals since a second adrenal tumor can frequently be diagnosed before it is clinically apparent.

The preoperative management of patients undergoing surgery for pheochromocytomas has consisted of a 2-week preparation with the alpha-receptor blocker phenoxybenzamine (40 to 200 mg. a day). Rarely beta adrenergic receptor blockade with propranolol (40 mg. per day) has been necessary when tachycardia develops with phenoxybenzamine. Intraoperative control of hypertension is best achieved with sodium nitroprusside or phentolamine. Bilateral adrenalectomy obviously requires long-term glucocorticoid and mineralocorticoid replacement therapy.

The surgical management of medullary carcinoma in patients with the sporadic type of disease is a total lobectomy of the lobe containing the solitary neoplasm. It has been our policy to do a subtotal lobectomy on the opposite side. Should involved lymph nodes be present then a neck dissection is required. In patients with MEN-II or MEN-IIb, it is absolutely essential that a total thyroidectomy be performed, leaving no remnant of thyroid tissue in the neck. This is necessary because in 100 percent of these patients the MCT is bilateral. The tumors grossly are almost always confined to the upper outer parts of the thyroid lobes, but in our experience four patients have developed recurrent disease following bilateral subtotal thyroidectomies where all gross disease was resected. In patients with familial MEN-II or MEN-IIb, it is recommended that the central nodes of the neck inferior to the hyoid bone and medial to both jugular veins be excised with the thyroid gland. Also, retrosternal nodes should be removed when possible. If hypercalcemia is present in patients with MEN-II, it is almost always due to parathyroid hyperplasia. It has

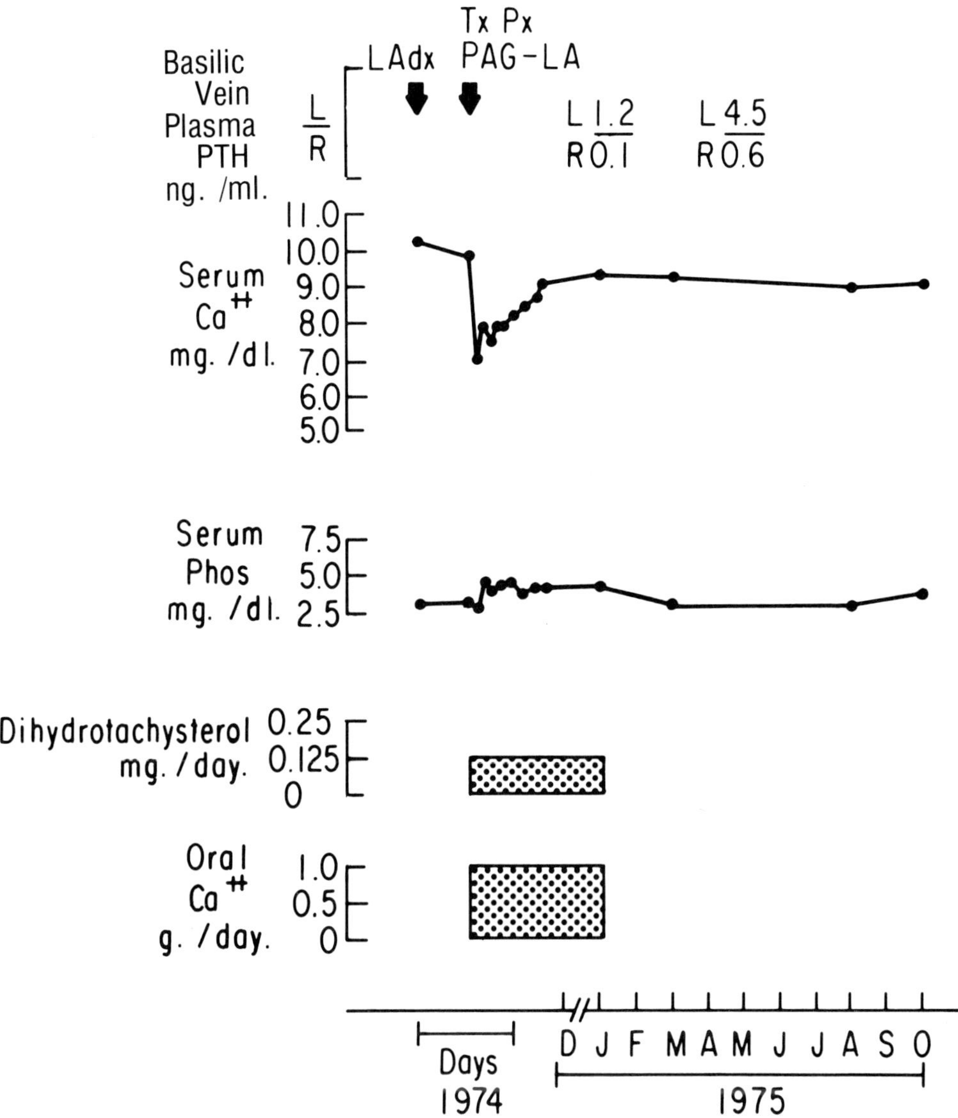

Fig 18-6. This graph depicts the clinical course of an MEN-II patient undergoing left adrenalectomy (LA dx) for pheochromocytoma and 7 days later a total thyroidectomy (TX), total parathyroidectomy (PX) and parathyroid autograft to the left arm (PAG-LA). After a brief course of replacement therapy (dihydrotachysterol and oral calcium), the autograft functioned, and the patient was normocalcemic subsequently. Plasma PTH was detectable in much higher concentrations in the left arm (L) compared to the right (R). (Wells, S. A., Jr., et al.: N. Engl. J. Med., *295*:60, 1976[14])

been our policy in these patients to manage this disease by removing all parathyroid tissue and autografting a portion of one gland to the forearm musculature.[14] This method has worked extremely well in our experience as demonstrated in Figure 18-6.

POSTOPERATIVE FOLLOW-UP

In MEN-II and MEN-IIb, the medullary carcinoma is the disease that is most frequently lethal for the host. This might be somewhat misleading since when one reviews a family history of a kindred with familial MEN-II, it is apparent that patients have occasionally met catastrophic deaths at a young age which might indicate the presence of a pheochromocytoma resulting in a cerebrovascular accident or myocardial infarction. The MCT in patients with MEN-IIb seems to be more virulent than in patients with MEN-II. In our experience, it is unusual for patients with MEN-IIb to live beyond 30 years of age. Even in patients with MEN-II, the disease course is very capricious, as some patients die at a young age whereas others live a normal life expectancy even into the 70's or 80's without complications developing from the thyroid tumor. With the radioimmunoassay for TCT a specific tumor marker can be followed, and invariably the detection of an elevated level of this hormone in the peripheral blood following surgery is indicative of recurrent or persistent MCT. Generally, patients should be followed at 6-month intervals after surgery with provocative testing. If an elevated TCT level is detected in the peripheral plasma of a patient following surgery whereas it had previously been undetectable, it is useful to perform simultaneous selective venous catheterization with pentagastrin stimulation to detect the site of tumor recurrence. This is achieved by simultaneously placing catheters into both innominate veins, the hepatic vein and a peripheral vein, and injecting pentagastrin intravenously. By sampling blood from these various sites at 1, 2, 3, 5 and 10 minutes, plasma TCT levels can be determined and foci of tumor metastases detected. An elevated level of TCT in the sample site indicates the presence of MCT. Obviously, detection of a markedly elevated level of TCT in a hepatic vein is diagnostic of metastatic MCT, and the patient is not then a candidate for further surgery. Should the disease be confined to the neck, however, the patient might be a candidate for a neck dissection if this were not done at the initial surgical procedure.

In patients with metastatic MCT who are not surgical candidates, it is unclear what the best systemic therapy is. These tumors are not thyroid tumors in the sense that they concentrate iodine, and radioactive iodine ablation has not been helpful. Also, the tumors are not responsive to thyroid replacement therapy and resultant suppression of TSH. The tumors appear to be radioresistant, and so far little data are available regarding their response to chemotherapeutic agents. Gottlieb and associates[2] have reported that some patients have responded to doxorubicin hydrochloride; however objective data regarding this response are not available. Responsiveness of MCT to chemotherapeutic agents could be readily assessed by measuring serial TCT levels during therapy.

The mortality rate for MCT is lower than for anaplastic thyroid neoplasms; however, it is higher than that for papillary or follicular tumors. The 10-year survival is approximately 50 percent.

Hill and his colleagues[5] have categorized the postoperative courses of MCT patients into three clinical groups. Group 1 patients underwent surgery for disease localized to the neck and remained disease-free thereafter, the average survival time being 111 months. Group 2 patients had surgery at a similar clinical stage but postoperatively exhibited disease progression with early signs of recurrent and/or residual tumor. Patients in the subgroup 2a had a more prolonged course with an average survival time of 75 months, whereas patients in group 2b progressed more rapidly, dying with disseminated disease at an average of 22 months. Group 3 patients had a latent period, often as long as 10 years or more between the time of surgery and the appearance of metastatic disease. The average survival time of this group was 107 months. There is no known method for predicting a patient's disease course.

REFERENCES

1. Carney, J. A., Sizemore, G. W., and Tyce, G. M.: Bilateral adrenal medullary hyperplasia in multiple endocrine neoplasia, type 2. Mayo Clin. Proc., *50*:3, 1975.
2. Gottlieb, J. A., and Hill, C. S.: Chemotherapy of thyroid cancer with Adriamycin. N. Engl. J. Med., *290*:193, 1974.
3. Hazard, J. B., Hawk, W. H., and Crile, G., Jr.: Medullary (solid) carcinoma of the thyroid—a clinico-pathologic entity. J. Clin. Endocrinol. Metab., *19*:152, 1959.
4. Hennessy, J. F., et al.: A comparison of pentagastrin injection and calcium infusion as provocative agents for the detection of medullary carcinoma of the thyroid. J. Clin. Endocrinol. Metab., *39*:487, 1974.
5. Hill, C. S., Jr., Ibanez, M. L., Samaan, N. A., Ahearn, M. J., and Clark, R. L.: Medullary (solid) carcinoma of the thyroid gland—an analysis of the M. D. Anderson Hospital experience with patients with the tumor, its special features and its histiogenesis. Medicine (Baltimore), *52*:141, 1973.
6. Keiser, H. R., et al.: Sipple's syndrome: Medullary thyroid carcinoma, pheochromocytoma and parathyroid disease. Ann. Intern. Med., *78*:561, 1973.
7. Manning, P. C., Molnar, G. D., Black, B. M., Priestly, J. T., and Woolner, L. B.: Pheochromocytoma, hyperparathyroidism and thyroid carcinoma occurring coincidentally. N. Engl. J. Med., *268*:68, 1963.
8. Melvin, K. E. W., Miller, H. H., and Tashjian, A. H., Jr.: Early diagnosis of medullary carcinoma of the thyroid by means of calcitonin assay. N. Engl. J. Med., *285*:1115, 1971.
9. Pearse, A. G. E.: The APUD cell concept and its implications in pathology. *In* Sommers, S. C. (ed.): Pathology Annual. pp. 27-41. New York, Appleton-Century-Crofts, 1974.
10. Schimke, R. N., and Hartmann, W. H.: Familial amyloid-producing medullary thyroid carcinoma and pheochromocytoma. A distinct genetic entity. Ann. Intern. Med., *63*:1027, 1965.
11. Sipple, J. H.: The association of pheochromocytoma with carcinoma of the thyroid gland. Am. J. Med., *31*:163, 1961.
12. Steiner, A. L., Goodman, A. D., and Powers, S. R.: Study of a kindred with pheochromocytoma, medullary thyroid carcinoma, hyperparathyroidism and Cushing's disease. Multiple endocrine neoplasia, type 2. Medicine, *47*:371, 1968.
13. Tashjian, A. H., Jr., et al.: Immunoassay of human calcitonin. Clinical measurement relation to serum calcium and studies in patients with medullary carcinoma. N. Engl. J. Med., *283*:890, 1970.
14. Wells, S. A., Jr., Ellis, G. J., and Gunnells, J. C.: Parathyroid autotransplantation in primary parathyroid hyperplasia. N. Engl. J. Med., *295*:57, 1976.
15. Wells, S. A., Jr., et al.: The early diagnosis of medullary carcinoma of the thyroid gland in patients with multiple endocrine neoplasia type II. Ann. Surg., *182*:362, 1975.
16. Williams, E. D.: A review of 17 cases of carcinoma of the thyroid and pheo-

chromocytoma. J. Clin. Pathol., *18*:288, 1965.

17. Wolfe, H. J., et al.: C-cell hyperplasia preceding medullary thyroid carcinoma. N. Engl. J. Med., *289*:437, 1973.

Selected Reading

Khairi, M. R. A., et al.: Mucosal neuroma, pheochromocytoma, and medullary thyroid carcinoma: multiple endocrine neoplasia type III. Medicine, *54*:89, 1975.

(This monograph discusses the most recently described variant of MEN-II. Most investigators speak of this syndrome as MEN-IIb. The authors have a large number of personal cases and have collected others from the literature. There is an excellent discussion of the clinical manifestations of this specific syndrome.)

Melvin, K. E. W., Tashjian, A. H., Jr., and Miller, H. H.: Studies of familial (medullary) thyroid carcinoma. Recent Prog. Horm. Res., *28*:399, 1972.

(This manuscript is devoted to the genetic aspects, pathophysiology, early diagnosis and treatment of multiple endocrine neoplasia type II.)

Steiner, A. L., Goodman, A. D., and Powers, S. R.: A study of a kindred with pheochromocytoma, medullary thyroid carcinoma, hyperparathyroidism, and Cushing's disease: multiple endocrine neoplasia, type II. Medicine, *47*:371, 1968.

(This was the first comprehensive study dealing with the entity of multiple endocrine neoplasia type II.)

EDITORIAL COMMENTARY

Although less than 10 percent of thyroid cancers are of the medullary type, this carcinoma has generated much interest because of its humoral capabilities and its genetic associations. The usual clinical presentation, excluding those instances when it is uncovered through family screening programs, is simply a mass in the neck, the palpable primary or metastatic tumor. Its humoral product, thyrocalcitonin, is a hypocalcemic agent, yet values of serum calcium below normal levels are not usually observed; on the contrary, hypercalcemia is more often encountered, which directs attention to parathyroid involvement in pluriglandular associations. There are polyhormonal capabilities of this tumor; approximately 30 percent of patients with clinically evident MCT may present with diarrhea due to tumor elaboration of either thyrocalcitonin, prostaglandins, serotonin (5-HT) or vasoactive intestinal peptide (VIP). Rarely patients with MCT actually present with a clinical picture compatible with Cushing's syndrome due to thyroid tumor elaboration of ACTH. These polyhormonal capabilities are complicated by the inherent propensity toward multiple endocrinopathy (MEN-II); this latter association is a clinical hallmark of genetic instigation of tumors of the APUD cell system, of which the parafollicular C cells of the thyroid are charter members. Therefore, MCT becomes involved in clinical syndromes when it is associated with pheochromocytoma (Sipple's syndrome) plus hyperplastic hyperparathyroidism (MEN-II), and with mucosal neuromas without hyperparathyroidism (MEN-IIb). In the latter syndrome, the neuromas are true neuromas; on the other hand, neurofibromas in Von Recklinghausen's disease (Schwann cell tumors of probable neural crest origin) are also sometimes associated with pheochromocytomas. In any instance the symptomatology related to pheochromocytoma(s) and/or hyperparathyroidism may dominate the clinical presentation and may be discovered in relatives of the patient. The syndrome of MEN IIb is probably the purest neurolymphoma of all the APUD-omas because each component in this constellation arises from cells definitely originating from the neural crest. By contrast, parathyroid cells, on the basis of comparative embryologic studies, are believed to arise from neuroectodermal placodes, not from the neural crest per se; this may account for the infrequency of hyperparathyroidism in the sub-syndrome of MEN-IIb.

In the MEN-II syndrome with MCT and pheochromocytoma(s) and hyperparathyroidism, it is not unusual for the patients to be eucalcemic, the effects of TCT and PTH having balanced or canceled each other. There is no uniformity of opinion as to whether the parathyroid abnormality is a manifestation secondary to TCT-induced hypocalcemia or whether the same genetic defect (single clone mutation) accounts for both the MCT and the parathyroid adenopathy which seems more likely since their association is not usually seen in MEN-II b or in sporadic MCT. Moreover, it has not been proven whether the parathyroid changes progress from hyperplasia to neoplasia (adenoma and carcinoma) as it is believed may occur in C-cell abnormalities.

Pathologically the thyroid gland may contain numerous minute calcifications as do other thyroid tumors, and the primary lesion(s) of medullary carcinoma may be small, multifocal and sometimes obscured in size by the enlarged lymph nodal metastases. Histologically, a diagnostic feature is the finding of amyloid in the thyroid stroma and it is considered that this material is composed of the prohormone of thyrocalcitonin synthesized by the tumor cells.

A significant elevation of basal plasma TCT in a patient with a thyroid mass is important in differentiating MCT from other thyroid neoplasms. In patients with no evidence of clinical disease, the detection of elevated plasma TCT levels either basally or following pentagastrin stimulation, allows one to diagnose this malignancy preclinically. Even higher plasma TCT levels can be measured in thyroid vein effluent following pentagastrin stimulation. Asymptomatic relatives of patients having MEN-II have been identified in this way and histologic examination of the surgically removed thyroid gland has confirmed the diagnosis of MCT.

S.R.F.

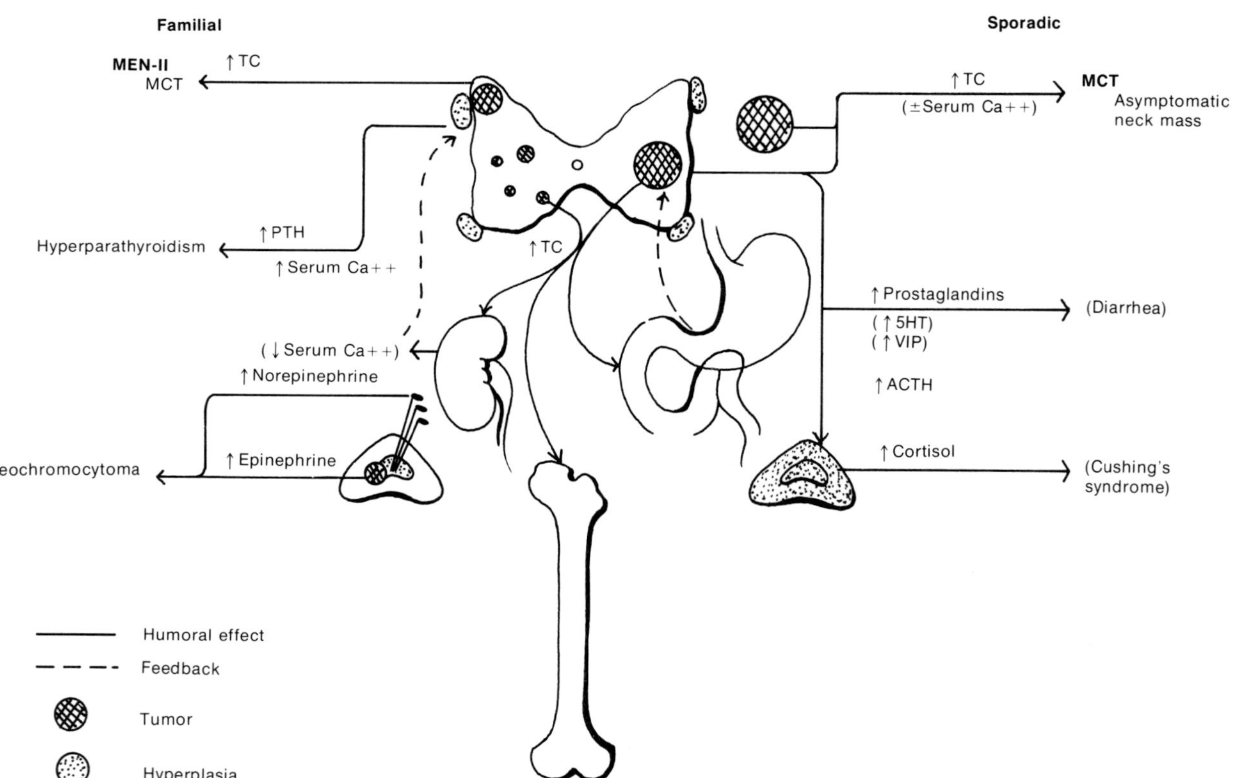

Fig. 18-7. Pathophysiology of medullary carcinoma of the thyroid and multiple endocrine neoplasia, Type IIa, syndrome.

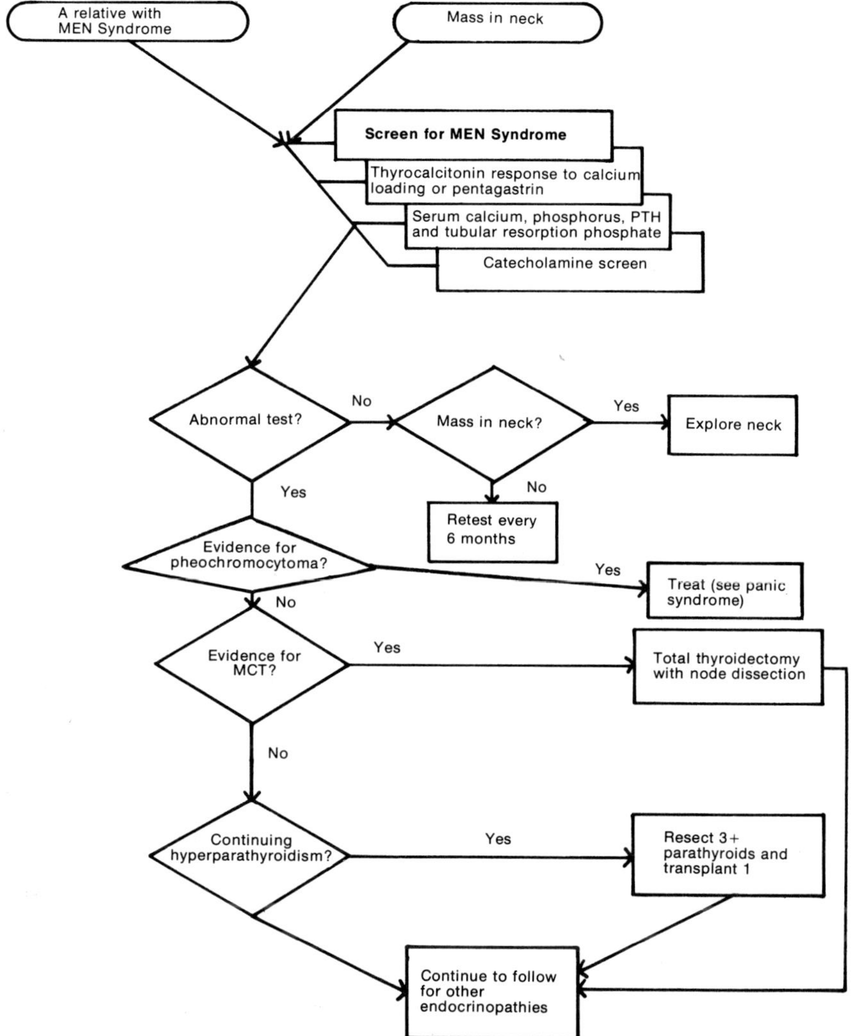

Fig. 18-8. Management flowchart of medullary carcinoma of thyroid and MEN-IIa syndrome.

19

Pituitary Syndromes

J. Blake Tyrrell, M.D., and Charles B. Wilson, M.D.

The pituitary syndromes discussed in this chapter include the somatogenic syndromes of acromegaly and gigantism (HGH); the galactorrhea-amenorrhea syndromes (PRL); Cushing's disease: pituitary-dependent hyperadrenocorticism (ACTH); the hyperpigmentation (Nelson's) syndrome (MSH). Pituitary adenomas account for approximately 10 percent of intracranial tumors and constitute the most frequent cause of pituitary dysfunction. These tumors are almost always benign and are readily amenable to treatment if the diagnosis is established prior to extrasellar extension. Clinical presentation is a consequence of local tumor growth or dysfunction of anterior pituitary hormone secretion. Recent development and availability of specific and accurate immunoassays for the major anterior pituitary hormones have allowed the diagnosis of anterior pituitary dysfunction at an early stage, and current neuroroentgenographic techniques permit the diagnosis of hypersecreting pituitary adenomas before they cause gross enlargement of the sella turcica. The development of microsurgical approaches to the pituitary gland permits selective resection of small pituitary tumors with minimal morbidity and the preservation of normal pituitary function in the majority of patients. The application of these techniques has led to diagnosis and effective treatment of pituitary tumors before the development of late manifestations such as visual loss and panhypopituitarism.

DIFFERENTIAL DIAGNOSIS OF HYPOTHALAMIC-PITUITARY LESIONS

Pituitary Tumors

Primary pituitary adenomas, the most frequent intrasellar mass lesion in adults, vary in size from a few millimeters to those very large tumors with extrasellar extension and visual impairment. Tumors less than 1 cm. in size do not cause gross sellar enlargement on plain roentgenographs but frequently cause minor degrees of sellar asymmetry on sellar tomograms. These small tumors, designated pituitary microadenomas, usually present with manifestations of either prolactin or corticotropin hypersecretion.[15,42,44,45] Larger tumors present with both local manifestations of tumor growth and variable degrees of excess or deficiency of anterior pituitary hormone secretion.

Classification of pituitary tumors by light microscopy reveals three major cell types: acidophilic, basophilic and chromophobe. However, by EM and immunofluorescent studies, chromophobe tumors that were previously thought to

Differential Diagnosis of Hypothalamic-Pituitary Abnormalities

Pituitary adenomas
- Somatotrophe (acidophil, chromophobe)
- Lactotrophe (chromophobe, acidophil, basophil)
- Corticotrophe (basophil, chromophobe)
- Mixed:
  - Somatotrophe/lactotrophe
  - Corticotrophe/lactotrophe
- Nonfunctional (chromophobe)
- Malignant (rare)

Empty sella syndrome

Suprasellar and intrasellar neoplasms
- Craniopharyngioma
- Primary CNS neoplasms:
  - Meningioma, chordoma, optic glioma, epidermoid and dermoid tumors
  - Pineal tumors (pinealoma and teratoma)
- Metastatic neoplasms

Intrasellar cyst

Carotid aneurysm

Inflammatory and infiltrative hypothalmic-pituitary lesions
- Meningitis
- Septic foci (blood-borne or direct extension)
- Tuberculosis
- Syphilis
- Mycoses
- Histiocytosis-X
- Hemochromatosis
- Sarcoidosis

Congenital or familial hypopituitarism
- Panhypopituitarism
- Isolated deficiency of pituitary trophic hormones

Adult hypopituitarism
- Sheehan's syndrome
- Traumatic
- Idiopathic

Nontumorous pituitary enlargement following primary endocrine failure
- Primary hypothyroidism
- Primary hypogonadism
- Adrenogenital syndromes

be nonfunctional may secrete prolactin, growth hormone, corticotropin and, rarely, thyrotropin and gonadotropins.[1,6,8,21,23,25,29,39] This older classification should now be abandoned and tumors should be classified by the type of hormone secreted (e.g., somatotropin, lactropin, or corticotropin).[8] Mixed tumors secreting both growth hormone and prolactin, or corticotropin and prolactin, may occur, and nonfunctional tumors now account for a minority of pituitary adenomas.[6,25,29] Malignant pituitary tumors are extremely rare. These present with rapidly progressive local invasion and may rarely metastasize to distant sites.

The Empty Sella Syndrome

The empty sella syndrome is the second most frequent cause of sellar enlargement, and failure to recognize this benign condition may result in the mistaken diagnosis of a pituitary adenoma.[30] The primary empty sella is caused by a congenital defect in the diaphragm sella allowing herniation of the arachnoid membrane into the sella with enlargement consequent to the transmission of cerebrospinal fluid pressure. This syndrome is commonly seen in middle-aged obese women who are often hypertensive. Headache is a common and possible coincidental symptom. The primary empty sella is also associated with conditions resulting in increased intracranial pressure, such as pseudotumor cerebri and chronic respiratory insufficiency. Secondary types of empty sella syndrome may follow surgery or radiation therapy for pituitary adenomas, spontaneous degeneration or infarction of pituitary adenomas and possibly rupture of pituitary cysts.

In the primary empty sella the sellar enlargement is classically symmetrical (i.e., the sella is ballooned) but varying degrees of asymmetry mimicking intrasellar mass lesions may be encountered. The diagnosis can be unequivocally established only by demonstrating air within the sella at pneumoencephalography, and this procedure should be carried out in every patient with sellar enlargement before surgical or roentgenotherapeutic intervention for a presumed tumor.

Pituitary function is normal in virtually all patients with the primary empty sella, and the findings of endocrine abnormalities should provoke a search for other causes. Amenorrhea and inadequate growth hormone responsiveness are the endocrine abnormalities most often associated with the empty sella and appear to be secondary to the obesity seen in this group of patients rather than to the empty sella per se. Occasionally a pituitary microadenoma secreting growth hormone or prolactin may coexist within a partially empty sella. The diagnosis of these small tumors is difficult and requires careful documentation of the endocrine abnormality.

Spontaneous cerebrospinal rhinorrhea occurs in less than 5 percent of patients with the empty sella syndrome with the consequent risk of meningitis. Rarely, there may be herniation of the optic chiasm into the sella with visual impairment.[30]

Craniopharyngioma and Other Intracranial Tumors

Craniopharyngioma is the most common tumor of the hypothalamic-pituitary region in childhood and adolescence, although one-third present in adulthood. They arise from remnants of Rathke's pouch epithelium and often present with both suprasellar and sellar manifestations. The tumors are usually cystic, and suprasellar calcification is seen in 70 percent of younger patients and approximately 40 percent of older patients. Increased intracranial pressure with papilledema is frequent in younger patients. Visual field deficits are common, and hypopituitarism and diabetes insipidus reflect pituitary and hypothalamic dysfunction. Therapy should be directed toward surgical removal of small tumors and partial removal and decompression of cysts in large tumors. Current studies indicate that postoperative radiotherapy will significantly decrease the incidence of tumor recurrence and prolong survival.[3]

Primary central nervous system tumors may present as intra- or suprasellar tumors including meningioma, chordoma, optic glioma, epidermoid and dermoid tumors, and pineal area tumors including teratomas and pinealomas. Manifestations are variable and may be secondary to mass effect with increased intracranial pressure or to a variety of endocrine disturbances including variable degrees of pituitary failure, diabetes insipidus or precocious puberty. Metastatic lesions to the pituitary gland are common, especially in disseminated breast carcinoma, but are an unusual cause of clinical hypothalamic-pituitary dysfunction.

Miscellaneous Pituitary Lesions

Pituitary adenomas, craniopharyngiomas and the empty sella syndrome account for the great majority of cases of pituitary lesions with enlargement of the sella turcica. Rare causes of sellar enlargement or pituitary failure are intrasellar cysts; carotid aneurysm; acute or chronic inflammatory lesions including meningitis, septic foci, tuberculosis, syphilis, and mycoses; and infiltrative lesions such as histiocytosis-X, hemochromatosis and sarcoidosis. Hypopituitarism as a consequence of these lesions may be secondary to either hypothalamic or pituitary involvement.

Congenital deficiencies of one or more anterior pituitary hormones occur and may be familial. Isolated deficiencies of growth hormone and gonadotropins are the most common and must be differentiated from acquired hypothalamic and pituitary lesions. In the adult, hypopituitarism in the absence of a pituitary tumor is most commonly secondary to postpartum pituitary necrosis following intra- or postpartum hemorrhage. Cerebral trauma sufficient to cause hypothalamic-pituitary damage is usually fatal, but some patients survive and may manifest hypopituitarism with diabetes insipidus and galactorrhea as a consequence of traumatic stalk section.

Nontumorous Pituitary Enlargement

Primary failure of the thyroid gland or gonads leads to hyperplasia of the pituitary cells secreting thyrotropin and gonadotropins, respectively, with concomitant hypersecretion of these pituitary trophic hormones.[26,48] In this setting of physiologic pituitary hyperfunction, minor degrees of sellar enlargement have been demonstrated roentgenographically. Pituitary enlargement may rarely occur in the adrenogenital syndromes in which deficient adrenal glucocorticoid secretion leads to corticotropin hypersecretion. These conditions may be differentiated from hypersecreting pituitary tumors in that the elevated pituitary trophic hormones are suppressed by physiologic replacement therapy with the appropriate end-organ hormone.

LOCAL MANIFESTATIONS OF PITUITARY TUMORS

Clinical Features

Headache is the most usual local manifestation of pituitary adenomas and occurs in the majority of patients who have enlargement of the sella turcica. The headache of pituitary tumors is variable in intensity and is nonspecific in both location and character.[8] Headache is frequently absent in patients with pituitary microadenomas who present with endocrine disturbances in the absence of overt sellar enlargement. Visual field defects, characteristically bitemporal, reflect pressure on the inferior aspect of the optic chiasm by pituitary tumors extending superiorly from the sella turcica.[16] With suprasellar extension of the tumor, vision is affected first in the superior temporal quadrants; later involvement of the inferior temporal quadrants leads to the typical bitemporal hemianopsia. The end result of unrelieved pressure on the optic chiasm is eventual blindness with optic atrophy. Atypical visual field abnormalities occur as a result of variations in the position of the optic chiasm and eccentric suprasellar extension of pituitary tumors.[16] Careful search for a pituitary lesion should be carried out in patients with atypical visual field abnormalities, since this is a potentially curable cause of visual loss. Compression of the cavernous sinuses by lateral tumor extension may cause impairment of third, fourth and sixth cranial nerve functions with extraocular muscle palsies. Rarely, major suprasellar extension of pituitary adenomas may produce hypothalamic dysfunction leading to diabetes insipidus and alterations in sleep, temperature and appetite regulation. Diabetes insipidus is unusual in intrasellar tumors, and its presence should arouse the suspicion of either a primary hypothalamic lesion or a major suprasellar extension of a pituitary adenoma.

Evidence of suprasellar and parasellar extension of pituitary tumors implies extensive tumor growth. With careful neuroroentgenographic and endocrine evaluation, it is now possible to detect many pituitary tumors at a time when they are purely intrasellar.

Pituitary apoplexy is a relatively uncommon local complication of pituitary tumors and occurs in 2 to 3 percent of patients as a consequence of infarction of, or hemorrhage into, a pituitary adenoma.[35] Symptoms are caused by sudden expansion of the intrasellar contents, with severe headache, rapid visual failure and extraocular motor palsies secondary to compression of the cavernous sinuses. Acute pituitary insufficiency with hypotension and hyperthermia may result, and rapid mental deterioration, coma and death may ensue. Emergency treatment with steroids and transsphenoidal decompression of the intrasellar contents may be lifesaving and prevent permanent visual loss. Occasional patients may undergo subacute infarction of pituitary adenomas with intermittent headache and transient ocular palsies without life-threatening consequences.

Diagnosis

Neuro-ophthalmologic Evaluation. A detailed visual field examination should be performed in every patient with a suspected intrasellar lesion. The earliest effect of inferior chiasmal compression is red desaturation of the superior temporal fields; subsequently, vision is lost, leading to superior temporal field defects and eventually to bitemporal hemianopsia. Surgical intervention in patients with early visual loss usually restores vision to normal and at least prevents further deterioration. Careful mapping of the visual fields will allow post-treatment evaluation of the extent of surgical decompression and provide a basis for future assessment of tumor recurrence.[16]

Neuroroentgenographic Evaluation. Lateral and anteroposterior roentgenographs of the sella turcica should be obtained in all patients with suspected pituitary lesions. Plain roentgenographs may show overall enlargement of the sella turcica, erosions of the floor, or destruction of the clinoid processes. Sellar tomography provides much clearer demonstration of sellar abnormalities and delineates unilateral sellar enlargement, sloping of the sellar floor, and focal erosion with extension into the sphenoid sinus.[44,45] Sellar tomography has led to the roentgenographic definition of pituitary microadenomas (i.e., pituitary tumors less than 1 cm. in diameter that do not cause gross enlargement of the sella turcica but which do cause focal anterior bulging, asymmetry or sloping of the floor). Since variations in sellar configuration may occur in normal individuals,[41] the diagnosis of pituitary microadenoma should be made only in the presence of both an abnormality of the sella on tomography and a definite abnormality of pituitary function such as hyperprolactinemia, acromegaly, or Cushing's disease. Suprasellar extension and panhypopituitarism are rare in pituitary microadenomas, and the absence of these late manifestations should not exclude the diagnosis. Patients with minor asymmetry of the sella who have normal anterior pituitary function may be safely followed with serial assessment of sella tomograms and endocrine function.

Pneumoencephalography is the only reliable method of defining suprasellar extension and should be performed in all patients with sellar lesions prior to therapy, since the extent of upward growth must be known to the surgeon and roentgenotherapist. Tomography of the suprasellar region during pneumoencephalography will delineate small degrees of tumor extension into the suprasellar cistern and will define eccentric suprasellar growth. Larger tumor extension will cause deformity and displacement of the anterior recesses of the third ventricle. Pneumoencephalography is the only means of excluding the empty sella syndrome, a condition that rarely requires sugical intervention.[30] Current techniques of performing computerized axial tomography (CAT and EMI scans) do not have sufficient resolution of the base of the skull to permit definition of intrasellar tumors and will only define lesions with gross suprasellar extension. At present, pneumoencephalography is the only technique that provides the surgeon with accurate definition of suprasellar anatomy and delineates minor degrees of suprasellar extension.

Lateral extension of pituitary tumors can be assessed by either carotid arteriography or cavernous sinus venography, thus directing the attention of the surgeon to these areas during pituitary exploration. Carotid arteriography will establish the rare diagnosis of intrasellar aneurysm and prevent a potential surgical disaster.

ASSESSMENT OF ANTERIOR PITUITARY FUNCTION

The major anterior pituitary hormones are now measurable by specific immunoassay. This permits accurate diagnosis of specific types of pituitary tumors and has made possible the diagnosis of pituitary adenomas before the development of overt enlargement of the sella turcica. Endocrine syndromes are often the earliest manifestation of pituitary tumors and may be a consequence of either hyper- or hyposecretion of one or more anterior pituitary hormones. Pre- and postoperative endocrine evaluation permits accurate assessment of the response to therapy and also the necessity for hormonal replacement therapy. In the evaluation of anterior pituitary function, reliance on basal hormone levels may be misleading, and the use of dynamic suppression and stimulation tests has enhanced the specificity of diagnosis.

Pituitary Hypersecretion

Hypersecretion of growth hormone, prolactin, and adrenocorticotropin (ACTH) by the anterior pituitary lead to the classic syndromes of acromegaly, gigantism, galactorrhea/amenorrhea and hyperadrenocorticism (Cushing's disease). Hypersecretion of thyrotropin (TSH) and the gonadotropins, follicle-stimulating hormone (FSH) and luteinizing hormone (LH), by pituitary adenomas has been reported but is quite rare.[4,17]

Growth Hormone Hypersecretion. Basal levels of human growth hormone (HGH) in the unstressed patient are less than 5 ng./ml.; however, higher levels are seen in acute illness, in anxious individuals and after exercise. Fasting HGH levels in patients with acromegaly or gigantism are usually greater than 10 ng./ml.; however, approximately 10 percent of patients will have lower levels. The diagnosis of acromegaly with HGH hypersecretion can be established in the presence of an elevated basal HGH level that is not suppressible to less than 2.5 ng./ml. 60 minutes after administration of 100 g. glucose p.o.[32] Acromegalic patients with normal or slightly elevated HGH levels characteristically do not show normal suppressibility with hyperglycemia. A paradoxic rise in HGH levels following oral glucose may be seen in as many as one-third of acromegalics and also in patients with renal failure, chronic liver disease and porphyria. In these latter conditions, the characteristic clinical features of acromegaly are absent.

Prolactin Hypersecretion. Prolactin is the hormone most frequently secreted by pituitary tumors and levels have now been shown to be elevated in the majority of the chromophobe tumors previously thought to be nonfunctional.[6,25,29] Prolactin levels are also elevated in patients with hypothalamic lesions in whom secretion of prolactin-inhibiting factor is deficient and in patients following pituitary stalk section. Immunoassays for prolactin are now available and levels should be measured in all patients who present with galactorrhea or sellar enlargement. Basal prolactin levels range from 5 to 25 ng./ml. in most laboratories, and elevated levels have been reported in the majority of conditions causing galactorrhea. Suppression tests of prolactin using L-dopa or water-loading have been described, but these tests do not clearly separate those patients with "functional" hyperprolactinemia from those with prolactin-secreting pituitary tumors.

Basal prolactin levels of more than 100 ng./ml. are usually indicative of a pituitary adenoma and in most cases will be accompanied by enlargement of the sella turcica. Many patients with moderate elevation of plasma prolactin levels in the range of 30 to 100 ng./ml., who were previously thought to have functional or idiopathic hyperprolactinemia, have been shown to harbor prolactin-secreting pituitary microadenomas.[5,15,44] Careful tomographic examination of the sella turcica should be carried out in all patients with galactorrhea and elevated prolactin levels.

ACTH Hypersecretion. Pituitary ACTH hypersecretion leading to bilateral adrenal hyperplasia and hypercortisolism is the most common form of spontaneously occurring Cushing's syndrome. The diagnosis is established by the findings of elevated plasma and urine corticosteroid levels that are not suppressible with low-dose dexamethasone but which show partial suppression with high dose dexamethasone (Chap. 20) in the presence of normal to moderately elevated plasma ACTH levels (50-200 pg./ml).[2] Pituitary-dependent Cushing's syndrome, known as Cushing's disease, must be differentiated from other forms of hypercortisolism such as primary adrenal tumors or the ectopic production of ACTH by nonpituitary tumors (Chaps. 20 and 23). Because ACTH secretion is episodic and plasma levels are variable in normal individuals and, frequently, are normal in patients with well-documented Cushing's disease,[2,42] basal levels are diagnostically reliable only in those patients with documented cortisol excess in whom the presence of normal ACTH levels is inappropriate.

Plasma ACTH levels are markedly elevated (500-20,000 pg./ml.) in those patients who develop a progressive ACTH-producing pituitary tumor after bilateral adrenalectomy for Cushing's disease (Nelson's syndrome)[2,31] and are characteristically nonsuppressible except with high doses of dexamethasone. Because plasma ACTH levels provide a reliable indicator of the presence of a pituitary tumor in these patients, regular follow-up determinations and sellar tomograms should be undertaken. Although pituitary secretion of β-melanocyte-stimulating hormone (β-MSH) is elevated in both Cushing's disease and Nelson's syndrome and is responsible for the pigmentation seen in these disorders, assays for β-MSH are not currently available for clinical use.

Pituitary Hyposecretion

Although the majority of patients with pituitary tumors are currently diagnosed before the development of panhypopituitarism, careful evaluation of pituitary trophic hormone function should be undertaken prior to, and at intervals following, therapy. Anterior pituitary hormones may be measured directly, and pituitary reserve may be accurately assessed by the use of appropriate stimulation tests. Current assays of pituitary hormones cannot distinguish low-normal from deficient levels of secretion; however simultaneous measurement of the pituitary hormone and its target-gland secretion can establish the diagnosis of pituitary deficiency in most instances. For example, the finding of normal to low levels of TSH in the presence of low circulating thyroid hormone concentrations clearly separates pituitary hypothyroidism from primary thyroid failure in which circulating TSH is elevated.

Compromise of anterior pituitary function is gradual in most cases and destruction of more than 80 percent of the anterior pituitary is required to produce panhypopituitarism. Deficiencies of growth hormone and gonadotropin secretion are the earliest manifestations of pituitary hypofunction and occur before TSH and ACTH deficiency.[32] Assessment of the reserve of these hormones provides a sensitive index of pituitary function. Post-therapeutic assessement of anterior pituitary function is useful in determining the need for hormonal replacement therapy, and subsequent deterioration in pituitary function suggests either tumor recurrence or radiation-induced injury to non-neoplastic anterior pituitary cells.

Growth Hormone Deficiency. Growth hormone deficiency is an early and sensitive index of pituitary dysfunction; however, HGH is secreted in low levels in normal children and adults, and current immunoassays cannot distinguish low-normal from subnormal levels. Measurement of basal levels is therefore not reliable in the diagnosis of HGH deficiency, and stimulation tests that measure HGH reserve are required. Insulin-induced hypoglycemia (insulin tolerance test) is the most consistent and sensitive stimulus of HGH secretion:[22,32] Hypoglycemia acts through the hypothalamic-pituitary axis to induce release of both HGH and ACTH and is a useful test of the pituitary reserve of these two hormones. Sufficient insulin (0.1-0.15 U/kg. in normal subjects; 0.2-0.3 U/kg. in acromegaly, hypercortisolism, or obesity) to reduce the plasma glucose to less than 40 mg./100 ml. is required to produce an adequate stimulus of HGH secretion. In response to hypoglycemia, plasma HGH reaches a maximum of more than 10 ng./ml. in normal subjects, whereas patients with HGH deficiency show no response. This test should not be performed in patients with seizure disorders, ischemic heart disease, or cerebrovascular insufficiency; in these, HGH responsiveness may be assessed with stimulation tests using either L-dopa or arginine.[22]

Gonadotropin Deficiency. Basal levels of both pituitary gonadotropins, FSH and LH, and gonadal steroids are extremely variable and, as is the case with HGH, stimulation tests may be required to establish the diagnosis of gonadotropin deficiency. The presence of deficient gonadal steroid secretion accompanied by low serum FSH and LH strongly suggests the diagnosis of hypogonadotropic hypogonadism of hypothalamic or pituitary origin. In male patients with suspected hypothalamic-pituitary lesions, measurements of plasma testosterone and gonadotropins are essential. In the patient with low circulating testosterone, concomitant low-normal or low FSH and LH is consistent with the diagnosis of gonadotropin deficiency. In female patients with oligo- or amenorrhea, plasma estrogen levels below the normal follicular phase with simultaneous normal or low FSH and LH are also highly suggestive of hypogonadotropic hypogonadism. In postmenopausal female patients, serum FSH and LH levels are normally elevated and the finding of normal or low gonadotropin levels is highly suggestive of impaired pituitary gonadotropin secretion.

Stimulation tests with clomiphene or LH-releasing hormone (LH-RH) may give further useful information regarding pituitary function.[28,32] Clomiphene is an anti-estrogen that acts at a hypothalamic level to cause release of FSH and LH, and patients with hypothalamic or pituitary hypogonadism will show impaired or absent responses. LH-RH is the hypothalamic-releasing hormone for FSH and LH and acts directly at a pituitary level to stimulate gonadotropin secretion. Although this test provides a rapid and direct measurement of pituitary gonadotropin reserve, experience has shown that it has not been as sensitive as expected in predicting early pituitary dysfunction and differentiating hypothalamic from pituitary hypogonadism.[28] The normal response to LH-RH is a rapid increase in serum LH to a maximal level two to three times greater than basal, with a lesser and more delayed FSH response. In patients with early pituitary tumors, the LH-RH test may be normal; however, with progressive loss of function, impaired, delayed or absent responses are seen.

Thyrotropin Deficiency. Deficient TSH secretion leads to secondary hypothyroidism. Measurement of serum TSH is useful but must be viewed in conjunction with circulating thyroid hormone levels. In the presence of low circulating thyroid hormones, low or low-normal serum TSH is consistent with TSH deficiency, and the low TSH level differentiates this condition from primary thyroid failure in which serum TSH levels are elevated. In euthyroid subjects, basal levels of TSH will offer no useful information concerning early pituitary dysfunction. Thyrotropin-releasing hormone (TRH) is a hypothalamic peptide that causes prompt stimulation of TSH secretion in normal individuals: 15 to 20 min. after intravenous injection, serum TSH reaches a peak of more than two to three times basal levels. In patients with hypothalamic or pituitary lesions, the TSH response is often impaired or delayed, although, in patients with small pituitary tumors, TSH reserve is often intact.[14,40]

ACTH Deficiency. Deficiency of ACTH leads to decreased production of adrenal glucocorticoids and androgens, but aldosterone secretion, which is primarily under the control of the renin-angiotensin system, remains intact. For this reason, signs of mineralocorticoid deficiency such as hypotension, dehydration, hyponatremia and hyperkalemia are absent, and the usual symptoms are nonspecific weakness and fatigue. Because of the lack of specific clinical features, accurate assessment of pituitary-adrenal reserve is necessary to determine the patient's ability to respond to stress. Low basal adrenal steroid levels in the presence of low plasma ACTH are consistent with pituitary hypoadrenalism, although normal levels may be present with partial ACTH deficiency. Insulin-induced hypoglycemia, the most specific test of pituitary-adrenal reserve, accurately predicts the ability to respond to stress and the need for corticosteroid replacement therapy.[11,32] The hypoglycemia stimulus is mediated by way of the central nervous system and the hypothalamus and, therefore, a normal response indicates that all elements of the hypothalamic-pituitary-adrenal axis are intact. Plasma cortisol reaches a peak level of more than 20 μg./100 ml. in normal individuals; in patients with hypothalamic or pituitary disorders, the response is subnormal or absent even though baseline levels may be normal. In patients in whom insulin-induced hypoglycemia is contraindicated, metyrapone may be used to assess the pituitary-adrenal axis.

Prolactin Deficiency. Prolactin is the pituitary hormone most resistant to damage and, therefore, hyposecretion usually occurs only in association with panhypopituitarism. Failure of prolactin secretion is of clinical importance in Sheehan's syndrome (postpartum pituitary necrosis) in which failure of lactation is a cardinal feature. Prolactin secretion is stimulated by TRH, and this test is useful in determining the pituitary reserve of both TSH and prolactin.[40]

SURGICAL MANAGEMENT OF PITUITARY TUMORS

Preoperative Management

Precise delineation of tumor size and extension, obtained with the neuro-ophthalmologic and neuroroentgenographic procedures previously detailed, permits the neurosurgeon to select the procedure of choice for each patient. Evaluation of anterior pituitary function establishes the presence of pituitary hypersecretion and the degree of compromise of anterior pituitary function. Prolactin hypersecretion is frequent in clinically "nonfunctioning" tumors, and the comparison of pre- and postoperative values provides a precise estimate of the completeness of surgical resection and the necessity for further therapy to eliminate residual tumor. Similarly, serial determination of anterior pituitary function provides an accurate assessment of the adequacy of surgical therapy in patients with HGH or ACTH hypersecretion.

All patients undergoing pituitary surgery should receive adrenal corticosteroid support in the form of a rapidly acting soluble preparation (hydrocortisone phosphate or hydrocortisone hemisuccinate). Parenteral hydrocortisone

(200-300 mg. in divided doses) should be given on the day of surgery and may be rapidly tapered to a maintenance dosage of 20 to 30 mg. orally by the fifth to seventh postoperative day without adverse consequences. The requirement for permanent endocrine replacement therapy is best determined 6 to 8 weeks postoperatively.

The Transsphenoidal Microsurgical Approach to Pituitary Tumors

Operative Procedure. The operative procedure is carried out with the patient under general anesthesia in a semi-sitting position facing the surgeon.[15,46] A fluoroscopic image intensifier is positioned to provide a lateral view of the sella on the television monitor. If the tumor extends above the sella, the third ventricle and suprasellar cisterns are filled with air through a lumbar subarachnoid catheter before the head is positioned in a skull fixation head frame. After injecting the nasal and gingival mucosa with epinephrine, the upper lip is elevated and a horizontal incision is made in the gingiva over the maxilla. The nasal spine and the projecting maxillary rim are removed and a submucosal plane is developed on the nasal floor and septum. The mucosa is reflected laterally by advancing a self-retaining speculum. Removal of the lower nasal septum exposes the rostral sphenoid. A high-speed air drill opens the sphenoid sinus and the sphenoidal mucosa is reflected and removed. Fluoroscopic monitoring and direct visualization with the operating microscope guide all further maneuvers. The anterior sellar wall is removed to expose the dural lining of the sella. The dura is coagulated and excised to visualize and remove the intrasellar and suprasellar tumor. Lumbar spinal air injection at the beginning of the procedure allows the surgeon to visualize (on the monitor) the dome of the suprasellar tumor. In addition to roentgenographic evidence, the operator must visualize the entire suprasellar portion of the tumor "capsule" before considering the operation complete. When the tumor is small (<2.0 cm. in diameter), and if the remaining cavity does not communicate with the subarachnoid space, Gelfoam saturated with absolute alcohol is placed within the cavity to destroy superficial microscopic nests of tumor cells. Following the intrasellar procedure, any defects in the sellar diaphragm are covered with fascia lata reinforced with either muscle or fat removed from the thigh, and the floor of the sella is reconstituted with a piece of nasal septal cartilage. The nasal cavities are packed with bacitracin-impregnated petrolatum gauze, which is left in place for 48 to 72 hours.

Indications and Contraindications. The transsphenoidal approach to pituitary adenomas has decided advantages in the operative treatment of pituitary microadenomas, larger adenomas confined to the sella turcica, tumors associated with cerebrospinal rhinorrhea, pituitary apoplexy and tumors with sphenoidal extension. Because of the procedure's low morbidity, it provides an attractive alternative to craniotomy for patients in suboptimal general health due to advanced age or concurrent serious medical conditions. In the treatment of adenomas with moderate suprasellar extension and visual impairment, transsphenoidal removal compares favorably with the transfrontal approach, and in our experience both major and minor complications have been fewer than with craniotomy.[46] Unless a contraindication exists, a transsphenoidal approach is selected in patients with untreated pituitary tumors and in those patients in whom an earlier therapeutic effort, surgical or nonsurgical, has failed.

Contraindications to the transsphenoidal approach are:

1. Dumbbell-shaped adenomas constricted at the diaphragma sellae, because visualization and safe sphenoidal delivery of a suprasellar mass require a wide sellar aperture.
2. Lateral suprasellar extensions, because, although rare, they cannot be visualized through a midline operative field and should be approached by craniotomy.
3. A massive suprasellar tumor which cannot be handled adequately with the limited exposure afforded through the sphenoidal sinus. The usual suprasellar mass causing chiasmal compression presents no problem because normal intracranial pressure, aided by the pulsation of surrounding cerebrospinal fluid, forces the suprasellar component downward into the expanded sella.

In our recent experience with 300 patients treated surgically for pituitary adenomas, only six required craniotomy and the remainder underwent transsphenoidal removal. The single death in this series resulted from postoperative pulmonary embolism, and serious surgical morbidity was unusual.[46] Transsphenoidal removal of pituitary adenomas is effective and experience with secreting adenomas has been excellent. Masses extending outside the sella, regardless of related endocrinologic abnormality, are best handled by operation followed by irradiation for incompletely removed tumors. Whereas anatomic considerations should dictate the type of approach used, in our own experience the great majority of pituitary tumors are admirably suited for transsphenoidal removal.

Postoperative Management

Recovery from transsphenoidal microsurgery is rapid and virtually all patients are ambulatory within 24 hours. Oral fluids are taken the evening of surgery and a progressive diet is undertaken on the following day. Headache is readily controlled by oral or parenteral codeine, and the nasal packs are removed in 48 to 72 hours. Hydrocortisone coverage is rapidly tapered to maintenance levels (20-30 mg. per day), and patients remain on this dosage until reevaluation of pituitary function is carried out at 6 to 8 weeks.

Subsequent management of patients surgically treated for pituitary adenomas should include a complete evaluation of pituitary function to determine the extent of surgical resection of hypersecreting adenomas and the need for permanent adrenal, thyroid, or gonadal replacement therapy. Postoperative roentgenotherapy is necessary only in those patients in whom microsurgical tumor removal is incomplete or in whom persistent tumor hypersecretion is demonstrated. All patients should be restudied annually for evidence of local tumor recurrence and endocrine dysfunction. Late hypopituitarism does not occur following pituitary surgery and, if present, suggests tumor recurrence or the delayed effect of pituitary irradiation.

SPECIFIC PITUITARY SYNDROMES

Acromegaly

Clinical Features (Table 19-1). Acromegaly is a chronic, disfiguring disease with a high incidence of late morbidity and mortality. After 45 years of age, the death rate in acromegalic patients from increased cardiovascular, cerebrovascular and respiratory disease is greater than twice that of the normal population. With adequate therapy, this excessive mortality rate can be reduced.[47]

The characteristic clinical manifestations are a consequence of prolonged growth hormone hypersecretion leading to progressive overgrowth of soft tissue, cartilage and bone.[8] Acral enlargement is present in all patients at the time of diagnosis and consists of the classic syndrome of coarse facial features, large nose, prominent supraorbital ridges, prognathism and widely spaced teeth.[38] The hands and feet are large, thick and bulky, with broad, blunt, spadelike fingers and toes, and progressive increases in ring, glove, and shoe size have usually occurred. Hyperhidrosis and heat intolerance are signs of hypermetabolism and suggest active growth hormone hypersecretion. The characteristic warm, moist, fleshy handshake reflects hypermetabolism, hyperhidrosis and soft-tissue proliferation.[38] Fatigue, weight gain, paresthesias secondary to carpal tunnel compression and arthralgias are present in greater than 60 percent of patients.

Local manifestations consist of headache in the majority of patients and enlargement of the sella in over 80 percent of cases.[24] In those patients with normal routine sellar roentgenographs, pituitary microadenomas can be demonstrated by sellar tomography.[24] Visual impairment was very common in older series,[9] but the fact that now only 20 percent of patients have visual field

Table 19-1. Clinical Features of Acromegaly

Local Manifestations	
Enlarged sella	>80*
Headache	65
Visual deficit	20
Manifestations of Growth Hormone Excess	
Acral enlargement	100
Soft-tissue overgrowth	100
Hyperhidrosis	88
Lethargy or fatigue	87
Weight gain	73
Paresthesias	70
Joint pain	69
Photophobia	46
Papillomata	45
Hyperthrichosis	33
Goiter	32
Acanthosis nigricans	29
Hypertension	24
Cardiomegaly	16
Renal calculi	11
Disturbance of Other Endocrine Functions	
Glucose intolerance	50
Hyperinsulinemia	70
Irregular or absent menses	60
Decreased libido or impotence	46
Hypothyroidism	13
Hypoadrenalism	4
Galactorrhea	13
Gynecomastia	8

*Percentage of patients in whom these features are evident.

deficits attests to the earlier recognition of the characteristic clinical manifestations of growth hormone hypersecretion.[46]

Alterations in other endocrine functions are extremely common in untreated acromegaly.[8,20,38] Glucose intolerance occurs in 50 percent of patients and hyperinsulinemia in 70 percent; however, clinical diabetes mellitus is present in less than 10 percent. Hypogonadism manifested by amenorrhea, impotence, or decreased libido occurs in over 50 percent of cases and is the most common indicator of pituitary hypofunction. In contrast, hypothyroidism and hypoadrenalism are unusual.[20,38,43] Galactorrhea occurs in approximately 15 percent of patients and is frequently accompanied by hyperprolactinemia.

Routine roentgenographic studies show sellar enlargement, enlarged frontal and maxillary sinuses, thickening of the calvarium and elongation of the jaw. Roentgenographs of the hands and feet reveal soft-tissue thickening, widening of joint spaces, arrowhead tufting of the terminal phalanges, and thickening of the heel pads due to soft-tissue overgrowth. Routine laboratory tests frequently show elevation of serum inorganic phosphate, and hypercalciuria is common.

Gigantism is a rare disorder in which the onset of growth hormone hypersecretion occurs in childhood or adolescence prior to fusion of the epiphyses. The characteristic feature is excessive skeletal growth with maintenance of normal body proportions. When the onset of growth hormone hypersecretion occurs at the time of puberty, features of both gigantism and acromegaly are often present.

Diagnosis. The diagnosis of acromegaly can be established by measurement of serum growth hormone in the basal state and following suppression with hyperglycemia. Basal levels are elevated by more than 10 ng./ml. in over 90 percent of patients with active acromegaly and may be as high as 50 to 500 ng./ml. In those few patients with normal or borderline elevation of growth hormone, nonsuppressibility with hyperglycemia establishes the diagnosis.[32] Evaluation of sellar size, visual fields and the special neuroroentgenographic procedures previously described should also be carried out to define tumor size prior to therapeutic intervention. Assessment of anterior pituitary function as previously described delineates the degree of compromise of the normal pituitary gland.

Treatment. The objective of therapy in acromegaly is to prevent the late cosmetic manifestations and increased mortality by achieving adequate reduction of excessive growth hormone secretion. If a post-treatment growth hormone level of less than 10 ng./ml. is achieved, clinical progression of acromegaly will be arrested. Hyperhidrosis and hypermetabolism are usually reversible and there is reduction in the degree of the soft-tissue component of acral enlargement in 80 percent.[38] Headache, paresthesias, carpal tunnel syndrome, joint pains and oily skin are reversible in over 65 percent of patients, whereas weight gain and symptoms of hypogonadism are less responsive to therapy. Glucose tolerance returns to normal in the majority of patients. The bone and cartilage overgrowth of acromegaly is irreversible, but further progression is prevented.

Acromegalic patients with primarily intrasellar tumors show excellent responses to therapy, but it is now clear that patients with markedly elevated growth hormone values ($>$50 ng./ml.) and those with large invasive tumors (i.e., with suprasellar, lateral or sphenoid sinus extension) respond less well.

In these patients, multiple therapies including both surgical and roentgenotherapeutic approaches are usually required.

Surgical Therapy for Acromegaly. Transsphenoidal selective microsurgical adenomectomy is the procedure of choice in the majority of patients with untreated acromegaly and in those with inadequate responses to other surgical procedures or radiation.[15,43] Transsphenoidal microsurgery is ideally suited for pituitary microadenomas and larger tumors within the confines of the sella turcica. It is the only effective approach for removal of tumor extension into the sphenoid sinus. It is also effective in those patients with mild to moderate suprasellar extension and chiasmal compression in whom the sellar aperture is wide enough to permit delivery of the tumor from below. In experienced hands, serious surgical complications including cerebrospinal rhinorrhea, meningitis and postoperative hematoma occur in fewer than 5 percent of patients and mortality is negligible. Diabetes insipidus occurs in approximately 15 percent but is virtually always transient and does not require prolonged therapy. Transient ocular palsies occur in approximately 5 percent of cases, expecially in those patients with lateral tumor extensions, but visual impairment is rare as a surgical complication.[46]

In our current experience with over 40 patients with previously untreated acromegaly, adequate reduction of growth hormone to less than 10 ng./ml. has occurred in 80 percent.[43] Reduction in growth hormone secretion is immediate and clinical reversal of soft-tissue bulk frequently begins in the first postoperative weeks. Since this procedure allows selective removal of the tumor with preservation of the normal pituitary gland, postoperative hypopituitarism is unusual and occurs in less than 10 percent of patients.

Transsphenoidal stereotactic cryohypophysectomy has been used extensively in acromegaly and is an effective form of therapy in 60 to 70 percent of patients.[20,38] It is less effective than transsphenoidal microsurgical removal and should not be used in patients with very large tumors or in those with suprasellar, lateral or sphenoid sinus extension. Surgical complications include cerebrospinal rhinorrhea, meningitis, transient visual field deficits and transient extraocular palsies in 10 to 15 percent. Diabetes insipidus and the inappropriate secretion of antidiuretic hormone are frequent but almost always transient, and surgical hypopituitarism requiring replacement therapy occurs in 20 percent of patients. Transfrontal craniotomy is an ineffective means of lowering growth hormone in the majority of patients and is still accompanied by significant mortality and serious surgical morbidity. For these reasons, craniotomy should be reserved for those few patients in whom extensive lateral or suprasellar extension precludes adequate tumor removal by way of the transsphenoidal route.

Other Therapeutic Approaches. Conventional external radiotherapy using dosages of 4,000 to 5,000 rad is effective in 60 to 70 percent of acromegalic patients—the major disadvantage being that the effect is slow and significant reduction of growth hormone levels may not occur for 3 to 6 years.[13] Serious complications are rare and, although hypopituitarism has been infrequently reported, current data suggest that with sensitive endocrine testing a much higher incidence of pituitary damage will be uncovered as a consequence of pituitary irradiation.[36]

Proton beam or heavy particle irradiation is effective in 70 to 80 percent of acromegalic patients with intrasellar tumors but is available at only a few centers.[19] Reduction in growth hormone levels occurs more rapidly than with conventional irradiation, but several years may be required to achieve full effectiveness. Damage to cranial nerves and adjacent neurologic structures occurs in a few patients and hypopituitarism develops in at least one-third.

Local roentgenotherapy with intrasellar implantation of radioactive isotopes achieves control of acromegaly in the majority of cases but is associated with a high incidence of rhinorrhea, meningitis and hypopituitarism.

Medical treatment of acromegaly has been attempted with estrogens, progesterone and chlorpromazine without significant success. Somatostatin, a hypothalamic peptide, effectively inhibits growth hormone secretion in acromegaly; however, current preparations are insufficiently long-acting for chronic use. Bromoergocryptine, an ergot alkaloid effective in the treatment of hyperprolactinemia, has been shown to reduce growth hormone secretion in acromegaly[7] and may be an effective form of therapy in some patients who have responded inadequately to other methods.

Prolactin-Secreting Pituitary Tumors

Clinical Features. The clinical application of prolactin assays has established that prolactin is the hormone most commonly secreted by pituitary tumors.[6,25] Hyperprolactinemia can be demonstrated in many patients who were previously thought to have nonfunctional chromophobe adenomas and is extremely useful in the evaluation and subsequent follow-up of these patients.[25] In addition, clinical awareness that hyperprolactinemia frequently accompanies the galactorrhea-amenorrhea syndromes has led to recognition of pituitary microadenomas in which galactorrhea or amenorrhea or both are the earliest manifestations.[5,15,44]

Pituitary prolactin secretion is under a tonic inhibitory effect of a hypothalamic peptide, prolactin-inhibiting factor, and hyperprolactinemia follows damage to the hypothalamus or pituitary stalk. However, EM and immunofluorescent techniques have shown that prolactin secretion directly by pituitary tumors is the usual cause of hyperprolactinemia in hypothalamic-pituitary disorders.

Although the classic manifestations of hyperprolactinemia are galactorrhea and amenorrhea, galactorrhea is absent in the majority of patients even in the presence of marked elevation of serum prolactin.[6,12,17,25,29] In addition, galactorrhea is generally mild, may be transient, or may never occur spontaneously. Manual expression is required to demonstrate galactorrhea in most patients. It is even less common in male patients and presentation is usually with decreasing libido or impotence. For these reasons, prolactin determinations should be performed in all patients with galactorrhea, enlargement of the sella turcica, or suspected hypothalamic-pituitary dysfunction. Current reports indicate that hyperprolactinemia may occur in significant numbers of patients presenting with amenorrhea in the absence of other pituitary manifestations, and a number of these patients have been shown to have functioning pituitary adenomas.[12,17,37] Consequently, plasma prolactin determinations should be included routinely in the evaluation of patients with unexplained amenorrhea, decreased libido, or impotence.

Differential Diagnosis of Galactorrhea. The principal disorders causing galactorrhea are shown in the list below, and in the majority of these conditions elevated prolactin has been demonstrated. Physiologic increases in prolactin occur during pregnancy and in the postpartum period; however, some pituitary tumors have become clinically evident after pregnancy and patients with galactorrhea and amenorrhea persisting for more than 1 year should be evaluated for pituitary dysfunction. Galactorrhea is common during or after oral contraceptive use, but patients with persistent galactorrhea and amenorrhea following discontinuance of therapy should be evaluated for pituitary adenomas.[5] Drug-induced galactorrhea is common with medications affecting catecholamine metabolism of the central nervous system and resolves rapidly after discontinuance of the drug. Primary hypothyroidism should be considered in patients with galactorrhea and may be present in association with precocious puberty in children. Excessive breast stimulation, chest-wall or spinal-cord lesions are less common causes of galactorrhea. Ectopic prolactin secretion from non-pituitary tumors has been described, but the incidence is currently unknown.

Diagnosis. There are no available suppression or stimulation tests that clearly separate patients with prolactin-secreting pituitary tumors from those with hyperprolactinemia of other origins. Measurement of basal prolactin levels and careful assessment of the sella turcica with polytomography will establish the

Causes of Galactorrhea

Physiologic
- Pregnancy
- Postpartum
- Neonatal

Hypothalamic-pituitary disorders
- Prolactin-secreting pituitary adenomas
- Pituitary adenomas secreting growth hormone or cortiocotropin
- Pituitary stalk scction
- Hypothalamic lesions:
  - Tumors
  - Inflammatory and infiltrative lesions

Drugs
- Oral contraceptives
- Estrogens
- Phenothiazines
- Antidepressants
- Haloperidol
- Alpha-methyldopa

Endocrine disorders
- Hypothyroidism
- Hyperthyroidism

Nonpituitary tumors
- Ectopic prolactin secretion
- Estrogen-secreting tumors
- Choriocarcinoma of the testis

Local and neurogenic factors
- Breast stimulation
- Chest-wall injury (surgery, trauma, burns)
- Herpes zoster
- Spinal-cord lesions

diagnosis in most cases.[5,44] As previously stated, prolactin levels greater than 100 ng./ml. usually indicate a pituitary tumor accompanied by enlargement of the sella turcica. Patients with prolactin-secreting pituitary microadenomas have mildly to moderately elevated prolactin levels (30-100 ng./ml.) and usually have seller tomographic abnormalities diagnostic of a microadenoma.[5,44] When these results are borderline, they should be serially reassessed.

Hypogonadism is frequent in prolactin-secreting pituitary tumors, resulting in low plasma estrogen and testosterone levels in female and male patients, respectively. Basal FSH and LH levels are usually normal but are accompanied by failure to respond to clomiphene in the majority of patients.[17] Gonadotropin responses to LH-RH are variable and range from hyper-responsiveness with small tumors to absence in patients with larger tumors.[5]

Treatment. The increasing recognition of prolactin-secreting pituitary microadenomas has raised questions as to the frequency of this disorder and whether all patients should undergo therapy since the natural history of these small tumors is not known. Tumors enlarging the sella turcica should be treated, and transsphenoidal microsurgery is the procedure of choice. Patients with persistent hyperprolactinemia postoperatively should be considered for pituitary irradiation.

Patients with microadenomas may be followed and therapy undertaken if progression occurs. If pregnancy is desired, selective microsurgical resection of the tumor by the transsphenoidal route should be carried out.[10] The incidence of hypopituitarism is minimal in experienced hands and relief of galactorrhea and amenorrhea is achieved in over 85 percent of patients.[5]

Bromergocryptine, an ergot alkaloid, is effective in suppressing hyperprolactinemia in patients with and without pituitary tumors,[17] and menstruation and ovulation are restored to normal in the majority; however, the question of tumor progression during long-term therapy has not been resolved. Patients with untreated pituitary tumors who desire pregnancy should not be treated with bromergocryptine nor should ovulation be induced, since rapid tumor progression with visual failure during pregnancy may occur.[10]

In the post-therapeutic period, serial prolactin determinations will assess the adequacy of surgical resection and predict tumor occurrence. Current experience is insufficient to determine the recurrence rate after transsphenoidal microsurgery and regular follow-up must be undertaken.

Pituitary ACTH Hypersecretion

Cushing's Disease. The diagnosis and management of Cushing's syndrome has been detailed in Chapter 20; the discussion in this chapter will be limited to the management of pituitary tumors in patients with Cushing's diesase (pituitary ACTH hypersecretion). Although the pathogenesis of this disorder is controversial, it is now established that pituitary tumors are present in the great majority of patients with Cushing's disease,[4,15,33,42] and successful correction of hypercortisolism after tumor resection is being reported.[15,18,42] Tumor size is small and enlargement of the sella on routine roentgenographs is rare; however, sellar polytomography reveals changes consistent with a pituitary microadenoma in 75 percent of cases.[15,42] In our own experience, pituitary microadenomas were identified at transsphenoidal exploration in 18 of 20 patients with Cushing's disease, and correction of hypercortisolism has been achieved in 17 patients.[42] Tumor size varied from 2 to 9 mm., with the majority being less than 5 mm. in diameter. Smaller tumors are frequently located within the body of a normal-appearing anterior pituitary gland and, in one case in which no gross tumor was found, total hypophysectomy revealed a 1.5-mm. basophilic adenoma with positive staining for ACTH by immunofluorescence. It is our recommendation that transsphenoidal microdissection by an experienced neurosurgeon should be the initial therapy for Cushing's disease because resection of a pituitary adenoma will obviate the necessity for adrenalectomy and prevent the subsequent development of Nelson's syndrome.

Nelson's Syndrome. Following bilateral adrenalectomy for Cushing's disease, 10 to 20 percent of patients will develop progressive enlargement of a pituitary tumor with increasing pigmentation as a consequence of ACTH and MSH hypersecretion.[27,31] Since it is now apparent that pituitary adenomas are present in the majority of patients with untreated Cushing's disease, Nelson's syndrome presumably is due to accelerated growth of these preexisting tumors.

These pituitary adenomas are the most invasive and aggressive of all pituitary adenomas, and the clinical course is characterized by severe hyperpigmentation, rapid sellar expansion and suprasellar extension occurring within several years after adrenalectomy. Hypopituitarism is frequent; there is a high incidence of pituitary apoplexy; and malignant transformation of these tumors with parasellar invasion has been reported.[34] An aggressive therapeutic approach should be taken and should include both surgical and roentgenotherapeutic intervention. Transsphenoidal microdissection is the procedure of choice in patients with intrasellar tumors; however, craniotomy is required in larger invasive tumors with extrasellar extension.

Although these aggressive tumors are the most dramatic manifestation of pituitary adenomas after adrenalectomy, the majority of the remaining patients can be shown to have pituitary microadenomas by ACTH measurement and sellar tomography.[45] The adenomas in this larger group of patients tend to be nonprogressive and noninvasive and the reasons for the difference in the behavior of these two clinical groups of patients are not clear. These patients should be followed with sellar tomography and plasma ACTH levels. If progression occurs, transsphenoidal exploration and tumor resection should be performed.

REFERENCES

1. Baylis, P. H.: Case of hyperthyroidism due to a chromophobe adenoma. Clin. Endocrinol., *5*:145, 1976.
2. Besser, G. M., and Edwards, C. R. W.: Cushing's syndrome. Clin. Endocrinol. Metab., *1*:451, 1972.
3. Bloom. H. J. G.: Combined modality therapy for intracranial tumors. Cancer, *35*:111, 1975.
4. Burke, C. W., et al.: Cushing's disease: treatment by pituitary implantation of radioactive gold or yttrium seeds. Q. J. Med. (New Series), *42*:693, 1973.
5. Chang, R. J., Keye, W. R., Young, J. R., Wilson, C. B., and Jaffe, R. B.: Detection, evaluation and treatment of pituitary microadenomas in patients with galactorrhea and amenorrhea. Am. J. Obstet. Gynecol., *128*:356, 1977.
6. Child, D. F., et al.: Prolactin studies in "functionless" pituitary tumours. Br. Med. J., *1*:604, 1975.
7. Chiodini, P. G., et al.: Stable reduction of plasma growth hormone (hGH) levels during chronic administration

of 2-Br-αergocryptine (CB-154) in acromegalic patients. J. Clin. Endocrinol. Metab., *40*:705, 1975.

8. Daughaday, W. H.: The adenophypophysis. *In* Williams, R. H. (ed.): Textbook of Endocrinology. ed. 5. Philadelphia, W. B. Saunders, 1974.
9. Davidoff, L. M.: Studies in acromegaly. II. Historical note. Endocrinology, *10*:453, 1926.
10. Editorial: Pituitary tumors and pregnancy. Lancet, *1*:404, 1976.
11. Edwards, C. R. W., and Besser, G. M.: Diseases of the hypothalamus and pituitary gland. J. Clin. Endocrinol. Metab., *3*:475, 1974.
12. Franks, S., et al.: Incidence and significance of hyperprolactinaemia in women with amenorrhoea. Clin. Endocrinol., *4*:597, 1975.
13. Gorden, P., and Roth, J.: The treatment of acromegaly by conventional pituitary irradiation. *In* Kohler, P. O., and Ross, G. T. (eds.): Diagnosis and Treatment of Pituitary Tumors. pp. 230-233. Amsterdam, Excerpta Medica (Int. Cong. Ser. No. 303), 1973.
14. Hall, R., Ormston, B. J., Besser, G. M., Cryer, R. J., and McKendrick, M.: The thyrotrophin-releasing hormone test in diseases of the pituitary and hypothalamus. Lancet, *1*:759, 1972.
15. Hardy, J.: Transsphenoidal surgery of hypersecreting pituitary tumors. *In* Kohler, P. O., and Ross, G. T. (eds.): Diagnosis and Treatment of Pituitary Tumors. pp. 179-194. Amsterdam Excerpta Medica (Int. Cong. Ser. No. 303), 1973.
16. Hollenhorst, R. W., and Younge, B. R.: Ocular manifestations produced by adenomas of the pituitary gland: analysis of 1000 cases. *In* Kohler, P. O., and Ross, G. T. (eds.): Diagnosis and Treatment of Pituitary Tumors. pp. 53-68. Amsterdam, Excerpta Medica (Int. Cong. Ser. No. 303), 1973.
17. Jacobs, H. S., et al.: Clinical and endocrine features of hyperprolactinaemic amenorrhoea. Clin. Endocrinol., *5*:439, 1976.
18. Lagerquist, L. G., Meikle, A. W., West, C. D., and Tyler, F. H.: Cushing's disease with cure by resection of a pituitary adenoma: evidence against a primary hypothalamic defect. Am. J. Med., *57*:826, 1974.
19. Lawrence, J. H., et al.: Treatment of pituitary tumors with heavy particles. *In* Kohler, P. O., and Ross, G. T. (eds.): Diagnosis and Treatment of Pituitary Tumors. pp. 253-262. Amsterdam, Excerpta Medica (Int. Cong. Ser. No. 303), 1973.
20. Levin, S. R., et al.: Cryohypophysectomy for acromegaly: factor associated with altered endocrine function and carbohydrate metabolism. Am. J. Med., *57*:526, 1974.
21. Lewis, P. B., and Van Noorden, S.: "Nonfunctioning" pituitary tumors. Arch. Pathol., *97*:178, 1974.
22. Lucke, C., Hoffken, B., and Morgner, K. D.: L-dopa induced growth hormone secretion. Comparison with insulin tolerance test, arginine infusion and sleep induced GH-secretion. Acta Endocrinol., *77*:241, 1974.
23. McCormick, W. F., and Halmi, N. S.: Absence of chromophobe adenomas from a large series of pituitary tumors. Arch. Pathol., *92*:231, 1971.
24. McLachlan, M. S. F., Wright, A. D., and Doyle, F. H.: Plain film and tomographic assessment of the pituitary fossa in 140 acromegalic patients. Br. J. Radiol., *43*:360, 1970.
25. Malarkey, W. B., and Johnson, J. C.: Pituitary tumors and hyperprolactinemia. Arch. Intern. Med., *136*:40, 1976.
26. Montgomery, D. A. D., and Welbourn, R. B.: Medical and Surgical Endocrinology. p. 32. London, Edward Arnold Ltd., 1975.
27. Moore, T. J., Dluhy, R. G., Williams, G. H., and Cain, J. P.: Nelson's syndrome: frequency, prognosis, and effect of prior pituitary irradiation. Ann. Intern. Med., *85*:731, 1976.
28. Mortimer, C. H., et al.: Luteinizing hormone and follicle stimulating hormone-releasing hormone test in patients with hypothalamic-pituitary-gonadal dysfunction. Br. Med. J., *4*:73, 1973.

29. Nader, S., Mashiter, K., Doyle, F. H., and Joplin, G. F.: Galactorrhoea, hyperprolactinaemia and pituitary tumours in the female. Clin. Endocrinol., *5*:245, 1976.
30. Neelon, F. A., Goree, J. A., and Lebovitz, H. E.: The primary empty sella: clinical and radiographic characteristics and endocrine function. Medicine, *52*:73, 1973.
31. Nelson, D. H., Meakin, J. W., and Thorn, G. W.: ACTH-producing pituitary tumors following adrenalectomy for Cushing's syndrome. Ann. Intern. Med., *52*:560, 1960.
32. Nelson, J. C., Kollar, D. J., and Lewis, J. E.: Growth hormone secretion in pituitary disease. Arch. Intern. Med., *133*:459, 1974.
33. Plotz, C. M., Knowlton, A. I., and Ragan, C.: The natural history of Cushing's syndrome. Am. J. Med., *13*:597, 1952.
34. Rovit, R. L., and Berry, R.: Cushing's syndrome and the hypophysis: a reevaluation of pituitary tumors and hyperadrenalism. J. Neurosurg., *23*:270, 1965.
35. Rovit, R. L., and Fein, J. M.: Pituitary apoplexy: a review and reappraisal. J. Neurosurg., *37*:280, 1972.
36. Samaan, N. A., et al.: Hypopituitarism after external irradiation: evidence for both hypothalamic and pituitary origin. Ann. Intern. Med., *83*:771, 1975.
37. Seppala, M., Hirvonen, E., Ranta, T., Virkkunen, P., and Leppaluoto, J.: Raised serum prolactin levels in amenorrhoea. Br. Med. J., *2*:305, 1975.
38. Seymour, R. J., Levin, S., Tyrrell, B., and Forsham, P. H.: Long term results of cryohypophysectomy for the treatment of acromegaly. *In* Proceedings of the European Workshop on Treatment of Pituitary Adenomas, [in press].
39. Snyder, P. J., and Sterling, F. H.: Hypersecretion of LH and FSH by a pituitary adenoma. J. Clin. Endocrinol. Metab., *42*:544, 1976.
40. Snyder, P. J., et al.: Diagnostic value of thyrotrophin-releasing hormone in pituitary and hypothalamic diseases. Ann. Intern. Med., *81*:751, 1974.
41. Swanson, H. A., and duBoulay, G.: Borderline variants of the normal pituitary fossa. Br. J. Radiol., *48*:366, 1975.
42. Tyrrell, J. B., et al.: Pituitary tumors in Cushing's disease: Reversal of hypercortisolism by selective transsphenoidal adenomectomy. Program of the Fifty-ninth Annual Meeting of The Endocrine Society, Chicago, Illinois, June 8-10, 1977, p. 142 (Abstr.).
43. U, H. S., Wilson, C. B., and Tyrrell, J. B.: Transsphenoidal microhypophysectomy in acromegaly. J. Neurosurg., *47*:840, 1977.
44. Vezina, J. L., and Sutton, T. J.: Prolactin-secreting pituitary microadenomas: roentgenologic diagnosis. Am. J. Roentgenol. Rad. Ther. Nucl. Med., *120*:46, 1974.
45. Weinstein, M., Tyrrell, B., and Newton, T. H.: The sella turcica in Nelson's syndrome. Radiology, *118*:363, 1976.
46. Wilson, C. B., and Dempsey, L. C.: Transsphenoidal microsurgical removal of 250 pituitary adenomas. J. Neurosurg., *48*: 1978.
47. Wright, A. D., Hill, D. M., Lowy, C., and Fraser, T. R.: Mortality in acromegaly. Q. J. Med., *39*:1, 1970.
48. Yamada, T., Tsukui, T., Ikejiri, K., Yukimura, Y., and Kotani, M.: Volume of sella turcica in normal subjects and in patients with primary hypothyroidism and hyperthyroidism. J. Clin. Endocrinol. Metab., *42*:817, 1976.

Selected Reading

Cushing, H., The Pituitary Body and its Disorders. Philadelphia, J. B. Lippincott, 1912.

Friesen, H. G., Guyda, H., Hwang, P., Tyson, J. E., and Barbeau, A., Functional evaluation of prolactin secretion: A guide to therapy. J. Clin. Invest., *51*:706, 1972.

Pearse, A. G. E., Peptides in brain and intestine. Nature, *262*:92, 1976.

EDITORIAL COMMENTARY

Harvey Cushing, in his book, *The Pituitary Body and its Disorders*, published in 1912, stated:

> It is conceivable that the day is not far distant when our present methods of dealing with hypophyseal enlargements with scalpel, rongeur and curette—new as these measures actually are and brilliant as the results may often be—will seem utterly crude and antiquated, for it is quite probable that surgery will in the end, come to play a less, rather than a more important role in ductless gland maladies. This Utopia, however, will be reached only when a sufficient understanding of the underlying aetiological agencies enables us to make more precocious diagnosis.

Today he surely would be heartened to know that RIA measurement of polypeptide hormones, stimulation and suppression tests, and computerized radiodiagnostic maneuvers now allow much earlier diagnoses of the dynamic functioning capabilities of small lesions before the development of "neighborhood pressure symptoms." Such biologic and technical advances, coupled with his "precocious" teachings may seem utopian now, particularly when it is realized that modern surgical treatment, still primarily indicated, is done with the aid of a binocular microscope and television-image intensification.

Cushing recognized, long before our time, that one object of surgical treatment was to "lessen the excessive secretion of a gland in a state of hyperpituitarism," and that the hyperfunctioning state could be due to either hyperplastic or adenomatous changes. He further described many clinical associations as "polyglandular syndromes." It was already known in his day that, "partial extirpation of the hyperplastic thyroid gland serves, in many cases, to alleviate the constitutional symptoms of hyperthyroidism, and it is a natural conclusion that similar measures might, in like fashion, modify the symptoms of hyperpituitarism." Following the suggestion of Schloffer, in 1906, that such treatment of the hypophysis might check the progress of acromegaly, he reported that his patient, Case XXVI, did indeed experience subjective relief of symptoms as well as marked amelioration of the acromegalic manifestations.

Whereas hypofunction or endocrine deficiencies of the pituitary-hypothalamic unit cause recognizable clinical entities from which much is learned concerning its normal functions, the presence of hypopituitarism is usually uncovered in the process of diagnosing enlarging pituitary tumors that compress the remaining gland within the rigid, bone-encased sella. Since low levels of circulating pituitary trophic hormones are difficult to evaluate, stimulation tests for "pituitary reserve" are important in the diagnosis of pituitary insufficiency. On the other hand, suppression tests are most useful in those clinical situations associated with hyperfunction. The excesses of central humoral elaboration of polypeptides produce classical clinical syndromes, either by their direct action (GH, MSH and PRL) on peripheral tissues, or indirectly by their trophic action (TSH, ACTH and gonadotropins) on the thyroid, adrenal cortex and the gonads, which in turn affect peripheral tissues by their elaboration of amines and steroids. This interdependence of the various components of the neuroendocrine system, evident in most endocrine syndromes, is seen here in the peripheral feedback mechanisms and the central hypothalamic and CNS controls of the pituitary. It is interesting to note also that both the hypothalamus and the gastrointestinal tract share identical polypeptide substances (gastrin, vasoactive peptide, somatostatin and substance P).

The term, Cushing's disease, signifies pituitary-dependent (ACTH instigated) hypercorticism and is but one variant of the clinical picture of Cushing's syndrome, which includes hypercorticism due to exogenous administration of corticosteroids, primary endogenous adrenocortical elaboration of them and nonpituitary ectopic elaboration of ACTH. One of the most unforgettable clinical pictures of a hypersecretory endocrinopathy is Nelson's syndrome (i.e.: that of a black-skinned individual with Caucasian features) due to excessive pituitary elaboration of MSH (with ACTH) after bilateral adrenalectomy. The pathogenesis of this syndrome is not proven, but there is evidence to support a concept of a primary hypothalamic abnormality, rather than a new autonomous disorder of the pituitary after bilateral adrenalectomy; inhibition of ACTH/MSH by hypothalamic somatostatin has been reported. In this hyperpigmentation syndrome the melanocytes of the skin are "ectocrine" APUD cells responsive to MSH; it is interesting to speculate that the opposite clinical picture of vitiligo, which is sometimes seen in association with thyrotoxicosis, achlorhydria, pernicious anemia or autoimmune endocrine disorders, may be due to either a receptor failure at the melanocyte or an abnormality in secretion of pituitary MSH or of hypothalamic inhibitory hormone (MRIH).

Since assay techniques for prolactin are now possible, it has been found that 20 to 50 percent of so-called "nonfunctioning" chromophobe adenomas are really prolactin-secreting pituitary tumors with serum PRL levels of 500 ng./ml. and above. The syndrome of galactorrhea with amenorrhea (Forbes-Albright syndrome or the Chiari-Frommel syndrome if in the postpartum period) is usually accompanied by elevated serum prolactin levels and occasionally depressed FSH levels. The hypothalamus elaborates an inhibitory hormone (PIF)but no stimulatory hormone for pituitary prolactin. The role of prolactin in hormone-dependent breast carcinoma may be of importance but certainly conjectural at this time; further investigations of hormone receptors on breast neoplastic cells are necessary. *S.R.F.*

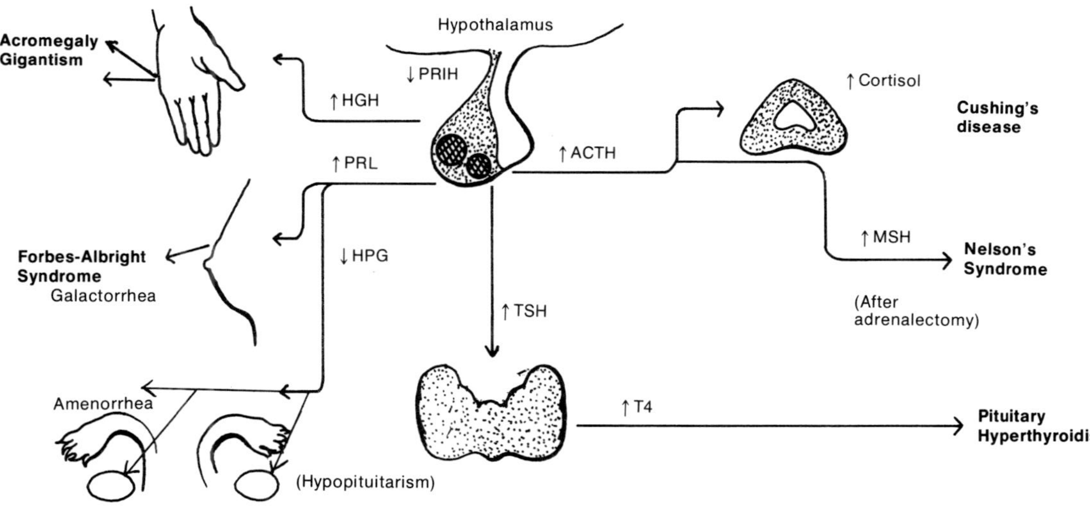

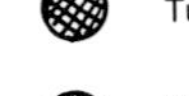

Fig. 19-1. Pathophysiology of the pituitary syndromes (acromegaly and gigantism; galactorrhea and amenorrhea; hyperpigmentation of Nelson's syndrome; pituitary hyperthyroidism).

(See overleaf for flowchart)

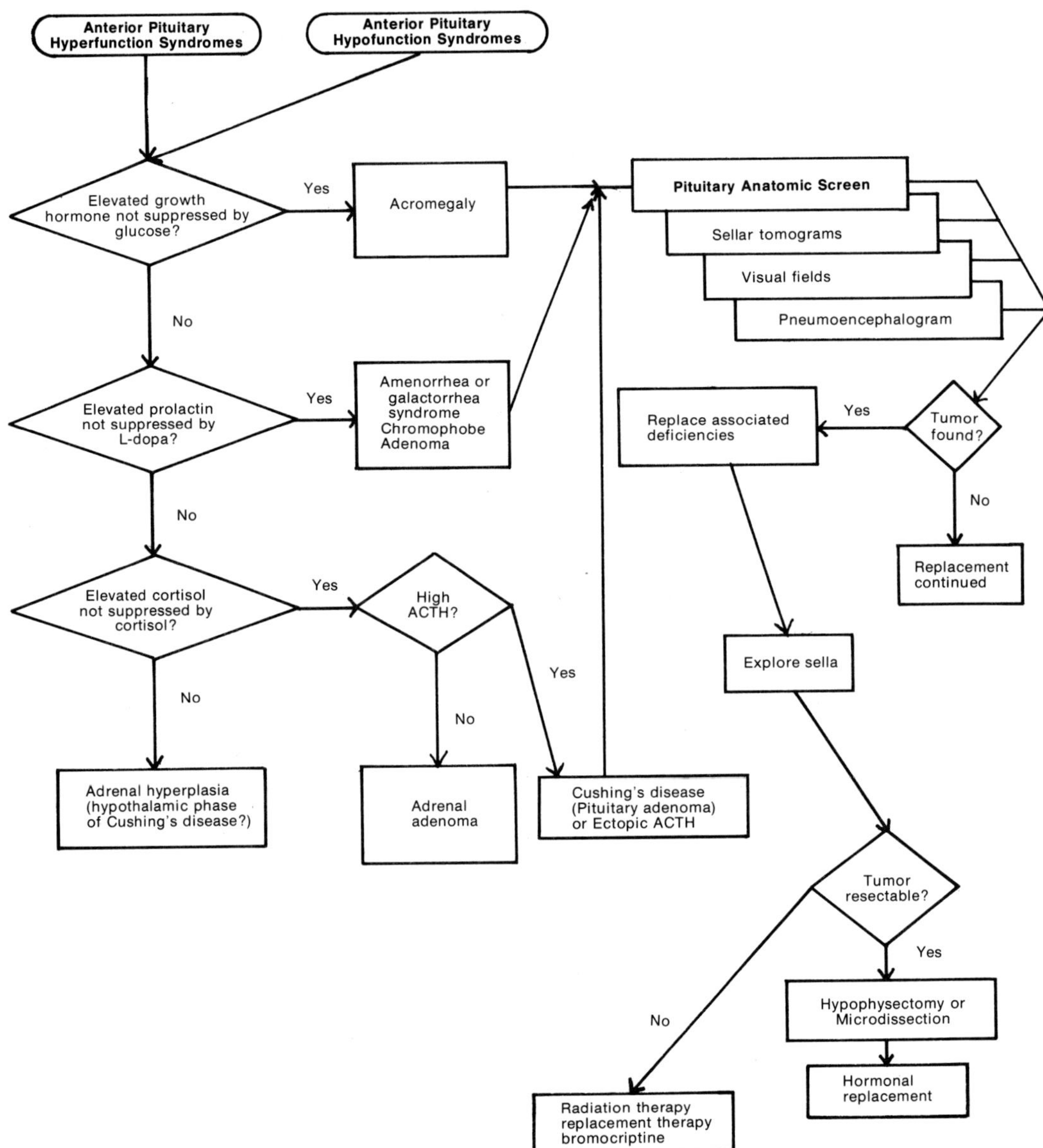

Fig. 19-2. Management flowchart of the pituitary syndromes.

PART 3
Steroids

20

Cushing's Syndrome: Hypercortisolism

Thomas K. Hunt, M.D., and J. Blake Tyrrell, M.D.

Cushing's syndrome (hypercortisolism) results from an excess of cortisol or corticosterone, which may be due to exogenous or endogenous sources of hormone. The three main causes are:

1. Exogenous corticoid administration
2. ACTH-stimulated bilateral adrenal hyperplasia from either pituitary tumors (Cushing's disease) or extrapituitary tumors
3. ACTH-independent adrenal tumors (adenoma or carcinoma)

Those types of Cushing's syndrome resulting from endogenous corticoid production occur about 10 times more frequently in women. The peak incidence is in the third and fourth decades, although the span ranges from infancy to old age, and the natural history of the disease varies widely from a mild indolent form to rapid progression and early death.[22,24] The diagnosis is complex and choice of treatment depends on a precise clinical and biochemical appraisal of the patient.

CLINICAL FINDINGS

The features of Cushing's syndrome include trunkal obesity, osteoporosis, hirsutism, moon facies, buffalo hump, purple striae, acne, arterial hypertension (and its sequelae) and diabetes (Table 20-1). The most striking single symptom is weakness, the next most common probably being psychologic change and sexual dysfunction. Common laboratory aberrations are hypokalemia, leukocytosis and lymphopenia. Since ACTH-producing pituitary tumors and others usually secrete melantropins (MSH) as well as ACTH, increased skin pigmentation may be present. Adrenal carcinomas frequently secrete androgens as well as cortisol or corticosterone, and signs of virilism point to a neoplasm of the adrenal.[9]

As in other diseases of the adrenals, hypercorticism is somewhat different in children. Here, the most consistent finding is the cessation of growth accompanied by obesity, and the most common cause is malignant adrenal tumor.[5,15] However, benign tumor and bilateral hyperplasia do occur.

For the surgeon, some of the important clinical findings are obesity (although weight rarely surpasses 90 kg.) and muscular weakness, both of which predict postoperative pulmonary complications. Other important features are acne and diabetes, which indicate susceptibility to infection, and atrophic skin and easy bruisability, both of which forecast a difficult operation due to tissue fragility and poor wound healing.

Table 20-1. Estimated Frequency of Manifestations of Cushing's Syndrome

Feature	*Frequency (%)*
Obesity	90
Hypertension	80
Evidence of diabetes with normal fasting blood glucose	80
Centripetal distribution of fat	80
Weakness	80
Muscle atrophy in upper and lower extremities	70
Hirsutism	70
Menstrual disturbance or impotence	70
Purple striae	70
Plethoric facies	60
Osteoporosis	50
Easy bruising	50
Acne or skin pigmentation	50
Mental changes	50
Edema	50
Headache	40
Poor wound healing	40
Leukocytosis with lymphopenia	Frequent

NATURAL HISTORY OF HYPERADRENOCORTICISM

Once the patient develops Cushing's syndrome, complications have either already begun or will soon follow.[22,24] Indeed, the major cause of death is cardiovascular complication. Hypertension, causing renal failure, strokes, and cardiac disease, is common, as is mental illness (especially with sleeplessness, manic activity, severe depression and even hallucinations). Diabetes becomes worse; hyperglycemia and infections appear. The hypercortisolism produces a debilitating muscular wasting and weakness that are frequently enhanced by hypokalemia.

Cancer of the adrenal metastasizes early to the liver and lungs, and is usually rapidly fatal.[9] Uncontrolled tumors of the pituitary may produce visual field changes, especially following bilateral adrenalectomy, but in modern practice tumors are rarely allowed to grow that large (see Chap. 19).

PATHOLOGY

The histologic features of adrenal disease are quite diverse, and even the gross changes of adrenal hyperplasia may be subtle. In patients with a confirmed diagnosis, adrenal weights may vary from normal (7-12 g. combined weight) to as much as 70 g. for both glands combined, although the average combined adrenal weight in hyperadrenocorticism is between 20 and 25 g.[18]

Microscopic examination may show fairly subtle micronodular changes of the zona fasciculata; and, on electronmicroscopic examination, most cases of hyperadrenocorticism originate in hyperplastic cells of the fascicular zone of the adrenal cortex.

The endocrine-active adrenal adenoma has a monotonous facade of fascicular-like adrenal cells. Benign pathology blends imperceptibly with that of malignancy until the obvious histologic features of multinucleated giant cells, mitoses and venous invasion plainly mark the malignant tumor. The dividing line between carcinoma and benign disease is obscure, and pathologists frequently hesitate to make a firm diagnosis in borderline cases.

Most adrenal malignancies are large and metastasize in the bloodstream, but metastases through the lymphatic system and by direct invasion are both common.[9]

In Cushing's *disease,* a pituitary tumor is responsible for the adrenal hyperplasia in the great majority of cases.[3,7,22,23] Contrary to the initial experience, these tumors may be basophilic, acidophilic, or chromophobic, and the majority of them are benign (see Chap. 19). This condition is much more frequently diagnosed now than in the past several decades, and these patients constitute the largest single group with hypercortisolism.

In a few cases, tumors or hyperplasia of ectopic adrenal tissue have been the source of excessive cortisol secretion. The ectopic tissue has been found in a variety of locations from the neck to the gonads, but the most common sources are near the abdominal aorta and represent remnants of neuroendocrine tissue involved in the embryogenesis of the adrenal, the organ of Zuckerkandl, and so on.

Cushing's syndrome is also caused by ACTH-secreting extrapituitary neoplasms. By far the most common example is cancer of the lung, but tumors of the pancreas, thymus, thyroid, prostate, esophagus, colon and other organs have been found to secrete ACTH. The majority of these tumors are highly malignant, and by the time that Cushing's syndrome has become significant to the patient, there is usually little to gain in operating either on the primary neoplasm or on the adrenals.

Cushing's syndrome sometimes results from ovarian tumors, which are usually malignant, are often associated with adrenal hyperplasia and are thought in most cases to represent a form of ectopic ACTH syndrome.

LABORATORY DIAGNOSIS

Unfortunately, the diagnosis is difficult. No one test is specific and a combination of findings must be used. In a normal patient, there is a daily rhythmic variation of plasma ACTH, which is paralleled by cortisol secretion: levels are highest early in the morning and decline gradually during the day, reaching their nadir in the evening. This variability of the normal levels is responsible for the inexactness of many of the testing procedures, and a precise analysis requires consideration of the circadian rhythm.

In Cushing's syndrome, total secretion of cortisol is increased and the circadian rhythm is abolished. In mild cases, the plasma cortisol and ACTH levels may be within the generally accepted limits of normal during much of the 24-hr. cycle, but serial testing will yield abnormally high results during at least part of the day. The excess circulating cortisol leads to elevated levels of plasma and urinary free cortisol, 17-hydroxycorticosteroids and 17-ketogenic steroids. For this reason, urinary free cortisol levels on a 24-hr. basis provide one of the most discriminating tests available.[2,4,19]

When Cushing's syndrome is suspected, the first goal is to establish the diagnosis and then to determine the ultimate cause. An algohithm for the diagnosis is found in Figure 20-1. The first abnormal finding will usually be an elevated urinary 17-hydroxycorticosteroid or plasma cortisol level. When these

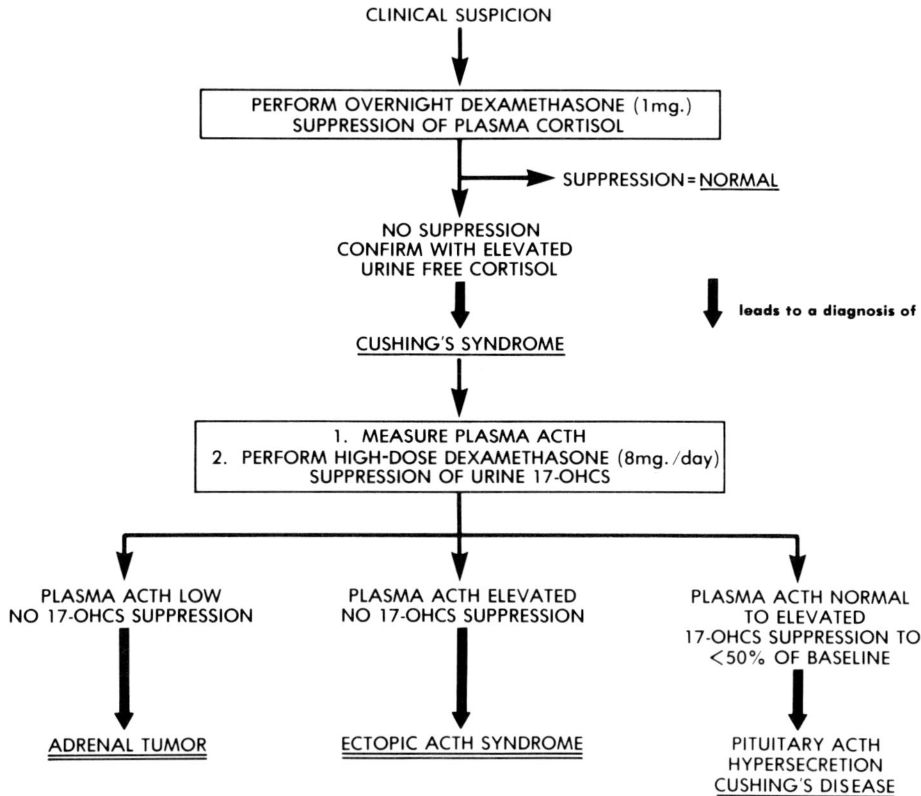

Fig. 20-1. An algorithm for the diagnosis of the causes of Cushing's syndrome.

are found, or simply when hyperadrenocorticism is suspected, an overnight dexamethasone suppression test is the first step in the diagnostic sequence. Normal, unstressed subjects produce about 30 mg. of cortisol a day. Dexamethasone, 1 mg. orally (equivalent to about 30 mg. of cortisol), will suppress ACTH secretion, and cortisol production will literally stop in normal subjects. This amount of dexamethasone, however, will not suppress pathologically excessive cortisol production from an autonomous adrenocortical tumor or an adrenal that is being driven by excessive ACTH secretion. Since 1 mg. of dexamethasone contributes almost nothing to the plasma cortisol level, suppression of endogenous circulating cortisol is easily demonstrated. The test is done as follows[21]: At exactly 11:00 p.m., the patient is given 1 mg. of dexamethasone and about 100 mg. pentobarbitol, both by mouth. (The sedative is added to ensure an unstressed night's rest.) A fasting plasma sample for cortisol determination is drawn the following morning. If the patient is receiving estrogen therapy, a basal plasma level, drawn previously, is required for evaluating suppression. A normal woman receiving estrogen (birth control pills, etc.) will have increased cortisol-binding globulin and thus will show a high basal plasma cortisol. In normal and obese subjects, the morning level will be suppressed to less than 5 μg./100 ml.; in normal subjects taking estrogens, the level will be 50 percent below baseline; in patients with Cushing's syndrome, it will not be suppressed below 10 μg./100 ml. This absence of suppression indicates fixed production of ACTH or cortisol (i.e., Cushing's syndrome). Although partial suppression may occur in patients with acromegaly or thyrotoxicosis, in patients who are chronically depressed, and in those who are chronically ill or who are under chronic physical stress, these conditions are usually clinically evident.

The results of the dexamethasone test can be confirmed with a measurement of urinary free cortisol—ordinarily the best test to follow an abnormal dexamethasone suppression test. It measures the physiologically active form of circulating cortisol directly and "integrates" the daily variations of cortisol production. This test is the most sensitive and reliable means of diagnosing Cushing's syndrome.[2,4] Only in hyperadrenocorticism will urinary free cortisol exceed 100 μg. per 24 hours.

The combination of overnight dexamethasone suppression of plasma cortisol and measurement of urinary free cortisol will establish the diagnosis of Cushing's syndrome in virtually all patients. Reliance on basal levels of plasma or other urinary steroids (17-hydroxycorticosteroids, 17-ketogenic steroids and 17-ketosteroids) may give misleading results.[19] The classic low-dose suppression test of Liddle (0.5 mg. dexamethasone every 6 hr. for 2 days) gives the same information as the overnight suppression test but is considerably more time-consuming and cumbersome since it requires 3 days of urine collections for 17-hydroxycorticosteroids.[13]

If the plasma cortisol level is not suppressed and urinary free cortisol is elevated, the diagnosis of Cushing's syndrome has been established. The next step is to determine the precise cause. Measurement of plasma ACTH levels will differentiate bilateral adrenal hyperplasia from primary adrenal tumors[1]—very high levels are found in the ectopic ACTH syndrome, whereas patients with Cushing's disease have normal to moderately elevated levels that are inappropriate for the degree of hypercortisolism. Adrenal tumors function autonomously, causing suppression of the hypothalamic-pituitary axis with consequent subnormal levels of plasma ACTH.

The high-dose dexamethasone suppression test can give further useful information regarding the cause of Cushing's syndrome.[13] Here, dexamethasone is given in a dose of 2 mg. every 6 hours for 2 days with concomitant 24-hour urine collection for 17-hydroxycorticosteroid values.

The algorhithm of Figure 20-1 is now complete. Hypercortisolism and nonsuppressibility with low-dose dexamethasone are diagnostic of Cushing's syndrome. Normal to elevated plasma ACTH levels and partial suppression of urinary 17-hydroxycorticosteroids with high-dose dexamethasone indicate Cushing's disease, whereas markedly high plasma ACTH and lack of suppression with high-dose dexamethasone are typical of the ectopic ACTH syndrome. Primary adrenal tumors, either adenoma or carcinoma, are characterized by subnormal plasma ACTH and failure of suppression with high-dose dexamethasone. Carcinoma is more likely if urinary 17-ketosteroid levels are elevated, although adrenal adenomas may also secrete some 17-ketosteroids. If compound S and aldosterone are present in excess, the chance of adrenal carcinoma increases still further. The metyrapone test is occasionally useful because it helps detect the bilateral hyperplasia due to overproduction of pituitary ACTH; in this case, there will be at least a doubling of urinary 17-hydroxycorticosteroid output following metyrapone administration.

Table 20-2. Iodocholesterol Adrenal Scans in Cushing's Syndrome

Bilateral hyperplasia	Both adrenals	Increased uptake
Adrenal adenoma	Affected adrenal	Increased uptake
	Opposite adrenal	No uptake (suppressed)
Adrenal carcinoma	Affected adrenal	No uptake
	Opposite adrenal	No uptake (suppressed)

LOCALIZATION OF UNILATERAL ADRENAL DISEASE

There are three good methods for localizing adrenal disease: $^{I-131}$iodocholesterol scan; tomograms (usually with intravenous pyelogram) and angiograms. A simple tomogram of the suprarenal area may disclose a unilateral adrenocortical tumor with typical contralateral adrenal atrophy.

$^{I-131}$Iodocholesterol scanning is proving very useful in localizing adenomas and demonstrating greatly enlarged glands[14]; however, it is not entirely reliable in detecting small adenomas. Hyperplastic glands usually give bilaterally enlarged images; atrophic glands usually give no image. Adenomas in Cushing's syndrome give very large images and are usually unmistakable because the contralateral adrenal is suppressed and gives no image. Carcinomas show no image; indeed, this lack is often a useful diagnostic feature. Adrenal scanning has removed the necessity for adrenal arteriography in most cases; however, an angiogram is occasionally necessary in order to find an ectopic source of cortisol (Table 20-2).

TREATMENT

Adrenal hypercortisolism can be treated by operation on or irradiation of the pituitary; operation on the adrenals; attempts to modify the synthesis of adrenal hormones with drugs; or attempts to destroy adrenal tissue with chemotherapeutic ablation of the adrenals through retrograde venous injection (see list below).[1,3,7,9–12,20,23,24]

Therapy of Cushing's Syndrome

Medical	**Surgical**
Metyrapone	Unilateral adrenalectomy
Aminoglutethimide	for adenoma or carcinoma
o,p′ D′D′D′	Bilateral total adrenalectomy
Cyproheptadine	for bilateral hyperplasia
Pituitary Roentgenotherapy	Transsphenoidal pituitary micro-
Conventional	surgery in Cushing's disease
Heavy particle	**Venous, Retrograde Infusion of Nitrogen Mustard**

Medical Therapy

Medical treatment includes temporary control with metyrapone or aminoglutethimide, both of which inhibit steps in steroid biosynthesis. Eventual escape from control is the rule in ACTH-dependent Cushing's syndrome, but temporary control (usually for a few months) may be advantageous in preoperative preparation. This treatment is often effective in patients with benign adrenocortical tumors when immediate surgery is contraindicated, as, for instance, in patients with recent myocardial infarction.

Mitotane (o,p′-D′D′D′), a DDT derivative toxic to the adrenal cortex, has been used with moderate success in the treatment of adrenal hypersecretory states, especially adrenal carcinoma.[9] Unfortunately, serious side effects, usually of the gastrointestinal tract and central nervous system, are common with effective doses.

Cyproheptadine has been reported to be helpful in treating hypercortisolism, but its effectiveness is still controversial.[10] Also controversial, because of reports of recurrence, is the retrograde chemical ablation method.

Pituitary Microsurgery

Pituitary ablation can be done with either radiation[12,20] or direct operation on the pituitary. Many medical centers are using transsphenoidal microsurgical excision of pituitary adenomas as the treatment of choice in Cushing's disease.[7,11,23] Relief of symptoms is rapid and the chance for normal residual pituitary-adrenal function is good. However, this treatment has been used only a few years, and the long-term chances for recurrence are not yet established (see Chap. 19). Results of pituitary surgery in our institution are shown in Table 20-3. So far, these are holding well, and most patients with pituitary-dependent hypercortisolism are having pituitary explorations (see Chap. 19).

There is no fixed method for selecting patients for pituitary operation. Proof of hypercortisolism with repeatedly elevated urinary free cortisol, no suppression with the low-dose dexamethasone test but suppression with the high-dose test, and an iodocholesterol scan showing bilaterally enlarged adrenals constitute adequate indication for pituitary exploration by way of the transsphenoidal route. Certainly, an enlarged sella turcica also helps make the decision.

Table 20-3. Pituitary Microsurgery in Cushing's Disease

	Number of Patients	*Correction of Hypercortisolism*
Surgical Results		
Total patients	20	
Technical failure	2	0
Tumor identified		
Definite (3-10 mm.)	14	13
Probable tumor (2-3 mm.)	3	3
Microscopic (total hypophysectomy)	1	1
Complications		
Transient diabetes insipidus	4	
Hypopituitarism (total hypophysectomy)	1	
Histology of Pituitary Tumors		
Gross tumor		
Basophil	1	1
Chromophobe	10	9
Mixed	3	3
Microscopic tumor		
(Basophil 1.5 mm.)	1	1
Inadequate or nondiagnostic specimen	3	3

Adrenal Surgery in Cushing's Syndrome

Patients with severe Cushing's syndrome are poor candidates for abdominal operation, and this is one reason why the pendulum has recently swung toward pituitary procedures. Nevertheless, bilateral adrenalectomy is the surest treatment of Cushing's syndrome due to bilateral hyperplasia, and unilateral adrenalectomy is the only feasible surgical treatment for adenoma or carcinoma of the adrenal.

Operative Procedures.[6,24] The transabdominal route is the best for relatively low-risk, lean patients who need bilateral adrenalectomy. The posterior approach is better for some poor-risk patients and for those with small, preoperatively localized adenomas. The lateral or flank approach is relatively rarely used, but is best in extremely obese or poor-risk patients in whom wound dehiscence represents an important consideration and in whom staged procedures are planned. The posterior and lateral approaches lend themselves best to unilateral adrenalectomy, but both can be used for bilateral adrenalectomy as well. Many technical details are graphically presented in other texts.[8]

The Transabdominal Approach. A bilateral subcostal or a long midline incision is used. In most patients, the former provides the best exposure. The approach to the right adrenal through the peritoneal cavity is relatively standard. The adrenal is located posterior and lateral to the vena cava well superior and medial to the right kidney. The lower pole of the adrenal is usually 5 to 10 cm. above the renal vein. To expose the right adrenal, it is necessary merely to incise the peritoneum at the lateral border of the vena cava, retract the liver upward and anteriorly, and gradually develop the adrenal from the retroperitoneal fat and the vena cava. Mobilization of the duodenum is not necessary. The safest plane for separating the adrenal from the vena cava is, of course, the surgical plane of the vein. If dissection is gentle, the right adrenal vein can be found before it is injured. The right adrenal vein enters the vena cava from almost directly posterior. It may be as much as a centimeter long but is usually 4 to 5 mm. long and may be as wide as or wider than it is long. There is rarely room enough on the vein for two standard surgical clamps. Therefore, the vena cava side of the vein is usually ligated in continuity and the vein is simply divided, thereafter. The adrenal vein must be treated very gently to avoid avulsion from the vena cava. Bleeding, especially in the anterior approach, can be very difficult to manage. If it does occur, it is best not to try to clamp the bleeding point but to tamponade it with the fingers or the sponge forceps and gain control of the vena cava with a side-biting vascular clamp. If this fails, the vena cava can be occluded above and below, but usually only after the right costal margin and the diaphragm are divided and the liver is displaced upward into the thoracic cavity. In this manner, the adrenal vein can be well visualized.

Rarely, the tip of the right adrenal may be imbedded in the liver, If so, some of the lower hepatic veins are endangered during removal. These veins are rarely large, and the adrenal can usually be "cored" out of the liver. If significant hemorrhage results, it can usually be controlled with suture ligatures.

Technically, the major problem in removing the right adrenal from the anterior approach is the poor exposure. One useful "trick" to improve it is to place a Penrose drain around the superior pole of the right kidney and clamp it under tension to the drapes below, thus pulling the kidney inferiorly. The kidney exerts traction on the renal vein, the renal vein on the vena cava and the vena cava on the adrenal. This will usually move the adrenal downward and anteriorly as much as 2 or 3 cm.

The left adrenal can be approached from the anterior side in any of four methods.

1. The transverse mesocolon can be incised just lateral to the disappearance of the inferior mesentery vein, and this plane can be developed across the renal vessels and on through to the left adrenal. This is an excellent approach.
2. The greater omentum can be separated from the colon for a distance of about 15 to 20 cm., or the lesser omentum can be divided for about the same distance. The lower border of the pancreas can then be seen across the lesser sac. The peritoneum at the lower border of the pancreas can be incised from lateral to the inferior mesenteric vein almost to the tip of the pancreas. (The tip of the pancreas should be left in place because, if it is mobilized, the spleen tends to fall medially and obscure vision.) Dissection immediately below the pancreas soon reveals the splenic vein. This can be retracted anteriorly and superiorly. The adrenal and the superior tip of the left kidney are now in view. A few thin layers of peritoneal reflections may separate this dissecting plane from the adrenal. This approach to the adrenal is much the same as that which would be used from the root of the colon mesentery. The advantages of this "transligamentous" approach are that the colon and its mesentery act as an effective retractor of the small bowel. The "transligamentous" approach is probably the most commonly used and probably the safest.
3. The splenic ligaments can be detached and the entire pancreas can be freed and the spleen and tail of the pancreas retracted medially. This gives a magnificent view of the adrenal. However, the incidence of splenic and pancreatic injury is far larger when compared to the preceding two methods.
4. The splenic artery can be dissected free and moved up or down and the pancreas moved downward to expose the left adrenal. We have not used this approach, but it has been used by many experienced surgeons.

The adrenal vein on the left is remarkably constant and is usually 2 to 2.5 cm. long, extending straight inferiorly to join the side of the left renal vein. It is easily controlled and divided. The major problems in removing the left adrenal are on its medial border where the phrenic vessels may release many small arterial branches to the adrenal. The very tip of the adrenal is so far away from the operator's point of vision that the last dissection often has to be done "blind." Fortunately, there are no major vessels in this area.

The lateral approach to the adrenal in Cushing's disease is usually done for patients who are so obese or represent such a severe risk of dehiscence that the anterior approach is out of the question. Furthermore, these patients will usually have large tumors making the posterior approach undesirable. Many incisions have been advocated. We place the patient in the anterolateral position with the side to be operated elevated forward approximately 45° by means of sandbags or pillows under the shoulders and buttocks. The leg and arm are supported with padded towels and tapes. One should remember that patients with severe Cushing's disease have osteoporosis and the surgeon should try to avoid rough handling on the operating table, which may cause bruised skin or broken bones.

We prefer to make an incision starting at the lateral border of the rectus muscle, going over the tip of the tenth rib, across the eleventh rib and curving up slightly to follow the course of the twelfth rib. When this incision is deepened into the latissimus dorsi and the oblique muscles, it will be found to be immediately superficial to the reflection of the pleura, which almost always is exactly perpendicular to the spine at the level of the L-1 spinous process. The distal third of the eleventh rib can be removed and most of the twelfth rib also. The periosteum of the twelfth rib is incised, and the twelfth neurovascular bundle is reflected downward. The incision is carried anteriorly to the eleventh neurovascular bundle, which is dissected a few centimeters above and below the line of the incision and is retracted upward. When the anesthesiologist gives a forced inspiration, the lung can be seen descending to the pleural fold. The fibers of the diaphragm can then be identified and detached from their attachments to the periosteum of the ribs. The above-described incision of the periosteum is made immediately below the pleural reflection. The pleural fold, therefore, is moved up about 1 to 1.5 interspaces. The deep fascia is divided, Gerota's fascia is divided and the kidney is found. A small or medium Finichietto retractor is very useful to move the lower ribs upward. The upper blade should be heavily padded to avoid damage to the eleventh and twelfth neurovascular bundles and subsequent hypesthesia in the groin.

With the patient in this position, the peritoneum falls away from the operator and the kidney is easily seen. On the right, the adrenal will be seen well medial and superior to the kidney. On the left, the adrenal will be seen immediately medial to the upper pole of the kidney. On the right, the vein is most easily seen through this approach. It is well to dissect out a small amount of vena cava around the area of the vein so that the vena cava can be clamped with a side-biting vascular clamp should the adrenal vein be torn. Patients with severe Cushing's disease, the ones most often operated through this approach, have such fragile tissues that the vein can easily tear. As in other approaches, I prefer to isolate small pedicles of tissue surrounding the adrenal with a right-angle clamp and divide them with the electrocautery. If a fairly large vessel is seen in them, a small stainless steel clip is often used for security. The right adrenal vein is often clipped before tying as a safety precaution.

The posterior approach has also been done in many different ways. As with the lateral approach, incisions have been made to go below the ribs, to take portions of ribs, or even to go transpleurally intentionally. I prefer a modification of the late Hugh Young's approach. The patient is placed prone on the operating table with suitable support under the hips and shoulders so that the abdomen does not touch the operating table. The knees and arms must be supported. The abdomen is kept from touching the operating table so that when the anesthesiologist gives the patient a deep breath, the abdomen falls anteriorly (downward), and the retroperitoneal fat moves inferiorly and anteriorly. If the abdomen is tightly in contact with the operating table, the retroperitoneal fat is pushed out of the incision and directly into the surgeon's vision each time the patient is given a deep breath.

A curvilinear incision is made starting over the tenth or eleventh rib at the lateral edge of the paraspinous muscle. The incision parallels the paraspinous muscles until the twelfth rib is crossed and it curves laterally below the twelfth rib to intersect and terminate at its tip. The subcutaneous tissue and the latissimus dorsi fascia are divided in the same line as the skin incision. This exposes the paraspinous muscles. They are detached from their lateral attachments and this often incurs a small hemorrhage from the neurovascular bundles. The muscle is retracted backward with a wide rake retractor, and the periosteum of the twelfth rib is incised with the electrocautery. The twelfth rib is removed intraperiostially. When the anesthesiologist gives the patient a deep breath, the lower edge of the pleura can be seen and, once again, the diaphragmatic attachment is loosened from below and the pleural fold is retracted up one interspace. Rarely, the pleural space is inadvertently opened and can be closed with a stitch or two taken during a forced inspiration.

Just as in the lateral approach, the various fascia are divided until the adrenal is located. In this case, however, the right adrenal vein is maximally hidden and the whole gland is literally dissected loose before it is truly safe to divide the vein. Once again, it is useful to dissect about 90° of vena cava so that, if the vein is wide, particularly short, or otherwise difficult, the vena cava can be controlled by a side-biting vascular clamp, and the adrenal vein orifice can be oversewn. The approach on the left is difficult only in that the kidney falls forward and, instead of the adrenal vein coursing inferiorly, directly parallel to the spinal column, the course is somewhat anterior and tends to lie deep in the field of dissection.

For closure of incisions, the layers are closed with either 2-0 Dexon or 2-0 silk, and the skin is closed with running nylon since tapes tend to blister patients with Cushing's disease. Staging for bilateral adrenal hyperplasia is rarely necessary anymore, but it is quite feasible.

Complications of Operation. Regardless of the approach, problems with wound healing and, to some extent, wound infection are fairly common in patients with Cushing's syndrome. In fact, all complications, ranging from splenic injury, to bleeding, to pancreatitis, to infection and dehiscence are all more common in Cushing's syndrome than in operations for aldosteronism or pheochromocytoma. The "transligamentous" approach is the safest of the anterior approaches. Despite the dissection of the pancreas, pancreatitis is rare.

For adrenalectomy, mortality rates have been given as 2 to 4 percent, but are probably lower now. Infectious complications in wounds, subphrenic spaces, pneumonia, and so on probably occur about 10 percent of the time, but these complications are all clustered in the severely cushingoid patients.[6,24]

There still is some discussion over whether total or partial adrenalectomy should be used to treat bilateral adrenal hyperplasia. The vast majority of surgeons prefer total adrenalectomy. Except in one series, the recurrence rate after subtotal resection is about 40 percent. Recurrence is seen, occasionally, even after allegedly total resections; the estimated frequency is 5 to 10 percent. In our experience, one patient with a total resection slowly gained adrenal function over a period of 10 years and eventually developed Cushing's syndrome again. Many technical details are graphically presented in other texts.[8]

Postoperative Maintenance Therapy. After removal of carcinomas and adrenal adenomas, one must recognize that the opposite adrenal has usually been chronically suppressed. Therefore, cortisol and occasionally aldosterone replacement are necessary. After total resections for hyperplasia, lifelong total replacement is necessary.

The following schedule is commonly used:

1. Do not give cortisol until the adrenals are removed during surgery; and give the first dose about the time the second adrenal vein is controlled. Giving cortisol earlier merely compounds the hypercortisolism the patient is already suffering.
2. On the first day, give 100 mg. hydrocortisone phosphate or hemisuccinate every 8 hours. In most cases, the intramuscular route can be used, but, if the patient is not doing well, give the drug intravenously. Electrolyte maintenance is much easier if the 300-mg. total dose is given in appropriate increments every 6 to 8 hours.
3. In the next 24 hours, 50 mg. given intramuscularly every 8 hours is usually sufficient. Thereafter, taper the dose downward as tolerated. If patients have had extremely high levels preoperatively, they may not tolerate rapid withdrawal. Although shock and sodium wasting are rarely seen, the patient may become depressed, sleepless and even psychotic if excessively rapid withdrawal is forced.
4. As the hydrocortisone dose is reduced below about 50 mg. per day, it is often wise to add fludrocortisone (0.1 mg. per day orally) to avoid excessive urinary electrolyte losses. The usual maintenance dose of hydrocortisone is about 20 to 30 mg., with two-thirds given in the morning and 0.1 to 0.2 mg. of fludrocortisone given once daily.

The above schedule can be used for maintaining any addisonian patient through any operation. If shock or hyperkalemia occurs despite cortisol, some saline solution or blood must be given. If salt losses not regulated by the adrenal are increased (e.g., diarrhea, gastric lesions), salt intake must be maintained and an increase in steroids should be considered. Fever, hypotension, hyperkalemia, and abdominal pain are the most common indications of adrenal insufficiency. In general, however, we see more complications of hyperaggressive cortisol treatment than of inadequate cortisol treatment.

PROGNOSIS IN CUSHING'S SYNDROME

The prognosis for patients with benign Cushing's syndrome is quite good after adrenalectomy or after resection of a pituitary adenoma. The clinical manifestations begin to subside in several weeks, and complete endocrinologic cure is the rule. The major long-term problem of recurrence due to retained adrenal is about 10 percent. Nelson's syndrome with hyperpigmentation and visual field loss due to an enlarging pituitary occur in patients with an ACTH-producing pituitary tumor after adrenalectomy, and occurrence is estimated at 10 to 20 percent.[16,17] Unfortunately, Cushing's syndrome leaves many irreversible changes; and, in the past, about 20 percent of patients have died of cardiovascular problems within about 2 to 3 years of operative "cure."[24]

When Cushing's syndrome is due to adrenal carcinoma, the prognosis is grave and only rare survivals of more than a few years are reported. Unfortunately, by the time Cushing's syndrome occurs secondary to ACTH-producing cancers, the tumor is almost always beyond surgical care, although palliation can rarely be achieved by adrenalectomy when Cushing's syndrome is the principal clinical problem.

REFERENCES

1. Besser, G. M., and Edwards, C. R. W.: Cushing's syndrome. Clin. Endocrinol. Metab., *1*:451, 1972.
2. Burke, C. W., and Beardwell, C. G.: Cushing's syndrome. An evaluation of the clinical usefulness of urinary free cortisol and other urinary steroid measurement in diagnosis. Q. J. Med. (New Series), *42*:175, 1973.
3. Burke, C. W., et al.: Cushing's disease: treatment by pituitary implantation of radioactive gold or yttrium seeds. Q. J. Med. [New Series], *42*:693, 1973.
4. Eddy, R. L., et al.: Cushing's syndrome: A prospective study of diagnostic methods. Am. J. Med., *55*:621, 1973.
5. Editorial: Cushing's syndrome in childhood. Lancet, *2*:267, 1972.
6. Egdahl, R. H.: Surgery of the adrenal gland. N. Engl. J. Med., *278*:939, 1968.
7. Hardy, J.: Transsphenoidal surgery of hypersecreting pituitary tumors. *In* Kohler, P. O., and Ross, G. T., (eds.): Diagnosis and Treatment of Pituitary Tumors. pp. 179-194. Amsterdam: Excerpta Medica (International Congress Series No. 303).
8. Hunt, T. K.: Adrenalectomy. *In* Surgical Techniques Illustrated. Vol. 3 [11], Jan., 1978.
9. Hutter, A. M., and Kayhoe, D. E.: Adrenal cortical carcinoma. Am. J. Med., *41*:572, 581, 1966.
10. Krieger, D. T., Amorosa, L., and Linick, F.: Cyproheptadine-induced remission of Cushing's disease. N. Engl. J. Med., *293*:893, 1975.
11. Lagerquist, L. G., Meikle, A. W., West, C. D., and Tyler, F. H.: Cushing's disease with cure by resection of a pituitary adenoma: evidence against a primary hypothalamic defect. Am. J. Med. 57:826, 1974.
12. Lawrence, J. H., et al.: Treatment of pituitary tumors with heavy particles. *In* Kohler, P. O., and Ross, G. T. (eds.): Diagnosis and Treatment of Pituitary Tumors. pp. 253-262. Amsterdam: Excerpta Medical (International Congress Series No. 303), 1973.
13. Liddle, G. W.: Tests of pituitary-adrenal suppressibility in the diagnosis of Cushing's syndrome. J. Clin. Endocrinol. Metab., *20*:1539, 1960.
14. Lieberman, L. M., Beierwaltes, W. H., Conn, J. W., Ansari, A. N., and Nishiyama, H.: Diagnosis of adrenal disease by visualization of human adrenal glands with ^{131}I-19-iodocholesterol. N. Engl. J. Med., *285*:1387, 1971.
15. McArthur, R. G., Cloutier, M. D., Hayles, A. B., and Sprague, R. G.: Cushing's disease in children. Findings in 13 cases. Mayo Clin. Proc., *47*:318, 1972.
16. Moore, T. J., Dluhy, R. G., Williams, G. H., and Cain, J. P.: Nelson's syndrome: frequency, prognosis, and effect of prior pituitary irradiation. Ann. Intern. Med., *85*:731, 1976.
17. Nelson, D. H., Meakin, J. W., and Thorn, G. W.: ACTH-producting pituitary tumors following adrenalectomy for Cushing's syndrome. Ann. Intern. Med., *52*:560, 1960.
18. Neville, A. M., and Mackay, A. M.: The structure of the human adrenal cortex in health and disease. Clin. Endocrinol. Metab., *1*:361, 1972.
19. Nichols, T., Nugent, C. A., and Tyler, F. H.: Steroid laboratory tests in the diagnosis of Cushing's syndrome. Am. J. Med., *45*:116, 1968.
20. Orth, D. N., and Liddle, G. W.: Results of treatment in 108 patients with Cushing's syndrome. N. Engl. J. Med., *285*:243, 1971.
21. Pavlatos, F. Ch., Smilo, R. P., and Forsham, P. H.: A rapid screening test for Cushing's syndrome. JAMA, *193*:720, 1965.
22. Plotz, C. M., Knowlton, A. I., and Ragan, C.: The natural history of Cushing's syndrome. Am. J. Med., *13*:597, 1952.
23. Tyrrell, J. B., et al.: Pituitary tumors in Cushing's disease: Reversal of hypercortisolism by selective transsphenoidal adenomectomy. p. 142 (Abstr.). Program of the Fifty-ninth Annual Meeting of The Endocrine Society. Chicago, June 8 - 10, 1977.

24. Welbourn, R. B., Montgomery, D. A. D., and Kennedy, T. L.: The natural history of treated Cushing's syndrome. Br. J. Surg., *58*:1, 1971.

Selected Reading

Cushing, H.: The basophil adenomas of the pituitary body and their clinical manifestations (pituitary basophilism). Johns Hopkins Hosp. Bull., *50*:137, 1932.

Stanton, M. E., and Thomson, E. H.: Harvey Cushing: From tallow dip to television. Surgery, *81*:284, 1977.

EDITORIAL COMMENTARY

The syndrome of truncal obesity, hypertension and diabetes with features of moon face, hirsutism, acne, buffalo hump and abdominal striae has become more readily recognizable since corticosteroids have been synthesized and administered to patients for diseases involving the autoimmune system. This sequence of events is similar to that of the recognition of endogenous hyperinsulinism after the use of exogenously administered insulin in overdosage of patients with diabetes mellitus. Nevertheless, Cushing's syndrome due to endogenous hypercortisolism was recognized and treated prior to the observations of the exogenous iatrogenic forms, but it has not always been a simple matter to determine whether the syndrome was due to a primary abnormality of the adrenal cortex (an autonomous cortisol-secreting adenoma or carcinoma), or to primary pituitary stimulation of adrenocortical hyperplasia (pituitary ACTH-dependent hypercortisolism—"Cushing's *disease*"), or to so-called ectopic ACTH-secreting tumors. Bilateral adrenocortical hyperplasia may be a consequence also of increased hypothalamic secretion of corticotropin-releasing factor (CRF) with consequent increase in ACTH secretion. Rarely, bilateral cortical hyperplasia may be primary in the adrenal (idiopathic) in which case the diagnosis requires the demonstration that circulating ACTH is not present in normal or increased amounts. In each of the clinical situations involving increased endogenous steroid production, the adrenal cortex is hyperfunctioning, either primarily or secondarily (to polypeptide stimulation), and the diagnosis of each patient requires differentiation (made easier now by assay and suppression tests) as to the source of the hypersecretion (hypothalamus, pituitary, adrenal or ectopic), and the management involves appropriate judgment as to the type of treatment (medical, roentgenologic or surgical).

The adrenal cortex inherently produces, from its different zones, steroids which can be classified functionally, generally, into the glucocorticoids, the mineralocorticoids and the adrenal androgens. In Cushing's syndrome the glucocorticoid effect is predominant and responsible for the gluconeogenesis that results in conversion of protein to carbohydrate and subsequent storage as fat. These metabolic changes produce the picture of muscle atrophy and weakness of the extremities, relative obesity of the trunk, neck and face and the diabeteslike chemistry. Some aspects of Cushing's syndrome, due to whatever cause, but more likely with tumors, may be related to the mineralocorticoid effects of cortisol and include hypertension, hypokalemia and metabolic alkalosis. The hirsutism sometimes seen is related to adrenocortical tumor secretion of androgens. The cause of the osteoporosis which requires gentle handling is unknown; experimentally the osteopenia is due to cortisol inhibition of bone formation independent of parathyroid activity.

Sometimes, particularly when the assay for ACTH is not easily available, the differentiation between pituitary and adrenal origin is more difficult; in such instances localization by scanning and selective venous sampling for cortisol might implicate unilaterality (i.e., one adrenal gland). A total lack of suppression by dexamethasone suggests an autonomous adrenocortical tumor whereas partial suppression indicates a pituitary tumor, which occasionally may be demonstrated on routine skull films.

The syndrome-disease which Cushing so brilliantly described and the mechanisms he conceived by 1932 are only now becoming clarified—again from a clinical scientific approach—and refinements of his "favored" surgical approach are now yielding important investigative information, safer operations and better clinical results. This renewed transsphenoidal approach to the anterior lobe of the pituitary gland, using binocular microscopic visualization and television monitoring, has led to the documentation of microadenomas in a much higher incidence than heretofore, so much so that the erstwhile concept of primary adrenocortical hyperplasia is disappearing. Furthermore, this microdissection technique has also allowed excision of the tumor without total excision of the gland or lobe. This means that some abridgement of replacement requirements is possible.

Bilateral adrenalectomy for hyperplasia remains a therapeutic approach for certain patients. Occasionally, bilateral excision of the adrenals may not actually be complete; if such is suspected, the detection of persistent hyperfunctioning cortical tissue is possible by supporting the patient with mineralocorticoid while discontinuing the glucocorticoid and then testing for the presence of endogenous plasma cortisol. Of all the hormones of the body, only one, cortisol, is absolutely essential for life. When it is necessary to eliminate all hyperfunctioning cortisol-secreting tissue or the corticotrophic polypeptide-secreting tissue by total excision of the adrenal glands or the pituitary gland tissue, as the case may be, such an operation commits the patient to lifetime substitution therapy of an adrenocorticosteroid (and thyroid hormone and sometimes testosterone, if hypophysectomy has been done). *S.R.F.*

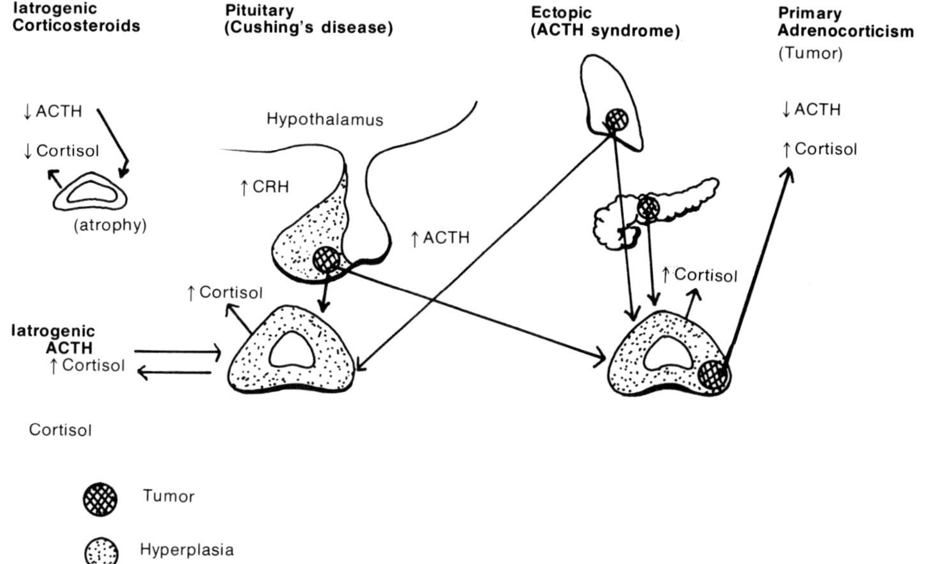

Fig. 20-2. Pathophysiology of Cushing's syndrome.

(See overleaf for flowchart)

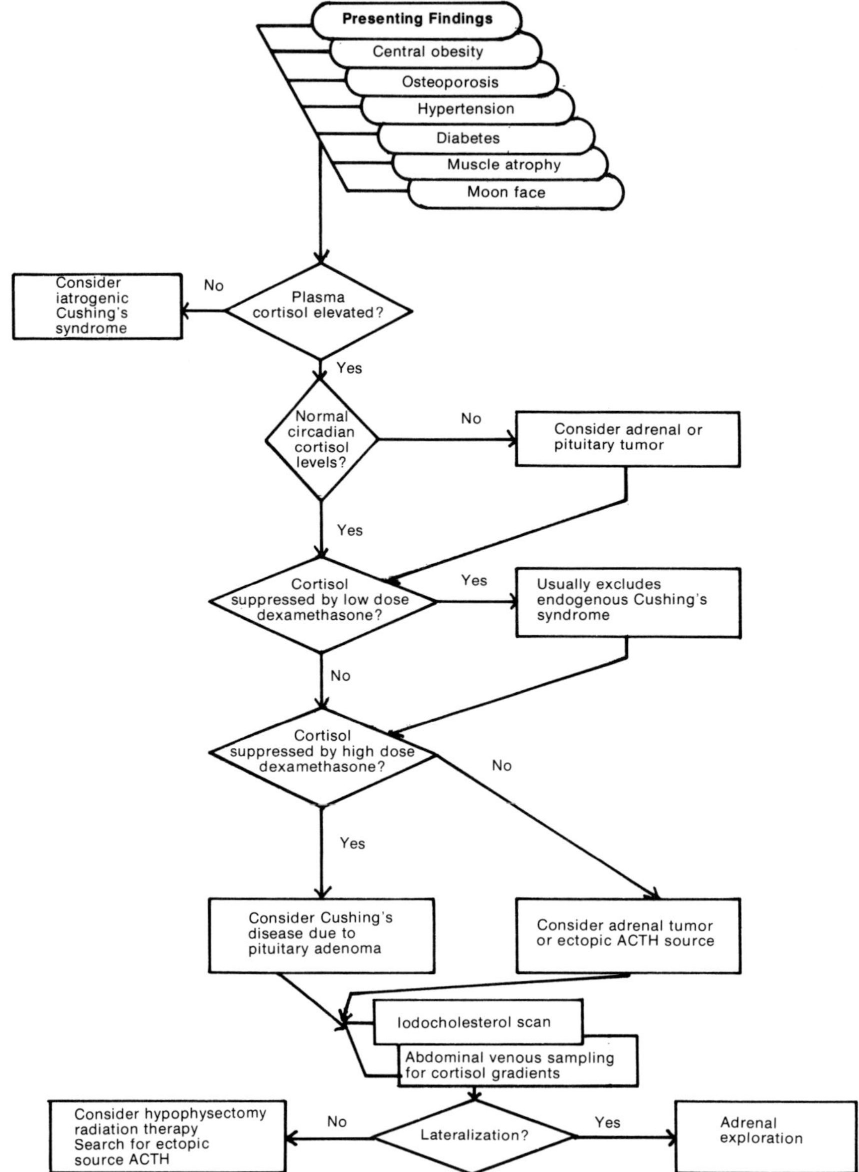

Fig. 20-3. Management flowchart of Cushing's syndrome.

21

Conn's Syndrome: Primary Aldosteronism

Bernard Zimmermann, M.D., Ph.D., and Walter H. Moran, Jr., M.D.

Although aldosterone is the most recent of the essential adrenocortical steroids to be characterized, clinical and experimental evidence for it existed for many years. The necessity of adrenal glands for sustaining life has been recognized since the description by Thomas Addison in 1885 of the disease which bears his name. The first active extracts of adrenal cortex shown to be capable of maintaining life in adrenalectomized animals were prepared in the 1920's. In 1943 Albright in his Harvey Lecture on Cushing's syndrome postulated the presence of an adrenal substance which caused a negative nitrogen balance (glucocorticoid), a second which caused positive nitrogen balance (androgen) and a third which regulated mineral and water metabolism (mineralocorticoid). The subsequent work of Kendall in the United States and Reichstein in Switzerland resulted in the isolation and characterization of substances related to cortisone, but residue from which these compounds had been extracted retained potent life-preserving and electrolyte-regulating properties. The first adrenal corticoid to be shown to have predominant electrolyte-regulating activity was desoxycorticosterone (DOC), but this was produced synthetically before it was demonstrated to be present in minute amounts in adrenal extracts. In 1952 Simpson and Tate in collaboration with Reichstein demonstrated the chemical nature of aldosterone, the electrolyte-regulating and life-maintaining hormone of the cortex. The difficulty in isolating and characterizing this substance was in part related to its unique aldehyde group at the C-18 position which is masked by the formation of the hemiacetal form of the compound (Fig. 21-1). Three years after the discovery of aldosterone Conn described the clinical syndrome associated with excessive aldosterone secretion.[3,4]

Initially biologic assays were employed to determine aldosterone in body

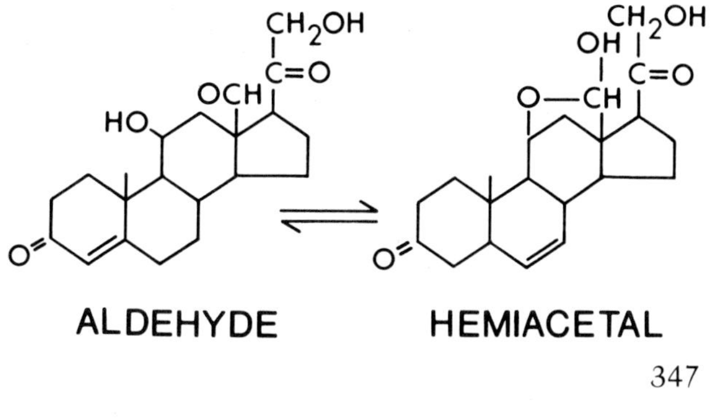

Fig. 21-1. Chemical structures of aldosterone.

fluids, particularly urine and adrenal vein blood, following which chemical methods not involving isotopes were developed. Subsequently aldosterone determinations in investigation and diagnosis of human disease have utilized modifications of the double-isotope method of Kliman and Peterson.[13] The procedure depends on labeling aldosterone in the extracted sample by forming its tritium-labeled acetate in the presence of a known amount of ^{14}C-labeled aldosterone diacetate. Refinement of the method has made possible the measurement of concentrations in peripheral blood, although at the present time such determinations are being carried out by radioimmune technique. In peripheral blood, aldosterone is present in extremely small concentrations such as 1 to 3 ng. (10^{-9} g.) per 100 ml.[23] In contrast to measurements in adrenal venous effluent methods modified for measurement of peripheral blood levels are tedious and most frequently employed for research purposes.

Through the release of aldosterone the adrenal gland maintains normal concentrations of sodium and potassium by stimulating resorption of sodium from the renal tubule which simultaneously rejects potassium ion. Under circumstances of challenge to normal homeostasis an even more important role is served. Deprivation of sodium ion results in increased aldosterone secretion as does flooding of the circulation with excess potassium.[22] Aldosterone is an essential ingredient for the normal reaction in which sodium loading produces potassium diuresis. In the presence of increased aldosterone levels this effect is accentuated and forms the basis for one of the tests for aldosteronism. Reduction in circulating volume also results in increased aldosterone output and retention of sodium along with water in isotonic proportion. This is a sensitive mechanism for preservation of effective circulation.

ACTION OF ALDOSTERONE

Present evidence indicates that the initial absorption of sodium from its isotonic position in the glomerular filtrate takes place without the action of special endocrine influence in the proximal tubule. The movement of water in a similar direction is passive and predicted by the necessity of osmotic equilibrium. Endocrine control of sodium resorption occurs by the action of aldosterone on the distal convoluted tubule. There is evidence that aldosterone may affect the collecting tubules as well. Here the fine adjustments are effected which maintain or readjust sodium balance after most of the water and electrolyte in the glomerular filtrate have been returned to the bloodstream. It should be emphasized that most of the resorption occurs without the participation of hormones, and the action of aldosterone and other mineral-active substances only accelerates a fundamental cellular process.

The mechanism of action of aldosterone on cells capable of sodium transport is a matter of considerable interest. The presently accepted concept conforms to the models of other steroid hormones which have been developed to explain the specificity of infinitesimal concentrations of substances which radically influence cell activity.[8,25] The hormone is active in an in vitro system consisting of two chambers separated by a toad bladder. The chemical events involved in its action have been explored in this system by utilizing radioactive-labeled aldosterone and known specific inhibitors of DNA and RNA functions.

The hormone combines with aldosterone-specific protein receptor in the cytoplasm of the cell. This complex acts on nuclear chromatin causing an increase in RNA-directed formation of messenger RNA and the coded synthesis of a specific aldosterone-induced protein (AIP).

The mechanism by which AIP stimulates the activity of cells capable of cation transport remains debatable. One theory holds that it makes ATP energy available to the "sodium pump." Another suggests that AIP is a component of a "permease" which enhances the entry of sodium through the mucosal membrane. Another possibility would involve increasing the efficiency of "sodium pumps" or the formation of new ones. Similarly the action of the aldosterone-produced protein on potassium transport is unsettled. Though it is possible to explain the reverse movement of potassium as being secondary to the electrochemical gradient produced by the changes in sodium movement, there is considerable evidence for a direct effect on potassium transport.

REGULATION OF ALDOSTERONE

Before the chemical structure of the individual steroids responsible for organic metabolism and electrolyte balance had been defined, histochemical studies on animals challenged with exogenous DOC and subjected to vigorous alterations in sodium and potassium intake indicated that the outermost layer of cells or zona glomerulosa of the adrenal cortex was responsible for regulation of sodium, potassium and water balance, and that in this capacity they could respond independently of pituitary corticotropic influence.[7,10] After aldosterone was discovered, it became apparent that in man more than one mechanism could be involved in the elaboration and output of this steroid. ACTH does produce a significant increase in aldosterone output concomitant with and in proportion to the stimulated production of cortisol from the zona fasciculata. However, the adrenals will respond with increased aldosterone output to sodium restriction or potassium loading in the absence of pituitary influence. Finally, the zona glomerulosa responds in a very sensitive manner to reduction in circulating fluid volume by releasing aldosterone which causes sodium retention and thereby protects the circulating blood volume. The elegant studies of Davis, Mulrow, Laragh, Genest, and others showed that the kidney itself is the receptor for this response and that angiotensin II, in addition to its vasoconstricture activity, is the "trophic hormone" for the zona glomerulosa.[6,14,15,17] Reduction in volume perfusing the kidney stimulates the production of renin by the juxtaglomerular cells to release renin, a proteolytic enzyme which acts on an alpha II globulin (angiotensinogen) to produce the decapeptide angiotensin I. Two amino acids are then split from the latter to produce the physiologically active angiotensin II. This in turn acts at an early stage of the synthesis of adrenal steroids from cholesterol and causes the output of aldosterone which in turn acts to maintain homeostasis in the vascular system. Interpretation of these steps is important because it provides the basis for distinguishing between primary and secondary aldosteronism and other causes of hypertension.

CLINICAL PICTURE OF CONN'S SYNDROME

In the syndrome described by Conn, hypertension is associated with hypokalemia and metabolic alkalosis resulting from excessive secretion of aldosterone. In contrast to other forms of hyperadrenalism, primary aldosteronism is not associated with any somatic abnormalities. Usually the hypertension is of considerable duration at the time the diagnosis is made and hypokalemia when severe causes profound muscular weakness and intestinal paralytic ileus. Carpopedal spasm, Trousseau's sign and, less frequently, Chvostek's sign may be seen since reduction in ionized calcium occurs in the presence of alkalosis. The accidental production of carpal spasm by the blood pressure cuff at the time the hypertension is recorded is a classic presentation of the syndrome.[29,31] Almost invariably a history of polyuria and polydypsia is obtained. The most frequent pathologic finding in primary aldosteronism is a benign cortical adenoma. These tumors are rather small compared to other functioning adrenal neoplasms. Adrenal carcinomas are fortunately much more rare since they tend to be highly malignant with a tendency toward rapid growth and metastasis. Conn's syndrome may also be associated with hyperplasia or adenomatous hyperplasia of the adrenal cortex, but whether these cases represent truly primary adrenal disease or the result of stimulation from some extra-adrenal mechanism is not clear and the term "idiopathic hyperaldosteronism" may be preferable for all cases not related to actual tumors.[16] The role of surgery in the management of these cases remains therefore debatable. Long-term follow-up of such patients who have undergone total or partial adrenalectomy have shown minimal or no permanent reduction of hypertension.[2,9,11] It has been our experience as well as that of others that improvement in electrolyte changes has been a more consistent result than reversal of hypertension in these cases. It is of interest that all of our cases of "adenomatous hyperplasia" had levels of blood urea nitrogen in the range of 30 to 40 mg./100 ml. and were found to have very small kidneys.

We have had experience with 15 cases of which 10 were caused by adrenal tumors.[30] Of these one was malignant and the other nine benign adrenal adenomata. There were two cases of diffuse hyperplasia and three of adenomatous hyperplasia. Of the benign tumors, eight originated in the left gland and only one in the right. This predilection for the left adrenal, interesting to note, appears in most reports. Larger series report similar distribution with 70 to 85 percent adenomata.[9,11,26] There is a definite predilection for the female in the adenoma group. The tumors are usually small (1 to 3 g.) and well encapsulated.

It is generally accepted that hypertension related to excessive aldosterone production can exist for a long time, perhaps years, before hypokalemia is recorded. It is reasonable to assume, therefore, that there are cases of normokalemic aldosteronism in which the diagnosis can be made only by the actual demonstration of increased circulating aldosterone in the presence of reduced renin.[5] The actual incidence of this disease in the hypertensive population is still not known.

DIAGNOSIS OF ALDOSTERONISM

Since it is not feasible to do direct determinations of aldosterone production in all patients with hypertension, attention is directed toward the group who display hypokalemia or inducible hypokalemia. A screening and diagnostic routine such as used by Melby* has been widely employed.[19,20] Prior to diagnostic investigation it is extremely important to eliminate the possibility of unrecorded use of diuretics, chronic cathartic use and habitual ingestion of substances such as licorice having mineralocorticoidlike activity. Hypertensive patients with persistent or episodic values of serum K^+ of less than 3.5 mEq./L. are the most readily recognized. The second group are those in whom hypokalemia occurs readily after institution of even minimal antihypertensive therapy since patients with primary aldosteronism are extremely sensitive to the hypokalemic effects of thiazide diuretics. The third group are those in whom hypokalemia can be induced by salt loading. Fifty mEq. of sodium chloride in excess of the normal diet are administered 4 times daily for a period of 4 days ("normal" diet = Na: 62.5 mEq. per 24 hr. and K: 50 mEq. per 24 hr.). Aldosteronism is strongly suspected if the serum potassium falls below 3.5 mEq./L. by the fifth day after institution of this regimen. Sodium loading almost never lowers the serum potassium in normal individuals.

Since spironolactone is the competitive antagonist to aldosterone, a therapeutic test utilizing this drug can be helpful in establishing the diagnosis. Unfortunately the blood pressure of a significant number of patients with other forms of hypertension will respond to this form of treatment and therefore spironolactone is used in cases which have been tentatively identified as primary aldosteronism and accelerated hypertension, and in which renal and renovascular disease have been ruled out. The response of blood pressure and metabolic alkalosis to 400 mg. of spironolactone daily after 2 to 3 weeks aids greatly in confirming the diagnosis and provides excellent preoperative preparation.

Chemical Confirmation of Excessive Aldosterone Production

Definitive confirmation of aldosteronism must be established by measurement of aldosterone and its metabolites in the urine or by the rate of secretion of the hormone from the adrenal.[19]

Excretion and secretory tests are performed on patients on a diet containing 120 mEq. of sodium and 50 mEg. of potassium per day, and thiazide diuretics and aldosterone antagonists should be discontinued for at least 3 weeks. Normally 30 to 140 mμ of aldosterone per day are secreted by the adrenal; 30 to 50 percent of this is excreted in the urine as tetrahydroaldosterone-3-glucuronide and 5 to 10 percent as the 18-monoglucuronide. The output is considered to be excessive if more than 16 μg. of monoglucuronide or 50 μg. of tetrahydroaldosterone is excreted in 24 hours.

Aldosterone secretion rate is carried out by isotope dilution, a tracer dose of 5 μCi. of tritium-labeled aldosterone (1, 2-H^3 aldosterone) is injected intravenously and the urine excreted in the subsequent 24 hours collected. The specific activity of a urinary metabolite is determined, divided into the injected dose and the secretion rate calculated.[19] Excretion rate of 150 μg. per 24 hours in an adult receiving 120 mEq. of sodium per day is considered elevated.

Blood Studies. Measurement of urinary aldosterone using the double-isotope methods remains the mainstay of tests for excessive aldosterone production.

*Personal communication.

Use of radioimmune assays makes possible the avoidance of urine collection by measurement of blood levels. Blood concentrations however change rapidly and are greatly influenced by pituitary corticotropic activity, and current experience suggests that they are diagnostic only in situations where aldosterone is very high and renin very low. Urinary excretion, on the other hand, integrates the "ups and downs" of blood level curves and gives a more sensitive index of minor degrees of hypersecretion.

Diagnosis of Primary Aldosteronism

Since autonomous production of aldosterone by the adrenal depresses renin output, the ability to measure circulating levels of renin makes possible the clear identification of aldosteronism of primary adrenal origin. Blood samples for plasma renin activity are drawn in the morning when the patient is recumbent and subsequently after the patient has assumed an upright posture at which time maximal levels are normally attained. Elevated aldosterone output in the presence of depressed renin activity provides clear evidence of primary hyperaldosteronism. In secondary aldosteronism such as is associated with renovascular disease, renin is expected to be high.

Unfortunately there is no single chemical or physiologic value which can be used to separate the group of patients with adrenal tumors from those with idiopathic hyperaldosteronism or "hyperplasia." Statistically, however, the deviation from the normal of the various parameters tends to be more extreme in the case of tumors. It has been possible therefore in the hands of some investigators to make reasonably accurate predictions by computer-assisted mathematical manipulation of several variables (i.e., pretreatment values for renin, aldosterone, sodium, potassium, mean systolic and diastolic blood pressure and age).[5,11] In most instances, however, the decision for surgical exploration will not be made until one or more of the methods discussed below for identifying tumors has been carried out.

LOCALIZATION OF LESION IN PRIMARY ALDOSTERONISM

Aldosterone-producing adenomata are characteristically small and may be difficult to identify at operation, and removal or serious damage to a normal adrenal gland in the process of searching for a tumor is to be avoided. Therefore, preoperative identification of the lesion or pathologic process is of great value. The small size of the tumors however has until recently seriously restricted the success of the usual angiographic techniques. At present, in units with experience in selective arteriography for this purpose, approximately 75 percent of studies are successful (i.e., at least two-thirds of each adrenal is adequately demonstrated) in tumors larger than 7 to 8 mm.[12] The arteriogram is of almost no value in the diagnosis of adrenal hyperplasia because of inadequate definition of normal size and the fact that hyperfunction occurs in glands which are apparently "normal" in size.

Selective phlebography is a relatively simple method of demonstrating the adrenals when the adrenal veins can be catheterized.[12] The quality of phlebograms varies because of the fine line between sufficient pressure to produce adequate reflux for filling of the adrenal veins and excessive pressure which can produce adrenal rupture. This complication is rather unpredictable and not only destroys the diagnostic usefulness of the procedure but has caused adrenal insufficiency in some instances. Adequate phlebograms are capable of demonstrating tumors in the range of 4 to 5 mm.

Selective adrenal venous sampling can be carried out if measurements of aldosterone blood levels are available. This has a diagnostic accuracy of 85 percent in the hands of those who have had excellent success in catheterizing both adrenal veins.[21] Aldosterone concentration ratios between the two glands in unilateral tumors are found in the 20:1 to 100:1 range. Renin activity can be determined at the same time and monitoring of plasma cortisol carried out to assure adequate specimen collection. As mentioned, however, success with this has been variable.[27]

The localization of adrenal tumors by photoscanning utilizing an iodinated precursor of adrenocorticoids has been utilized recently and promises to become a very valuable clinical technique.[18] ^{131}I-19-iodocholesterol administered to the patient becomes concentrated in a functioning adenoma and results in a high level of radioactivity. Recent experience with this method has shown it to be specific and very valuable for preoperative localization. The technique, of course, requires special computerized scanners.

TREATMENT

Patients identified as outlined above as having primary aldosteronism represent 0.5 to 7.5 percent of the hypertensive population and must be considered at least potential candidates for surgical exploration.

Preoperative Treatment

Patients with suspected primary aldosteronism are placed on a regimen of 400 mg. of spironolactone per day which should correct the hypokalemic-metabolic alkalosis and restore the blood pressure to normal. If this dose is not effective, adenomatous hyperplasia should be suspected. Although aldosterone inhibition will normally reverse the potassium deficit, it may be useful to add 50 to 60 mEq. per day of potassium supplement. Reduction of blood pressure is of obvious benefit in enhancing the safety of surgical procedures on these patients. Similarly correction of the potassium deficit greatly decreases the instance of metabolic complications, untoward reactions to anesthetic and muscle-relaxing drugs, cardiac arrhythmias and paralytic ileus.[31]

Surgical Approach

Before any methods were available for reliably localizing aldosterone-producing tumors, bilateral exploration of the adrenals through a transabdominal approach and a transverse upper abdominal incision was recommended. A posterior approach to the individual adrenal glands through the twelfth rib is however more direct, simpler and associated with fewer complications. Though it is particularly suited for patients in whom at least tentative lateralization of a tumor has been accomplished, separate posterior incisions with exposure of both glands can also be done. The left side is usually explored first since the left adrenal is more frequently the sight of an adenoma. If no adenomata are found and the diagnosis of primary hyperaldosteronism has been confidently made, bilateral total adrenalectomy may be justified.

Whether this is the best procedure for idiopathic primary hyperfunction is still open to question. Current opinion is in the direction of indefinite treatment with spironolactone as preferable to total removal of both glands. This clearly applies to patients with other serious diseases and those who cannot be relied upon to manage a replacement regimen to compensate for total lack of adrenal function.

Postoperative Care

In the patient in whom bilateral total adrenalectomy has been carried out, a replacement regimen designed to support the patient during operation and tapering off to maintenance level is required. This usually necessitates the administration of glucocorticoid and a mineral-regulating steroid such as desoxycorticosterone acetate or 9-α-fluorohydrocortisone. The regimen utilized in our institution has been outlined in detail elsewhere.[30] In patients with unilateral adenomata who have undergone preoperative treatment with spironolactone, no special postoperative regimen is required.

CONCLUSION

Since the incidence of recurrence of tumor or hyperfunction over a period of years is not known, more long-term follow-up studies on the course of patients with primary aldosteronism are in order. Though amelioration of hypertension may not be immediate, the results of surgical extirpation for autonomous aldosterone-secreting tumors are clearly superior to those of nonsurgical forms of therapy and therefore further refinements of methods for predicting the pathologic process responsible for hypersecretion should be pursued. Preoperative reversal of the effects of excessive aldosterone secretion is very effective, however, and deleterious effects of an exploration in which no tumor is found should not be feared. The most significant problem to be solved is the mystery of the nature and etiology of so-called hyperplasia or idiopathic hyperaldosteronism. Understanding of this entity will unquestionably lead to significant enhancement of knowledge of the physiology of blood pressure and electrolyte regulation, as well as of the background for treating these fascinating syndromes.

REFERENCES

1. Aitchison, J., et al.: Quadric analysis in the preoperative distinction between patients with and without adrenocortical tumors in hypertension with aldosterone excess and low plasma renin. Am. Heart J., *82*:660, 1971.
2. Biglieri, E. G., Schambelan, M., Slaton, P. E., and Stockigt, J. R.: The intercurrent hypertension of primary aldosteronism. Circ. Res., [Suppl. I, vols. 26 and 27] *1*:195, 1970.
3. Conn, J. W.: Part I: Painting background. Part II: Primary aldosteronism, a new clinical syndrome. J. Lab. Clin. Med., *45*:3, 1955.
4. ——: Progress report: Primary aldosteronism. J. Lab. Clin. Med., *45*:661, 1955.
5. Conn, J. W., Cohen, E. L., Rovner, D., and Nesbit, R. M.: Normokalemic primary aldosteronisn. JAMA, *193*:200, 1965.
6. Davis, J. O.: A critical evaluation of the role of aldosterone secretion and sodium excretion. Prog. Cardiovasc. Dis., *4*:27, 1961.

7. Deane, H. W., Shaw, J. H., and Greep, R. O.: The effect of altered sodium or potassium intake on the width and cytochemistry of the zona glomerulosa of the rat's adrenal cortex. Endocrinology, *43*:133, 1949.
8. Edelman, I. S., and Fanestil, D. D.: Mineralocorticoids. *In* Litwack, G. (ed.): Biochemical Actions of Hormones. vol. 1. New York, Academic Press, 1970.
9. Ferriss, J. B., et al.: Results of adrenal surgery in patients with hypertension, aldosterone excess, and low plasma renin concentration. Br. Med. J., *1*:135, 1975.
10. Greep, R. O., and Deane, H. W.: Cytochemical evidence for the cessation of hormone production in the rat's adrenal cortex after prolonged treatment with desoxycorticosterone acetate. Endocrinology, *40*:417, 1947.
11. Hunt, T. R., Schambelan, M., and Biglieri, E. G.: Selection of patients and operative approach in primary aldosteronism. Ann. Surg., *182*:353, 1975.
12. Kahn, P. C., Kelleher, D. M., Egdahl, R. H., and Melby, J. C.: Adrenal arteriography and venography in primary aldosteronism. Radiology, *101*:71, 1971.
13. Kliman, B., and Peterson, R. E.: Double isotope derivative assay of aldosterone in biological extracts. J. Biol. Chem., *235*:1639, 1960.
14. Laragh, J. H., and Stoerk, H. C.: On the mechanism of secretion of the sodium-retaining hormone (aldosterone) within the body. J. Clin. Invest., *34*:913, 1955.
15. Laragh, J. H., et al.: Renin, angiotensin and aldosterone system in pathogenesis and management of hypertensive disease. Am. J. Med., *52*:633, 1972.
16. Liddle, G. W.: Discussion of "secondary hyperaldosteronism and reduced plasma renin in hypertensive disease." Trans. Assoc. Am. Physicians, *80*:182, 1962.
17. Liddle, G. W., Duncan, L. E., and Bartter, F. C.: Dual mechanism regulating adrenocortical function in man. Am. J. Med., *21*:380, 1956.
18. Lieberman, L. M., Beierwaltes, W. H., and Conn, J. W.: Diagnosis of adrenal disease by visualization of human adrenal glands with ^{131}I-19-iodocholesterol. N. Engl. J. Med., *285*:1387, 1971.
19. Melby, J. C.: Primary Aldosteronism. Practitioner, *200*:519, 1968.
20. ——: Assessment of adrenocortical function. N. Engl. J. Med., *285*:735, 1971.
21. Melby, J. C., Spark, R. F., Dale, S. L., Egdahl, R. H., and Kahn, P. C.: Diagnosis and localization of aldosterone-producing adenomas by adrenal vein catheterization. N. Engl. J. Med., *277*:1050, 1967.
22. Moran, W. H., Rosenberg, J. C., and Zimmermann, B.: The regulation of aldosterone output: significance of the potassium ion. Surg. Forum, *9*:120, 1959.
23. Moran, W. H., Martinson, A., and Zimmermann, B.: Estimation of aldosterone in small peripheral venous samples. Surg. forum., *12*:21, 1961.
24. Moran, W. H., Goetz, F. C., Melby, J., Zimmermann, B., and Kennedy, B. J.: Primary aldosteronism without adrenal tumor. Am. J. Med., *28*:638, 1960.
25. O'Malley, B. W.: Unified hypothesis for early biochemical events in steroid hormone action. Metabolism, *20*:981, 1971.
26. Rhamy, R. K., et al.: Primary aldosteronism: experience with current diagnostic criteria and surgical treatment in fourteen patients. Ann. Surg., *167*:718, 1968.
27. Silen, W., and Egdahl, R. H.: Discussion of paper by T. K. Hunt, et al. Ann. Surg., *182*:353, 1975.
28. Simpson, S. A., and Tait, J. F.: Recent progress in methods of isolation, chemistry, and physiology of aldosterone. Recent Progr. Horm. Res., *11*:183, 1955.
29. Zimmermann, B., and Moran, W. H.: Aldosterone. Am. J. Surg., *99*:503, 1960.
30. ——: The adrenal glands. *In* Artz, C. P., Cohn, I., and Davis, J. H. (eds.): Brief Textbook of Surgery. Chap. 19. Philadelphia, W. B. Saunders, 1976.

31. Zimmermann, B., Moran, W. H., Jr., Rosenberg, J. C., Kennedy, B. J., and Frey, R. J.: Physiological and surgical problems in the management of primary aldosteronism. Ann. Surg., *150*:653, 1959.

Selected Reading

Conn, J. W.: Aldosteronism and hypertension: Primary aldosteronism versus hypertensive disease with secondary aldosteronism. Arch. Intern. Med., *107*:813, 1961.

——: The evolution of primary aldosteronism: 1954-1967. Harvey Lectures, *62*:257, 1968.

Davis, J. O.: The regulation of aldosterone secretion. *In* Eisenstein, H. B. (ed.): The Adrenal Cortex. Chap. 6, p. 203. Boston, Little, Brown & Co., 1967.

Harrison, T. S., Gann, D. S., Edis, A. J., and Egdahl, R. H.: Surgical Disorders of the Adrenal Gland. New York, Grune & Stratton, 1975.

Laragh, J. H., and Sealy, J. E.: The renin—angiotensin—aldosterone hormone system and regulation of sodium, potassium and blood pressure homeostasis. Handbook of Physiology. Sect. 8, Chap. 26, p. 8301. Washington, American Physiological Society, 1973.

Mulrow, P. J.: The adrenal cortex. Ann. Rev. Physiol., *34*:409, 1972.

Tepperman, J.: Metabolic and Endocrine Physiology. ed 3, Chap. 8. Chicago, Yearbook Medical Publishers, 1973.

EDITORIAL COMMENTARY

The clinical syndrome of hypertension with hypokalemic alkalosis which is caused by the effects of excessive circulating adrenocortical aldosterone upon the renal tubules, described by Conn, is associated with relative hypernatremia, suppressed renin activity, reduced formation of the renal polypeptide angiotensin II, but increased levels of aldosterone. The clinical picture may include symptoms of muscle weakness and paralytic ileus (hypokalemia), headache (hypertension), polydypsia and nocturnal polyuria (sodium retention) and carpopedal spasm (hypocalcemia of alkalosis). The adrenocortical elaboration of an excess of its mineralocorticoid from the zona glomerulosa overrides the delicate homeostasis between the adrenal and the kidney in the regulation of electrolyte (cation) balance and blood pressure. Although release of the potent sodium-retaining steroid, aldosterone, is partially regulated by the pituitary polypeptide, ACTH, the principal control of its release is mediated by the renin-angiotensin mechanism of the kidney. Within this axis, the cation concentration is influential; sodium deprivation, for instance, stimulates the release of renin, an enzyme at the juxtaglomerular apparatus; by a series of steps a polypeptide, angiotensin II, is formed in the blood of the pulmonary circulation and acts as the trophic hormone to stimulate adrenal aldosterone release; aldosterone then acts humorally at the collecting tubules to retain sodium and excrete potassium and hydrogen ion. Intracellularly aldosterone acts at the cytoplasmic and nuclear levels to induce protein synthesis of an enzyme which increases membrane permeability and the efficiency of the sodium pump of tissues in order to maintain the sodium/potassium ratio across cell membranes. Aldosterone was once appropriately called "electrocortin."

The key to the diagnosis of primary hyperaldosteronism is the measurement not only of increased aldosterone or its metabolites but also of the low suppressed renin activity. Normally, hyponatremia or hypotension stimulate renin release, but when aldosterone is secreted persistently by the adrenal tumor, the resultant sodium retention turns off or suppresses the renin release and is thus diagnostic of adrenocortical release of the sodium-retaining mineralocorticoid.

Once having determined that primary aldosteronism is present, the decision must be made whether the elaboration is from an autonomous tumor (usually a small benign adenoma on the left side) or hyperplasia.

The bilateral adrenocortical hyperplasia is called idiopathic hyperplastic aldosteronism (IHA) for good reason since it is not known what causes the hyperplasia (i.e., if there is a humoral stimulus or a genetic basis for the hyperplasia). Why hyperplasias occur at all with any of the endocrinopathies raises the question as to whether such changes are responses to an environment or to a genetic coding.

The determination of the histologic basis of the aldosteronism is not only an important surgical technical consideration, but also a prognostic one, because the results of surgical excision of the adenoma are much better than subtotal or total adrenalectomy for hyperplasia. Parameters for the diagnosis of the pathologic type include computerized evaluation of all clinical and laboratory data and lateralization or localization techniques such as selective sampling of adrenal vein aldosterone, cortisol and renal vein renin determinations and also radioiodinated cholesterol scanning for unilaterality. A promising feature in differentiation between adenoma and hyperplasia includes the observation that in patients with tumor, an upright posture after baseline levels during recumbency usually leads to a fall in the plasma aldosterone levels; in patients with idiopathic hyperplasia there is still an elevated response to an upright position.

Long-term follow-up information is revealing increasing rates of recurrence of hypertension and therefore some dissatisfaction with tumor excision as the ultimate surgical treatment for aldosteronomas (similar to the current unrest about the surgical treatment for parathyroid adenomas). The association of hyperplasia with adenomas, the return of hypertension in both groups, and the lack of knowledge of what constitutes the stimulus for adrenocortical hyperplasia, make firm decisions as to the best mode of surgical treatment seem difficult. Certainly, until more is known of the complexities of these mineral interrelationships (adrenal, kidney, thyroid, parathyroid) and their propensity for tumor development from hyperplasias, the best course is for excision of the adenoma and the occasional carcinoma, and prospective observations of the adrenocortical hyperplasias. Fortunately, spironolactone, not only as preoperative treatment, but for more definitive treatment of the bilateral hyperplasias, is available; the use of this antagonist of aldosterone makes the surgical treatment of Conn's syndrome exceedingly safe. *S.R.F.*

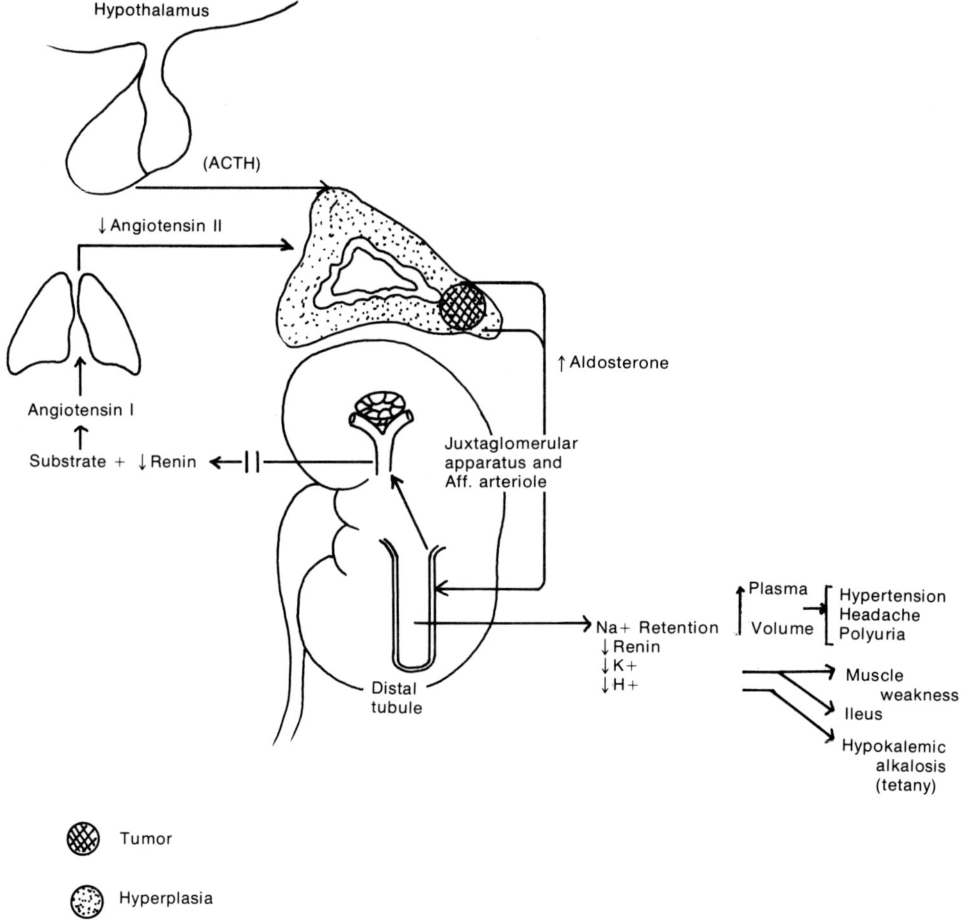

Fig. 21-2. Pathophysiology of primary aldosteronism (Conn's syndrome).

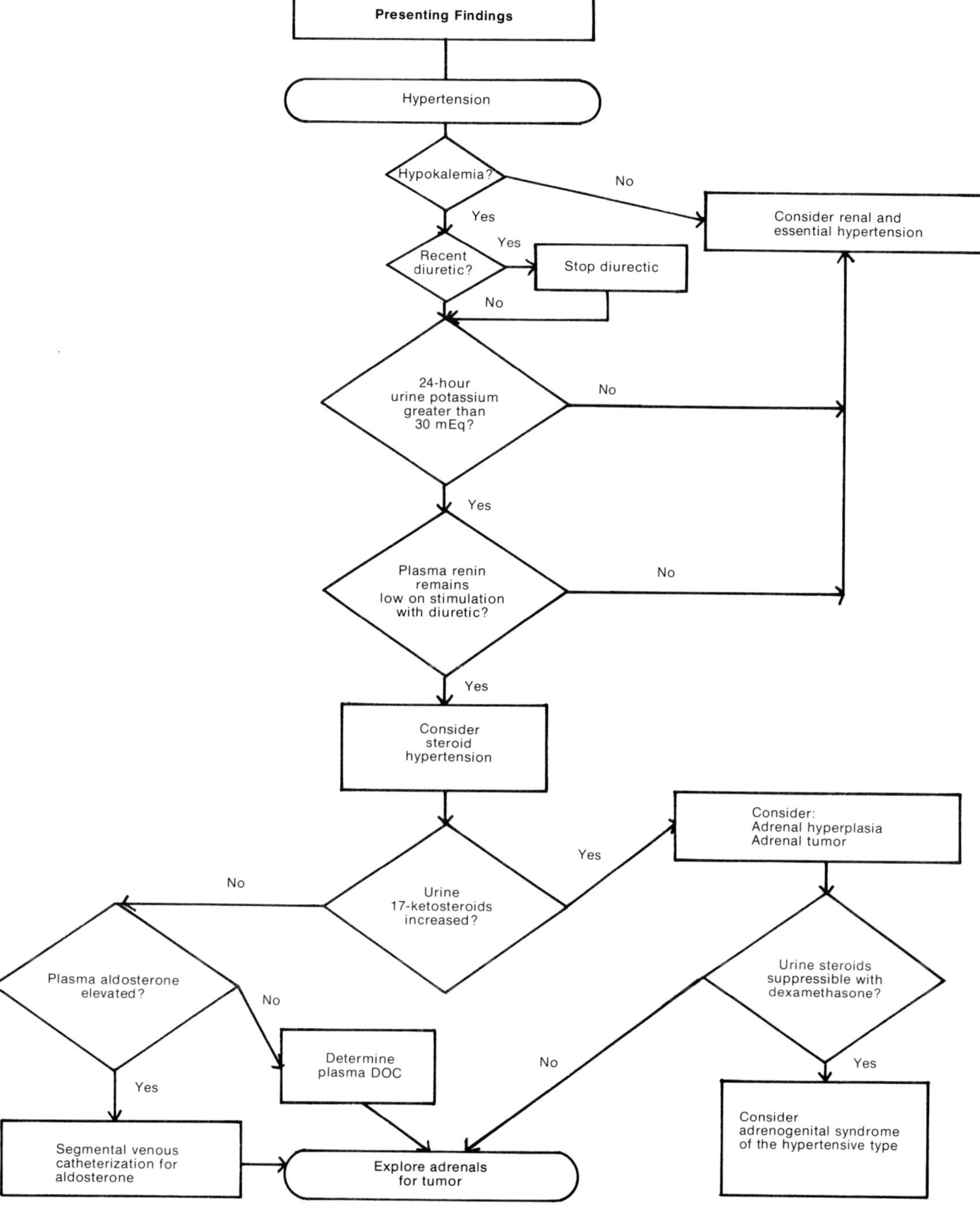

Fig. 21-3. Management flowchart of primary aldosteronism (Conn's syndrome).

22

Masculinizing and Feminizing Syndromes

Keith W. Ashcraft, M.D., and Thomas M. Holder, M.D.

Endocrine syndromes of masculinization or feminization may be manifest in several ways. The most dramatic are the disorders which affect sexual development in utero to produce genital ambiguity. Precocious puberty may be the first sign of an endocrine malfunction. Failure of normal secondary sex traits to develop at puberty is another manifestation of several endocrine-related sexual syndromes. Last, a normally developed and functioning child or adult may undergo isosexual or heterosexual changes as a result of functioning endocrine tumors.

Endocrine intersex disorders are distinguished from the chromosomal malformations by the fact that males are 46-XY, lack chromatin bodies and have testes. Females are 46-XX and are generally capable of reproduction.

The syndromes resulting from endocrine abnormalities may roughly be divided into five groups, the first one having two subgroups (see below).

Masculinizing-Feminizing Syndromes of Endocrine Etiology

1. Familial incomplete male pseudohermaphroditism (partial feminizing syndromes)
- *Type I*
  - Rosewater's syndrome
  - Reifenstein's syndrome
  - Lub's syndrome
  - Gilbert-Dreyfus syndrome
  - Hashem variations
- *Type II*
  - Pseudovaginal perineoscrotal hypospadias (PPSH)

2. Complete testicular feminization syndrome

3. Adrenogenital syndromes (congenital adrenal hyperplasia)
- Enzyme deficiencies of:
  - 21-Hydroxylase (female ambiguity and precocious puberty) or
  - 21-Hydroxylase (female ambiguity and salt-wasting)
  - 11-Hydroxylase (female ambiguity and hypertension)
  - 3β-HSD—Bongiovanni's syndrome (bisexual ambiguity and salt-wasting)
  - 17-Hydroxylase (male ambiguity and hypertension)
  - Cholesterol desmolase (male ambiguity and salt-wasting)

4. Sexual ambiguity due to maternal influences (exogenous androgenic syndromes)
- Maternal hormone ingestion
- Maternal endocrine disorders

5. Masculinizing-feminizing syndromes due to functioning tumors in normally developed children and adults
- Isosexual virilizing syndromes (males)
- Heterosexual virilizing syndromes (females)
- Isosexual feminizing syndromes (females)
- Heterosexual feminizing syndromes (males)

The first group is called familial incomplete male pseudohermaphroditism (incomplete feminization syndromes) of which there are types I and II. This term was suggested by Wilson and coworkers in 1974[15] to cover the rather broad spectrum of disorders in which patients obviously have male gonads but present with variable features of feminization, either at birth or at the time of puberty. The familial male pseudohermaphrodites (type I) include the syndromes reported by Rosewater, Reifenstein, Lubs, Gilbert-Dreyfus and probably the variations reported by Hashem. Although the syndromes were initially described as distinct, genetically determined disorders they are probably manifestations of the same lesion. In other words, in type I incomplete pseudohermaphroditism the familial pattern is established as a single gene, probably X-linked recessive trait which may be expressed as severe or mild in a particular patient. The type I patients heretofore discovered and reported have all been sterile.

The type II familial incomplete male pseudohermaphrodite subgroup comprises a disorder known as pseudovaginal perineoscrotal hypospadias or PPSH. The PPSH patients are generally mistaken for and raised as females. This is thought to be an autosomally carried defect with sex limitations.

The second group of patients are those with the complete testicular feminization syndrome. These patients have unquestionably female external genitalia except that the labia minora are underdeveloped. Transmission of testicular feminization appears also to be X-linked recessive but may well be autosomal recessive. Neither theory can be proven.

A third group of patients are the adrenogenital syndromes in which metabolic blocks in the synthesis of adrenal cortical hormones result in sexual ambiguity, precocious puberty and metabolic disorders which may be life-threatening. This constitutes probably the largest group of patients with intersex problems and certainly the majority of masculinizing problems in infancy. Inheritance is known to be autosomal recessive with equal sex prevalence. The severity of the lesion (i.e., its expression) is constant in a given family.

The fourth group of patients are those children whose mothers ingest androgens or have virilizing tumors affecting fetal external genital development. Usually the female infant is virilized and the male has hypospadias of varying degree.

The final group are the syndromes of masculinization or feminization due to functioning tumors in otherwise normally developed males or females. Elaboration of sex hormones may be primarily from adrenal or gonadal tumors or may be stimulated by a hormone intermediary from intracranial, adrenal or gonadal tumors.

EMBRYOLOGY AND BASIC UNDERLYING ABNORMALITIES

In the early fetus the gonad is an undifferentiated organ which takes female or male direction according to the chromosomal pattern. In the group of endocrine disorders under discussion in this chapter, all of the patients have chromosomal sex, chromatin and gonads which are concordant. Alterations in endocrine function produce masculinizing and feminizing disorders.

In the male the mullerian structures which are present in the embryo normally are inhibited by either testicular androgens, a local testicular inducer or mullerian inhibitor substance. The wolffian structures must be stimulated to develop by testes or an inducer substance. Testicular androgens probably cause the primordial external genitalia to develop in the male direction with an enlarged phallus, a fused scrotum and a urethra which extends out to the end of the penis.

In the female the ovaries develop, but it is the absence of testes and their inhibiting substances which allow mullerian structures to develop. The wolffian anlagen are not stimulated and regress. Without androgens the external genitalia develop into female structures.

Exogenous androgenic substances produced by or ingested by the mother during early stages of embryogenesis may alter the appearance of the female genitals to the point of ambiguity. The same hormones produce hypospadias in the male. Enzymatic blocks in the adrenal production of glucocorticoids in congenital adrenal hyperplasia often result in overproduction of androgens. In the male with testicular feminization syndrome there is a deficient target organ response to the androgens produced so that the external genitals develop into very nearly normal female structures.

Sexual ambiguity due to abnormal external genitalia is a cause for extreme anxiety on the part of the parents. The question by family and friends as to the sex of the newborn is one that cannot long be put off. Vascillation leads to rumors which may be a cause of considerable embarrassment for the child later in life. It is necessary to accurately and quickly diagnose the cause of ambiguity and assign a sex of rearing which will be compatible with adult sexual function. A change in gender after the age of 18 months is psychologically disturbing for the child.[10]

Sexual ambiguity may be due to endocrine disorders in which females are masculinized, males are incompletely masculinized or virtually completely feminized. In some forms of the adrenogenital syndrome early recognition of salt-wasting and prompt medical therapy may be required to save the life of the child. Although surgical procedures are almost always postponed until a much later time, the potential for corrective or cosmetic surgery must be realized. Accurate information and reassurance of the parents will help the entire family through this difficult time. Ultimately this support will affect the family's relationship with the child and his psychosexual orientation.

Excessive elaboration of sex hormones from tumors of the endocrine system is usually sporadic in occurrence without obvious genetic basis.

FAMILIAL INCOMPLETE MALE PSEUDOHERMAPHRODITISM

Type I—Incomplete Male Pseudohermaphroditism

This covers a spectrum of disorders previously thought to be relatively distinct but which may well be a variable expression of the same mutant gene.[15] This includes the syndrome described by Rosewater wherein the patient is thought to be an entirely normal male until puberty when gynecomastia develops and normal virilization does not take place. Reifenstein's syndrome finds the patient somewhat more toward the feminized end of the spectrum in which a bifid scrotum, mild hypospadias and small phallus accompany cryptorchism in infancy. At puberty gynecomastia develops and masculinization is deficient. The Gilbert-Dreyfus syndrome is a step further toward complete feminization of a male in that a miniscule phallus, bifid scrotum, perineal hypospadias and incomplete wolffian development are noted initially and with gynecomastia at puberty. Patients with Lub's syndrome are mistaken as female but almost always have testes located in the labia. They have incomplete wolffian development and yet no mullerian structures are recognizable. Wilson has brought all of these together in a very fine study of one family in whose affected member's manifestations of all of these syndromes have been found.[15] This would indicate that the lesions are X-linked recessive and the clinical variability is in the expression of the disorder.

Endocrine Pathology. The careful hormonal evaluation of this family of patients described by Wilson, et al., have demonstrated that plasma testosterone levels in all affected men postpuberty are elevated above the normal males in this same family. The disorder is thus not explained by a deficiency in testosterone synthesis. Luteinizing hormone (LH) levels were considerably higher than in the normal relatives of matched age whereas follicle-stimulating hormone (FSH) levels were not significantly lower than the normal controls. Attempted suppression of LH with Depo-Provera was unsuccessful, indicating that the feedback regulation of LH production by circulating androgen is not normal. They therefore conclude, as do others, that the feminization of these otherwise genetic males is probably due to a deficiency in androgen action. Federman suggests that the defect occurs in the inclusion of testosterone in the nucleus of body cells normally forming a protein-steroid chromatin complex necessary for the hormone to have effect.[5] In the incomplete forms of male pseudohermaphroditism some, but inadequate, androgenic effect is postulated, whereas in the testicular feminization syndrome this nuclear event appears to fail completely.

Diagnosis. The separation of these lesions from complete testicular feminization (see below) is possible by examination of the external genitalia. Patients with type I male pseudohermaphroditism are much more likely to have a hypospadias appearance. Testes may be palpable in labioscrotal folds with an inguinal hernia.

In the infant with ambiguous genitalia the possibility of congenital adrenal hyperplasia (CAH) must be excluded. In addition to family history of siblings with CAH, the urinary 17-ketosteroids, 17-OH, pregnanetriol and aldosterone are normal in type I male pseudohermaphrodites. Determination of serum testosterone, LH and FSH in these patients will not be fruitful in infancy since these hormones are only elevated postpuberty.

Differentiation of the virilized female or hypospadic male due to maternal androgenic influence is usually possible by history of ingestion or determining signs of virilization in the mother.

It may be difficult to differentiate the otherwise endocrinologically normal male with hypospadias and bilateral undescended testes from patients with much more serious endocrine malformations. Familial history will tend to support the diagnosis of male pseudohermaphroditism.

Treatment. These patients do not require hormonal substitution in any manner. Since these males do not respond to male hormones the penile development will be predictably inadequate. Surgical therapy is therefore directed toward conversion to a functional female status. This need not be done immediately after birth but the capabilities of reconstructive procedures must be kept in mind so that the female gender is assigned at birth. Parents must be reassured that although reproduction is impossible (as either sex), satisfactory sexual function can occur only as females. Testes probably do not need to be removed in these patients (in contrast to the complete testicular feminization syndrome) because testicular tumor development has not been reported. Cosmetically, however, testes in the inguinal canal or labia might not be desirable. If the male gender is assigned it is wise to remove the excessive breast tissue for cosmetic reasons but this is done near puberty.

Type II—Incomplete Male Pseudohermaphroditism

This is also designated as pseudovaginal perineoscrotal hypospadias (PPSH) and apparently is the only abnormal feature of this group of disorders.[14] Testes are present, virilization occurs at puberty, spermatogenesis is apparently the rule and there is no gynecomastia.

It is thought that PPSH is inherited as a sex-limited autosomal trait as opposed to an X-linked dominant for the type I incomplete male pseudohermaphroditism and the testicular feminization syndrome. First cousin consanguinity has been reported in several families with this disorder.

Endocrine Pathology. The mechanism for development of genital ambiguity is now known. Either inadequate testicular androgen influence at the embryonic stage of genital development or inadequate response may be the cause. Probably the former is the best explanation, for at puberty testicular androgen production and response are normal.

Diagnosis. PPSH is a familial lesion and therein lies its hope for early and correct diagnosis. The small penis and severe hypospadias may be confused with a female with clitoromegaly. Testes in the rugated labioscrotal folds may help in sex determination.

If raised as a female, at puberty the young "girl" undergoes masculinization. The clitoris will enlarge further and the blind short vagina will be discovered.

Treatment. Ideal treatment of these patients depends upon their being recognized at birth as males. Although excision of the pseudovagina and correction of the hypospadias may be done, there may be a problem of penile inadequacy with which to contend. An assessment of probable shaft length must enter into the decision to operate upon and raise the child as a male. Some of those who may be mistaken for females and raised accordingly to puberty obviously should not have gender assignment changed to male without a great deal of consideration. A well-adjusted, sterile female in whom breasts may be implanted is perhaps preferable to a confused young male with all the real or imagined performance hurdles.

No substitution therapy is necessary. Testes must be removed if the female role is maintained because at puberty androgen production and response will occur.

COMPLETE TESTICULAR FEMINIZATION SYNDROME

Complete testicular feminization syndrome is the most extreme form of male pseudohermaphroditism. Externally these males appear as normal females. Often they are not diagnosed until amenorrhea is investigated. This disorder can be recognized considerably earlier than puberty by the underdeveloped labia minora and testis-containing inguinal hernias. In the female infant with gonads in inguinal hernias, the absent labia minora should be an indication for gonadal biopsy and vaginoscopy at the time of hernia repair. Careful examination of the infant or young child with this syndrome will reveal a short blind-ending vagina and no mullerian structures. At puberty breast development may be marked but the breasts are composed mostly of fat with pale areolae and very small nipples. There is very scanty body hair, including the axillary and pubic areas. Some patients have been found to have epididymis and immature vas deferens but wolffian development certainly has been inadequate. There is no evidence of spermatogenesis in the testes, and when biopsied they show mostly stromal tissue. There is a predilection for testicular tumor development, malignant germinomas or benign tubular adenomas being the most frequent lesions.

Endocrine Pathology. The endocrinology in this form of male pseudohermaphroditism has probably been investigated better than any of the others.[3] Urinary ketosteroids (as a measure of androgen metabolites) were found to be normal or frequently elevated, suggesting that fetal androgen response was deficient. Urinary estrogens are noted usually to be in the midrange between male and female. Pituitary gonadotropins are normal or somewhat elevated. Adults with this syndrome have normal male levels of plasma testosterone. Determinations of androgen and estrogen biosynthesis have been made and found to be intact. These facts suggest that the testes are capable of producing androgen which for some reason does not stimulate the primordial external genitals to produce maleness. It is the local testicular inducer substance rather than androgens which are thought to be responsible for mullerian suppression. Wolffian development which does depend upon testosterone is incomplete in these patients.

Diagnosis. The diagnosis of complete testicular feminization rests not upon chemical tests but upon physical examination and the obtaining of a familial history. Since this defect is thought to be inherited in a dominant manner, one-half of the males at risk will be affected. Frequently there will be a history of an aunt who was amenorrheic or there will be a disparity between the number of uncles and aunts on the maternal side (some aunts being genetic males). Whether this is a sex-limited autosomal dominant trait or an X-linked dominant is impossible to determine. It is known that testicular feminization and color blindness are separately inherited indicating that either the gene for testicular feminization is located on an autosome as opposed to the X-linked color blindness gene or that the loci are widely separated allowing crossover in meiosis.

Careful examination of the external genitalia in a female with palpable gonads in the labia can lead to early diagnosis of this lesion. Otherwise most are diagnosed at puberty when amenorrhea is noted.

Treatment. It is necessary to remove the testes in these patients because of the propensity for tumor development, although the actual incidence of tumor development is unknown. Attempts to raise these children as males is completely out of the question.

Table 22-1. Adrenogenital Syndrome (CAH)*

Enzyme Deficiency	**Clinical Features**					**Laboratory Features**				
	Genital Ambiguity at Birth		*Salt Loss*	*BP*	*Precocious Puberty*	*Urine*		*Pregnanetriol*	*Aldosterone*	*Plasma Testosterone*
	♀	♂				*17-KS*	*17-OH*			
21-Hydroxylase (mild)	+	0	0	0	+	⇈	N or ↓	⇈	N	↑
21-Hydroxylase (severe)	+	0	+	0	+	⇈	↓	⇈	↓	↑
11-Hydroxylase	+	0	0	+	+	⇈	⇈	↓	↓	↑
3β-HSD	+	+	+	0	0	↑	⇊	↓	↓	↓
17-Hydroxylase	0	+	0	+	0	⇊	⇊	⇊	↓	⇊
Cholesterol Desmolase	0	+	+	0	0	⇊	⇊	⇊	⇊	⇊
18-Hydroxylase	0	0	+	0	0	N	N	N	⇊	—
18-OH Dehydrogenase	0	0	+	0	0	N	↑	N	⇊	—

*The clinical and laboratory diagnostic features of the various adrenogenital syndromes are shown. The responsible enzyme deficiency is listed at the left. The 18-hydroxylase and 18-OH-dehydrogenase are included for completeness, although these syndromes do not include features of masculinization or feminization. (Adapted from New, M. I., and Levine, L. S.: Adv. Human Genet., *4*:251, 1973)[11]

CONGENITAL ADRENAL HYPERPLASIA (ADRENOGENITAL SYNDROMES)

Probably the most common cause of sexual ambiguity or problems with masculinization and feminization are those associated with enzymatic blocks in the adrenel cortex.[11] Enzymatic blocks alter the production of mineralocorticoids, glucocorticoids and sex steroids from cholesterol (Fig. 22-1). Derangements in sexual development are due either to excessive or insufficient androgen production. The most common block, that of 21-hydroxylase, if mild will affect only the conversion of 17-hydroxyprogesterone to compound S. If severe, the conversion of progesterone to desoxycorticosterone (DOC) is also affected and a more serious clinical manifestation will occur. The 3β-HSD enzymatic block affects all three pathways.

The primary stimulus for adrenocorticol steroid production is adrenocorticotropic hormone (ACTH) from the pituitary. The production of adequate amounts of compound F (cortisol) will cause the pituitary to shut off or markedly reduce ACTH production. This feedback to the adrenal cortex then results in lower production of mineralocorticoids, glucocorticoids and sex steroids. If compound F, however, is not produced in normal amounts, this negative feedback is lost and excessive production of ACTH stimulates adrenocortical hyperplasia, and unrestricted production of steroids in the unblocked pathways takes place. Thus, with most of the enzymatic blocks under discussion, excessive androgens are produced and the female fetus will be masculinized. In the case of 3β-HSD block, however, the accumulation of dehydroepiandrosterone (DHEA) will act as an androgen for the female fetus but not a potent enough androgen to completely masculinize the male. There will be, in this instance, paradoxic ambiguity for both sexes. The 18-hydroxylase and 18-hydroxydehydrogenase enzymatic deficiencies which occur late in the mineralocorticoid pathway will cause no alteration in sex steroid production because the production of compound F is normal and the pituitary feedback mechanism is intact. As can be seen from Table 22-1 the sexual ambiguity or normalcy of the patient is a clue to the diagnosis of the particular enzymatic disorder.

Of major importance is the severe 21-hydroxylase block which will block the conversion of progesterone to DOC. Aldosterone production is deficient as a result and the ability to retain salt by the kidney is lost. Death from dehydration and electrolyte imbalance will result if the condition is not promptly recognized and treated. This sudden disastrous event generally occurs at about 2 to 3 weeks of age. Salt-loss to varying degrees can occur with other enzymatic deficiencies including the 3β-HSD.

Hypertension may result from accumulation of excess DOC in the 11-hydroxylase deficiencies. In males with mild 21-hydroxylase block the only clue to the presence of the congenital adrenal hyperplasia may be precocious puberty occurring at approximately 2 years of age with the onset of pubic hair, acne and enlargement of the phallus. These children have a growth spurt at this time and will be considerably larger than their peers, although ultimately because of early epiphyseal closure they will be of short stature. The normally formed male with high blood pressure and precocious puberty will result from 11-hydroxylase block. The various combinations of clinical manifestations, therefore, will allow sorting out of the enzymatic blocks to a great degree.

Confirmation of the disorder usually depends upon the laboratory features

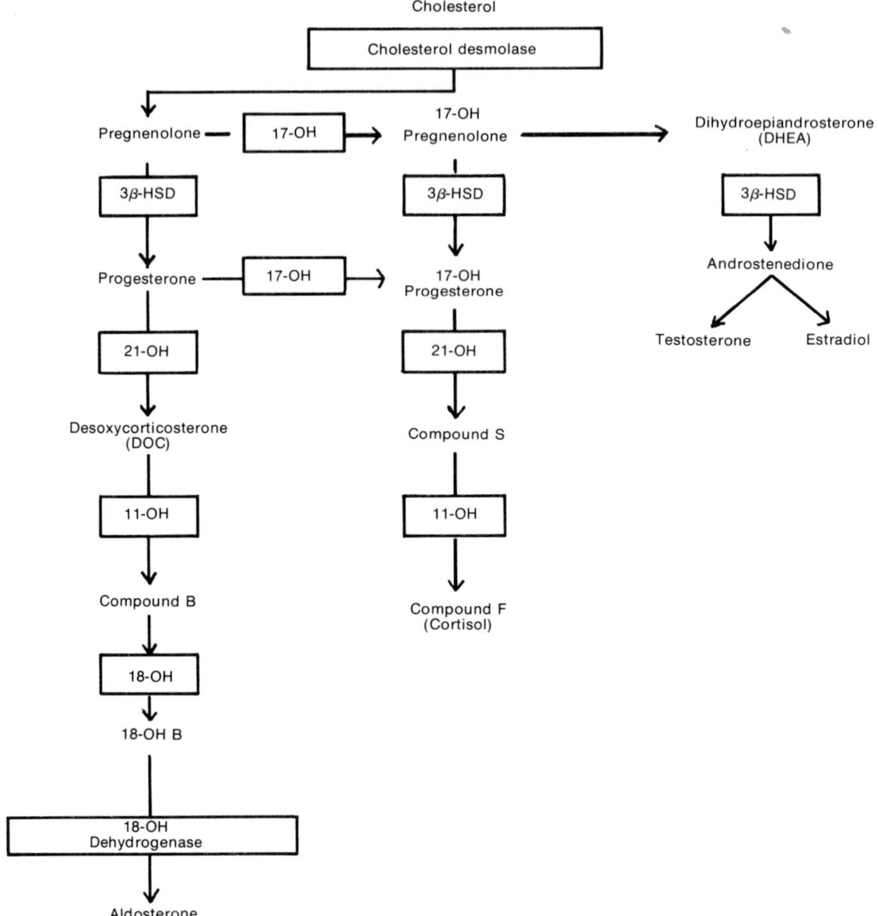

Fig. 22-1. This schematic of the adrenal cortical pathways for steroid synthesis shows the mineralocorticoids on the left, the glucocorticoids in the center column and the sex steroids on the right. The enzyme responsible for conversion of one compound to another is shown in the box between each compound. Absence of a particular enzyme will effectively block normal pathways although in some instances metabolic detours may be possible. Compound F is probably the major feedback end product to the pituitary. If low levels of compound F are perceived by the pituitary the ACTH is stimulated and the adrenal signaled to produce more. Thus functional overactivity occurs in the adrenal cortex and actual hyperplasia of the cortex results.

which can be seen from the right half of Table 22-1. Urinary ketosteroids, primarily DHEA, androstenedione and androsterone are included in this group of steroids. The 17-hydroxycorticosteroids are primarily tetrahydro compound S and tetrahydro compound F. The pregnanetriol is a measure of ketogenic steroid, an excretion form of 17-hydroxypregnenolone and 17-hydroxy-progesterone. The urinary aldosterone is a measure of mineralocorticoid production. In addition, plasma testosterone will give some clue as to which disorder is present, although determination of the four urinary metabolites generally are enough. It is to be emphasized that the adrenogenital syndrome, if properly treated, is perfectly compatible with the normal sexual life, including reproduction.

21-Hydroxylase Deficiency

The most common of the enzymatic blocks in congenital adrenal hyperplasia is 21-hydroxylase deficiency **(female ambiguity and precocious puberty).** Because compound F production is deficient the pituitary feedback mechanism is not active and production of mineralocorticoids and androgens is stimulated. Females may be virilized to the point where they have a penile urethral opening but they also have normal uterus, tubes, ovaries and vagina. Males, generally speaking, are not noted to be abnormal until 2 to 3 years of age when secondary sex characteristics develop. They are always larger than average babies and the genitals often are heavily pigmented. The family history of another sibling with the disease may be of extreme importance in recognizing the male early and in diagnosing the female at birth.

Treatment. Corticosteroid substitution started early allows normal growth and development with fertility. If not started until late in life short stature results because of early epiphysial closure. In the untreated male, sterility may occur because the testes do not develop normally.

About 30 percent of patients with 21-OH insufficiency will manifest the severe or "salt-wasting" form **(female ambiguity and salt-wasting)**. Severe salt-wasting is the clinically most prominent feature in males and females. Females, of course, are masculinized but both sexes at 2 to 3 weeks of age will vomit, become dehydrated, develop prostration and coma. The serum sodium will often be in the range of 100-mEq. per L. with elevated serum potassium. If recognized early as adrenogenital syndrome because of ambiguity, careful measurement of the electrolytes for the first several weeks will allow a detection of the salt-wasting before severe salt depletion has occurred. Measurements of urinary aldosterone production in the salt-wasters, of course, will reveal subnormal levels. It is also to be emphasized that the degree of severity of 21-hydroxylase deficiency appears to be constant in a given family.

In addition to treatment by glucocorticoid substitution, DOCA or 9-α-fluorohydrocortisone will compensate the block and allow the adrenal cortex to produce aldosterone. Adequate early treatment will allow normal life and fertility, whereas failure to treat may result in death from salt loss.

11-Hydroxylase Deficiency

The enzymatic disturbance next most common to 21-hydroxylase deficiency is the 11-hydroxylase block **(female ambiguity and hypertension).** In addition to continued ACTH stimulation of androgen production, an accumulation of desoxycorticosterone (DOC) is thought to be responsible for hypertension. The mechanism of hypertension due to DOC is probably mediated through the renin-angiotension system. It has been observed with 21-hydroxylase deficiency of the salt-losing type that hypertension follows onset of DOC therapy.

Diagnosis. Females with this disorder are virilized and the males are normal. There is no salt-losing. The blood pressure may be considerably elevated. If untreated, the male undergoes pubertal changes at about 2 years of age. Urinary ketosteroids are abnormally elevated and measurement of urinary steroid 17-hydroxysteroids in the form of THS may be as much as 100 times normal. Pregnanetriol is increased, aldosterone is diminished and plasma testosterone is increased.

Treatment. Treatment consists of the administration of cortisol which in turn shuts off ACTH. The stimulus for androgen and mineralocorticoid production is thus diminished. This will effectively control the hypertension as well as ameliorating other symptoms. If untreated the child will experience rapid somatic growth, early epiphyseal closure and precocious puberty. Untreated females are further virilized.

3β-HSD Deficiency

Deficiency of 3β-HSD **(bisexual ambiguity with salt-wasting or Bongiovanni's syndrome)** affects all three metabolic pathways in the adrenal cortex. Pregnenolone is not converted to progesterone, 17-hydroxypregnenolone is not converted to 17-hydroxyprogesterone and DHEA is not converted to androstenedione. Because DHEA is a very weak androgen male infants affected with this syndrome are incompletely masculinized. Because, however, DHEA is an androgen, females with this syndrome are mildly virilized. Thus the child with ambiguous genitalia may have 3β-HSD, 21-hydroxylase or 11-hydroxylase deficiencies.[1] A normal-appearing male with salt-loss, however, cannot be other than a 21-hydroxylase deficiency.

Most of the infants affected with this syndrome demonstrate such profound adrenal insufficiency that they die in infancy. A few patients, however, have reached puberty at which time testes seem to produce a bit of virilization. Gynecomastia is probably due to failure of fetal testosterone to inhibit the breast anlage. Unopposed by adequate androgens at puberty these breasts develop. Completely inadequate development of secondary sex characteristics at puberty, however, is the rule.

Diagnosis. Diagnostic criteria for this disorder are ambiguous genitalia (both male and female) and salt-wasting. There will be elevated urinary ketosteroids in the urine (as DHEA) but low 17-hydroxycorticosteroids, pregnanetriol and aldosterone. Plasma testosterone is lower than normal.

Treatment. Treatment of this lesion consists of cortisol and 9-α-fluorohydrocortisone. Although few patients have lived to puberty, perhaps androgens would be indicated in the male with this disorder.

17-Hydroxylase Deficiency

A complex and fortunately rare disorder, 17-hydroxylase deficiency **(male ambiguity and hypertension)** blocks the production of 17-OH-pregnenolone and 17-OH-progesterone from their precursors resulting in excessive intermediate mineralocorticoids and deficient glococorticoids and androgens.

Diagnosis. This disorder as described by New and Levine is one of female sexual infantilism in which mullerian structures are noted. The males are pseudohermaphrodites in whom prominent breast development occurs as the only secondary sex characteristic at puberty. On the other hand, pubertal females have virtually no breast development.

Females are not generally ambiguous when newborn but the males are. Salt-losing is not a feature of this syndrome but hypertension may very well be. Urinary 17-ketosteroids, 17-hydroxysteroids, pregnanetriol and aldosterone are low as is the plasma testosterone. Measured aldosterone, however, has not been above normal levels.

Treatment. It is postulated that renal tubular resorption of sodium is increased due to excess DOC suppressing renal renin production. The renin stimulation of the adrenal zona glomerulosa is lost and aldosterone synthesis diminished. By giving dexamethasone to suppress ACTH the production of DOC is shut off. Renin will then stimulate the glomerulosa to secrete aldosterone. Thus dexamethasone treats the mineralocorticoid deficiency.

Cholesterol Desmolase Deficiency

This cholesterol desmolase disorder (**male ambiguity and salt-wasting**) interferes with the conversion of cholesterol to pregnenolone and also the conversion of 17-hydroxypregnenolone to DHEA. Although the defects appear to be nearly universally fatal, one patient has been reported by Camacho with a mild form of the disorder.

Diagnosis. Severe salt-wasting is a prominent finding. There is incomplete masculinization of males but females appear to be normal at birth. Urinary 17-ketosteroids, 17-hydroxysteroids, pregnanetriol and aldosterone as well as plasma testosterone are diminished.

Treatment. The lesion theoretically is treatable by 9-α-fluorohydrocortisone, cortisol and perhaps androgen for the pubescent male.

EXOGENOUS ANDROGENIC SYNDROMES

A number of progestational agents may be ingested during pregnancy to help prevent abortion. Unfortunately, the effect of these drugs upon the developing fetus is sometimes quite deleterious. It is interesting to note that the ingestion of the same material may produce in the female infant extreme degrees of virilization and yet tend to produce in the male infant feminization (i.e., hypospadias).[1] Given this history of such ingestions, the sex of the child is usually not difficult to determine.

In addition to exogenous sex steroids which may influence the fetus there are the hormone-producing maternal tumors[9] either of gonadal or adrenal origin which may adversely affect the fetus. These are much more difficult to diagnose unless the signs of virilization on the part of the mother are incontrovertible. Again, the degree of masculinization in the fetus is usually less than one would see with congenital adrenal hyperplasia or the derangements of androgen response in the male pseudohermaphrodite. There are instances reported, however, where a penile urethra has been formed in the female by a virilizing tumor in the mother and instances of penoscrotal hypospadias following ingestion of maternal progestational agents.

The history will allow differentiation of these lesions from the others.

MASCULINIZING-FEMINIZING SYNDROMES DUE TO FUNCTIONING TUMORS

Isosexual Virilizing Syndromes

Several lesions may produce a syndrome of precocious puberty in the male child or a further increase in virilization in the older male. These include CNS lesions which produce interstitial cell-stimulating hormone (ICSH) causing the testicle to produce abnormal amounts of androgens. There may be a pineal tumor stimulating the pituitary to in turn stimulate testosterone production by the adrenal cortex. Primary lesions of the testes such as Leydig cell tumors and testicular choriocarcinoma may result in isosexual masculinization. Finally some adrenal cortical tumors may produce large amounts of testosterone without stimulation from a CNS lesion.[8] The diagnosis of these lesions may be difficult. Treatment of testicular and adrenal tumors is often futile for most are malignant. Localization and control of CNS tumors even when benign may be difficult.

Heterosexual Virilizing Syndromes in Females

There are several ovarian and adrenal lesions other than congenital adrenal hyperplasia which will produce masculinization in the otherwise normally developed female. Ovarian lesions include the luteoma of pregnancy,[13] arrhenoblastoma,[4] lipid cell tumors[12] and polycystic ovarian syndrome of Stein-Leventhal.[6] Adrenal lesions may be hyperplasia, benign or malignant tumors.[8] Determination of the source of hormone excess is a combination of history, physical examination and laboratory determinations.

Ovarian tumors which produce virilization often occur in the child-bearing group of postmenopausal women. The evidences of such a tumor are deepening of the voice, development of facial hirsutism and clitoromegaly. None of the tumors is very common. Although few of these tumors are histologically malignant, even fewer are biologically malignant. Being usually unilateral, these tumors may be removed with or without the ipsilateral fallopian tube, leaving the woman capable of reproduction. In the postmenopausal woman there is probably a great deal more support for bilateral oophorectomy along with removal of tubes and uterus.

The polycystic ovary of Stein-Leventhal is not a tumor disorder but does delay menarche and may be the etiology for sterility in a number of young patients. This lesion is sometimes responsible for inadequate female pubescent changes but is probably more often found as a cause for secondary amenorrhea or sterility in somewhat older women. Actual virilization may result from the Stein-Leventhal ovary.

A group of adrenal tumors which may produce abnormal sexual characteristics include both benign and malignant adrenocortical tumors. Carcinomas of the adrenal cortex which produce masculinization in the female can usually be differentiated from adrenal hyperplasia by failure to suppress with dexamethasone. Autonomously functioning benign or malignant tumors similarly will not respond to ACTH stimulation. Therefore the determination of hormone levels and their response to ACTH and dexamethasone suppression will usually differentiate hyperplasia from benign or malignant tumors. Sometimes determination of malignancy in adrenal cortical tumors must be made on the basis of capsular invasion, since the cellular structure of adenomas and carcinomas frequently is similar.

Isosexual Feminizing Syndromes (in Females)

One of several extremely unusual lesions may produce precocious puberty or evidence of further feminization of an adult female. The hormone estrogen may be produced by an ovarian lesion such as a granulosa cell tumor.[12] Abnormal production of estrogen by a normal ovary may result from luteinizing hormone (LH) by a pituitary tumor or from chorionic gonadotropin produced by a choriocarcinoma.

Heterosexual Feminization Syndromes (in Males)

When an adult male develops feminizing characteristics, the lesion is almost always a malignant adrenal cortical tumor.[7,8] Treatment is most often ineffectual.

OPERATIVE PROCEDURE FOR AMBIGUOUS GENITALIA

The sex assignment of normal infants is based on the appearance of the external genitalia. In the infant with ambiguous genitalia the sex assignment should in fact be based on what can be done operatively to make the genitalia appear and function as a reasonably normal male or female. In general a more satisfactory female can be constructed than a male. Although a penis which can act as a conduit for urine can be constructed, there is no way to produce erectile tissue which has a satisfactory sexual function. Standard procedures for correction of hypospadias and orchiopexy are employed for the child to be raised as a male.

For the female with congenital adrenal hyperplasia and masculinization of the external genitalia there is an adequate vagina although there is fusion of the labioscrotal folds of varying degree. Usually all that is required for these girls is a perineal vaginoplasty to open the introitus and allow the urethra to open directly to the outside without having the vagina fill with urine every time the child voids.

If the clitoral enlargement is not marked and the patient is treated adequately from birth usually nothing need be done for the phallus. If the clitoris remains moderately enlarged a clitoral recession should be performed during the second year of life.[2] If the phallus approached penile size a clitoridectomy with removal of the corpora from their origin along the pubic bone is done before 2 years of age.[10] It is probably best to preserve as much clitoral tissue as possible provided the recession does not produce distortions which will be painful at erection.

REFERENCES

1. Aarskog, D.: Intersex conditions masquerading as simple hypospadias. Birth defects. Original Article Series, 7:122, 1971.
2. Boix-Ochoa, J., and Martinez-Mora, J.: Nuestra experiencia y technica quirurgica en los estados intersexuales. Rev. Quir. Espanola, *1*:268, 1974.
3. Crawford, J. D., et al.: Syndromes of testicular feminization. Clin. Pediatr., 9:165, 1970.

4. Cruikshank, D. P., and Chapler, F. K.: Arrhenoblastomas and associated ovarian pathology. Obstet. Gynecol., *43*:539, 1974.
5. Federman, D. D.: His and hers. [Editorial] N. Engl. J. Med., *290*:1137, 1974.
6. Givens, J. R., Andersen, R. N., Umstot, E. S., and Wiser, W. L.: Clinical findings and hormonal responses in patients with polycystic ovarian disease with normal versus elevated LH levels. Obstet. Gynecol., *47*:388, 1976.
7. Greenwood, R. H.: Selective feminization due to an adrenal carcinoma. Proc. R. Soc. Med., *67*:671, 1974.
8. Harrison, J. H., Mahoney, E. M., and Bennett, A. H.: Tumors of the adrenal cortex. Cancer, *32*:1227, 1973.
9. Haymond M. W., and Weldon, V. V.: Female pseudohermaphroditism secondary to a maternal virilizing tumor. J. Pediatr., *82*:682, 1973.
10. Hendren, W. H., and Crawford, J. D.: The child with ambiguous genitalia. Curr. Probl. Surg., Nov., 1972.
11. New, M. I., and Levine, L. S.: Congenital adrenal hyperplasia. Adv. Human Genet., *4*:251, 1973.
12. Norris, H. J., and Chorlton, I.: Functioning tumors of the ovary. Clin. Obstet. Gynecol., *17*:189, 1974.
13. Polansky, S., DePapp, E. W., and Ogden, E. B.: Virilization associated with bilateral luteomas of pregnancy. Obstet. Gynecol., *45*:516, 1975.
14. Simpson, J. L., New, M. I., Peterson, R. E., and German, J.: Pseudovaginal perineoscrotal hypospadias (PPSH) in sibs. Birth defects. Original Article Series, *7*:140, 1971.
15. Wilson, J. D., Harrod, M. J., Goldstein, J. L., Hemsell, D. L., and MacDonald, P. S.: Familial incomplete male pseudohermaphroditism, Type I. N. Engl. J. Med., *290*:1097, 1974.

Selected Reading

Federman, D. D.: Abnormal Sexual Development. Philadelphia, W. B. Saunders, 1967.

EDITORIAL COMMENTARY

There are some masculinizing and feminizing syndromes of endocrinologic basis in which the surgeon is likely to be involved. Such involvement may take the form of participation in decisions regarding sex selection in genital ambiguity of the infant and child and subsequent surgical alteration of genital anatomy and function. The surgeon's participation is more obvious when intervention is necessary in the diagnosis and operative treatment of tumors which elaborate sex hormones. For these reasons, some genetic, chromosomal abnormalities not involving surgical considerations are not included here.

The endocrine role in sex differentiation of the external genitalia is evident when it is realized that in intrauterine development of the fetus the presence or absence of androgenic stimulation is all-important to genital development. For instance, male development will occur only in the presence of androgenic stimulation during the first 12 fetal weeks; absence of testicular androgen results in the inherent tendency to feminize. The Leydig cells of the testes, after the fetal functioning stage, revert to mesenchymal cells by the first post-gestational month without resuming functional importance until the age of puberty, at which time the cells mature back into testosterone-secreting Leydig cells. The ability of the testes to virilize the patient at adolescence is frequently a recapitulation of their performance in masculinizing the external genitalia in utero. In male pseudohermaphroditism (chromatin-negative individuals) in which there is normal embryonic differentiation of testes, the defective male development must be ascribed to a more specific failure of the fetal testes to overcome the inherent tendency to feminize. This failure may stem either from a secretory failure of the testes themselves during this critical fetal period of sex differentiation, or from an abnormality of the physiologic action of androgen, or from a failure of the target tissues to respond normally. The spectrum of the clinical appearance of male pseudohermaphroditism then, may include at the one end the individual simulating a female and at the other end a male with only mild hypospadias or cryptorchidism.

Another spectrum of sexual ambiguity results from abnormalities in cholesterol metabolism in the adrenal cortex, commonly called the adrenogenital syndrome(s). It can be generally stated that enzyme deficiencies which produce **early** blocks in the metabolic pathways result in ambiguity of the male genitalia due to deficiencies in androgenic (testosterone) secretion without the occurrence of precocious puberty. On the other hand, if the enzyme deficiency produces a block which occurs **late** in the matabolic pathway (i.e., after androgen is synthesized) there will be no male ambiguity (just female ambiguity), with elevated androgen levels, and precocious puberty may develop.

Finally, clinical virilization and feminization due to tumor elaboration of hormones are not such subtle changes. Tumors of the pituitary, gonads, placental tissues and the adrenal glands produce both isosexual and heterosexual clinical abnormalities. Carcinomas produce the more dramatic changes, and if the tumor is of the adrenal cortex, the usual clinical picture is a change toward the opposite sex. If these tumors are diagnosed correctly and early in the course of the disease by specific determinations of humoral substances in the blood and urine, surgical excision is the usual mode of treatment. Humoral suppression for the treatment of hyperplastic endocrinopathies, on the other hand, may be all that is necessary. It has been recognized for some time that assays of certain gonadotropic hormones are not only diagnostic, but that such determinations are of additional value for prognosis after treatment. *S.R.F.*

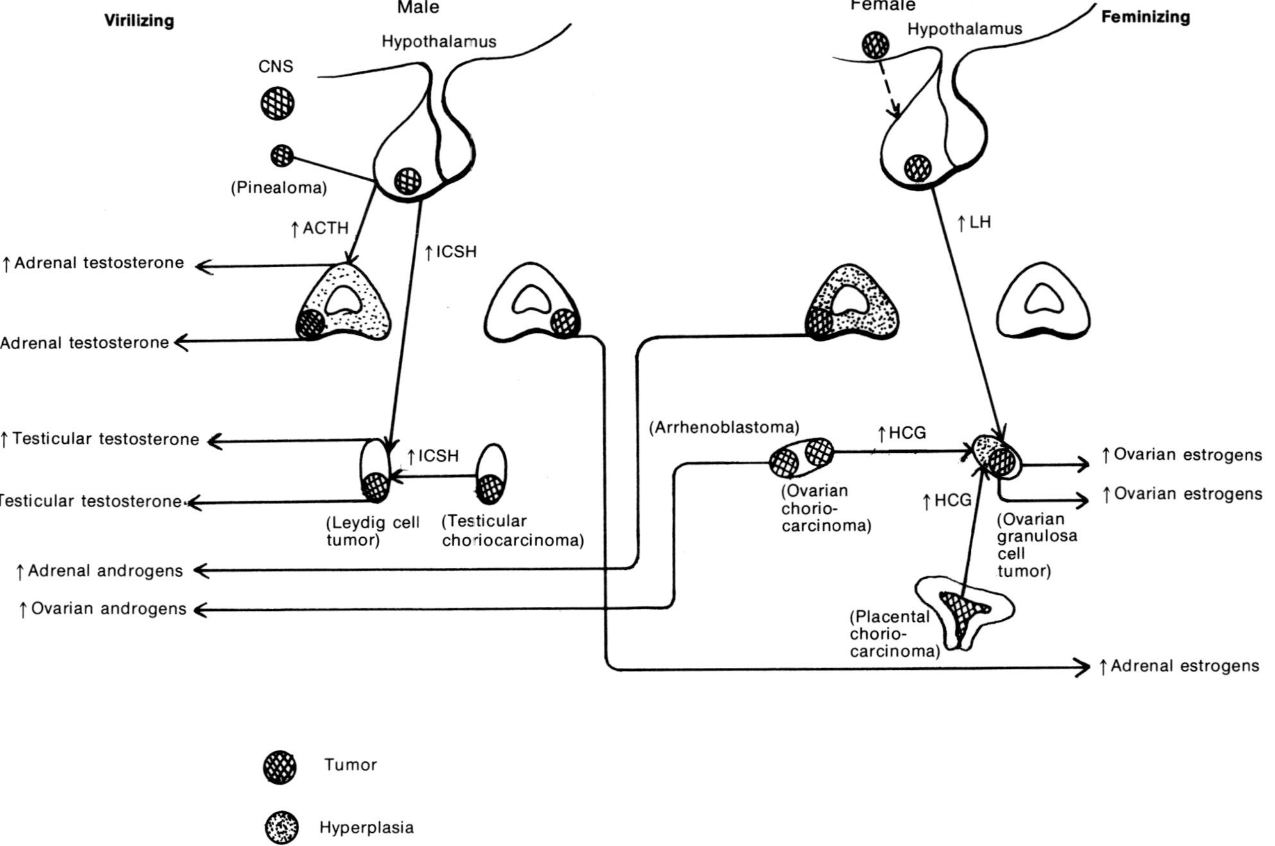

Fig. 22-2. Pathophysiology of the masculinizing and feminizing syndromes.

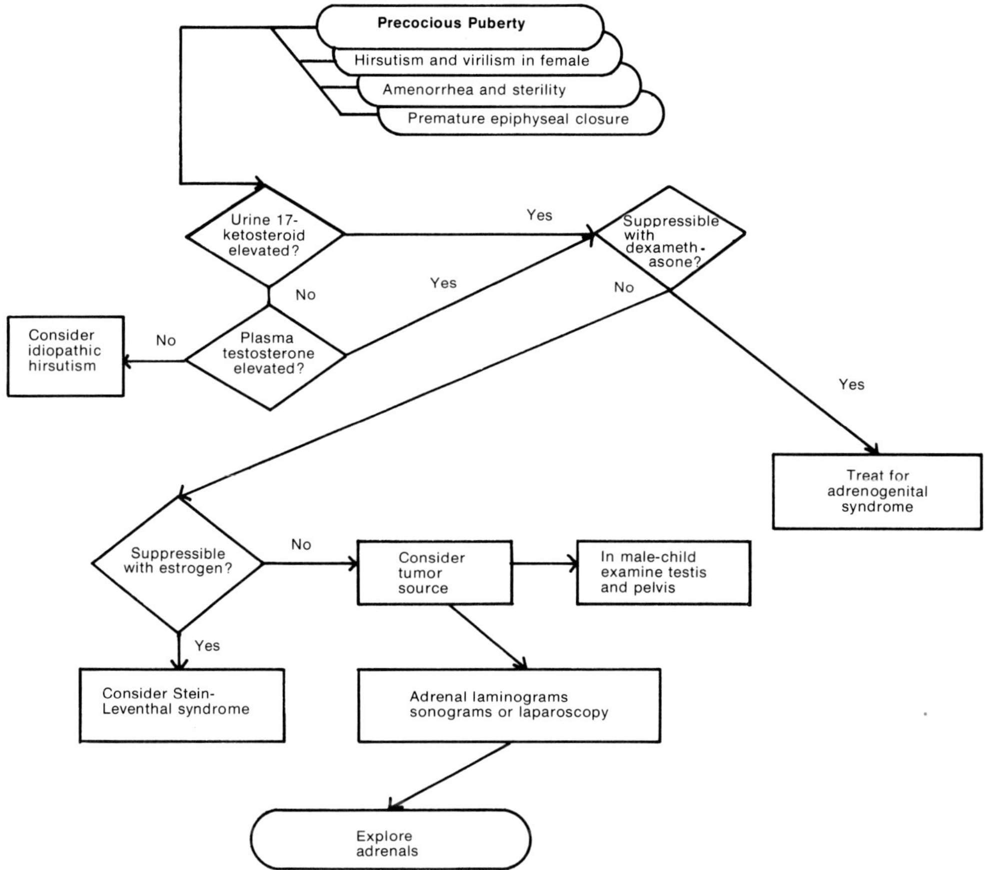

Fig. 22-3. Management flowchart of masculinizing and feminizing syndromes.

PART 4
Miscellaneous Syndromes

23

Syndromes Due to Ectopic Hormone Production

Laurence H. Smith, M.D.

"Ectopic hormone production" is a term introduced by Liddle in 1962. It refers to the production of hormones by a tumor which has arisen from tissue not usually considered "endocrine" or to the release of a hormone by a tumor which arises within an endocrine gland but that hormone being one not associated with that organ.[9]

The terms "ectopic," "endocrine" and "nonendocrine" must be regarded as arbitrary. For example, both erythropoietin secretion by the kidney and gastrin release by the gastric antrum surely demonstrate the process of internal secretion of hormones; however, the kidney and the stomach are not usually considered members of the classically defined endocrine system.

Should a gastrin-producing islet cell tumor of the pancreas be regarded as an example of an ectopic hormone syndrome? According to conventional wisdom, yes. The physiologic source of gastrin is the antrum, not the pancreas. The questionable presence of gastrin-producing D cells in the normal pancreas illustrates the deficiencies of attempts at absolute classification.

THEORIES OF ECTOPIC HORMONE PRODUCTION

Genetic regression is one reasonable theory to explain the ability of tumors to produce hormones. It is obvious that at one point in the development of an organism, a single cell has complete and full totipotentiality, (i.e., the fertilized ovum). Daughter cells necessarily lose functions as they differentiate. Certain cellular activities are "repressed"; others are maintained and augmented. The final cell is known by the function it carries out. Reversal of the process of repression (derepression) could explain hormone production by a tumor.

Another theory postulated concerns the presence of "hidden clones." This theory proposes that within any given tissue there are clones of cells which are less differentiated than those which surround them. These cells have never lost the ability to elaborate and release hormones, but as their numbers are few, the amount of hormone produced is small, and their presence cannot be detected. Specific neoplasia of this group of cells results in a tumor capable of secreting hormones.

Another consideration among the theories of ectopia concerns aberrant release of hormones from tumors of APUD cells, those normal secretory cells which develop from the neural crest. Cells of this line disperse and mature to become much of what is designated the endocrine system.[6,10] The APUD group consists of 24 cells (so far identified) sharing the characteristics of common ancestry, similarity of amine metabolism, the microscopic presence of storage granules, and the synthesis of amine and polypeptide hormones. It is the presence of APUD cells within various organs which allows that organ to be classified as a member of the endocrine system.[7] Note, however, that not all tissues capable of internal secretion contain APUD cells. For example, thyroxine and parathyrin are produced by cells which have no known close relationship to the APUD family. Similarly, the adrenal cortex and the gonads develop from the mesonephric ridge, not from the neural crest. The hormones released by them are steroids and steroid hormones are not typical of APUD cells.

Ectopic hormone syndromes are always the result of overproduction of amine or polypeptide hormones. The tumor syndromes of hyperthyroidism, hyperadrenal corticotropism or gonadal steroid hormone excess occur by the secondary stimulation of these organs, not by the primary elaboration of their hormones. For example, Cushing's syndrome effected by a carcinoma of the lung occurs as a consequence of ACTH release, **not** by tumor synthesis of cortisol or a similar substance. This is in accord with the assumption of a single-step derepression allowing the expression of a latent protein-producing mechanism. Steroid hormone production, on the other hand, is a complex, multistaged process which is not likely to be accorded by any such simple regression.

The concept of tumor derepression permits a classification of such activity as suggested (with modification) by Baylin[1] and Levine.[4]

1. **Simple Hyperfunction.** Tumor hyperfunction requires only autonomy by escape from feedback constraints. The hormone released is indigenous to that tissue. Hyperinsulinemia by a beta-cell islet tumor of the pancreas and hyperparathyroidism from a parathyroid adenoma are good examples.
2. **First Order Regression.** This level of genetic alteration results in the production of a hormone not characteristic of the tissue from which the tumor arises, but appropriate to other tissues derived from the same cell line. This phenomenon is most clearly illustrated with the APUD family (e.g., ACTH release by a bronchial carcinoid). In this instance a Kulchitsky cell is releasing the hormone normally produced by the anterior pituitary corticotroph. Both of these cells are members of the APUD group.
3. **Second Order Regression.** Further loss of DNA suppression could result in the release of a hormone by a tumor with cellular origins not related in any obvious way to the cells which normally produce this hormone. Examples of this group could include parathyrin synthesis by an oat cell carcinoma and chorionic gonadotropin production by an adenocarcinoma of the lung.
4. **Primitive Expression.** Tumors which have regressed biologically to a great extent may produce and release hormones, enzymes and other protein segments which are normally found only in the fetus. Common examples here include circulating carcinoembryonic antigen in a patient with an ileal carcinoid and alphafetoprotein in one with hepatoma.

It is reasonable to assume that of the tumors exhibiting hormone production, those of the APUD cell line do not require the "large step" backward required of tumors arising from tissues which normally produce no hormones. Since the regressive step should be smaller, it could be predicted that APUDomas would behave clinically in a less malignant fashion than other tumors exhibiting hormonal ectopia. Generally, this is true. A noteworthy exception to this clinical observation is the oat cell carcinoma. This APUDoma is one of the most aggressively malignant tumors encountered. However, its very behavior suggests that it is a tumor which has undergone extensive derepression. Any such cancer so free from biological constraints could be expected to grow rapidly and to cause bizarre clinical manifestations.

It should be emphasized that tumor hormone synthesis is only part of the broader implications of aberrant protein metabolism. Those polypeptides with structural similarities to native hormones and produced in sufficient quantity are recognized as being involved in endocrinopathies. Other protein units, as yet unidentified, may result in one of the varieties of the "paraneoplastic syndrome." Still other peptides are discovered only because they have been looked for and give no systemic indication of their presence. Highly sensitive tests, such as radioimmunoassay, have shown this to be true. Furthermore, not all patients with hormone-producing tumors have recognizable endocrinopathies. In these patients it is possible that the hormone produced is incomplete and therefore biologically inactive. In many instances, hormone syndromes develop only after prolonged exposure to the hormone. A cancer patient may be killed by his malignancy before the syndrome has had time to appear.

CRITERIA FOR DIAGNOSIS OF ECTOPIC HORMONE SYNDROMES

A tumor should not be implicated as the cause of a specific clinical state unless certain criteria are met including: (1) Demonstration of nonsuppressible high blood levels of hormone appropriate to the syndrome, (2) high tumor levels of hormone in the blood with an arteriovenous difference across the tumor, (3) disappearance of the syndrome upon removal of the tumor, and (4) reproduction of the syndrome by injection of tumor extract into experimental animals. Without the application of at least some of these "Koch's postulates of ectopic hormones," the diagnosis of a tumor hormone syndrome is only a presumption. For example, hypoglycemia may occur in some patients with large mesenchymal tumors. Tumor release of insulin cannot be assumed until excessive levels of this hormone have been demonstrated. In fact, in this particular situation hyperinsulinemia has rarely been found.

Obviously, eradication of the tumor is the most direct method of correcting an ectopic hormone syndrome. Failing the cure, means of alleviating the symptoms must be sought. Now follows a brief description of tumor-hormone diseases and the means of treatment or palliation.

ECTOPIC HORMONE SYNDROMES

Ectopic ACTH Syndrome (Ectopic Cushing's Syndrome; ACTH) and Hyperpigmentation (MSH)

Cushing's **disease** is a primary malfunction of the hypothalamic-pituitary control of ACTH which results in bilateral adrenal cortical hyperplasia. Cushing's **syndrome** is simply the effect of glucocorticoid excess from any cause. Tumors may induce this syndrome most commonly by production of

ACTH, or rarely, by synthesis and release of corticotropin-releasing factor (CRF). Either way, the circulating ACTH levels are high and the adrenal cortices are stimulated. Tumor ACTH is biologically, if not structurally, identical to pituitary ACTH. Tumors which have been reported to induce ectopic Cushing's syndrome by the elaboration of ACTH (and hyperpigmentation by MSH secretion) include neoplasms of the lung, pancreas, thymus, thyroid (medullary), adrenal, parathyroid, gonads and liver.

Typical cushingoid features may be absent in patients with ACTH-active tumors. Less than half of patients with demonstrable elevation of ACTH can be clinically recognized. Signs of hyperadrenalcorticoidism develop only after prolonged exposure to such hormones; most patients with these functioning tumors simply do not live long enough to manifest, clinically, the typical Cushing's syndrome. The sudden onset of muscular weakness, fatigue and edema are suggestive features. All patients with tumors and who develop hypokalemic alkalosis should have the diagnosis pursued.

Dexamethasone suppression may be used to distinguish ectopic ACTH production from other forms of ACTH excess. With two exceptions, ACTH-secreting tumors are not suppressed. One is those patients with CRF-releasing tumors. Presumably, high levels of glucocorticoids can inhibit pituitary ACTH release despite continued ectopic production of CRF. Another exception is found in patients with ACTH-producing bronchial carcinoids. These tumors are often suppressed by high-dose dexamethasone.

Melanocyte-stimulating hormone (MSH) is normally released by the same cell which produces ACTH. This genetic linkage persists even through neoplastic change. Hypersecretion of MSH apart from the production of ACTH has not been reported. It is likely that elevated MSH levels could be found in every instance of ectopic ACTH syndrome. Cutaneous pigmentation requires a sufficient time of exposure and this probably explains its absence in most cases. The cell which produces melanocyte-stimulating hormone as well as the melanocyte itself have their cellular origins in the neural crest. The phylogenetic questions raised by this observation are largely speculative but certainly hint at the evolutionary purpose of such cells, one regulating the function of the other by means of neurotransmitter secretion.

Unfortunately, cure of patients with tumor-caused Cushing's syndrome is infrequent. About half of such patients have carcinoma of the lung and, therefore, carry with them the high mortality rate associated with that disease. Tumors of the pancreas and thymus are the next most common carcinoma sites and also have few survivors. Therefore, means of palliation are foremost considerations. Patients with incurable but controlled and slowly growing tumors may, under highly selected circumstances, be candidates for bilateral adrenalectomy. The possibilities for palliation are demonstrated by the several reports of patients who have undergone adrenalectomy for presumed Cushing's **disease** only to have an ACTH-secreting tumor discovered several years later. Shrewd clinical judgment must balance the intensity of symptoms, the rate of tumor growth and the operative risk on the one hand against the possible benefits of surgery on the other.

Two drugs may be useful in the treatment of patients who are not candidates for surgery. Metapyrone specifically inhibits adrenal 11-hydroxylase activity. Aminoglutethimide blocks conversion of cholesterol to pregnenolone. Both drugs have reported efficacy in the symptomatic relief of the ectopic ACTH syndrome. It should be noted that neither drug in any way affects the growth or metabolism of the primary tumor, but rather alters the function of its **normal** target organs, the adrenals.

Ectopic Hypercalcemic Syndrome (PTH)

Alterations in serum calcium elicited by tumors have numerous possible mechanisms including (1) bone metastasis, (2) vitamin D-like sterol production, (3) vitamin D-enhancing factors, (4) prostaglandin release, (5) elaboration of osteoclast activating factors, (6) parathyroid gland stimulation, or (7) parathyrin production.

Tumor hypercalcemia is at least as common as primary hyperparathyroidism. It therefore becomes prudent to distinguish between the two if a small inapparent tumor is not to be missed and if unnecessary neck exploration is to be avoided. Parathyrin causes a fall in serum phosphate whereas the hypercalcemia of bone metastases is usually associated with hyperphosphatemia. The secondary signs of hyperparathyroidism (e.g., bone resorption and renal calculi) are almost never noted in examples of the ectopic parathyrin syndrome. Finally, radioimmunoassay has demonstrated that tumor PTH elevates calcium more than native PTH for equivalent levels of hormone. This greater response is the result of fewer inactive segments in the tumor-released hormone. The test assays the biologically inactive segment of the hormone and is accurate to within 8 percent for differentiating true hyperparathyroidism from ectopic parathyrin production.[2]

Most tumors demonstrating this syndrome have been cancers of the lung and kidney or lymphomas. Carcinoma of the breast is the tumor most often associated with hypercalcemia, but it is doubtful that this neoplasm has even been demonstrated to release parathyrin. Other tumors reported to have been associated with hypercalcemia include those of the pancreatic islets, adrenal cortex, gonads, intestines and liver.

The clinical signs of hypercalcemia can be easily mistaken for the common manifestations of terminal carcinoma. Patients exhibiting fatigue, lethargy, anorexia or even coma should have serum calcium determinations. Significant palliation may be lost by simply overlooking the possibility of tumor-induced hypercalcemia.

Treatment may be directed at the tumor itself (surgical excision, roentgenotherapy or chemotherapy) or by combating the effects of hypercalcemia. Serum calcium may be lowered by saline and sulfate infusions, chelating agents, oral and intravenous phosphate, hemodialysis and mithramycin. Depression of serum calcium correlates well with patient improvement.

Ectopic Hyperglycemic Syndrome (Glucagon)

Radioimmunoassay has revealed the presence of two types of circulating glucagon, pancreatic and enteric. Both complete, molecule for molecule, for hepatic binding sites to activate adenylcyclase. Pancreatic glucagon is the more potent of the two. Pancreatic glucagon also suppresses intestinal motility and is in turn suppressed by oral glucose. Enteroglucagon release is inhibited by hypoglycemia. Normally, the two hormones are physiologically complementary in the maintenance of normal interprandial glucose levels. Histologically, the two cells which elaborate glucagon (pancreatic "A" cells and intestinal "EG" cells) appear to be identical.

Few patients with functioning "glucagonomas" have been identified. Tumors of the pancreas causing hyperglycemia, dermatitis and distinctive painful glossitis have been reported. Ectopic tumors include those of the lung and liver. A renal tumor causing inhibition of intestinal motility has been described. Extracts from this tumor were found to contain large quantities of enteric glucagon.

Ectopic Hypoglycemic Syndrome (Insulin)

A considerable body of information has been compiled as to what is **not** the cause of tumor hypoglycemia. Radioimmunoassay has shown that the condition is rarely the result of insulin release. Arteriovenous difference of glucose indicates that tumor glucose consumption is not the cause. Normal or decreased insulin levels rule out pancreatic stimulation.

Several observations are true of the tumor hypoglycemia state. It most often occurs in patients with large mesenchymal tumors. It has also been reported with carcinoma of the lung. Excessive insulin levels have been demonstrated in patients with carcinoids, carcinoma of the stomach and carcinoma of the uterine cervix. A polypeptide, somatomedin, has been shown to possess insulinlike activity and could be the active agent. Proinsulin, a normal intracellular precursor, has hypoglycemic action and if released, might account for some of the cases reported.

Whatever the cause, excision of the tumor relieves the symptoms. When cure is not possible, palliation becomes difficult. Glucose administration will alleviate symptoms but only while it is being given. Steroids and long-acting glucagon may be used to promote glycogenolysis.

Ectopic Ulcerogenic Syndrome (Gastrin)

The opening remarks of this chapter noted that the production of gastrin by a pancreatic islet cell tumor (the Zollinger-Ellison syndrome) may be, strictly speaking, an ectopic hormone syndrome. It is now considered unlikely that pancreatic "D" cells normally produce gastrin. However, other tumors, including islet and carcinoid tumors of the duodenum and lung, may produce identical symptoms. Ectopic hypergastrinism has also been reported in patients with thyroid medullary carcinoma, parathyroid adenoma, gastric and mesodermal tumors.

It has been demonstrated that the physiologic activity of gastrin resides in two molecules, one large and one small. There is evidence to implicate the release of "large gastrin" in patients with Z-E syndrome.

A pharmacologic effect of gastrin is to increase the tone of the lower esophageal sphincter and physiologically to increase gastric acid output. Pathologically elevated levels of gastrin, typical of tumors producing it, result in massive hypersecretion by the stomach. The result is extensive ulceration of the upper gastroinestinal tract, often extending into the jejunum. All patients with a particularly virulent return of ulceration after adequate gastric surgery or with unusual complications from such surgery (e.g., gastrocolic fistula) should be held suspect.

Many patients with this syndrome exhibit significant diarrhea. The etiology of this symptom may be simple irritation of the gastrointestinal tract by acid excess or it may be from the concomitant release of other polypeptides, prostaglandins or kinins.

Ideally, simple excision of the tumor should be adequate treatment. However, the frequency of occult functioning metastases has evolved total gastrectomy as the treatment of choice. Patients so treated suffer no ill effects from hypergastrinemia and are saved the complications of recurrent ulceration. Furthermore, Friesen[3] has postulated a tumor end-organ stimulatory effect and reports occasional tumor regression by the removal of the stomach. This suggests some sort of tumor-to-stomach feedback mechanism. This observation will require further investigation to test its validity. There is no doubt that the progress of the tumor and the patient's response to therapy can be followed by serial gastrin determinations. Calcium-stimulated gastrin may be more consistent in reflecting actual tumor mass.

Patients with Z-E tumors may develop medullary carcinomas of the thyroid. It is known that infused gastrin will elevate serum calcium and many patients with Z-E syndrome have hypercalcemia. It is possible that prolonged stimulation of thyroid C cells (which produce calcitonin), in an attempt to lower the calcium, might eventually lead to neoplasia. This aspect of the MEA syndrome might represent the occurrence of one tumor elicited by another, rather than the simultaneous appearance of two. This possibility is, however, conjectural.

Ectopic Diarrheogenic Syndrome (Secretin, VIP)

The watery diarrhea, hypokalemia, achlorhydria (WDHA) syndrome may be caused by tumors of the lung, pancreas, the adrenal medulla, sympathetic ganglia and kidneys. When the primary tumor arises in the pancreas, the disease is called "pancreatic cholera" or the Verner-Morrison syndrome (see Chap. 15). Such patients suffer severe fluid loss and consequent electrolyte imbalance. The associated achlorhydria is reversible upon removal of the tumor, suggesting that a hormonal acid-suppressing factor is present.

Experimentally, the infusion of secretin will cause diarrhea and increase pancreatic secretion six- to eightfold. Said and Faloona[8] have detected a secretinlike polypeptide in the serum of 93 percent of patients suffering from the WDHA syndrome and elevated tissue levels in all of the specimens examined.

Vasoactive intestinal polypeptide (VIP) is normally secreted by colonic "D" cells, although in animals it has been separated from lungs and pancreas. Pancreatic polypeptide (PP) and the prostaglandins have also been implicated as associated humoral substances.

Patients with the WDHA syndrome may also have associated hyperglycemia and hypercalcemia. Calcium elevation may result from parathyroid stimulation secondary to magnesium loss.

Excision of the primary tumor will allow a fall in the level of VIP and alleviation of symptoms. Previously achlorhydric patients often display "rebound" gastric hyperacidity.

"Inappropriate ADH Syndrome" (Water Intoxication Syndrome, Ectopic Hyponatremic Syndrome; ADH)

ADH is normally synthesized and released by the posterior pituitary. Its action is one part of the normal mechanism of fluid homeostasis. ADH increases the permeability of the renal collecting ducts. Water return to the renal medulla is increased, urine output is decreased and water is conserved.

The hormone has been produced by tumors of the lung, kidney, brain, pancreatic islets, anterior pituitary, breast and gastrointestinal tract. Studies have revealed the ectopic hormone to be essentially the same as pituitary ADH.

ADH is secreted by tumors in great excess of normal requirements and the physiologic effects are greatly exaggerated. The result is the "inappropriate ADH syndrome." Patients in this state retain large amounts of fluid and display the signs and symptoms of water intoxication. Serum sodium and osmolality fall drastically. In response to increased intravascular and extracellular volume, large amounts of sodium are excreted, thereby worsening the situation.

Eradication of the tumor is an ideal not often realized; most patients with this syndrome are victims of bronchogenic carcinoma. Attempts to correct hyponatremia by saline infusion are futile, since excessive sodium excretion by the kidney is a feature of the disease. Palliation is not difficult, however. The only effect of ADH is renal. Therefore, restriction of water intake allows the electrolytes and serum tonicity to return to normal and symptoms are relieved.

Ectopic Gonadotropism (HCG, FSH, LH)

Tumors may produce gonad-stimulating hormones which are similar to those normally released by the pituitary or the placenta. Thus, human chorionic gonadotropin (HCG), follicle-stimulating hormone (FSH) or luteinizing hormone (LH) may be produced. Tumors releasing gonadotropin include those of the liver, ovary and lung. Often the pulmonary neoplasm is of the "large cell" variety.

All gonadotropic hormones (as well as thyroid-stimulating hormone) are composed of two units, alpha and beta chains. The hormone is biologically inert unless both chains are present. The alpha chain is identical among all four hormones (HCG, FSH, LH, TSH). Alteration of the beta chain dictates the physiologic action. Specific immunoassays for both chains are available and afford a biologic marker for assessment of treatment effectiveness in patients with tumors releasing one or more of these subunits. Odell[5] has emphasized that standard tests for pregnancy are not sufficiently sensitive for the screening of patients suspected of demonstrating ectopic gonadotropin production.

Patients with gonadotropin-releasing tumors have included children and adults. Ectopically-produced gonadotropin more closely resembles HCG or LH than FSH in its biologic activity. Since LH, in the absence of FSH, has no effect in girls, it is not surprising that all instances of tumor-induced precocious puberty have occurred in boys. Adult males most commonly manifest mild gynecomastia. Females with this syndrome present with amenorrhea or menometrorrhagia.

The origin of excess gonadotropin is usually not occult. Most of the tumors releasing this hormone have been obvious. However, if the site is not obvious, a test analogous to the dexamethasone suppression test does exist. The patient is given a short course of estrogen in high doses. Pituitary gonadotropin will be suppressed by the normal feedback mechanism. Ectopically-produced gonadotropin is usually not suppressed.

Ectopic Thyrotoxicosis Syndrome (TSH)

There normally exist two thyroid-stimulating hormones, one from the anterior pituitary and one from the placenta. Another thyroid stimulator is found in patients with Graves' disease, the long-acting thyroid stimulator (LATS). TSH secreted by tumors most closely resembles that produced by trophoblastic tissues.

Few patients have been reported with symptomatic thyrotoxicosis secondary to tumors. In all of such patients, large amounts of gonadotropin have been simultaneously produced. As described before, TSH, FSH, LH and HCG all have a similar structure differing only by the configuration of the beta chain. It is not surprising that concomitant production of two closely related hormones might occur.

Excluding tumors which arise from trophoblastic tissues, most tumors giving rise to ectopic TSH syndromes have been gonadal choriocarcinoma, teratocarcinoma or bronchogenic carcinoma. Most patients have displayed few symptoms; when symptoms are present they usually include tachycardia, nervousness, weight loss and fatigue.

Ectopic Carcinoid Syndrome (Serotonin)

The prototype cell of the APUD family is the Kulchitsky cell. This cell was first discovered in the intestinal tract and has long been known to synthesize and to store serotonin. The neoplastic counterpart of this cell is the carcinoid. Carcinoid tumors arise along the length of the alimentary canal and within structures which have derived from it. Williams and Sandler[12] have noted that the biologic activity of such tumors is generally related to the anatomic position of the tumor. Hindgut carcinoids are slow-growing, nearly always benign and functionless. Midgut carcinoids are more likely to be invasive and may metastasize, giving rise to the typical "carcinoid syndrome." Foregut carcinoids are aggressive. They often metastasize and may exhibit bizarre endocrinologic behavior, releasing not only serotonin but kinins, vasoactive amines and a variety of polypeptide hormones.

Among the foregut-derived tumors of the APUD type may be placed the small cell anaplastic carcinoma (oat cell carcinoma). There is much direct and inferential evidence to suggest that this cancer has its origins from the Kulchitsky cell and, therefore, can be considered a highly undifferentiated carcinoid.

OTHER TUMOR-HORMONE MANIFESTATIONS

Secondary Polycythemia Syndrome (Erythropoietin)

Erythropoietin is normally released by the kidney in states of anemia or hypoxia. It stimulates the bone marrow and as a result the red cell mass is selectively increased. Tumors which elaborate this hormone may cause varying degrees of secondary polycythemia, which is reversible by excision of the tumor. Most of such tumors reported have been renal and as such cannot be regarded as ectopic hormone syndromes. Other tumors associated with polycythemia include cerebellar hemangioblastomas, uterine fibroids and pheochromocytomas.

Precise identification of the hormone has, in the case of cerebellar tumors, shown it to be quite similar to normal, endogenous erythropoietin. Other patients with tumors and polycythemia have had no erythropoietin detectable by bioassay. Obviously, however, something is being released with sufficient bioactivity to stimulate erythrogenesis. Sensitive radioimmunoassays are only now being developed.

Von Hippel-Lindau's disease is angiomatosis of the retina associated with hemangioblastoma of the cerebellum. Pheochromocytomas may also be discovered in such patients. A diffuse neural crest dysplasia, as suggested by Weichert[11] is certainly suspected.

Osteoarthropathy (Growth Hormone)

Growth hormone has been the suspected etiologic agent behind both osteoarthropathy and clubbing of the fingers in patients with various tumors. Consistent evidence for this observation is lacking. Clinical manifestations of excessive growth hormone require long periods of exposure. This probably accounts for the infrequency of symptoms attributable to its ectopic production.

Bronchogenic carcinoma of the lung and adenocarcinoma of the stomach are the usual tumors of origin. The hormone has been identified within and released from cells of lung adenocarcinoma growth in tissue culture.

Calcitonin Elaboration

Some of the neural crest cells migrate to the pharynx of the embryo to enter the ultimobranchial body. Later maturational development places these cells diffusely throughout the thyroid gland. These are the thyroid "C" cells which produce calcitonin and were one of the first characterized by Pearse as members of the APUD family.

Medullary carcinomas of the thyroid produce calcitonin and represent the malignant degeneration of such cells. This occurrence cannot be regarded as an ectopic hormone syndrome, however, since the thyroid normally produces calcitonin. Sensitive immunoassay has demonstrated that calcitonin synthesis is very common in human tumors, particularly among apudomas. In fact, it has been suggested that the detection of calcitonin within a tumor is prima facie evidence of the neural crest origin of that tumor.

Despite the frequency of tumor calcitonin, hypocalcemia from tumor release of calcitonin is extremely rare.

Common tumors in which significant levels of calcitonin have been found include carcinoids, pheochromocytomas, melanomas and oat cell carcinomas.

Prostaglandins

Prostaglandins comprise a family of physiologic substances with a variety of effects. The effects are manifested systemically when they are ectopically produced. In truth, it is difficult to state with certainty whether a particular prostaglandin is ectopic or not, since so many tissues normally produce them.

Prostaglandin E_2 may cause hypercalcemia and inhibits intestinal adenylcyclase. Prostaglandin E_{G2} inhibits gastric hydrochloric acid and pancreatic secretion.

Various prostaglandins have been implicated in the watery diarrhea, hypokalemia, achlorhydria (WDHA) syndrome.

Prostaglandin A is a potent vasodilator. A hypertensive patient is reported to have become normotensive when he developed a prostaglandin A-producing renal cell carcinoma.

MULTIPLE HORMONE PRODUCTION

Several examples of multiple hormone production have already been given (ACTH and MSH, gonadotropin and TSH). This may occur by means of obligatory genetic linkage of protein production sites or by the simultaneous release of several repression mechanisms. It is highly probable that multiple hormone production is frequent. The nearly uniform production of calcitonin among APUD tumors has been mentioned. In a given instance, the more biologically active hormone would define the particular clinical syndrome. Only by arbitrarily selecting the appropriate assay might a second hormone, produced in small quantity, be discovered. Uniform application of tissue analysis could ascertain the true incidence of multiple hormone production.

Foregut neoplasms are particularly notorious for this behavior. Such tumors may release (in various quantities and combinations) insulin, glucagon, gastrin, ACTH and MSH, catecholamines, kallikrein, bradykinins and other kinins.

SUMMARY

Ectopic hormone production is a small part of the more general phenomenon of abnormal protein synthesis in tumors. The APUD-cell concept offers a rational system of tumor relationships based on their common ancestry. The concept gives order to an otherwise obscure or seemingly accidental manifestation of cancer. The investigation of such a system gives insight into the genetic structure of tumors which are endocrinologically active and yet have no known close ties to the neural crest.

REFERENCES

1. Baylin, S. B.: Ectopic production of hormones and other proteins by tumors. Hosp. Prac., *10*:117, 1975.
2. Benson, R. C., Riggs, B. L., Pickard, B. M., and Arnaud, C. D.: Radioimmunoassay of parathyroid hormone in hypercalcemic patients with malignant disease. Am. J. Med., *56*:823, 1974.
3. Friesen, S. R.: A gastric factor in the pathogenesis of the Zollinger-Ellison syndrome. Ann. Surg., *168*:483, 1968.
4. Levine, R. J., and Metz, S. A.: A classification of ectopic hormone producing tumors. Ann. N.Y. Acad. Sci., *230*:633, 1974.
5. Odell, W. D.: Humoral manifestations of non-endocrine neoplasma-ectopic hormone production. *In* Williams, R. H. (ed.): Textbook of Endocrinology. p. 1105. Philadelphia, W. B. Saunders, 1974.
6. Pearse, A. G. E., and Polak, J. M.: Endocrine tumors of neural crest origin: Neurolophomas, Apudomas and the APUD cell concept. Med. Biol., *52*:3, 1974.
7. Pearse, A. G. E., Coulling, I., Weavers, B., and Friesen, S. R.: The endocrine polypeptide cells of the human stomach, duodenum and jejunum. Gut, *11*:649, 1970.
8. Said, S. I., and Faloona, G. R.: Elevated plasma and tissue levels of vasoactive polypeptide in the watery diarrhea syndrome. N. Engl. J. Med., *293*:155, 1975.

9. Smith, L. H.: Ectopic hormone production. Surg. Gynecol. Obstet., *141*:443, 1975.
10. ——: The APUD cell concept. J. Surg. Oncol., *8*:137, 1976.
11. Weichert, R. F.: The neural ectodermal origin of the peptide-secreting endocrine glands. Am. J. Med., *49*:232, 1970.
12. Williams, E. D., and Sandler, M.: Classification of carcinoid tumors. Lancet, *1*:238, 1963.

EDITORIAL COMMENTARY

The rare and interesting phenomena of clinical endocrinopathies produced by circulating humoral agents that are elaborated from unexpected sites has opened a gamut of conceptual considerations and investigations. Normal and abnormal hormones have been found to emanate not only from unusual locations of endocrine and neural elements but also from organs which are not generally considered to be endocrine in function (the paraneoplastic syndromes) and from mesothelial tumors not associated with an organ of any kind.

In one sense there should be no surprise in finding "ectopic" function from "ectopic" locations. If one considers that many of the endocrine cells, within the APUD concept, have similar cytochemical properties and embryologic origins from the neural crest and neuroectoderm, and have been dispersed diffusely, the principles of ectopia may be more understandable. The capacity of these APUD cells, primitive but totipotential, to be reactivated by derepression to again synthesize proteins, is a possibility wherever these cells reside at the time of the onset of neoplasia. Moreover, functioning tumors that are present in mesothelial areas may be explained by a developmental arrest during the migration of these cells; such a circumstance, for instance, could account for the relatively frequent observation of gastrinomas found near or on the surface of the pancreas, and insulinlike "somatomedin"-secreting mesotheliomas in retropleural and retroperitoneal areas. Within this concept it is doubtful that any unusual endocrine type of secretory tumor should be termed "ectopic" at all. This is especially true if secretory granules are observed on electron microscopy of the tumor cells indicating an endocrine cell origin of the ectopic tumor. It has been suggested that the pancreatic gastrinoma represents an ectopic phenomenon because adult islets do not normally secrete gastrin; the finding, however, that the islets of the fetal pancreas do contain gastrin-secreting cells is evidence for an entopic, rather than an ectopic, origin. The lung is a frequent site for tumors which elaborate polypeptides and amines "ectopically," yet cells having APUD cytologic characteristics are normally present there. The sympathetic nervous system can be the site of neural (ganglionic) tumors which elaborate a diarrheogenic polypeptide (VIP). Breast carcinoma is a relatively frequent cause of hypercalcemia; in such instances care must be taken to rule out skeletal metastases before assuming that the breast tumor is an "ectopic" cause of the hypercalcemic syndrome with elaboration of a heterogeneous parathyrinlike hormone. Almost every conceivable possibility in the spectrum of ectopic phenomena has been reported in the literature; some of the more common of these rare clinical conditions are illustrated in Figure 1-3.

Several important generalizations can be made which are common to "ectopia." First, the "ectopic" tumors are almost always malignant, either histologically or by virtue of metastases. Second, the cells of at least the ectopic endocrine malignancies contain secretory granules on EM, some of which have also been observed by immunofluorescent studies. Third, associated hyperplasia of other endocrine cells is rather common. Fourth, the substances which are elaborated by these neoplasms are biologically active, but frequently not immunologically active, at least by current assay technology. Fifth, the humoral substances themselves are frequently heterogeneous, composed of larger forms of the normal polypeptide molecule such as "big gastrin," and sometimes consist of prohormones, such as proinsulin. The heterogeneous larger polypeptide molecules usually require very specialized techniques for their selective detection in the plasma by RIA or in tissues by immunofluorescence, although some, like proinsulin, are measured together with insulin in the measurement of immunoreactive insulin. The determination of the concentration of circulating heterogeneous parathyrinlike activity from ectopic tumors is sometimes possible, and great care must be taken to differentiate such humoral activity from the measurable immunoreactive parathyrin from the normal parathyroid glands. In point, in a patient with a pancreatic islet cell carcinoma and hypercalcemia, the normal parathyroid parathyrin may be suppressed and undetectable until the hypercalcemia is corrected, at which time the assayable endogenous parathyrin will return to normal values. Such a patient may actually have elevated levels of the heterogeneous parathyrin from the ectopic tumor, capable of being measured only by very special techniques.

In patients with clinical evidence of ectopia, it is obviously important not only to measure the abnormal exocrine abberations, but also to determine, within the limits of availability of assays, the levels of radioimmunoassayable polypeptides, amines and the prostaglandins, systemically and selectively. Furthermore, routine and special radiologic techniques for the demonstration of the unsuspected tumor itself are necessary to locate the "abnormal locus."

S.R.F.

24

Rare Endocrine Tumors and Syndromes

William H. ReMine, M.D., M.S.(Surg.), D.Sc., and Jonathan A. van Heerden, M.B., Ch.B. (Cape Town), M.S., F.R.C.S.(C)

MASTOCYTOSIS SYNDROME—DIFFUSE APUDOMA

Clinical Features[4,15,24]

The symptoms of the mastocytosis syndrome listed below are in essence due to the systemic release of histamine by the mast cells. Although heparin is released as well, it is seldom of sufficient quantity to produce symptoms.

Common Symptoms
1. Flushing and tachycardia
2. Episodic severe diarrhea
3. Headaches

Rare Symptoms
1. Intestinal malabsorption
2. Hepatosplenomegaly
3. Telangiectatic skin lesions
4. Bone lesions (localized or diffuse sclerosis or porosis)
5. Bronchial spasm
6. Peptic ulceration
7. Pruritus and dermatographia

In children mastocytosis usually occurs as a localized skin lesion with mast cell infiltration. This is benign and self-limiting. In adults it most often takes on a systemic pattern with mast cell invasion of the reticuloendothelial system (liver, spleen, bone marrow, lymph nodes and skin). In rare instances, this usually benign disease behaves in a malignant fashion (pseudoleukemic phase).

It is worth noting that the symptomatology of mastocytosis is closely akin to that of carcinoid syndromes. They are, however distinct entities both in their etiology and pathogenesis.

Diagnosis

The diagnosis of this syndrome is based on clinical suspicions, determination of excessive histamine or its metabolites in the urine and histologic verification by representative biopsies.

Treatment

Treatment has by and large been highly experimental with no controlled studies. The following modalities have been entertained:

1. Antihistamine drugs
2. Chemotherapy, in particular cyclophosphamide
3. Dietary restriction of glutin and magnesium intake

4. Avoidance of histamine-releasing drugs (e.g., steroids and morphine alkaloids)
5. Local bone irradiation
6. Appropriate treatment of secondary hypersplenism, peptic ulceration and thrombocytopenia

Prognosis

Usually the prognosis for mastocytosis is excellent.

CATECHOLAMINE-SECRETING PARAGANGLIOMA OF THE GLOMUS-JUGULARE REGION RESEMBLING PHEOCHROMOCYTOMA

Catecholamine-producing tumors arising from tissue outside the adrenal medulla have long been recognized as causes of sustained or paroxysmal hypertension. Their origin has been attributed to neural crest derivatives occurring as nests of chromaffin tissue in the autonomic ganglions and "organs of Zuckerkandl" or as independent bodies adjacent to these ganglions or their nerves (paraganglions).

Until recently, most reported cases of nonchromaffin-reacting paraganglioma, including distinctive tumors of the carotid body, vagal body, glomus-jugulare complex, aortic and ciliary bodies and even tumors occurring as minute subpleural pulmonary nodules, have been considered to be a completely separate group of neoplasms arising from the chemoreceptor system. Beside differing in location from pheochromocytoma, paragangliomas are usually considered readily separable on the basis of lack of significant catecholamine production and nonchromaffin status, although histopathologically there may at times be considerable similarity. Some doubt has been cast on the complete separation of these two types of neoplasms in all cases because it has been shown that normal carotid bodies contain catecholamines and display neurosecretory granules on EM and are, therefore, another potential source of functioning paragangliomas. Furthermore, a few carotid body tumors and glomus-jugulare tumors have been reported to produce hypertension through increased secretion of catecholamines, predominantly norepinephrine. Three paragangliomas of the carotid body region, studied by Grimley and Glenner[12] by EM, displayed dense-cored neurosecretory granules of the catecholamine type in chief cells, similar to the granules seen in the normal carotid body.

The search for the cause of a patient's pheochromocytomalike symptoms must include the various sites of chemoreceptor glomera as rare potential locations for catecholamine-producing tumors. We reported such a case of a catecholamine-secreting paraganglioma of the glomus-jugulare region in 1969.[14]

The glomus-jugulare complex is composed of at least four minute glomera of chemoreceptor tissue located in and about the temporal bone: along the tympanic branch of the glossopharyngeal nerve, along the auricular branch of the vagus, in the adventitia of the jugular bulb, and in the jugular ganglion of the vagus nerve. Chemodectomas arising from these sites are similar histopathologically to those arising at any location in the chemoreceptor system and therefore are usually designated anatomically (e.g., carotid body tumor). In the case presented the tumor was first detected in its intracranial portion and by its involvement of the jugular foramen; only later was there a demonstrable cervical component that extended along the vagus nerve. Such a distribution of tumor would be in keeping with origin from the jugular glomus of the vagus.

Chemoreceptor structures have been classified as non-chromaffin-reacting paraganglionic tissue to differentiate them from the catecholamine-containing, chromaffin-reacting, paraganglionic tissue such as the adrenal medulla and autonomic nervous system. The chromaffin reaction is evidence that a phenolic substance has formed a colored polymer (adrenochrome or noradrenochrome) as the result of a chromate-mediated oxidative dehydrogenation. The chromaffin reaction itself, however, does not specifically identify catecholamines because serotonin and other phenolic amine compounds will give a positive result. Moreover, within the last few years the role of the chromaffin reaction has been further challenged because chromaffin-negative paraganglionic structures and tumors of them (paragangliomas) have been shown to contain catecholamines by various assay techniques. It is not always possible[11] to differentiate histologically a chemodectoma from a tumor of the cervical sympathetic chain or even a pheochromocytoma by light microscopy.

The presence of both norepinephrine and epinephrine in human carotid bodies was demonstrated by Hamberger, et al. in 1966.[14]

It now seems clear that the normal paraganglionic structures of the neck and the tumors of these structures contain and may secrete physiologically active catecholamines. The inclusive term "catecholamine-secreting paraganglioma" is now used to describe these tumors, whether reported to be chemoreceptor or other neurosecretory origin.

TUMOR HYPOGLYCEMIA

Hypoglycemia is an abnormality of glucose homeostasis which arises from an imbalance between glucose production and utilization.

Pathology[23]

The most common non-islet cell tumors causing hypoglycemia are hepatomas, retroperitoneal fibrosarcomas and mediastinal mesotheliomas.

The shared characteristic of all of these tumors is their large size—usually more than 1 kg.

Mechanisms[6]

The following mechanisms have been postulated to explain this secondary hypoglycemia: (1) Excessive uptake of glucose by the tumor, (2) tumor secretion of insulin, (3) development of an acquired glycogen-storage disease as occurs in hepatomas, (4) tumor production of substance that may inhibit gluconeogenesis, (5) release of an insulin potentiator and (6) elaboration of somatomedin.

Diagnosis

The hypoglycemia occurring in the fasting state may be severe, with blood sugar levels below 25 mg./100 ml. The clinical picture may in every way resemble that in patients with insulinoma, including a prompt ameliorative response to oral or intravenous administration of glucose. The finding of elevated or inappropriate levels of plasma immunoreactive insulin, however, is usually not present with these nonpancreatic tumors, even though bioassays of insulinlike activity in the tumor may be found.

Treatment

Excision of these large tumors has been reported to eliminate the hypoglycemia and its symptomatology.[17]

THYMOMAS

In 1939, Blalock, et al. first reported remission of myasthenia gravis following the removal of a thymic tumor.[3] The syndromes occurring in association with thymic tumors are well documented. Their cause remains an enigma.

Syndromes Associated With Thymic Tumors

Myasthenia Gravis. Whereas 15 percent of patients with myasthenia gravis have thymic tumors, Bernatz, et al. found that 46 percent of a series of patients with thymic tumors had myasthenia gravis.[2] Approximately 30 percent of patients who undergo thymectomy can anticipate a regression of their myasthenia.

Acquired Agammaglobulinemia. Although it has been postulated that the thymus is an important source of a protein such as gamma globulin, the association is extremely rare and poorly understood.

Agenesis of Erythrocytes. The association of this syndrome with the spindle cell variety of thymoma is well documented but not understood. The remaining hematopoietic elements are undisturbed whereas reticuloytes are markedly reduced.

Cushing's Syndrome. Castleman first emphasized the epithelial predominance of thymic tumors when associated with Cushing's syndrome.[5]

Surgical Approach

The anterior approach by way of a median sternotomy is preferred. If pulmonary resection is anticipated, a posterolateral thoracotomy is utilized. Especially in the myasthenic patients, tracheostomy with ventilatory mechanical support may decrease postoperative morbidity.

Pathology

Approximately 30 percent of thymomas are invasive. Histological identification of malignancy, as with many endocrine tumors, is difficult. One in four patients with myasthenia gravis will have malignant thymomas.

Treatment

The treatment for thymomas may be aggressive surgical resection and ancillary roentgenotherapy in nonresectable or partially resectable instances.

Prognosis

Sixty-three percent of patients with thymomas may expect a 5-year survival and 50 percent may be expected to survive for 10 years.

NELSON'S SYNDROME

Definition

This clinical syndrome consists of an ACTH-producing tumor of the pituitary gland that occurs in some patients who have undergone bilateral adrenalectomy for Cushing's syndrome associated with pituitary ACTH-dependent adrenocortical hyperplasia (Cushing's disease).[19]

Clinical Features[21]

The syndrome usually manifests itself about 3 years following adrenalectomy. Current data suggest that the incidence is roughly 15 percent. The outstanding clinical features are cutaneous hyperpigmentation; sellar expansion with ocular defects, usually an incongruous homonymous hemianopsia; and elevated ACTH levels.

Pathology

Most of the pituitary tumors are chromophobe adenomas. Rarely are they malignant (± 10%).

Diagnosis

More pituitary tumors are currently being discovered in patients with Cushing's disease prior to adrenalectomy as well as postadrenalectomy with the use of spinal sellar tomography and/or selective angiography.

Any patient who becomes very darkly pigmented following bilateral total adrenalectomy for Cushing's disease in spite of full replacement dosage of cortisol (or any potent synthetic glucocorticoid) should be suspected of having Nelson's syndrome. The finding of greatly elevated levels of plasma ACTH with the patient on full glucocorticoid replacement therapy supports the diagnosis and is an indication for not only standard roentgenographic examination of the head but also spinal tomograms of the sella and carotid arteriography with roentgenographic views of the sellar area using magnifications and subtraction techniques and looking for a vascular blush or other vascular abnormalities. Careful examination of the vesical fields is also indicated in these patients.

Importance

This syndrome does not appear to occur following adrenalectomy for an adrenocortical tumor. This supports the concept that the primary abnormality in Cushing's disease resides in the anterior pituitary or the hypothalamus. It is hoped that with more effective procedures for evaluating the anterior pituitary and hypothalamic status in patients with Cushing's disease, a better form of therapy can be developed—one that corrects the hypercortisolism and leaves the patient with normal anterior pituitary adrenocortical function.

VON HIPPEL-LINDAU SYNDROME

This syndrome consists of central nervous system hemangioendothelioma and ocular (usually cerebellar hemangiomas with a significant incidence of associated benign cysts of the intra-abdominal solid organs) hypernephromas (in 10-35% of cases), paragangliomas and rarely pheochromocytomas.[7]

Polycythemia occurs in 10 to 20 percent of patients with this syndrome and is thought to be caused by an increase in erythropoietin activity.[25] It is more frequent with solid hemangioendotheliomas rather than cystic. The reasons given for erythrocytosis in association with cerebellar hemangioblastomas are:

1. These highly vascular tumors might be an active site for erythropoiesis. (This has not been accurately proven.)
2. Medullary compression might lead to arterial hypoxia causing a secondary erythrocytosis. (This is unlikely since cerebellar hemangioendotheliomas comprise only 6 percent of cystic cerebellar tumors yet they are the only posterior fossa neoplasms associated with erythrocytosis.)
3. Production by the tumor of a humoral substance which stimulates erythropoiesis by the bone marrow. (Erythropoietin has been isolated from these tumors and appears to be the most plausible etiologic factor. The association of polycythemia with hypernephroma and other tumors has similarly been shown to be on the basis of the tumor's production of erythropoietin.)[9]

Clinical Features

This syndrome is transmitted as an autosomal-dominant trait with variable penetrance and delayed expression. It occurs predominantly between the third and fifth decades of life.

The outstanding clinical presentations are those of cerebellar dysfunction and increased intracranial pressure due to posterior fossa tumors.

Diagnosis

The diagnosis must be determined by neurologic signs, computerized tomography of the brain with contrast and cerebral angiography with subtraction technique.

A combination of the above modalities has led to a high degree of diagnostic accuracy.

Treatment

The only treatment for von Hippel-Lindau syndrome is surgical removal of tumors.

HYPOTHALAMIC TUMOR AND PRECOCIOUS PUBERTY

Clinical Features[18]

Presenting features of hypothalamic tumor include sexual precocity; mental and physical lethargy; and water, carbohydrate or fat abnormalities.

Physiology

The neurohypophysis (posterior pituitary lobe) is under the direct control of the hypothalamus with humoral factors being transmitted down the supraoptico hypophyseal tract.

The adenohypophysis (anterior lobe of the pituitary), in contrast, receives its hypothalamic influence by way of the portal system between the hypothalamus (pars tuberalis and the tubercinereum) and the anterior pituitary lobe. It has been demonstrated that stimulation of the region of the pars tuberalis and the tubercinereum results in gonadotropic secretion.

Site of Lesion

Less than 10 percent of pineal tumors cause pubertas praecox. This might be due to the fact that the majority of pineal tumors do not directly impinge on the hypothalamus. Those that enlarge anteriorly, however, do impinge—all intracranial lesions causing pubertas praecox involve the hypothalamus.

Type of Lesion

A diversity of pineal tumors has been associated with this entity. Although the pineal dysgerminoma has been implicated most often, tumors such as true pinealomas and astrocytomas have been encountered. The site of the tumor would then appear to be more important than the pathologic nature thereof.

Mechanism[22]

That the lesion of the posterior part of the hypothalamus releases the adenohypophysis from the inhibiting control of the hypothalamus has been postulated but is doubtable. It seems more plausible that when the hypothalamus is destroyed, its function is taken over by other parts of the brain and then carried by way of the portal system to the adenohypophysis.

Laboratory

Findings from laboratory procedures are increased 17-ketosteroids, testosterone and gonadotropin.

Treatment

Since most tumors in this region cause early obstruction of the aqueduct and since the most commonly encountered tumor (dysgerminoma) is radiosensitive, the mainstays of treatment are shunting procedures and roentgenotherapy.

Surgical excision, with its morbidity and great technical difficulty, is reserved for progressive lesions and is becoming more feasible with the use of microsurgical techniques.

POLYPOID HAMARTOMAS OF BRUNNER'S GLANDS

Wepfer[13] in 1679 first mentioned the presence of duodenal glands, but Brunn[13] (Brunner) in 1688 first described them in detail. The glands develop during the sixth month when the cells at the base of the crypts of Lieberkühn extend into the submucosa. In maturity the glands achieve a compound tubular form, arranged in lobules, 0.5 to 1 mm. in diameter. They generally are most numerous in the first portion of the duodenum, gradually decreasing in number distally, the number and distribution varying among individuals. In some, the glands extend distally into the jejunum; they may even occur ectopically near the tail of the pancreas. The cells are columnar or cuboidal, containing a pale mucoid or finely granular cytoplasm and at the base a somewhat flattened nucleus. The branched and coiled ducts penetrate the muscularis mucosae and empty into the bases of the crypts of Lieberkühn; at the point of juncture the cell type abruptly changes to the normal columnar epithelium of the gut. The glands more or less continuously secrete a small amount of viscid, alkaline mucus; secretion can be increased by injections of cholecystokinin, natural secretin, synthetic secretin and the decapeptide cerulein.

In 1876, the first "adenoma" of Brunner's glands was reported by Salvioli.[13] This discrete type of tumor, as opposed to Brunner's gland hyperplasia, remains sufficiently rare to make a single case worth reporting.

The label of "adenoma" or Brunner's gland tumor has been in dispute, and other terms such as adenomatous or hamartomatous polyp have been suggested. Some consider the lesion to be a hamartoma, for the tumor is neither encapsulated nor clearly demarcated from anatomic Brunner's glands. Furthermore, it has all the normal anatomic constituents, being predominantly made up of lobulation of ductular and acinar elements, and to a lesser extent smooth muscle, blood vessels and fat are seen. Ducts from the lobulations extend to the surface mucosal crypts similar to those seen in the anatomic glands. Some Peutz-Jeghers polyps contain Brunner's glands.

The most common location is the posterior wall of the duodenum near the junction of its first and second portions. Most frequently these tumors are discovered in patients in the fourth to sixth decades of life, though the age in reported cases ranges from 11 days to 80 years.

The symptoms presented by the patient are usually attributable to some coexisting condition or to some functional disturbance. An exception is the occurrence of melena or other symptoms of gastrointestinal bleeding, even to the point of exsanguinating hemorrhages. Another but very infrequent exception is the occurrence of obstructive symptoms. Malignant change in such a tumor has never been proven, though adjacent adenocarcinoma has been reported.

Hamartoma of Brunner's glands is so rare that it deservedly is near the bottom of the list in any differential diagnosis of upper gastrointestinal symptoms. Roentgenographic signs, however, permit one to suspect such a lesion promptly. These signs include the presence of a rather smooth, round or oval, polypoid or nodular tumor attached by a stalk or broad base to an otherwise normal duodenal wall. Differential diagnosis includes lipoma, leiomyoma, adenomatous polyp, the other rare benign tumors and carcinoma. We reported six such patients in 1970.[20]

We strongly urge operative treatment of any polypoid lesion of the duodenum. Though the risk of malignancy is low and the risk of obstruction seems little greater, the rather high risk of bleeding and the unknown cell type of the lesion indicate the need for such therapy.

HETEROTOPIC PANCREATIC TISSUE

Variously called heterotopic pancreatic tissue, accessory pancreas or aberrant pancreas, this entity may be defined as the presence of pancreatic tissue that lacks anatomic and vascular continuity with the main body of the pancreas.

The frequency of heterotopic pancreatic tissue in autopsy material ranges from 0.55 percent to 13.7 percent. Most series have reported the lower range. Clinically, it has been determined to occur about once in every 500 operations in the upper abdomen.

Several theories have been advanced to explain the origin of heterotopic pancreatic tissue. Perhaps the most accepted is that suggested by Horgan[1]: Before coalescing, small buds of the branching ends of the anterior and posterior pancreatic anlagen become attached to the gut wall at various locations and are carried with it as the gland pulls away from the gut in its normal pattern of growth and development. Warthin[1] suggested that accessory pancreatic tissue develops from the lateral budding of rudimentary pancreatic ducts as they penetrate the bowel wall.

Possibly the first reported example of pancreatic heterotopia was presented by Jean Schultz in 1727.[8] It remained for Klob in 1859[16] to present histologic confirmation of this condition in two cases.

The gross appearance of islands of aberrant pancreas is usually that of firm, yellow irregular nodules, varying in size from 2 mm. to 4 cm., that are intramural and often described as being submucosal or subserosal. Their mucosal surface frequently possesses a central umbilication. Their histologic appearance varies from that of perfectly formed pancreatic lobules with ducts, acini and islands with a normal appearance to that of a few widely separated ducts.

The roentgenographic and gastroscopic features are sometimes characteristic. The lesions appear as well-delineated submucosal filling defects with, classically, a central umbilication. This appearance is sometimes difficult to differentiate from that of a leiomyoma. When the central umbilication is larger than usual, it can be confused with the base of a gastric or duodenal ulcer. In our series, 80 percent of lesions in the stomach were located in the prepyloric region on the greater curvature.

The relationship of aberrant pancreas to diverticulum formation has been noted both clinically and experimentally. Diverticula have been produced in the small bowel of the dog by the implantation of pancreatic tissue, the probable result of weakening of the wall musculature by pancreatic enzyme. In our series, aside from those in Meckel diverticulum, only one example was found in a duodenal diverticulum, and a second was found in a duodenum that elsewhere possessed a diverticulum.

No particular symptom complex can be attributed to this condition. Symptoms noted are abdominal distress, distention, gaseous eructation, nausea, vomiting, diarrhea, constipation and epigastric pain. Others concluded that pancreatic heterotopia may mimic symptoms of duodenal ulcer, diaphragmatic hernia or gallbladder dysfunction. Malignant degeneration, cyst formation, pancreatitis, insulinoma, hemorrhage, intussusception and obstruction have been reported. This condition apparently has been held responsible for almost any symptom complex that might warrant investigation of the upper part of the gastrointestinal tract. It may be that it is a diagnosis made by serendipity.

The mechanism whereby this tissue could produce these various symptoms is not clear. It has been suggested that the heterotopic pancreatic tissue is stimulated to secrete and, in so doing, produces inflammation, spasm or hyperirritability. This seems rather unlikely. Why, if these lesions are antenatal in development, do they not produce symptoms from the very beginning? Moreover, pancreatic tissue has occurred in similar locations without producing any symptoms.

The cause of gastrointestinal tract hemorrhage is another interesting problem. When there is ulceration in the overlying mucosa, the association is obvious. The relationship is much less clear when the mucosa is intact.

We can then infer that heterotopic pancreatic tissue was not responsible for the initial features in the majority of cases. It appears also that remission of symptoms can be expected as frequently with expectant observation as with surgical intervention, though an obvious exception might be valid in the case of patients such as the three in our series of 212 patients[10] who had suspected gastrointestinal tract blood loss and who had no such difficulties after operation.

REFERENCES

1. Barbosa, J. deC., Dockerty, M. B., and Waugh, J. M.: Pancreatic heterotopia: review of the literature and report of 41 authenticated surgical cases, of which 25 were clinically significant. Surg. Gynecol. Obstet., *82*:527, 1946.
2. Bernatz, P. E., Harrison, E. G., and Clagett, O. T.: Thymoma: A clinicopathologic study. J. Thorac. Cardiovasc. Surg., *43*:4, 1961.
3. Blalock, A., et al.: Myasthenia gravis and tumors of the thymic region. Ann. Surg., *110*:554, 1939.
4. Broitman, S. A., et al.: Mastocytosis and intestinal malabsorption. Am. J. Med., *48*:382, 1970.
5. Castleman, B.: Tumors of the thymus gland. Armed Forces Institute of Pathology, Sect. 5, Fasc. 19, 1955.
6. Chowdbury, F., et al.: Studies of tumor hypoglycemia. Metabolism, *22*:5, 1973.
7. Coulam, C. M., et al.: Hippel-Lindau syndrome. Semin. Roentgenol., *11*:1, 1976.
8. Derbyshire, R. C.: Studies of accessory pancreas. [Thesis] Mayo Graduate School of Medicine, University of Minnesota, Rochester, 1940.
9. DeWeerd, J. H., and Hagedorn, A. B.: Hypernephroma associated with polycythemia. J. Urol., *82*:1, 1959.
10. Dolan, R. V., ReMine, W. H., and Dockerty, M. B.: The fate of heterotopic pancreatic tissue. Arch. Surg., *109*:762, 1974.
11. Glenner, G. G., Crout, J. R., and Roberts, W. C.: A functional carotid body-like tumor secreting levarterenol. Arch. Pathol., *73*:230, 1962.
12. Grimley, P. M., and Glenner, G. G.: Histology and ultrastructure of carotid body paragangliomas: Comparison with the normal gland. Cancer, *20*:1473, 1967.
13. Kaplan, E. L., Dyson, W. L., and Fitts, W. T., Jr.: Hyperplasia of Brunner's glands of the duodenum. Surg. Gynecol., Obstet., *126*:371, 1968.
14. Levit, S. A., Sheps, S. G., Espinosa, R. E., ReMine, W. H., and Harrison, E. G.: Catecholamine-secreting paraganglioma of glomus-jugulare region resembling pheochromocytoma. N. Engl. J. Med., *281*:805, 1969.
15. McBride, T. I., et al.: Mast cell disease. Postgrad. Med. J., *43*:176, 1967.
16. Martinez, N. S., et al.: Heterotopic pancreatic tissue involving the stomach. Ann. Surg., *147*:1, 1958.

17. Miller, D. R., Bolinger, R. E., Janigan, D., Crockett, J. E., and Friesen, S. R.: Hypoglycemia due to non-pancreatic mesodermal tumors; report of two cases. Ann. Surg., *150*:684, 1959.
18. Morley, T. P.: Hypothalamic tumor and precocious puberty. J. Clin. Endocrinol. Metab., *14*:1, 1954.
19. Nelson, D. H., et al.: ACTH producing tumors following adrenalectomy for Cushing's syndrome. Ann. Intern. Med., *52*:560, 1960.
20. ReMine, W. H., Brown, P. W., Jr., Gomes, M. R., and Harrison, E. G., Jr.: Polypoid hamartomas of Brunner's glands. Arch. Surg., *100*:313, 1970.
21. Salassa, R. M., et al.: Pituitary tumors in patients with Cushing's syndrome. J. Clin. Endocrinol. Metab., *19*:12, 1959.
22. Schonberg, D. K.: Dynamics of hypothalamus-pituitary function during puberty. Clin. Endocrinol. Metab., *4*:1, 1975.
23. Service, J. F.: Comp. Ther., *2*:7, 1976.
24. Vaidya, A. B., et al.: Failure of epinephrine to provoke flushing in patients with systemic mastocytosis. Ann. Intern. Med., *74*:711, 1971.
25. Waldmann, T. A., et al.: The association of polycythemia with a cerebellar hemangioblastoma. Am. J. Med., *31*:318, 1961.

EDITORIAL COMMENTARY

It is reasonable to assume that the more familiar endocrine tumors and syndromes already presented are themselves rare and uncommonly seen in an active hospital and surgical experience. The even more rare clinical situations that are presented in this chapter, however, need to be mentioned if for no other reason than for completeness in differential diagnoses. Some of these are also discussed by association in previous chapters.

One of the more interesting syndromes (mastocytosis syndrome with apudosis) is that due to histamine release from proliferating mast cells in mastocytosis. The tissue mast cells are APUD cells which synthesize (from histadine), store (in secretory granules) and secrete histamine as a local amine "hormone." When these cells proliferate to form diffuse or nodular infiltration of the skin and other organs, characterized by hyperplasia rather than tumor formation, the lesion is called diffuse apudoma or apudosis; the symptoms are due to increased elaboration of histamine similar to that observed in the atypical carcinoid syndrome of foregut origin. Although it is possible that heparin should also be released, such has not been observed clinically. Metiamide, an H-2 receptor antagonist, has been reported to abolish the gastric acid hypersecretion due to increased histamine secretion in a patient with systemic mastocytosis.

The paragangliomas which secrete catecholamines are apudomas, cytochemically, and are neuroendocrine in origin and in function. These benign tumors may be classified, based on location or histologic criteria, as chemoreceptor or neurosecretory types, but functionally they act as pheochromocytomas in unusual locations. Paragangliomas of the duodenum without discernable endocrine function have been described. Vagal body tumors in families with associated multicentric paragangliomas have been reported. The tumors contained neurosecretory-type granules on ultrastructural study and were malignant and metastasizing. A single extremely unusual case has been reported in which "nerve growth factor" has been isolated by bioassay from the blood and tumor (liposarcoma) of a patient with abnormal nerve growth (neuroma at the site of cholecystectomy) apparently secondary to humoral stimulation from a tumor.

"Nerve growth stimulating activity" has been implicated in the development of von Recklinghausen's neurofibromatosis, tumors of totipotential Schwann cells (special glial elements) of probable neural crest (neuroectodermal) origin. These familial tumors have been reported in association with pheochromocytomas and acoustic neuromas. The cells of the tumors and of the café au lait areas contain pigmented granules in the melanocytes, and the tumors also contain mast cells with secretory granules and cholinesterase which are characteristics of APUD cells.

Rarely, hypoglycemia of organic origin is not caused by a pancreatic insulinoma, but is associated with tumors of mesothelial origin or of the liver. The characteristic massive size of these tumors produces the typical symptomatology described as Whipple's triad. The elaboration of insulinlike activity, measurable by bioassay but not usually by radioimmunoassay of insulin, produces the hypoglycemia; the mediator is probably a somatomedin.

An endocrine role for the thymus is not yet fully established, even though a thymic humoral factor, thymosin, is probably involved in immunologic competence. The DiGeorge syndrome of immunoincompetence is due to congenital absence or dysfunction of the thymus in infants. The humoral function of the thymus is probably under the control of growth hormone which is thymotropic from the anterior pituitary, thus relating the thymus indirectly to the APUD system. Evidence for APUD cells in the thymus includes the fact that the gland is the occasional ectopic site for APUD endocrinopathies such as those due to tumor elaboration of ACTH and 5-HT. In myasthenia gravis an unknown humoral substance, tentatively called thymin, may be secreted by a thymic tumor and cause the inhibition of neuromuscular transmission, but the association of the tumor with the clinical condition is not constant. A humoral factor in the pathogenesis is supported by the reported observation that plasma exchange improved the muscle weakness and fatigability in three patients with acquired myasthenia gravis. The myasthenic neuromuscular blockade may, however, be due to abnormal antibody at the neuromuscular acetylcholine receptor whose immune response is correctable in some instances by thymectomy or by high-dose glucocorticoid therapy or anticholinesterases.

A rare, but nonhumoral, tumor of the thymus and substernal parathyroid gland is the "parathyroid cyst," having the appearance of a substernal "bag of fluid." Remnants of thymic and clear cell parathyroid tissue, of the same embryologic origin, may coexist in the thin walls of the "cyst"; in such instances the cyst may be of thymic origin in which the parathyroid tissue may be hamartomatous, probably representing dilatation of remnants of the ducts of Kursteiner.

Nelson's syndrome of hyperpigmentation after bilateral adrenalectomy may become even more uncommon with time because of the more frequent use of the transsphenoidal approach for microscopically controlled excision of tumors of the anterior pituitary gland in Cushing's disease, rather than bilateral adrenalectomy for the secondary adrenocortical hyperplasia. Increased pigmentation of the skin in this syndrome is due to the stimulation of melanocytes by pituitary MSH. Hyperpigmented melanomas of the skin and the eye are not rare tumors. Although the cells of these tumors are members of the APUD family, no endocrine manifestations are known. Absence of pigmentation, vitiligo, occurs in patients with disorders of autoimmunity and endocrinopathies such as hyperthyroidism, thyroiditis, adrenal insufficiency, and pernicious anemia, and in patients with melanomas who have strong immunity against malignant melanocytes. Whether the vitiligo is due to an inhibition of MSH elaboration or to immunologic or cytotoxic destruction of melanocytes is unknown. There is evidence for a genetic etiology.

The hereditary von Hippel-Lindau syndrome is a type of the paraendocrine (ectopic) syndromes in which angioblastoma of the retina is associated with cerebellar hemangioblastoma, hypernephroma and rarely, pheochromocytoma. Erythrocythemia may be due to the excessive elaboration of erythropoietin, a polypeptide hormone from one or more of these tumors. The cerebellar and pressure symptoms due to the intracranial tumor predominate over the systemic effects. Erythrocythemia and increased erythropoietin secretion may occur also secondarily to chronic hypoxia. Such findings may occur in chronic renal disease, renal tumors and pulmonary tumors; in the latter situation, clubbing of the fingers (hypertrophic pulmonary osteoarthropathy, perhaps due to growth hormone elaboration) may be an associated finding in which the symptoms promptly disappear after excision of the pulmonary tumor.

Hypothalamic and cerebral tumors produce rare syndromes due to their effect on hypothalamic and pituitary function. The pineal gland, which originates from the roof of the third ventricle, receives its nerve supply from the brain and from sympathetic nerve fibers which allows the autonomic nervous system to control the secretory tissue of the pineal gland. Parenchymatous tumors of the pineal gland (pinealomas) have an endocrine effect by hyperfunction which produces delayed puberty due to secondary gonadal failure; nonsecretory hypofunctioning tumors are related to precocious puberty. The pineal secretory amine, melatonin, which affects skin color of amphibia but not of mammals, affects pituitary and gonadal function. Specifically it appears to inhibit gonadal function; therefore, hypersecreting pinealomas delay puberty whereas hypofunctioning tumors are no longer able to synthesize the inhibitory hormone, and precocious puberty ensues. On the other hand, nonfunctioning pineal tumors may produce precocious puberty by impinging pressure on the hypothalamus.

The justification for including Brunner's gland tumors of the duodenum among endocrine abnormalities rests with the observations that hyperplasia of Brunner's glands is sometimes associated with the hypergastrinemia of ulcerogenic tumors. This hyperplasia is believed to be a cause of the duodenal nodularity seen radiographically in the Zollinger-Ellison syndrome; such nodularity has also been ascribed to "isletization" of the duodenal mucosa. Whatever the cause, the differential diagnosis of duodenal nodules in endocrinopathies includes Brunner's gland tumors, carcinoid tumors, duodenal gastrinomas, polyps, carcinomas and Crohn's disease.

Heterotopic pancreatic tissue contains islet tissue as well as acinar and ductile pancreatic tissue, and insulinomas have been reported in such ectopic tissue. Heterotopic pancreatic rests of the prepyloric area should be differentiated from leiomyoma and rare gastrinomas of the stomach. *S.R.F.*

Appendix

ABBREVIATIONS USED IN THIS TEXT

A	Adrenalin
ACTH	Adrenocorticotrop(h)in, corticotrop(h)in
ADH	Antidiuretic hormone, vasopressin
AIP	Aldosterone-induced protein
APUD	Amine, precursor uptake, decarboxylation
ATP	Adenosine triphosphate
AVP	Arginine vasopressin
BAC	Basal acid concentration
BAO	Basal acid output
BBS	Bombesin
BPG	Big plasma glucagon
CAH	Congenital adrenal hyperplasia
cAMP	Cyclic 3′,5′—adenosine monophosphate
CAT	Computerized axial tomography
CCK-(PZ)	Cholecystokinin—pancreozymin
CG	Chorionic gonadotrop(h)in
CHD	Congenital heart disease
CRH (CRF)	Corticotrop(h)in-releasing hormone (factor)
CTSH	Chorionic thyrotrop(h)in
DA	Dopamine
DHEA	Dehydroepiandrosterone
DNA	Deoxyribonucleic acid
DOC	Desoxycorticosterone
DOCA	Desoxycorticosterone acetate
DOPA	Dihydroxyphenylalanine
DPH	Diphenylhydantoin
E	Epinephrine
EC	Enterochromaffin
EDTA	Ethylenediaminotetra acetic acid
ELISA	Enzyme-linked immunosorbent assay
EM	Electron microscopy
EPS	Exophthalmos-producing substance
ERCP	Endoscopic retrograde cholangiopancreatography
ESR	Erythrocyte sedimentation rate
FBC	Free binding capacity
FIF	Formaldehyde-induced fluorescence

FRH (FRF)	Follicle-stimulating hormone—releasing hormone (FSH-releasing factor)
FSH	Follicle-stimulating hormone
FTI	Free thyroxine index
GEP	Gastroenteropancreatic system
GH (STH)	Growth hormone, somatotrop(h)in
GIP	Gastric inhibitory peptide
GRH (GHRF) (SRF)	Growth hormone-releasing hormone, GH-releasing factor, Somatotrop(h)in-releasing factor
GRIH (SST) (SRIF)	Growth hormone release-inhibiting hormone (factor), Somatostatin
H	Histamine
HCG	Human chorionic gonadotrop(h)in
HGH	Human growth hormone
5-HIAA	5-Hydroxyindoleacetic acid
HPG	Human pituitary gonadatrop(h)in
HPL	Human placental lactogen
HPP	Human pancreatic polypeptide
HPT	Hyperparathyroidism
5-HT	5-Hydroxytryptamine, serotonin
5-HTP	5-Hydroxytryptophan
HVA	Homovanillic acid
ICSH	Interstitial cell-stimulating hormone
IHA	Idiopathic hyperplastic aldosteronism
ILA	Insulinlike activity
IRI	Immunoreactive insulin
JGA	Juxtaglomerular apparatus
LATS	Long-acting thyroid stimulator
LGI	Large glucagon immunoreactivity
LH	Luteinizing hormone
LPH	Lipotrop(h)in, lypolytic hormone
LVP	Lysine vasopressin
MAC	Maximal acid concentration
MAO	Maximal acid output
MCT	Medullary carcinoma of the thyroid
MEA	Multiple endocrine adenopathy, adenomatosis
MEN	Multiple endocrine neoplasia
MES	Multiple endocrine syndromes
MRIH (MIF)	Melanocyte-stimulating hormone release-inhibiting hormone (factor)
mRNA	Messenger ribonucleic acid
MSH (MRF)	Melanocyte-stimulating hormone, melanotrop(h)in-releasing factor
MT	Melatonin
NA	Noradrenalin
NE	Norepinephrine
n.g.f.	Nerve growth factor

NME	Necrolytic migratory erythema
OT	Oxytocin
PAO	Peak acid output
PBI	Protein-bound iodine
PES	Paraendocrine syndromes
PG	Prostaglandin
PIF	Pituitary inhibitory factor
PL	Placental lactogen
PP	Pancreatic polypeptide
PPSH	Pseudovaginal perineoscrotal hypospadias
PRIH (PIF)	Prolactin release-inhibiting hormone (factor)
PRL	Prolactin
PTH	Parathyrin, parathyroid hormone
RIA	Radio immunoassay
RNA	Ribonucleic acid
SRF (SRH, GHRF, GRH)	Somatotrop(h)in-releasing factor (hormone), growth hormone-releasing factor (hormone)
SST (SRIF, GRIF)	Somatostatin, Somatotrop(h)in release-inhibiting factor (hormone), growth hormone release-inhibiting factor (hormone)
STH (GH)	Somatotrop(h)in, growth hormone
Subs. P.	Substance P
T	Tryptamine
T_3	Triiodothyronine
T_4	Thyroxine
TBG	Thyroid-binding globulin
TCT (TC)	Thyrocalcitonin, calcitonin
TG	Thyroglobulin
TRH (TRF)	Thyrotrop(h)in-releasing hormone, TSH-releasing factor
TRP	Tubular resorption of phosphate (ratio)
TSH	Thyrotrop(h)in, thyroid-stimulating hormone
VIP	Vasoactive intestinal peptide
Vit. D	Vitamin D
VLP	Vasoactive lung peptide
VMA	Vanillylmandelic acid
VP	Vasopressin
WDHA	Watery diarrhea, hypokalemia, achlorhydria
Z-E	Zollinger-Ellison

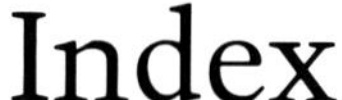

Index

Index

Numerals in *italic* indicate a figure; "t" indicates a table.